Multimodality Imaging for Cardiac Valvular Interventions, Volume 1 Aortic Valve

Francesco Maisano • Philipp Kaufmann
Hatem Alkadhi • Michel Zuber
Alberto Pozzoli • Edwin Ho
Editors

Multimodality Imaging for Cardiac Valvular Interventions, Volume 1 Aortic Valve

From Diagnosis to Decision-Making

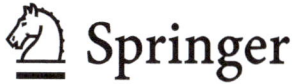 Springer

Editors
Francesco Maisano
University of Zurich
Zurich
Switzerland

Hatem Alkadhi
University Hospital of Zurich
Zurich
Switzerland

Alberto Pozzoli
Heart Surgery Unit
Zurich University Hospital
Zurich
Switzerland

Philipp Kaufmann   ·
University of Zurich
Zurich
Switzerland

Michel Zuber
Cardiology Unit
Zurich University Hospital
Zurich
Switzerland

Edwin Ho
Heart Center
University of Zurich
Zurich
Switzerland

ISBN 978-3-030-27583-9   ISBN 978-3-030-27584-6   (eBook)
https://doi.org/10.1007/978-3-030-27584-6

This Springer imprint is published by the registered company Springer Nature Switzerland AG
The registered company address is: Gewerbestrasse 11, 6330 Cham, Switzerland

Preface

"We live in an era of great innovation and technological evolution, which is expressed at its best in the cardiovascular field. The cross-fertilization between surgical and endovascular treatments, which are functioning complementary, stimulates the constant improvement of both the techniques (e.g., classic cardiac surgery itself entered a new phase of enrichments).

This new frontier translates into new needs and new demands, in which a proper understanding of cardiovascular imaging becomes fundamental.

Technological evolution has led the world of cardiac imaging to technical possibilities considered unexpected a few years ago. We have moved from two-dimensional diagnostic imaging to the current landscape, which consists of several very sophisticated imaging modalities to be combined. Integration of preoperative echocardiographic and multislice computed tomography (MSCT) information, nuclear radiology, fusion of intraprocedural echocardiographic, and MSCT imaging with angiography is part of an education that has become necessary today.

This book originates from an innovative editorial concept, which offers the reader a structured and complete overview of multimodality imaging related to the aortic valve. The five chapters illustrate diagnosis of different aortic valve diseases, criteria of preoperative screening, surgical and transcatheter planning, intraprocedural imaging, and the related postoperative follow-up.

Multimodality imaging is one of the most stimulating and enriching steps that will lead to a common language of cardiac surgeons and interventional cardiologists in the near future. This knowledge is nowadays essential, as well as the next frontier to be dominated by those who will have to deal with cardiovascular therapies."

Zurich, Switzerland   Francesco Maisano
Zurich, Switzerland   Philipp Kaufmann
Zurich, Switzerland   Hatem Alkadhi
Zurich, Switzerland   Michel Zuber
Zurich, Switzerland   Alberto Pozzoli
Zurich, Switzerland   Edwin Ho

Contents

Diagnosis, Indication and Timing

1

Edwin Ho, Alberto Pozzoli, Mizuki Miura, Shehab Anwer,
Philipp Haager, Hans Rickli, Gudrun Feuchtner,
Thomas Senoner, Fabian Morsbach, Hatem Alkadhi,
Gräni Christoph, Buechel Ronny, Philipp Kaufmann,
Michel Zuber, and Felix Tanner

1.1 Introduction

The global burden of aortic valve disease is significant and has been estimated to be as high as 4.8% in those over 75 years old in North American epidemiologic studies [1]. As population demographics are expected to age in most developed countries, this burden will continue to increase.

E. Ho
Heart Center, Zurich University Hospital, Zurich, Switzerland

Division of Cardiology, St. Michael's Hospital, Toronto, ON, Canada

Division of Cardiology, Montefiore Medical Center, Bronx, NY, USA
e-mail: edwin.ho@unityhealth.to

A. Pozzoli
Heart Surgery Unit, Zurich University Hospital,
Zurich, Switzerland
e-mail: alberto.pozzoli@usz.ch

M. Miura · S. Anwer
Heart Center, Zurich University Hospital, Zurich, Switzerland
e-mail: mizuki.miura@usz.ch; shehab.anwer@usz.ch

P. Haager · H. Rickli
Cardiology Unit, Kantonsspital St. Gallen, St. Gallen, Switzerland
e-mail: philipp.haager@usz.ch; hans.rickli@kssg.ch

G. Feuchtner · T. Senoner
Radiology Unit, Innsbruck University Hospital, Innsbruck, Austria
e-mail: gudrun.feuchtner@i-med.ac.at; thomas.senoner@i-med.ac.at

F. Morsbach · H. Alkadhi
Radiology Unit, Zurich University Hospital, Zurich, Switzerland
e-mail: fabian.morsbach@usz.ch; hatem.alkadhi@usz.ch

G. Christoph · B. Ronny · P. Kaufmann
Nuclear Medicine Unit, Zurich University Hospital,
Zurich, Switzerland
e-mail: christoph.Graeni@usz.ch; buechel.ronny@usz.ch; pak@usz.ch

M. Zuber (✉) · F. Tanner
Cardiology Unit, Zurich University Hospital, Zurich, Switzerland
e-mail: michel.zuber@usz.ch; felix.tanner@usz.ch

The most commonly cited guidelines for the diagnosis and management of valvular heart disease have been published by the American Heart Association and the European Society of Cardiology [2–4]. Both have specified that multimodality imaging plays a crucial role in the detection, evaluation and management of aortic valve disease. For example, the American Heart Association guidelines consider transthoracic echocardiography a class I indication for the initial evaluation of patients with suspected or known valvular heart disease [3]. The European Society of Cardiology guidelines specify that cardiac MRI is indicated for quantification of aortic regurgitation when echocardiography measurements are equivocal and may be helpful in the setting of aortic stenosis by evaluating myocardial fibrosis [4]. Several additional recommendations on the use of multimodality imaging in the diagnosis of valvular heart disease will be discussed in greater detail throughout this chapter.

Imaging society guidelines, such as those published by the European Association of Cardiovascular Imaging (EACVI) and American Society of Echocardiography (ASE), describe in greater detail the technical aspects of conducting a good quality study in order to properly evaluate the etiology and severity of aortic valve disease [5–8].

Echocardiography is the predominantly the imaging modality of choice to evaluate aortic valve disease. In addition to being widely available, it is also relatively inexpensive and less time consuming than some other imaging techniques. This allows for easier and generally faster access to an initial study for diagnosis and for serial follow up studies to evaluate for disease progression. It also has the advantage of not exposing patients to ionizing radiation. The EACVI and ASE have both published guidelines outlining the important aspects of evaluating aortic valve stenosis, regurgitation and mixed aortic valve disease [7–9]. These parameters, once properly assessed, can be applied to the recommendations on the management of valvular disease.

Within the realm of echocardiography, transthoracic echocardiography is generally able to provide all the relevant

© Springer Nature Switzerland AG 2020
F. Maisano et al. (eds.), *Multimodality Imaging for Cardiac Valvular Interventions, Volume 1 Aortic Valve*,
https://doi.org/10.1007/978-3-030-27584-6_1

pieces of information about valve anatomy and function. This is particularly true for the evaluation of aortic valve stenosis. The orientation of the valve plane and blood flow acceleration can typically be aligned well enough to allow for an accurate and reliable assessment of blood flow velocities to understand mean and peak gradients as well as estimate aortic valve area using the continuity equation. Worldwide, it is recognized that practical thresholds for the diagnosis of severe aortic stenosis include a mean gradient of 40 mmHg, peak velocity of 4 m/s and calculated aortic valve area of less than 1 cm^2 [9]. International guidelines also recognize that there are limitations to transthoracic echocardiography, especially in the calculation of aortic valve area by continuity equation due to variability in measurements of the left ventricular outflow tract, assumptions made in the shape of the left ventricular outflow tract and anatomic variability that can result in underestimated Doppler velocities. These sources of error may result in discordant findings in some cases. Alternative imaging modalities can then play an important role in clarifying the degree of aortic valve disease in question. In the setting of aortic regurgitation, pressure half time, semi-quantitative and quantitative Doppler evaluation can usually be performed easily. However, important limitations exist that reduce the accuracy of these measures. Some are related to concurrent cardiac disease, such as multiple valve disease, which is independent from the quality of the echocardiographic study. In these situations, again, the use of additional imaging modalities is recommended to clarify the severity of aortic valve disease (Fig. 1.1).

For example, transesophageal echocardiography can provide additional information due to the increased spatial resolution achieved by the proximity of the transducer probe to the aortic valve. This is of particular relevance in the setting of congenital aortic valve disease or in the assessment of endocarditis. However, due to the orientation of the aortic valve plane relative to the esophagus, Doppler assessment of blood velocity across the valve is often suboptimally assessed for aortic stenosis, but may be possible if good quality transgastric views are obtained. Quantification of aortic valve regurgitation may be more accurate compared to transthoracic echocardiography if image quality was a limitation for the transthoracic study (Fig. 1.2).

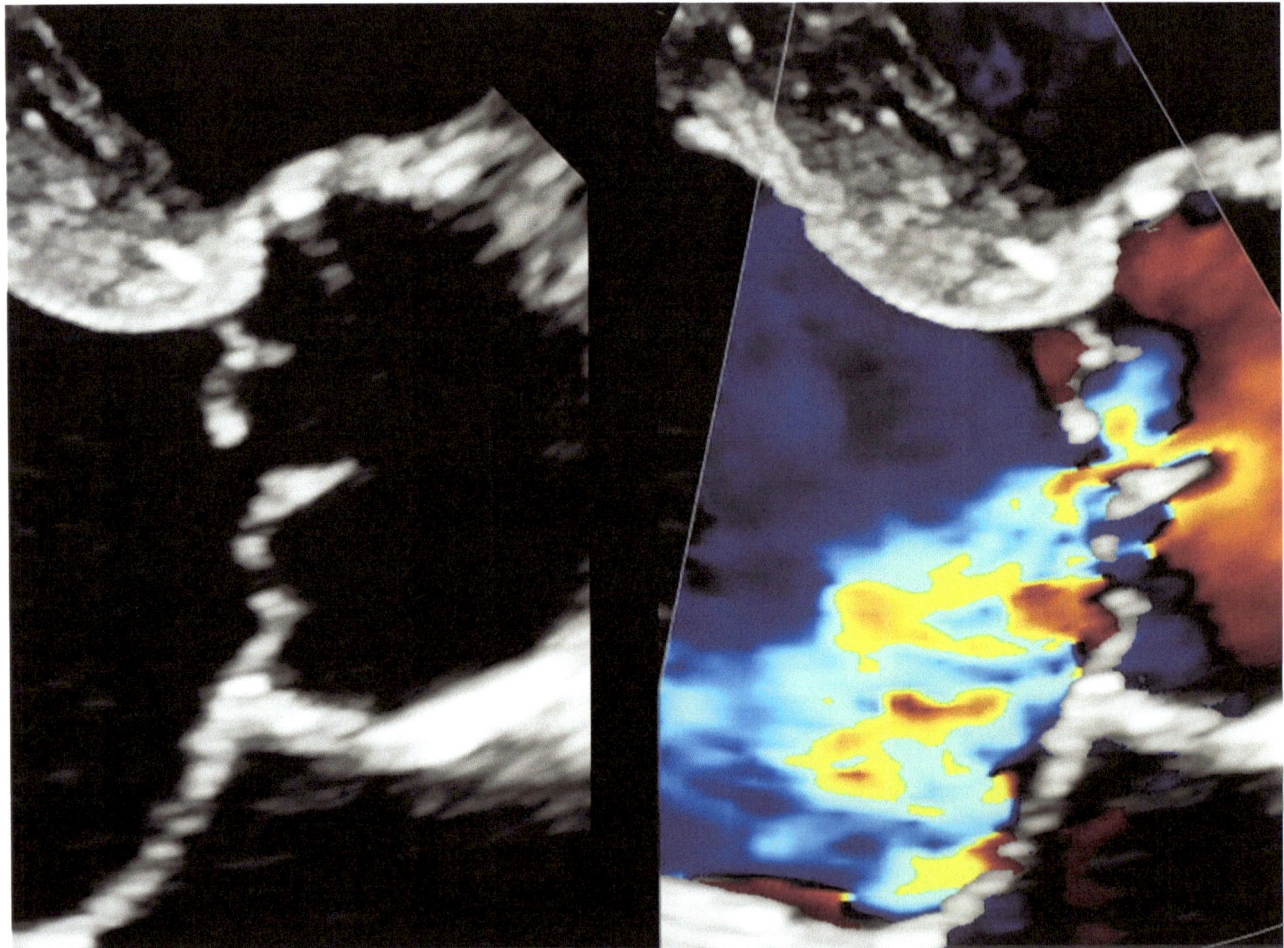

Fig. 1.1 Flail aortic valve leaflet with severe eccentric aortic regurgitation on transthoracic echocardiography

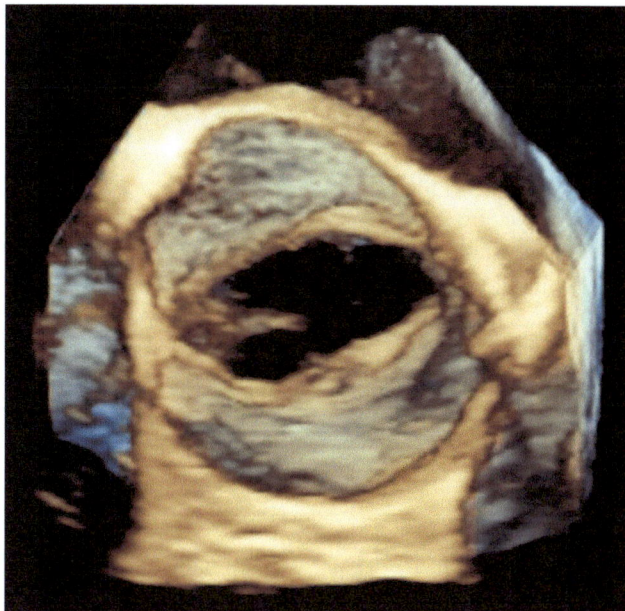

Fig. 1.2 Bicuspid aortic valve seen with 3-dimensional transesophageal echocardiography

Computed tomography can also play a role in the evaluation of aortic valve disease, especially in the assessment of aortic stenosis. Calcium burden has been recognized as having good correlation to the aortic valve area and is related to clinical outcomes [10, 11]. Thus, it provides useful additional information when echocardiography yields internally discordant findings or a conclusion that does not fit with the clinical status of a patient. Additional anatomic features of the aortic valve such as cusp configuration and the anatomy of the aortic root and ascending aorta are easily evaluated [12]. Lastly, if surgical or transcatheter intervention is indicated, computed tomography plays an important role in procedure planning since it is able to visualize the surrounding cardiac structures, estimate optimal fluoroscopic angles, provide the most accurate dimensions of the left ventricular outflow tract and aortic annulus, assess the access vessels, and indicate if there are potentially important anatomic features that may increase the complexity of an intervention or increase the risk of complications [13].

Cardiac magnetic resonance imaging can also be useful in the evaluation of valvular heart disease, and in the setting of aortic valve disease, especially for regurgitant lesions. In addition to providing detailed anatomic data, phase contrast evaluation allow for quantification of flow volumes across a defined cross sectional planar area. These values can therefore provide regurgitant volume as well as regurgitant fraction. More accurate left ventricular volumes and calculated ejection fraction can also better evaluate the consequence of the volume overload state [12].

The individual strengths of each imaging modality are recognized in global imaging society guidelines, which have recommended an integrated approach utilizing multi-modality imaging when needed to accurately diagnose disease severity [7]. This approach also highlights the importance of the cardiac imaging specialist in Heart Valve Teams, who should have familiarity with all imaging modalities and the specific information the can be obtained from each.

1.2 Quantification of Aortic Stenosis

1.2.1 Is the Gradient Severe?

1.2.1.1 Introduction

The major reason for aortic stenosis in developed countries is aortic valve degeneration with fibrosis and calcification of both anulus and leaflets. Less frequent causes are rheumatic and congenital heart disease [14]. Patients usually become gradually symptomatic and exhibit dyspnea, angina, or syncope. Clinical examination reveals a spindle-shaped systolic murmur, usually best heard over the right upper parasternal region, with extension of the murmur in both carotid arteries, eventually a systolic thrill, and a low pulse amplitude with a slow rise and a late peak. When the diagnosis is suspected clinically, it should be confirmed by echocardiography [15].

The echocardiographic evaluation of aortic stenosis severity can be difficult, as over- or underestimation may occur depending on the individual situation. However, accurate assessment of the severity of aortic valve stenosis is very important for clinical decision making. Understanding the fluid dynamics of valvular stenoses is helpful for troubleshooting in unclear situations and may improve correct grading of aortic stenosis [15].

The hallmark of valve stenosis is the transvalvular pressure difference occurring across the stenotic orifice. Within the stenosis, the pressure difference is associated with flow convergence resulting in flow acceleration; hence, potential energy is converted into kinetic energy. Besides convective acceleration there is some energy required for accelerating the blood flow and for overcoming viscous friction [16–18].

The stenosis jet is composed of a proximal convergence zone just proximal to the stenotic orifice, vena contracta, central jet, and distal turbulences resulting from penetration of the central jet into an almost immobile blood column. Maximal flow velocity is reached in the vena contracta, which is the narrowest part of the jet as measured by colour Doppler [16, 17].

Distal to the stenosis, there are variable degrees of flow expansion with flow deceleration and turbulence. During deceleration of blood flow between the aortic valve and the ascending aorta, part of the kinetic energy is converted back to potential energy in a process called pressure recovery. The latter can occur at a variable extent which is determined by the ratio of valve orifice area and the cross-sectional area of the proximal ascending aorta. Pressure recovery is particularly relevant in individuals with severe aortic stenosis and small aortic roots, while it is negligible in those with a dilated proximal ascending aorta. The part of the energy not recovered distal to the stenosis is lost due to turbulences and converted into heat [19].

1.2.1.2 Echocardiography and Doppler Echocardiography

Echocardiography is the noninvasive method of choice for determining the severity of aortic valve stenosis. Due to various pitfalls discussed below it is advisable to evaluate a stenotic aortic valve with particular care.

Comprehensive evaluation of aortic valve stenosis includes key clinical information including symptoms and signs of the patient. The echocardiographic examination should always be complete because a severe aortic stenosis is known to induce cardiac remodeling; hence, it should not only analyze the aortic valve but provide data on size and function of all the cardiac cavities as well. Myocardial hypertrophy, ejection fraction, longitudinal systolic strain, and diastolic function of the left ventricle are particularly important parameters in this context.

Before any hemodynamic measurements are taken, the aortic valve is assessed morphologically including the left ventricular outflow tract, aortic anulus, aortic leaflets, and aortic root with particular emphasis on the extent and distribution of calcified or fibrosed areas. Next the mobility of aortic valve leaflets is examined, in particular the location and extent of leaflet motion. Valve opening is evaluated in the context of left ventricular size and function, taking into account that stroke volume influences the extent of leaflet motion. Image quality and frame rate should be optimized by different projections, narrow sector, and zoom mode.

Functional evaluation of the aortic valve is based on the Doppler method, confirms the morphological assessment, and completes the analysis. This is achieved by colour Doppler, pulsed-wave Doppler, and continous-wave Doppler, all of which are applied in a complementary manner [15, 20].

Colour Doppler is useful for determining the level of flow acceleration, the direction of the stenosis jet, and the presence of an accompanying aortic regurgitation [21]. The aliasing velocity should be set between 50 and 70 cm/s or eventually higher values under high output conditions. To define the level of flow acceleration is essential because an aortic stenosis may be subvalvular such as in membraneous subaortic stenosis or subaortic septal hypertrophy, valvular such as in degenerative aortic stenosis, and supravalvular such as in genetic disease like Williams-Beuren syndrome. The direction of the stenosis jet is usually central but may be affected by the presence of an aneurysmatic ascending aorta,

by the aorto-mitral angle, and by the configuration of the degenerated aortic valve which may display distorted or fused leaflets. The latter is particularly important in bicuspid aortic valve, which is often associated with an eccentric jet leading to hurricane-like flow phenomena in the proximal ascending aorta [15, 22].

The systolic flow velocity in the left ventricular outflow tract is measured by pulse-wave Doppler. This information is useful in all conditions with increased proximal flow velocity such as fixed or dynamic subvalvular obstruction, moderate to severe aortic regurgitation, or any form of high output. As a rule of thumb, the velocity in the left ventricular outflow tract should be considered for calculations of aortic stenosis severity when it is higher than 1 m/s [15].

Maximal systolic flow velocity across the aortic valve is obtained by continuous-wave Doppler and determined at the vena contracta. The velocity profile of blood flow in the vena contracta is relatively flat and thus easy to measure and well reproducible. When stroke volume is small, however, this profile is more parabolic and associated with a larger distribution of values; therefore, the maximal velocity of blood flow may be missed when the probe is not carefully placed in the center of the jet [15, 18]. Another even more relevant problem is the angle between the echocardiography probe and the aortic stenosis jet. As the Doppler signal is strongly influenced by the angle between the direction of the probe and the jet via a cosinus function, careful alignment of the echocardiography probe is essential. Accordingly, it may be necessary to determine flow velocity from various views including suprasternal and right parasternal projections. This is particularly advisable in patients with bicuspid aortic valve, but is recommended in all the patients with aortic stenosis, because the direction of the jet is unpredictable and can be difficult to visualize by colour-Doppler [15, 20].

A reliable continuous wave Doppler spectrum is smooth and exhibits a well demarcated dense border indicating a homogenous maximal flow velocity in the vena contracta. In contrast, a soft border of the spectrum suggests an incomplete Doppler signal, particularly when it is combined with a low density of the spectrum. Similarly, relevant velocity signals on both sides of the baseline indicate an incomplete alignment of the probe and should not be used for analysis. A good Doppler spectrum allows to evaluate the shape of the signal, which is more rounded in severe aortic stenosis, as well as the timing of the peak velocity, which occurs later in systole in severe aortic stenosis.

According to the current guidelines, a maximal systolic flow velocity equal to or higher than 4 m/s as well as a mean systolic pressure gradient equal to or higher than 40 mmHg are consistent with severe aortic stenosis. These values are obtained by tracing the border of the Doppler spectrum and converting the resulting flow velocities into pressure gradients using the modified Bernoulli equation. In contrast to invasively determined pressure gradients, the maximal Doppler gradient represents the maximal instantaneous gradient as opposed to the peak-to-peak gradient obtained invasively. The peak systolic pressure gradient over the aortic valve and in the left ventricle do not occur simultaneously, so that the peak-to-peak gradient does not reflect a physiological measurement and is lower than the maximal instantaneous pressure gradient. Nevertheless, the echocardiographic method has been validated against invasively determined pressure gradients and has become the gold standard for clinical routine applications [4, 15].

Over a stenotic valve, there is acceleration of blood flow with conversion of potential into kinetic energy. Distal to the stenosis, flow decelerates again, and part of the kinetic energy which has not dissipated into heat can be converted back into potential energy. This process is called pressure recovery and is related to the ratio of effective orifice area of the aortic valve and the dimension of the proximal aorta. As turbulence is reduced in small aortic roots, pressure recovery is of importance in individuals with diameters of the sinotubular junction below 30 mm. Under such conditions, the severity of aortic stenosis is overestimated by the Doppler method and the continuity equation because the continuous-wave Doppler signal ignores pressure recovery completely. Hence, in such patients, it may be reasonable to calculate the energy loss index, which corresponds to the effective orifice area corrected for pressure recovery [19].

1.2.1.3 Magnetic Resonance Imaging

Magnetic resonance imaging (MRI) allows accurate and reliable assessment of aortic stenosis, which is particulary helpful in situations where echocardiography results are inconsistent or image quality is impaired and therefore a correct echo beam alignment through the stenotic jet is difficult to assess.

The main advantage of MRI is that it allows a comprehensive evaluation of patients with aortic stenosis by assessing not only valve morphology and function, but also LV volumes, mass and function as well as aortic pathology.

For the qualitative assessment of aortic stenosis, cine images are used. The cine images are planed in the standard long-axis (2-,3- and 4- chamber) views, the perpendicular LVOT view as well as a complete stack of sequential short-axis cine images (8–10 mm from base to apex) with an excellent signal-to-noise ratio and a typical in-plane spatial resolution of 1.5–2.0 mm. They allow one to differentiate between subvalvular, valvular and supravalvular aortic stenosis and gives a first impression of the aortic stenosis severity by visualization of the turbulent flow jet. Gradient echo may be preferred as it can visualize high flow stenosis with less artifacts in comparison to the standard SSFP images. However, SSFP images appear to correlate better with tran-

soesophageal echocardiography in the assessment of aortic valve area [23].

For the quantitative assessment of aortic stenosis, antegrade peak velocity, pressure gradient as well as planimetry of the aortic valve area are used routinely [24]. The transvalvular velocity is measured directly by phase-contrast velocity mapping. These phase-contrast pulse sequences are based on the property that protons moving within a magnetic field gradient acquire a shift in the phase of their rotational spin compared with stationary protons [25]. These sequences are a unique advantage of CMR as they are not dependent on derivation from complex calculations as with forumlas used in echocardiography and invasive catheterization [24]. From the peak velocity, the pressure gradient can be estimated by using the modified Bernoulli equation. It is important to plane a through-plane velocity map in the short-axis orientation parallel to the aortic stenosis jet to achieve correct measurements (Fig. 1.3). Any velocity >4 m/s should be considered as severe aortic stenosis unless there is relevant combined aortic regurgitation, which significantly increases the antegrade flow across the valve. Any misalignment might lead to an underestimation due to partial volume effects with the narrow stenosis. However, even with through plane, MRI tends to underestimate the peak velocity, most likely because of a lower temporal resolution (typically 25–45 ms) in comparison to continuous wave Doppler echocardiography (~2 ms), partial volume effects within the vena contracta of very high velocity jets as well as artifacts from turbulent jets [24–26]. In addition, it is prerequisite for optimal measurements in phase contrast sequences, that the expected maximum velocity is provided as otherwise aliasing artefacts may occur. The latter appears in the centre of the flow area, as the opposite color to forward flow. Beside the technical issues, one of the other main limitations of CMR in the flow assessment of patients with aortic stenosis is the lack of specific thresholds. The current thresholds for aortic valve stenosis are derived from echocardiography. Due to the described limitations of direct flow assessment in aortic stenosis, planimetry of the aortic valve area should be the technique of choice as described in one of the following chapters.

In addition to the assessment of the aortic valve itself, it is fundamental to comprehensively assess patients with aortic stenosis. In this context, MRI has been proven to be a very good option for assessing LV volumes, function and LV mass [27, 28]. The key strengths include its accuracy, reproducibility and unrestricted field of view. In addition, MRI has the ability to characterize myocardial tissue, in particular to evaluate for the presence of fibrosis. The techniques may include inversion recovery images acquired late after contrast administration, diffuse fibrosis assessment with T1 mapping and extracellular volume (ECV) measurement. Fibrosis has been shown to correlate with disease severity and to be an independent predictor of mortality [29, 30].

Fig. 1.3 Maximal velocity assessment: Projection plane in 3 chamber view (**a**) and LVOT view (**b**) orthogonal to the aortic stenosis jet. Velocity time curve (**c**) with a maximal velocity of 4.2 m/s in a patient with severe aortic stenosis due to a bicuspid aortic valve

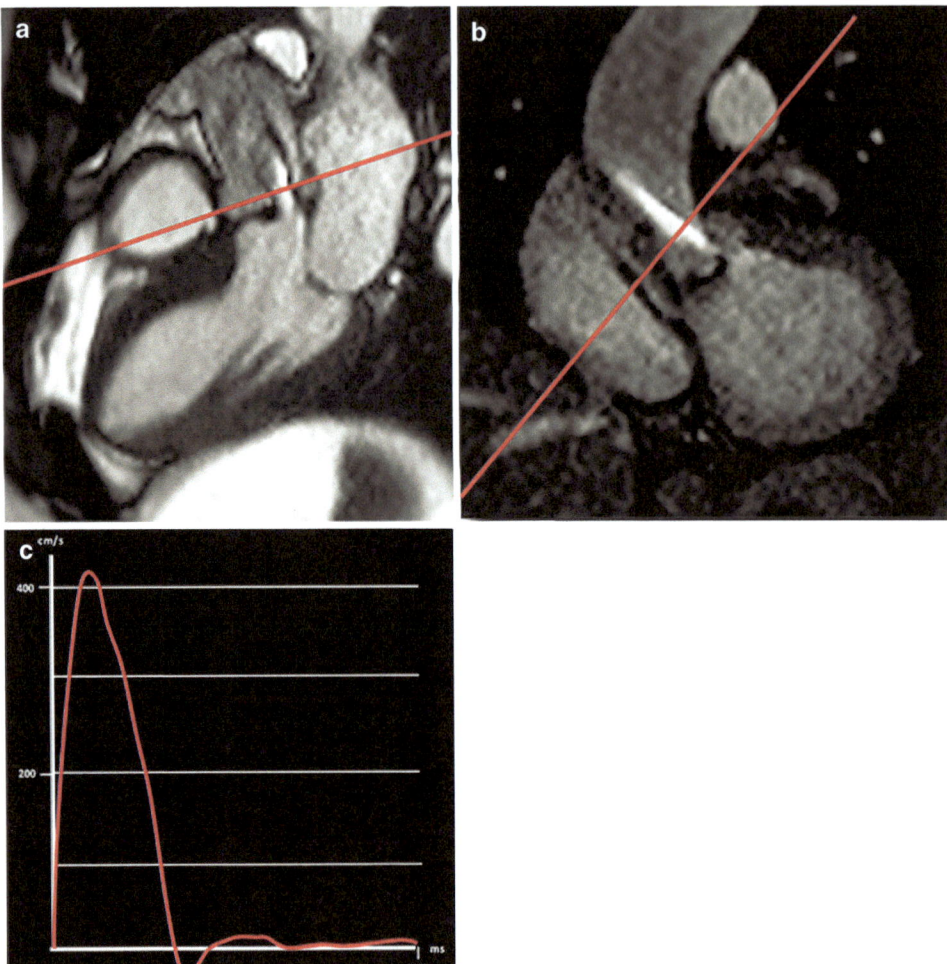

Currently, two-dimensional phase-contrast imaging is used in the evaluation of pulsatile blood flow in clinical routines. Further advances in technology with 4D flow offers the opportunity to assess flow-encoding in all three spatial dimensions and along the cardiac cycle [31]. Besides advantages for the recording, visualization and analysis of blood flow, in a post hoc analysis, 4D flow provides additional information about shear stress, pressure differences and turbulent kinetic energy [32–34]. These new parameters might further improve our understanding in patients with aortic valve stenosis and its related effects on the aorta [35]. However, robust software solutions and clinical outcome studies are important to implement this technique in our daily work.

1.2.1.4 Catheterization
Direct measurement of both the left ventricular (LV) cavity pressure and the ascending aortic pressure is the most accurate grading of the pathophysiology entity of aortic stenosis: the pressure drop due to the stenosis, labelled as the pressure gradient.

Most cases can be accurately diagnosed today using noninvasive echocardiography imaging. Unnecessary crossing of the stenotic aortic valve has a small risk of embolization and is therefore not indicated if the diagnosis of severe aortic stenosis is already made [36]. Therefore, its routine use is given a class III recommendation (not indicated and possibly harmful) in the actual guidelines [2].

But in some cases, there is a discrepancy between clinical findings, 2D echocardiography and Doppler measurements, resulting in an unclear diagnosis. In this circumstance, a class I recommendation is given for invasive hemodynamics (indicated and beneficial). Cardiac catheterization involves directly measuring the difference in pressure between the LV and aorta over time, providing both instantaneous and mean pressure gradients (Fig. 1.4). This can be done easily with 2 pressure lines and the use of a double lumen pigtail in a retrograde fashion with the same accuracy as 2 separate lines would provide. Micromanometer transducer tipped catheters are used when high-fidelity pressures are necessary in research applications, such as to generate pressure-volume curves. Due to

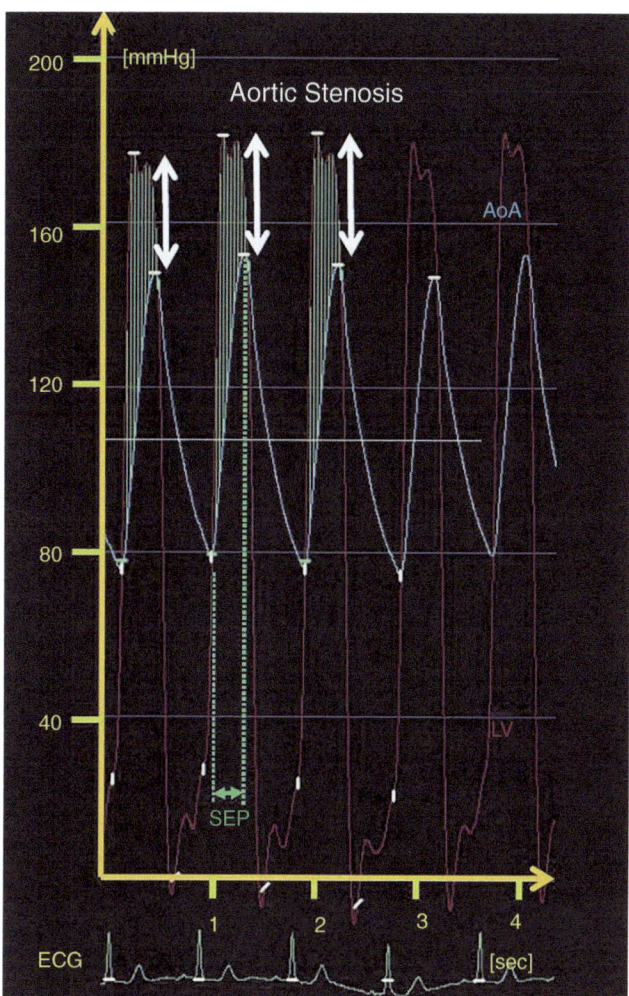

Fig. 1.4 Catheterization: Simultaneous Measurement of Aortic (blue) and left ventricular (red) pressure. White arrows demonstrate Peak-to-Peak Gradients. Green hatched area demonstrates mean gradient. *SEP* systolic ejection period between opening and closing of the aortic valve. Simultaneous ECG recordings are given below

surements. If not, careful troubleshooting is mandatory before additional data collection. Measurements using peripherial access and pressure measurement as a substitute for central aortic pressure is not accurate due to the temporal delay of the pressure wave and peripheral amplification, reducing the observed gradient.

Pullback of a single lumen pigtail from the LV cavity to the aorta allows only the calculation of peak-to-peak difference measurements. They correlate well with the mean gradient only in the setting of severe aortic stenosis. Therefore, this measurement technique does not offer much value in the uncertain cases where invasive measurements are meant to clarify the severity of stenosis.

Limitations of catheterization include the fact that temporal resolution of invasive measurements being defined by the equipment used. Additionally, a pigtail and a double lumen pigtail have multiple holes over a length of at least one centimeter at the tip of the catheter and at the shaft. The distance between the distal pigtail loop and the second lumen at the aortic side for a double lumen catheter is more than 5 cm. Therefore, it can be very difficult to differentiate true aortic valve stenosis from any other cause of an elevated gradient, such as subvalvular stenosis or a combination of both subvalvular and valvular stenosis. If one or more holes of the distal lumen are positioned falsely above the aortic valve, the pressure measurements become inaccurate, and may even mimic severe aortic valve regurgitation due to the erroneously high end diastolic pressures.

1.2.2   Is the Valve Area Critically Small?

1.2.2.1 Introduction

Aortic valve area determines the resistance of the valve to blood flow and hence is an important parameter with regard to symptoms of the patient as well as prognostic implications. In principle, the aortic valve area can be determined morphologically by planimetry and functionally by the calculated effective orifice area. Both methods have their advantages and limitations and should be applied in a complementary manner. An aortic valve area below 1 cm^2 is associated with adverse outcome and considered one of the hallmarks of a severe aortic stenosis. This value may be indexed to body surface area of the patient with a cut-off value for severe aortic stenosis of below 0.6 cm^2 per m^2. However, this is controversial because the currently applied parameter for assessing body size, body surface area, does not always accurately reflect aortic valve area and because aortic valve area does not increase with excess body size. Despite these limitations, aortic valve area should be indexed in small adults to avoid the false interpretation of a small aortic valve area in such individuals [15].

increased cost, they are normally not used in routine clinical scenarios.

Care must be taken using double lumen pigtail to avoid any damping of the small aortic pressure line not to overestimate the pressure gradient. Ensure that both lines are properly flushed, free of air and any kinks in the system. Before measurements begin, careful leveling of the zero pressure reference has to be done. Exact positioning of the system is mandatory: the distal end of the pigtail is placed in the middle of the LV cavity, avoiding the left ventricular outflow tract and any entrapment within the chordae of the mitral valve. The aortic outlet is placed above the sinotubular junction. After pullback of the pigtail into the aorta, exactly superimposed pressure curves from both proximal and distal ports demonstrate correct zero settings and pressure mea-

1.2.2.2 Echocardiography

Blood flow velocity and systolic pressure gradient increase with flow rate for a given aortic valve orifice area. Hence, the latter is a useful parameter for evaluation of aortic stenosis severity when flow rate is either very high or very low. However, it should be kept in mind that effective orifice area is not independent of flow rate, which is particularly important in patients with reduced ejection fraction.

Effective orifice area of the aortic valve is calculated by the continuity equation. This equation is based on the principle that the stroke volume, which passes the left ventricular outflow tract, also passes the aortic valve; hence, the two stroke volumes are equal. Stroke volume is calculated by the product of cross-sectional area and velocity time integral; hence, aortic valve effective orifice area can be determined from the cross-sectional area and the velocity time integral of the left ventricular outflow tract devided by the velocity time integral of the aortic valve [37–39].

Calculation of stroke volume therefore depends on the accurate measurement of cross-sectional area and velocity time integral of the left ventricular outflow tract. The current standard approach for determining the cross-sectional area of the outflow tract is done by measuring its diameter in a zoomed view and calculating the area of a circle with half of the diameter as the radius. The outflow tract diameter is obtained from the parasternal long axis view and should be measured in midsystole by the inner edge to inner edge method. Ideally, the diameter should be determined at the same location that the pulsed-wave Doppler sample volume is placed for obtaining the velocity time integral. As the latter is done in the apical 3-chamber or 5-chamber view, this location is not always easy to identify in an exact manner. Some authors recommend measuring the left ventricular outflow tract diameter at the level of the aortic anulus instead of a few millimeters into the left ventricle; this is reasonable in patients with congenital aortic stenosis and a doming valve. In most patients with degenerative aortic stenosis, however, flow acceleration occurs proximal to the aortic anulus, and the pulse-wave Doppler sample volume should be placed in the area of laminar flow just proximal to the beginning of flow acceleration. Therefore, most authors recommend measuring the left ventricular outflow tract diameter within 10 mm proximal to the aortic anulus, and fortunately, the diameter shows very little variability in this region assuming the imaging plane is in the center of the left ventricular outflow tract [15, 40–44].

While the Doppler measurements of velocity time integral in both left ventricular outflow tract and across the aortic valve display a relatively low variability, the diameter of the left ventricular outflow tract is less reproducible. For this reason, this diameter should be obtained by transoesophageal echocardiography if image quality in the transthoracic approach is not sufficient [15, 45]. In addition, there is a systematic error in calculation of the outflow tract area, because it is not actually circular but rather elliptical in most individuals. Because the echocardiographic parasternal long axis view visualizes only the short diameter of the ellipse in most cases, application of the continuity equation leads to underestimation of effective orifice area in these individuals [45–47]. Nevertheless, echocardiography remains the standard method of choice for quantification of aortic stenosis severity, not only because of its widespread availability and cost-effectiveness, but also because the parameters derived from echocardiography are strong predictors of outcome in patients with aortic stenosis [38, 48, 49].

An alternative approach for quantification of aortic stenosis severity closely related to the continuity equation is the dimensionless index. This parameter reflects the ratio of the velocity integrals or peak velocity values from the left ventricular outflow tract and aortic valve and is consistent with severe aortic stenosis when lower than 0.25. It is independent of the outflow tract diameter and also independent of body size, which represent major advantages; however, it also ignores the variation in left ventricular outflow tract dimension occurring independent of body size [15, 37].

Anatomic aortic valve area can also be visualized and quantified by planimetry. Unfortunately, artifacts such a reverberations and attenuation, mostly occurring due to fibrosis and calcification of the valve, make exact planimetry of the valve orifice difficult in many patients. Most of the literature on aortic valve orifice planimetry has been done by transoesophageal echocardiography and revealed good correlation between the planimetered valve area with Gorlin-derived values. Even in the transoesophageal approach, however, it can be difficult to assure that the minimal valve area is planimetered, because the valve often displays the shape of a dome, such as in congenital aortic stenosis, or of a funnel, such as in degenerative aortic stenosis. The best method for taking care of this problem is the 3-dimensional transoesophageal method, because it allows one to identify the minimal valve area by imaging plane reconstruction of the 3-dimensional dataset. If the aortic valve still exhibits some compliance, the orifice area is affected by stroke volume such that a small stroke volume leads to smaller opening of the valve; this issue is completely ignored when the anatomic valve orifice is determined [50–54].

In an integrative approach, aortic valve area should be determined by combining different echocardiographic methods [15]. The continuity equation should be applied and can be combined with the dimensionless index. If there are doubts regarding the effective orifice area determined by this approach, the left ventricular outflow tract area should be planimetered in 3-dimensional transoesophageal echocardiography or, alternatively, in MDCT, and the planimetered value should be used for the continuity equation. If stroke volume is normal and a 3-dimensional transoesophageal echocardiography is performed, planimetered aortic valve area can be assessed as well [45–47, 55, 56].

1.2.2.3 Stress Echocardiography

When left ventricular systolic function is impaired, stroke volume decreases. As a consequence, the aortic valve exhibits reduced opening during systole as long as the valve is not completely calcified and has retained some compliance. Hence, the severity of aortic stenosis is overestimated by both the continuity equation and the planimetric approach.

To differentiate a true severe from a pseudo-severe aortic stenosis, dobutamine stress echocardiography can be performed. If the left ventricle exhibits a contractile reserve, the systolic pressure gradient will increase, while the effective orifice area will remain small. If the maximal systolic flow velocity reached a value equal to or higher than 4 m/s or the mean systolic pressure gradient is above 30 mmHg while the effective orifice area never exceeds 1 cm^2 during the examination, the aortic valve stenosis is considered to be true severe. If these values are not reached, the aortic stenosis is pseudo-severe or, alternatively, the left ventricle does not have a significant contractile reserve. The latter two situations can be distinguished via the increase in stroke volume and ejection fraction during the dobutamine infusion [57–60].

1.2.2.4 Magnetic Resonance Imaging

MRI provides different tools in the assessment of aortic stenosis, i.e. transvalvular peak velocity and pressure gradient by direct flow assessment. However, flow assessment by phase-contrast velocity mapping tends to underestimate aortic valve severity due to several reasons, such as low temporal resolution, misalignment of the velocity maps, partial volume effects or artifacts due to turbulent jets [24–26]. The most reliable and robust technique in the assessment of aortic stenosis by MRI at this time appears to be the direct quantitative evaluation of the orifice area by planimetry as MRI-based planimetry does not rely on blood flow velocity quantification, pressure gradients, or complicated calculations [24].

To achieve detailed anatomical information of the aortic valve the images are planned in a stack of sequential short-axis cine images through the valve. Parallel to the valve tips multiple, thin (4–5 mm) slices should be acquired without the use of a gap or even using an overlap between the consecutive slices. Planimetry is then performed precisely at the level of the valve tips in systole (Fig. 1.5). The smallest maximum visible aortic valve area of all measurements should be used.

In contrast to conventional gradient echo, SSFP images have a superior contrast to noise and signal to noise ratio. Therefore, the SSFP signal intensity is widely independent of blood flow and haemodynamic status, which makes it robust against turbulence [61, 62]. As a consequence, SSFP images appear to correlate better with transoesophageal echocardiography in the assessment of aortic orifice area as conventional Doppler gradient echocardiography [23]. Moreover, with the use of SSFP sequences, susceptibility to artifacts due to valvular calcifications are significantly

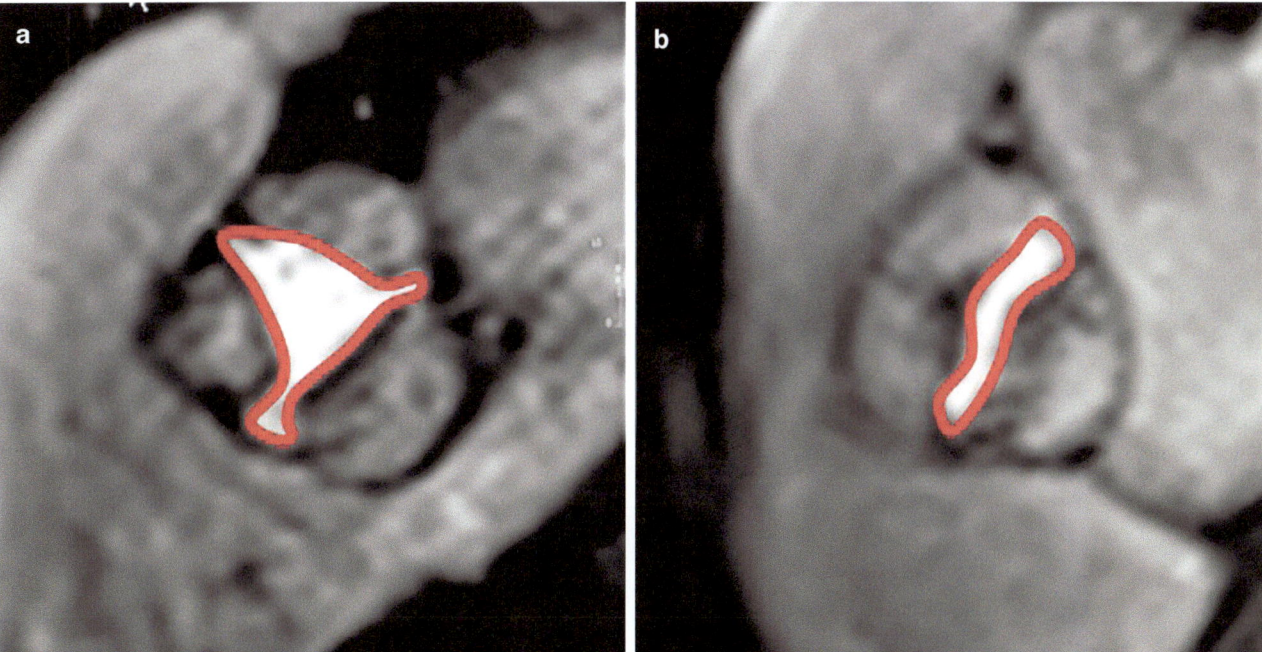

Fig. 1.5 SSFP MRI planimetry in patients with (**a**) tricuspid aortic valve and mild stenosis (aortic valve area 1.7 cm^2) and (**b**) bicuspid aortic valve and moderate stenosis (aortic valve area 1.2 cm^2)

reduced in comparison to conventional Doppler echocardiography [62]. Whereas echocardiography is mainly limited by the acoustic shadow of the usually severely calcified aortic valve, aortic valve area planimetry with SSFP imaging is widely independent of these limitations and makes it highly suitable for the visualization of valvular structures.

Beside a very high reliability and reproducibility, MRI planimetry has shown to have an even higher sensitivity and specificity than transthoracic and transoesophageal echocardiography in comparison to cardiac catheterization [63, 64], although MRI slightly overestimates aortic valve area as compared with catheterization [64]. Moreover, it correlates well with direct measurement of autopsy specimens [65].

Although SSFP imaging provides less susceptibility artifacts, heavy calcified aortic valves may still lead to suboptimal measurements due to signal void and turbulences [26]. The main limitations of planimetry by MRI, however, are the contraindications to MRI in general.

1.2.2.5 Computed Tomography

The anatomical aortic valve area (AVA) is the key parameter for defining aortic stenosis (AS) severity, in addition to the transvalvular pressure gradient and velocity. An AVA of less than 2 cm^2 is regarded as "stenotic" and classified as mild if 1.5–2 cm^2, moderate if 1.0–1.5 cm^2 and "severe" if <1 cm^2, "severe-critical" if less than 0.7 cm^2.

In patients with typical high-flow high-gradient aortic stenosis, the AVA alone plays a less critical role in the diagnostic pathway. However, for a special subtype of AS, the low –flow-low gradient AS, the AVA becomes much more important for defining stenosis severity.

Cardiac Computed Tomography (CT) has shown to be a reliable tool for sizing the anatomic AVA in numerous studies [10, 66, 67], with a trend of minor overestimation of AVA size as compared to flow dependent techniques such as transthoracic echocardiography and invasive measurements. Multiphase datasets over the entire cardiac cycle from 0 to 100% of the R-R interval (including systolic phases) are mandatory for measurement of the AVA.

Accurate sizing of the AVA by cardiac CT is obtained by using 3-D multiplanar reconstruction in 3 planes: Left oblique sagittal, left oblique coronal and then, the corresponding orthogonal axial view of the smallest valve orifice should be generated (Fig. 1.6). After this, the systolic phase (between 0 and 45% of R-R interval) of maximal leaflet opening, with best image quality (minimal artifacts) should be selected. Most commonly, the best phase with maximal opening is found around 25% of the R-R interval, but variations depending on heart rate and cardiac cycle time interval are normal. Then, the valve orifice should be reviewed on multiple 1 mm thin MRP axial reconstruction, and the image with smallest AVA area selected for measurement. Finally, the inner AVA is traced with a digital caliper (Fig. 1.7).

1.2.2.6 Catheterization

Until Doppler echocardiography entered the field in the 1980s, invasive hemodynamics were the standard to evaluate cardiac hemodynamics.

To evaluate the gradient across the aortic valve, a simultaneous measure of the pressure within the left ventricle and the ascending aorta has to be obtained as mentioned previously. Unfortunately, pressure gradients vary with flow.

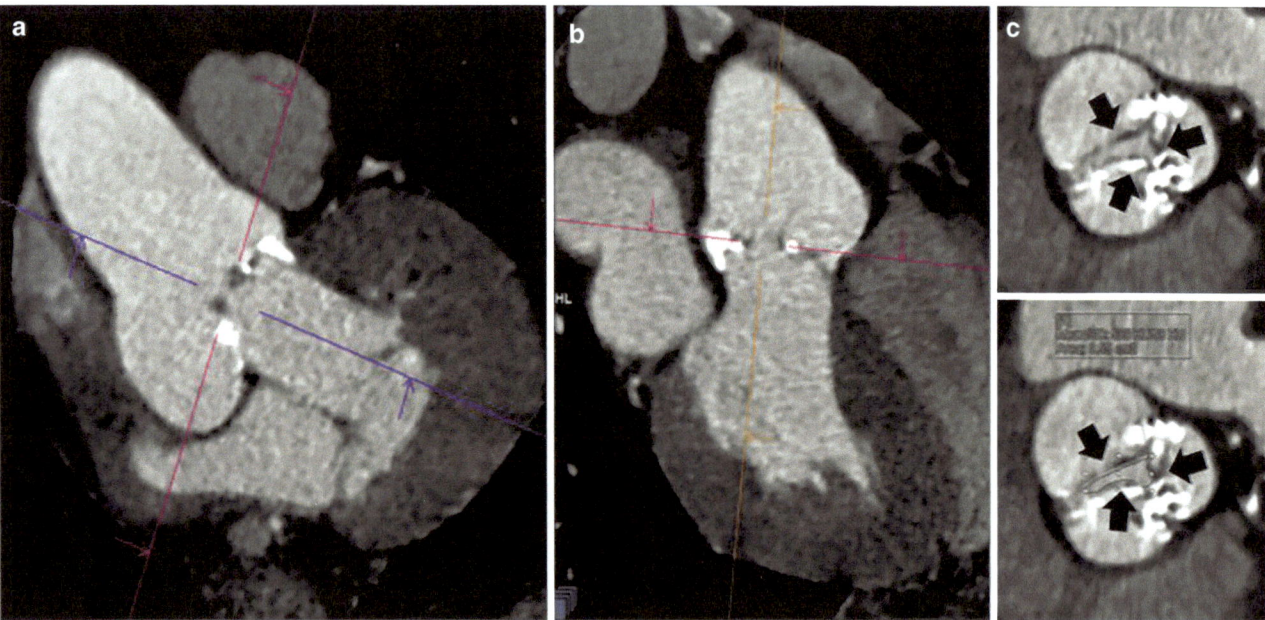

Fig. 1.6 AVA (aortic valve area) sizing of a tricuspid aortic valve

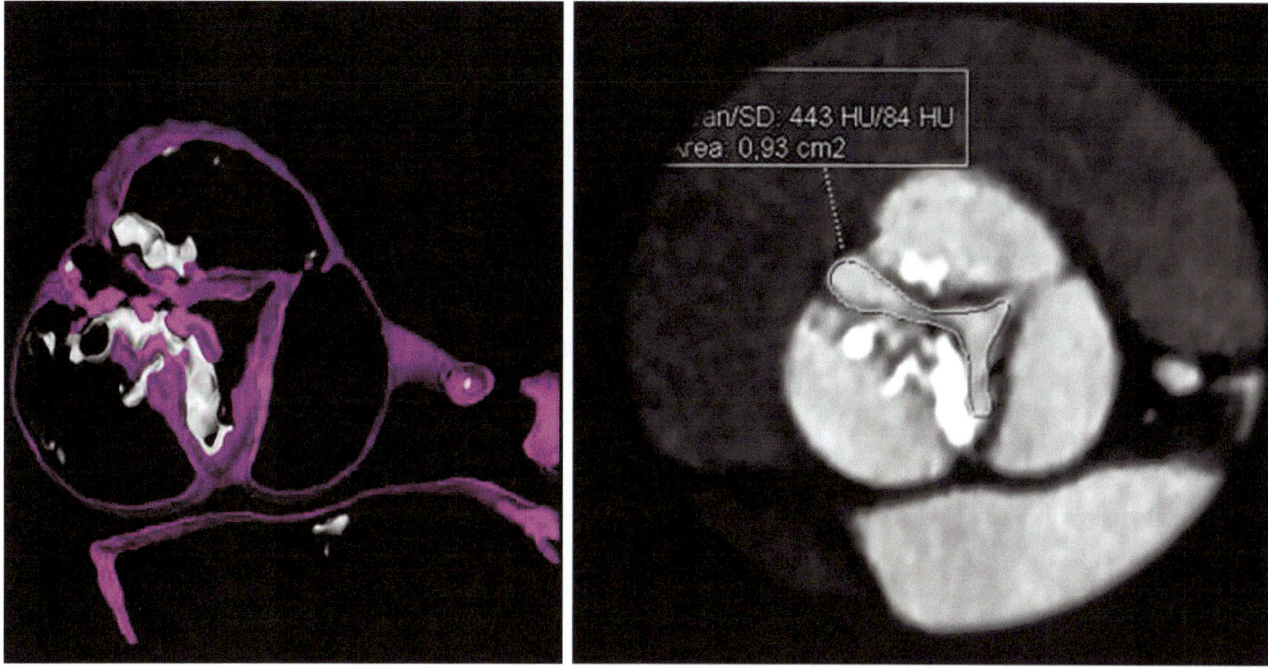

Fig. 1.7 Examples bicuspid valve with a typical "fish—mouth" opening appearance

Therefore, it is essential to accurately determine mean pressure gradients, cardiac output and the right formula for calculation of the aortic valve area to get the full picture about the grade of valve stenosis.

The most accurate method to obtain cardiac output is the Fick principle: oxygen consumed by the body is the product of O_2 delivery (cardiac output) and O_2 extraction by the tissue. Accurate measurement of hemoglobin, simultaneous measurement of the central venous and arterial oxygen content is needed as well as the oxygen consumption of the body at the same time. For this, a calm and controlled steady state is necessary without supplemental oxygen. Oxygen consumption can be measured directly in some situations, or more commonly, estimated from standardized charts. Significant errors can occur if all these steps are not performed properly [68].

Alternatively, the thermodilution method uses cold saline injected rapidly into the right atrium and measures the change in down-stream blood temperature over time at the pulmonary artery. Some pitfalls of this method exist. Very low cardiac output leads to errors due to passive warming of the cold saline over time in the right atrium and ventricle that is not flow related. Intracardiac shunts and relevant tricuspid regurgitation must also be excluded.

After obtaining these measurements, Aortic valve area can be calculated from the mean aortic transvalvular gradient and cardiac output using the Gorlin formula:

$$A = \frac{CO / SEP \times HR}{44.3 \times C \times \sqrt{mdP}}. \tag{1.1}$$

Equation (1.1): Gorlin Formula to calculate Aortic valve area (A) using Cardiac Output (CO), Systolic ejection period (SEP), Heart Rate (HR), empirical constant (C) to adapt the measured area to the true area (still 1.0, not yet verified) and the mean pressure gradient (mdP) across the aortic valve

The formula was primarily developed by the Gorlins in 1951 to calculate mitral valve area compared to autopsy findings or surgical specimens. It was adapted to the aortic valve using a correction factor C [69]. In the beginning, it was assumed C = 1.0 and should be calculated as soon as data became available. At that time, it was not done due to the fact it was considered malpractice to cross the aortic valve in a retrograde fashion. Unfortunately, this work has never been completed.

The limitation of the Gorlin formula for calculating aortic valve area is its flow dependency. This was nicely shown within the TOPAS trial [57]. If the gradient is below 40 mmHg and cardiac output is <5.0 L/min some cautions have to be addressed regarding the initial results: if the LV is weak and aortic valve area increases with positive inotropic drugs, it is in fact a "pseudo-aortic stenosis". This is in contrast to "true severe, critical aortic stenosis" characterized by an increase in Cardiac output and gradient with a constant valve area. The Easiest way to differentiate within the cath lab is to use a dobutamine challenge similar to stress echocardiography starting with 5 µg/kg/min up to 20 or 30 µg/kg/min. Further limitation occurs in low flow states (Cardiac Output <2.5 L/min). Gorlin Formula overestimates the severity of valve stenosis. Therefore, this forumula should be used with caution in these situations [70].

1.3 Quantification of Aortic Valve Regurgitation

1.3.1 Introduction

Aortic regurgitation occurs due to different reasons, which apart from the valve itself, may involve the sinus portion of the aortic root and the ascending aorta. At the level of the aortic valve, degenerative valve lesions or bicuspid valves account for the majority of cases. Dilatation of the aortic root and ascending aorta secondary to atherosclerosis, aortitis, or connective tissue disease is another important reason for aortic regurgitation [14]. Regarding the clinical presentation of patients with significant aortic regurgitation, the time course is crucial ranging from slowly developing lesions often resulting in minor symptoms to the development of acute severe aortic regurgitation with pronounced symptoms, pulmonary oedema, and cardiogenic shock. The latter clinical course is typically associated with rapidly progressive destruction of the valve by endocarditis or by acute aortic dissection.

Prior to imaging, a comprehensive clinical examination should be performed, including measurement of blood pressure at both arms and possibly at the lower extremity to assess signs of aortic coarctation associated with bicuspid valves, with a high pulse pressure indicating severe aortic regurgitation. Furthermore, a palpable wide pulse amplitude ("Corrigan's pulse") may be associated with significant aortic regurgitation, as well as a decrescendo diastolic murmur usually best heard over Erb's point. Of note, in severe aortic regurgitation with equilibration of aortic and end diastolic left ventricular pressures, the murmur may be very short, faint or even absent. Another murmur associated with significant aortic regurgitation is the Austin Flint murmur, possibly resulting from vibrations of the anterior mitral leaflet and mitral subvalvular apparatus from to the regurgitation jet directed at the leaflet, or due to relative mitral stenosis resulting from restricted opening of the mitral valve.

1.3.2 Echocardiography

Echocardiographic assessment of aortic regurgitation always starts with the evaluation of the valve's morphology, including assessment of the sinus portion, sino-tubular junction, ascending aorta and possibly the aortic arch and the proximal descending aorta [8, 71]. A comprehensive 2D echocardiographic description of the valve includes the number and relative size of the cusps (which should be symmetrical in a normal valve), the morphologic appearance (fibrosis, calcification, raphes, additional structures like valvular strands or other floating structures/endocarditic vegetations) and the movement of the valves (normal movement, restrictions or prolapse). For this purpose, every single cusp should be assessed and described separately, with distinct 2D loops also being taken in fundamental imaging to better assess native valve morphology. Special attention should be drawn to specific conditions associated with severe aortic regurgitation, i.e. restriction or prolapse of one or more cusps leading to a visible coaptation gap. These assessments are typically performed in the parasternal long and short axis views. The apical long axis, 5-chamber view or subcostal views can provide additional information, particularly regarding additional floating structures in heavily calcified valves. After description of the valve itself, additional information especially about the size of the sinus portion, the ascending aorta and the aortic arch must be gathered, and—especially in patients with bicuspid aortic valves—aortic coarctation should be excluded. A floating membrane, possibly seen in the ascending aorta or the aortic arch (both structures should be visualized in long and short axis), possibly in addition to a (new) pericardial effusion, may suggest acute aortic dissection.

Following a comprehensive 2-dimensional echocardiographic assessment, different Doppler-parameters help to assess the presence and grading of aortic regurgitation [8]. Colour Doppler imaging from the parasternal long and short axis views as well as from the apical long axis and 5- chamber views provide information about the presence and direction of an aortic regurgitation jet. Furthermore, the number of jets with their corresponding origin within the valve should be described, preferably from the parasternal short axis view. Special care must be applied during this step, as jet morphology and direction in addition to morphologic appearance of the valve help to understand the etiology of the aortic regurgitation. In addition, a semi-quantitative approach will be added, with the assessment of a vena contracta being the simplest. The jet width relative to the LVOT-width may also be easily calculated (approx. 5 mm proximal to the valve leaflets). From the apical or parasternal views (depending on jet direction), a Doppler spectrum of the regurgitant jet using the continuous wave (CW) Doppler technique may be acquired, with special care being applied to its acquisition and interpretation. Depending on image quality, an effective regurgitant orifice area (EROA) using the proximal isovelocity surface area (PISA) may be calculated. Finally, pulsed-waved (PW) Doppler spectra are being

LVOT   AV

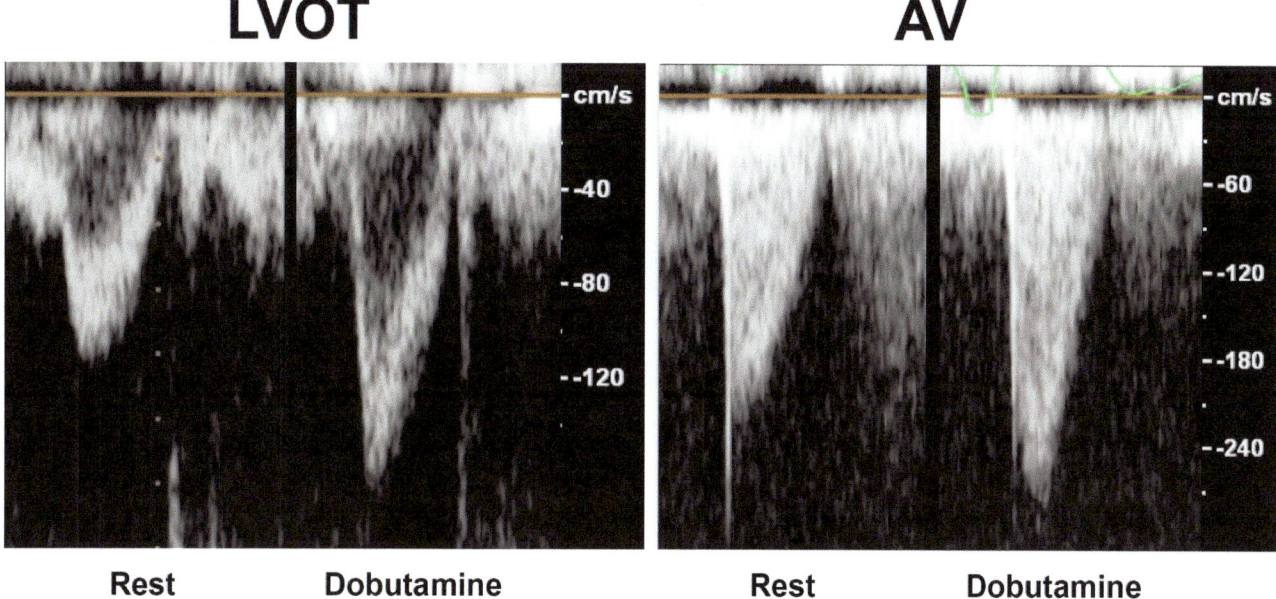

Rest   Dobutamine   Rest   Dobutamine

Fig. 1.8 Low Flow Low Gradient Aortic Stenosis and Dobutamine∗ Stress Echocardiography. ∗ Dose: 20 μg/kg/min. *LVOT* left ventricular outflow tract, *AV* aortic valve

acquired in the distal aortic arch and the abdominal aorta, where again special care should be taken to acquire good quality spectra, as sometimes very low flow velocities must be assessed (Fig. 1.8). Finally, the comprehensive cardiac assessment for aortic regurgitation concludes with measurement of size and volume of the left ventricle as well as the left ventricular ejection fraction. The American Society of Echocardiography provides an algorithm to further grade the severity of the aortic regurgitation depending on the available measurements [7].

1.3.3 Magnetic Resonance Imaging

Although echocardiography is the primary imaging tool for the assessment of aortic regurgitation (AR) severity, cardiac magnetic resonance (CMR) imaging has the advantage of not being limited by acoustic windows. Further, echocardiographic measurements may be hampered by eccentricity of the regurgitant jet and flow convergence shape. Quantification of AR by CMR relies on through plane phase-contrast velocity-encoded assessment of anterograde and retrograde flow at the sinotubular junction, thereby allowing accurate quantification of regurgitant volume and regurgitant fraction [72]. In order to receive correct measurements, it is important that the phase contrast slice is perpendicular in two orthogonal cine images to the aorta (Fig. 1.9). Oblique deviation of the slice from the orthogonal plane of the aorta may cause significant error in the peak flow and flow rate measurements [73]. CMR is the gold standard technique for evaluation of ventricular size and function and dimensions

of the thoracic aorta [28] and the 2014 American Heart Association/American College of Cardiology (AHA/ACC) guidelines give CMR a Class I recommendation for the assessment of left ventricular volume, function, and also AR severity [74]. The most recently published 2017 European Society of Cardiology (ESC) guidelines indicate that CMR should be used to quantify the regurgitation fraction when echocardiographic measurements are inconclusive [4]. However, both guidelines lack specifications on how to exactly quantify and grade AR by CMR [4, 74], possibly due to a lack of established cutoff values for identifying hemodynamically significant AR. Furthermore, little is currently known about the prognostic value of CMR in AR. A study investigated the diagnostic and prognostic utility of CMR in a large prospective AR cohort [75]. In 113 patients with echocardiographic moderate or severe AR undergoing CMR, progression to symptoms or other indications for surgery was monitored. AR quantification identified outcome with high accuracy: 85% of the subjects with regurgitant fraction >33% progressed to surgery in comparison with 8% of subjects with regurgitant fraction ≤33% (P < 0.0001); the area under the curve on receiver operating characteristic analysis was 0.93 (P < 0.0001). CMR-derived left ventricular end-diastolic volume >246 mL had good, although lower, discriminatory ability (area under the curve 0.88), but the combination of this measure with regurgitant fraction provided the best discriminatory power [76]. A recent study evaluating 232 patients with chronic AR suggests that in a significant proportion of patients, AR severity as determined by echocardiography may be reclassified based on CMR assessment. Furthermore, holodiastolic flow in the descend-

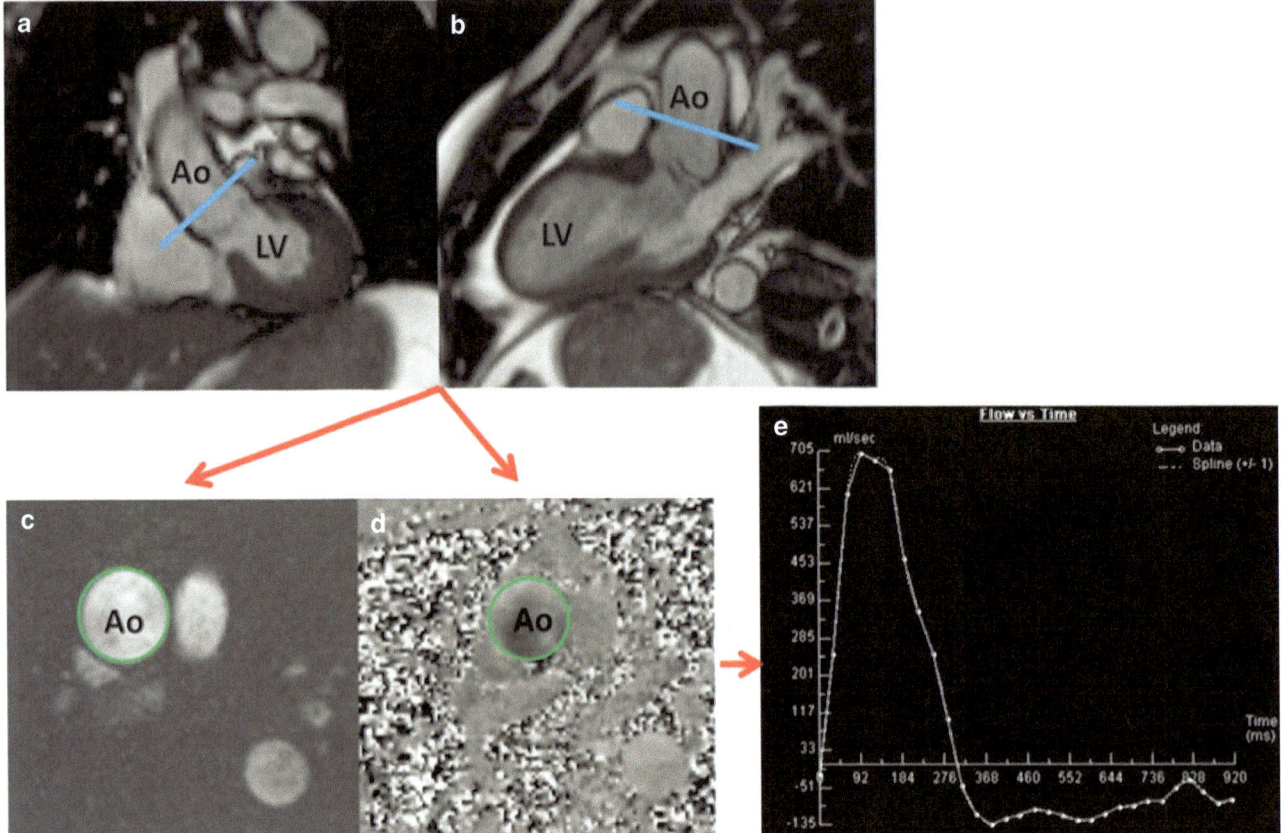

Fig. 1.9 With the use of a coronal and 3-chamber cine view for reference (**a**, **b**), a phase-contrast CMR slice is positioned above the aortic valve in the aortic root (blue lines). Two sets of images are acquired: (**c**) The magnitude image provides details of the anatomy, contour, and shape of the aorta. (**d**) The phase velocity map depicts the velocity and direction of the flow within the aorta. By outlining the contours of the aorta throughout each phase (green contours) in the cardiac cycle, a flow curve can be generated (**e**) to determine aortic flow and reverse stroke volume and flow. The forward volume is 127 mL and the reverse volume 57 mL, resulting in an AR fraction of 45% in this patient. Ao indicates aorta; AR, aortic regurgitation; CMR, cardiac magnetic resonance; and LV, left ventricle. Adapted with permission from Lee JKT et al. Circulation. 2018;137:184–196

ing aorta measured in CMR was strongly and independently associated with event-free survival and therefore CMR has the potential to add important diagnostic and prognostic information. Differentiation between severe and nonsevere AR by CMR should complement echocardiographic AR assessment, especially in cases with impaired examination quality or when more information is needed for clinical decision making [77].

1.3.4   Aortography and Catheterization

Invasive assessment of lesion severity in aortic regurgitation is more difficult and less accurate compared with stenosis evaluation. This is true for non-invasive tests as well and therefore invasive testing is performed more often to get additional information in doubtful clinical scenarios.

Aortography has to be performed using an unusually large amount of contrast in order to fully opacify the aortic root (Fig. 1.10). It is recommended to use 50–60 mL of con-trast and an injection speed of 20 mL/s. Grading of aortic regurgitation is done by evaluation of the opacification of the left ventricle as described by Sellers et al. In mild aortic regurgitation (AR grade 1) contrast fails to opacify the whole left ventricle (LV). Moderate (AR grade 2) regurgitation is stated when contrast enters the whole left ventricle but is less dense as compared with the aorta. AR grade 3 is present, when opacification of LV equals opacification of the aorta. Severe AR (grade 4) is present, when opacification of the LV exceeds that of the aorta. Still, this method is limited to image quality and is a subjective qualitiative method to grade severity [78].

Frick et al. compared in post TAVI implantation evaluation the value of angiography compared with MRI Assessment in 69 patients. There was a great overlap between Sellers class 1 and 2 as assessed by MRI. Sellers class 3 was only recognized in 3 patients, 4 in none. Schultz has used the Sellers method and compared it with a videodensitometric method to quantify the amount of regurgitation volume. Both methods correlated very well and the new method allows a

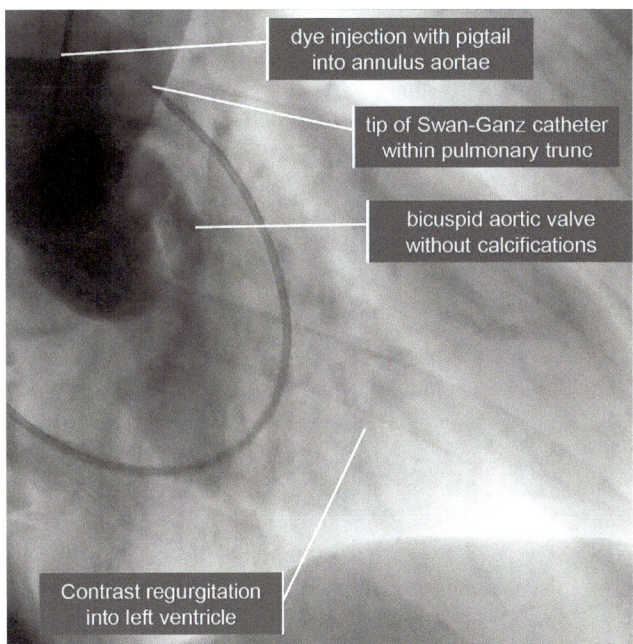

Fig. 1.10 Selective contrast injection into the aortic root with 40 cc at a rate of 20 mL/s from the right anterior oblique position. Aortic root and ascending aorta are completly filled with contrast. A bicuspid aortic valve can easily be detected due to the missing third sinus. Regurgitation is present but the left ventricle is not fully opacified (Sellers class I). A Swan-Ganz catheter is seen in the pulmonary artery, demonstrating that a complete hemodynamic study was performed

highly reproducible measurement. They used 30 cc contrast at 15 mL/s or 40 cc at 20 mL/s [79].

Hemodynamic assessment offers additional information. Aortic pressure measurements show the characteristic wide pulse pressure which is even more pronounced when using the femoral pressures. Compared with simultaneous left ventricular measurement, peripheral pressure is up to 50 mmHg higher [80] with no difference between femoral or brachial pressures.

In very severe aortic regurgitation, diastolic aortic pressure and LV end-diastolic pressure equalize (diastasis). LV diastolic pressure rises rapidly due to the volume contribution of the regurgitation. Peripheral pulse pressure (difference between systolic and diastolic pressure) is very large due to the increased stroke volume. A systolic gradient is typical missing in pure aortic regurgitation during invasive measurements (which in contrast can be seen in Doppler echocardiography due to the increased stroke volume).

Sinning et al. proposed a new index for hemodynamic evaluation of aortic valve regurgitation: diastolic blood pressure (aorta, DBP) minus left ventricular end diastolic pressure (LVEDP) divided by systolic blood pressure (aorta, SBP) multiplied by 100: $[(DBP-LVEDP)/SBP]\times100$. When this index was added to standard echocardiographic assessment of AR (AR none/mild or moderate/severe), patients with an AR Index

of <25 have a much higher 1-year mortality as compared with those >25 [81].

In conclusion, it is necessary to perform accurate injections with correct flow velocities for angiographic assessment of AR. Echocardiographic and hemodynamic measurements help to improve the grading of severity for clinical decision making. Videodensitometrie may offer additional value but is not commonly available within the cath-lab. MRI is limited by the fact that it cannot be used during a procedure.

1.4 Anatomical Assessment

1.4.1 Introduction

An important component of assessing the aortic valve in determining functional abnormalities and potential options for intervention is a detailed anatomic evaluation of the valve. This is recommended in international guidelines including those published by the European Association of Cardiovascular Imaging and American Society of Echocardiography [7–9]. For example, in the setting of a stenosed valve, cusp mobility restriction is expected to be concordant with the degree of stenosis detected by Doppler echocardiography. Anatomic valve abnormalities such as a bicuspid or unicuspid valve are also important to note.

In the setting of aortic regurgitation, the etiology is only understood by evaluating the anatomic features of the valve. This has both diagnostic and therapeutic implications. Regurgitation due to a prolapsing or flail leaflet is repaired in a different way than pure aortic root dilation, whereas repair is often not possible with rheumatic valve changes or sclerosis [82–84].

Understanding the morphology of a specific valve and the surrounding structures is especially important if an intervention is being considered. As already mentioned, some bicuspid aortic valves with significant regurgitation can be repaired [82, 84]. This avoids the need for a valve prosthesis and is generally associated with good clinical outcomes [85–87]. Additionally, in the era of transcatheter valve implantation, anatomic variations in the underlying valve should be assessed because of the specific design limitations of certain valves. This is clinically relevant because the likelihood of complications or a suboptimal final result may be affected. For example, bicuspid aortic valves have been associated with worse procedural outcomes, although this is improving with newer generation transcatheter valves [88–92].

Anatomic valvular assessment can be performed using different imaging modalities. Echocardiography is generally best because of the excellent temporal resolution and lack of radiation exposure. This allows the valve to be well visualized throughout the cardiac cycle. However, it may be difficult to evaluate leaflet configuration in the presence of significant thickening or calcification with 2-dimensional or 3-dimensional echocardiography [93]. In these situations, computed tomography or magnetic resonance imaging can provide additional information [10, 12, 63]. Valve calcification is seen with all imaging modalities but quantification is only standardized with computed tomography and has been linked to procedural and clinical outcomes [94–98]. Methods to perform echocardiographic calcium quantification is investigational at this time [99–101].

1.4.2 Bicuspid, Tricuspid, and Other Morphologies of the Aortic Valve and LVOT

1.4.2.1 Introduction
A normal aortic valve has 3 nearly symmetric leaflets and open triangularly to a near circular orifice during systole without any restriction.

Congenital abnormalities of the aortic valve represents the most common congenital lesion, affecting approximately 0.5 to 2% of the population [102]. The most common abnormality of these is a bicuspid aortic valve by far. A two leaflet aortic valve can take on many morphologies, including equal sized leaflets with no raphe (a thickened band representing a fused commissure) or asymmetric leaflets with a raphe if two of the three usual cusps are congenitally fused. The orientation of these morphologies can also vary. The most commonly used classification systems are the Schaefer and Sievers classification schemes [103, 104]. The Schaefer classification describes a bicuspid aortic valve based on which of the three usual leaflets are fused. A type 1 represent left and right coronary cusp fusion, type 2 right and non-coronary cusp fusion and type 3 is left and non-coronary cusp fusion [103].

The Sievers classification is based on the number of raphe present, anatomic appearance of the leaflets, and functional consequences to the valve [104]. For example, a Sievers 0 represents a true bicuspid valve with symmetric leaflets and is then subcategorized as "AP" (anterior-posterior) or "lat" (lateral) depending on the position of the cusps relative to the single commissure. Sievers 1 describes a single raphe and is followed by letters representing the location of the raphe, and is the same as the fused leaflets ("LR" for left-right fusion, "RN" for right-non fusion and "NL" for non-left fusion). A third component of this classification shceme describes the functional consequence, with an "S" for stenosis, "I" for insufficiency, "B" for both stenosis and insufficiency (mixed disease), or "No" for normal function. Two advantages of the three-block Sievers classification system is that it covers a wider range of anatomic variants and includes a description of any functional abnormalities.

Unicuspid and quadricuspid aortic valves can also be observed but are much rarer [105–109]. Associated anatomic abnormalities, such as an enlarged left ventricular outflow tract, dilated aorta or coarctation of the aorta, are associated with congenitally abnormal aortic valves [106, 107, 110].

The anatomic morphology of the aortic valve and left ventricular outflow tract are well assessed by all imaging modalities, including 2-dimensional and 3-dimensional echocardiography, computed tomography and cardiac magnetic resonance imaging (Figs. 1.11, 1.12, 1.13, 1.14 and 1.15).

1.4.2.2 Echocardiography
The aortic valve and left ventricular outflow tract morphology is easily assessed by transthoracic echocardiography [5]. The best windows to visualize the valve are the parasternal long axis and parasternal short axis views. A normal trileaflet aortic valve should open without any restriction on the short axis view and demonstrate three mobile cusps and three commissures that open all the way to the valve edge.

Congenital abnormalities of the aortic valve such as a bicuspid valve, or rarely a unicuspid or quadricuspid valve, is usually first suspected due to restricted opening and "doming" of the valve tip during systole in the parasternal long axis view. There may also be an enlarged left ventricular outflow tract seen on this view.

A parasternal short axis view at the level of the valve cusps is then able to visualize the number of cusps, orientation and shape of the orifice and its commissures, as well as presence or absence of raphes. A normal, trileaflet valve should appear symmetric when closed in diastole. It should then open triangularly into a circular orifice during systole.

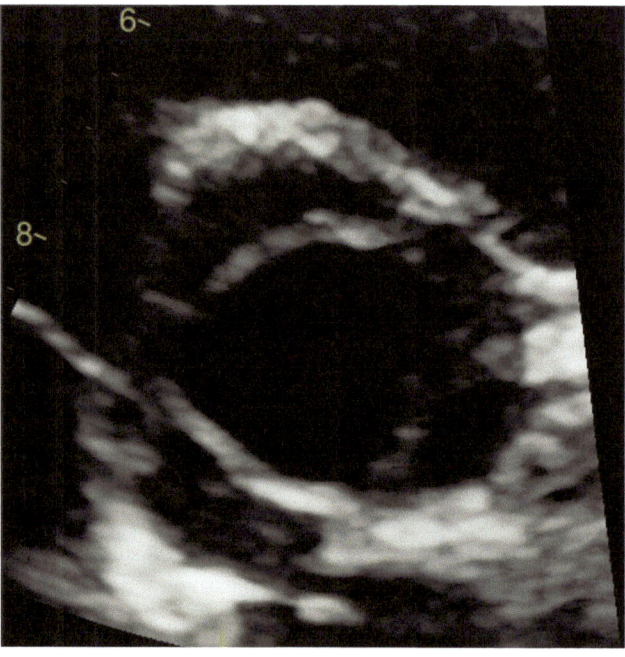

Fig. 1.11 A tricuspid aortic valve seen en-face by echocardiography in systole

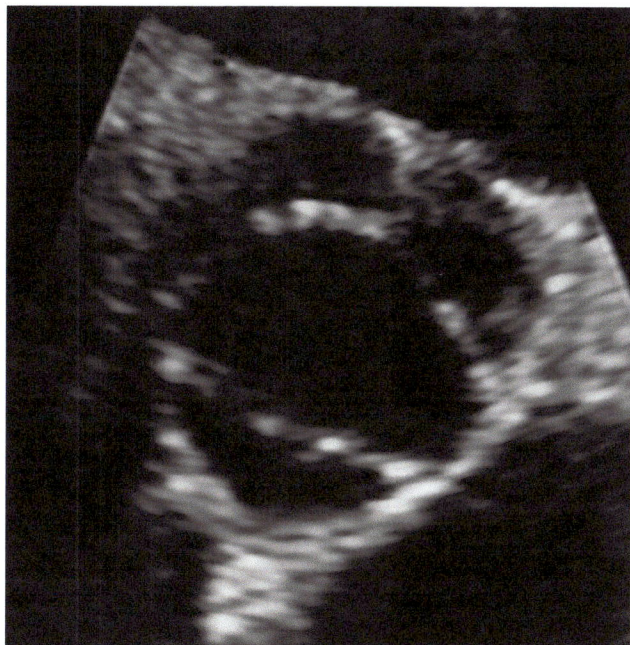

Fig. 1.12 A bicuspid aortic valve (Sievers 1 L/R) seen en-face by echocardiography in systole

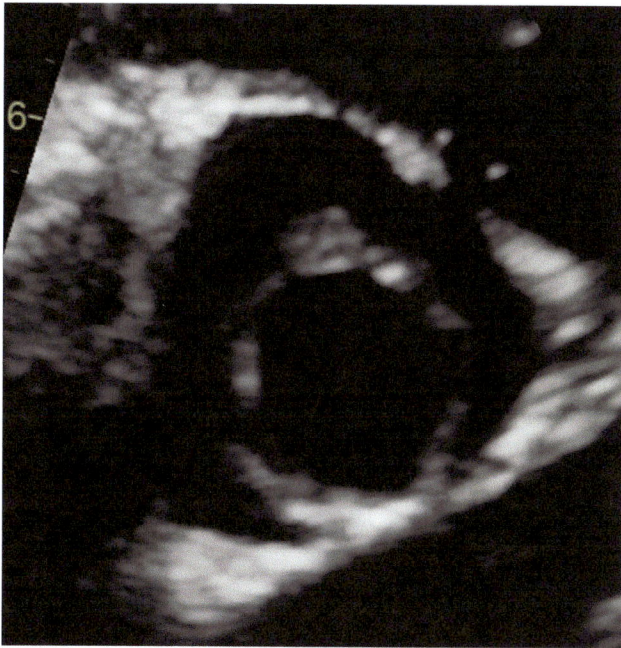

Fig. 1.14 A unicuspid aortic valve seen en-face by echocardiography in systole

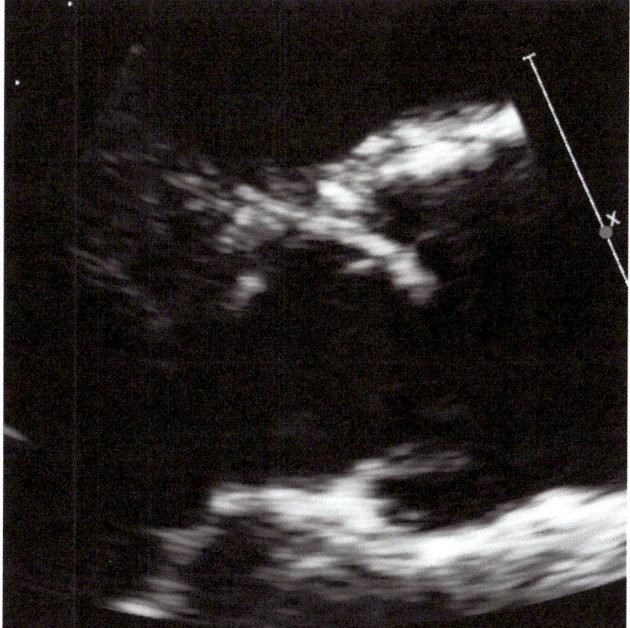

Fig. 1.13 Systolic doming of the aortic valve leaflet seen on the zoomed parasternal long axis view on a transthoracic echocardiogram, suggesting the presence of a bicuspid aortic valve

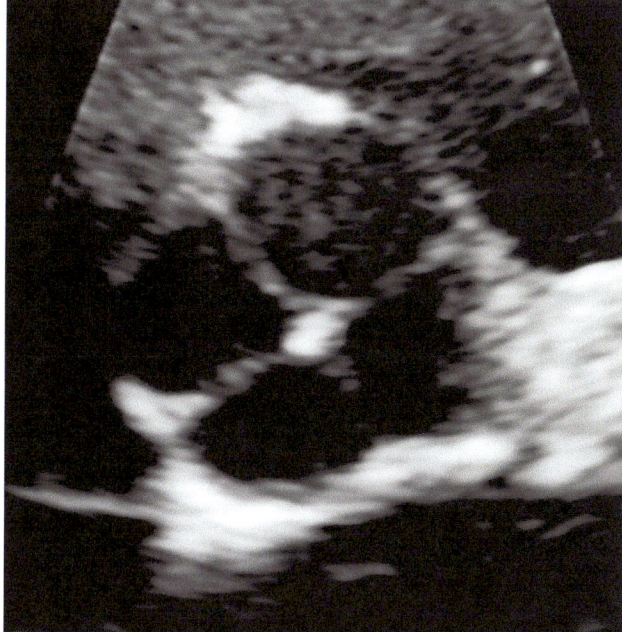

Fig. 1.15 A quadricuspid aortic valve seen en-face by echocardiography in diastole

Bicuspid aortic valves, however, have a much different appearance. When closed they may appear to still have "three" cusps due to the presence of a raphe, but generally still demonstrates some degree of asymmetry. Alternatively, they may appears to have two symmetric leaflets [104]. In systole, these valves will open in a slit-like fashion and appear more as an ellipse when fully open.

Unicuspid aortic valves can have no or a variable number or raphe [106]. The key differentiating factor is that the valve orifice is a single commissure and will open to the edge of the aortic annulus at only one location, rather than two in the case of a bicuspid valve or three in the case of a trileaflet valve. The systolic appearance of the open orifice can be circular or ellipsoid, but will not reach the edges of the annulus.

The parasternal plane axis appearance is variable depending on the location of the unicuspid commissure and imaging plane. Generally, symmetric leaflet closure is not seen and there will be difficulty in identifying distinct leaflets.

Quadricuspid aortic valves have four cusps and generally no raphe [107–109]. In the parasternal short axis view, four commissures are seen in the closed position. The valve opens in a star and then square shape. The maximally opened valve orifice may be circular if leaflet mobility is not restricted.

In addition to 2-dimensional echocardiography, a 3-dimensional view of the valve by echocardiography can be helpful when the parasternal short axis appearance is unclear. This can occur when there is significant motion of the leaflet tip plane during the cardiac cycle or due to respiration.

The left ventricular outflow tract can also be examined for abnormalities. A large left ventricular outflow tract is often seen in conjunction with a bicuspid aortic valve. Subvalvular membranes or shelves may also be visualized on the parasternal long axis, apical 5 chamber and apical 3 chamber views. 3-dimensional echocardiography with multiplanar reconstruction can allow for better understanding of the true cross-sectional shape and dimensions of the left ventricular outflow tract. This can be used to increase the accuracy of aortic valve area calculation and may be beneficial for planning interventions.

Transoesophageal echocardiography may also be used to further assess for structural abnormalities of the aortic valve or left ventricular outflow tract [111]. The midoesophageal window provides better spatial resolution of the aortic valve compared to transthoracic imaging, making details of the leaflets easier to see. Similarly, the left ventricular outflow tract is also generally well visualized by transoesophageal echocardiography. 3 dimensional echocardiography can be used during a transoesophageal study to view the valve en face if leaflet configuration is unclear on 2 dimensional imaging.

Echocardiography remains a primary imaging modality to assess for aortic valve structural abnormalities as well as the morphology of the left ventricular outflow tract. However, some important limitations remain. The leaflets of the aortic valve may be obscured by dense calcification of the leaflets or annulus, which can result in shadowing or blooming artifact. When transoesophageal echocardiography is not possible or is also inconclusive, other imaging modalities can be useful if the morphology is unclear and needs further assessment [112].

1.4.2.3 Computed Tomography

1.4.2.3.1 Diagnostic Value of CT

Echocardiography is the method of choice to screen for bicuspid valves. However, the bicuspid aortic valve can be visualized accurately by computed tomography (CT) as well if echocardiography fails to make the diagnosis or further investigation (e.g. for treatment planning) is warranted. CT has a high sensitivity and specificity in determining how many functional leaflets are present and if there is a raphe (Fig. 1.16). Additionally, valve calcifications can be accurately assessed and quantified. CT is also the method

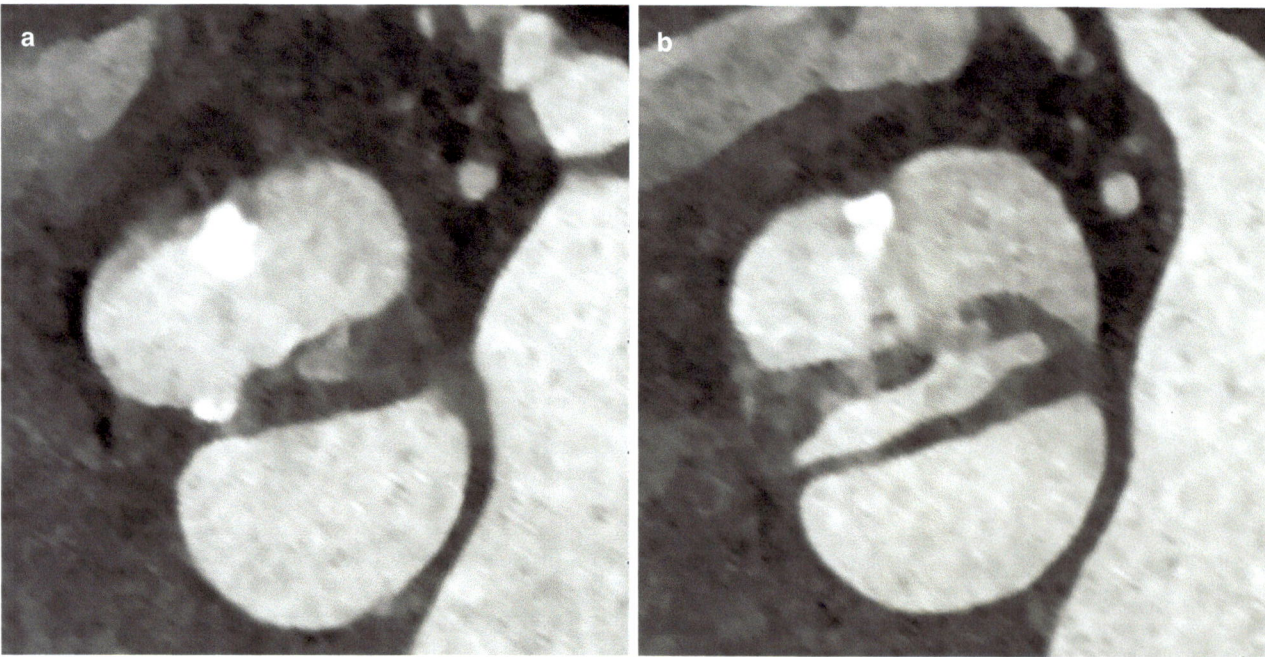

Fig. 1.16 46 year old patient with a bicuspid aortic valve with fusion between the coronary cusps and associated calcifications shown in (**a**) diastole and (**b**) systole

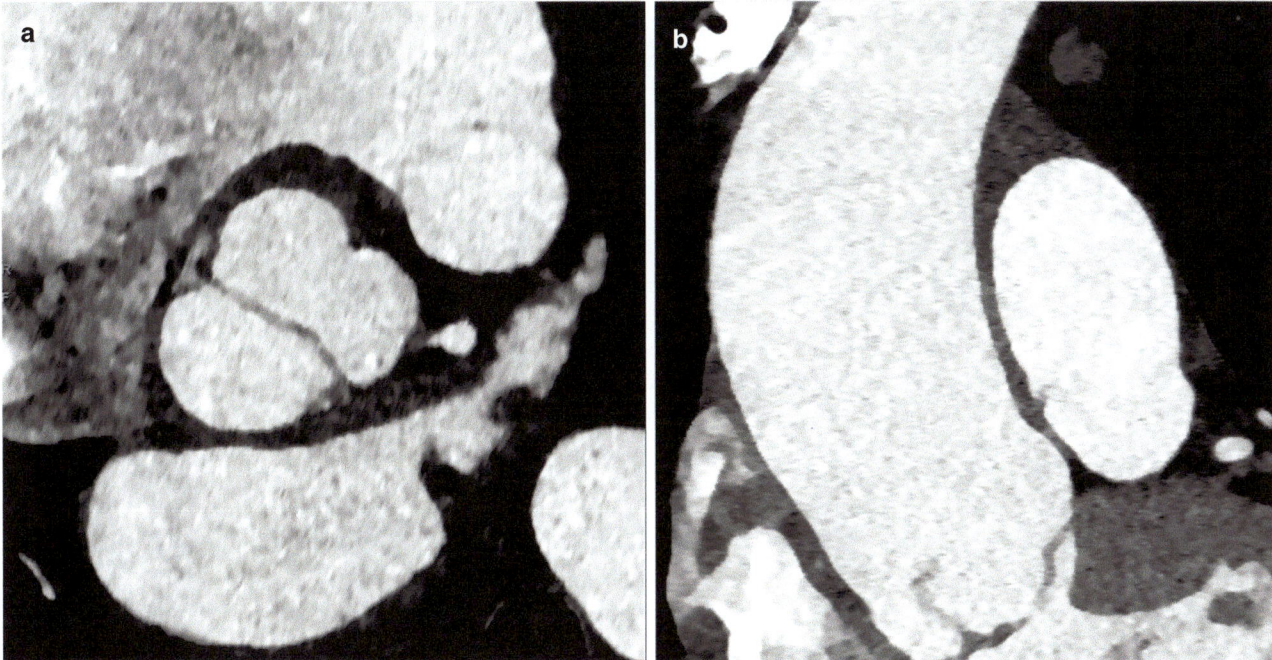

Fig. 1.17 39 year old patient with a bicuspid valve without raphe (**a**) and associated dilation of the aorta (**b**)

of choice to evaluate aortic dimensions and to exclude further associated aortic pathologies, as bicuspid aortic valves are associated with dilatation of the aortic root (Fig. 1.17) and with coarctation.

1.4.2.3.2 Image Acquisition
Contrast-enhanced, ECG-triggered CT is the modality of choice to further investigate aortic valve morphology. Data acquisition on CT must be ECG-triggered, including systolic phases of the heart cycle, to correctly see the opening of the leaflets during systole. It is important to note that the systolic phase must be acquired, as state-of-the-art low dose CT protocols usually acquire images only in the diastolic phase (in order to lower the radiation dose). CT should also include an unenhanced CT of the heart to enable accurate quantification of valve calcifications using the Agatston scoring system.

To evaluate associated pathologies of the aortic root and thoracic aorta, CT angiography of the entire thoracic aorta should be usually included in the evaluation of the aortic valve. Also, CT angiography can accurately guide further procedure planning. If endovascular treatment options are considered, CT angiography of the abdominal aorta, iliac and femoral arteries, to evaluate possible access sites, can be included.

1.4.2.4 Magnetic Resonance Imaging
The main advantage of magnetic resonance imaging (MRI) in the assessment of congenital malformations of the aortic valve in comparison to other non-invasive imaging modalities is its ability to comprehensively evaluate cardiac anat-

omy and function. This includes the assessment of left and right ventricular size, mass and function, visualization of valvular, sub- and supravalvular aortic pathology, the quantification of aortic stenosis and regurgitation by flow assessment and planimetry as well as angiography of the aorta.

In patients with bicuspid aortic valve, MRI allows for excellent characterisation of different valve morphologies with low inter-observer variability [113, 114], which is helpful to guide management, particular in situations where image quality by echocardigography is suboptimal. In addition, MRI can clearly detect associated aortic dilatation [114].

Left ventricular outflow tract (LVOT) obstruction is most often seen in patients with asymmetric hypertrophic cardiomyopathy and systolic anterior motion of the mitral valve. MRI can visualize flow acceleration across the LVOT, however flow quantification by velocity encoding may be inaccurate due to turbulent jets and misalignment [115, 116]. CMR planimetry of the LVOT area and the LVOT/aorta valve diameter ratio, however, enable identification of the presence and absence of a resting LVOT gradient [115, 116].

1.4.2.5 Angiography
It is necessary to identify the 3 sinuses (right, left- and non-coronary) of the aortic root to decide wheather it is a bi- or tricuspid aortic valve. Using rotational angiography or biplane imaging during contrast injection it is feasible in most cases to differentiate between both morphologies. The LVOT can examined during LV injection using the right anterior oblique and left anterior oblique projections.

1.4.3 Evaluating the Repairability of a Regurgitant Valve and Aorta

1.4.3.1 Introduction

When there is significant aortic regurgitation due to aortic root disease or aortic leaflet pathology, it may be preferable to repair the valve rather than replace it with a prosthesis, especially in the setting of younger individuals [82]. Mechanical prosthetic valves carry with them a not insignificant risk of thromboembolism [117, 118]. If anticoagulation is required, there is also an associated risk of bleeding [118, 119]. Mechanical valves also limit the performance of procedures that need to cross the valve and do not offer a transcatheter valve-in-valve option should repeat intervention be required due to prosthetic valvular degeneration. Bioprosthetic valves, on the other hand, may have a shorter lifespan prior to degeneration and require multiple interventions in a person's lifetime [120].

The surgical technique used to repair a regurgitant bicuspid aortic valve depends on the underlying mechanism of regurgitation. Strategies may include remodeling of the sinotubular junction, subcommissural annuloplasty, patch repair, prolapse plication and resuspension or shaving and decalcification for leaflet repair [82–84]. Therefore, a proper understand of the exact leaflet and aortic root pathology is essential in planning such an intervention.

Multimodality imaging is able to perform this pre-intervention assessment. Parameters derived from echocardiography, computed tomography and magnetic resonance imaging will demonstrate any intrinsic problems of the leaflets and the geometry of the aortic root [7, 8, 12, 121]. Findings may also be predictive of a durable repair and help determine the extent of surgery needed for the rest of the aorta [85–87, 122–125]. Details regarding the information from each imaging modality will be outlined in this section.

1.4.3.2 Echocardiography

Echocardiographic assessment of a regurgitant aortic valve is helpful in determining the likelihood of a successful repair. First, the leaflet morphology can be assessed in detail. This includes differentiating between a normal trileaflet valve with isolated root disease, which may be treated by repair of the aortic root or ascending aorta alone with valve preservation or reimplantation to improve valve coaptation. In this situation, the basal annular diameter is important to measure because a larger diameter (≥ 28 mm) is associated with recurrent aortic regurgitation [125].

If there is a bicuspid aortic valve, the size and orientation of the two cusps and commissures should be assessed. Raphes and the degree of thickening or calcification should also be noted. Cusp prolapse or billowing should be evaluated and commissural orientation angle and effective cusp height should be measured. The effective cusp height is measured as the distance from the aortic valve annulus to the most distal point of coaptation [123]. Similar to trileaflet valve repair, the annular dimension is important.

Due to the high spatial resolution needed to make these measurements, it is generally best to perform a transesophageal echocardiogram. This should ideally be done in the pre-operative setting but a detailed assessment under general anesthesia in the form of a peri-operative transesophageal echocardiogram is also useful to verify the surgical strategy at the time of a potential repair.

Symmetric cusps or a valve without significant calcification may be easier to repair. For example, valves with significant calcified raphe may need more extensive tissue excision and reconstruction using a pericardial patch. Degree of cusp prolapse should also be measured, since this may be repaired using free margin plication or resuspension [83, 86].

Specific anatomic criteria that have been found to be related to aortic valve repair durability. An annular diameter of over 30 mm is associated with recurrent aortic regurgitation in follow up in one study [124]. Another found factors predictive of reoperation include larger annular diameter (>28 mm), smaller effective cusp height (<9 mm), commissural orientation (<160°) and use of a pericardial patch [85].

In a third study, billowing, defined as prolapse of the nadir of the cusp but not the free edge of the leaflets, was associated with recurrent significant aortic regurgitation following surgical repair. These authors noted other echocardiographic findings in the immediate post-procedure setting that were predictive of worsening regurgitation in follow up were lower effective height (<8 mm), lower coaptation length (<4 mm), more than minimal aortic regurgitation and an eccentric aortic regurgitation jet [122].

Echocardiographic predictors of a successful repair include an eccentric regurgitant jet direction, no cusp thickening, no cusp calcification and absence of commissural thickening [87].

In addition to the aortic valve and annulus, the proximal ascending aorta and aortic root are well visualized by echocardiography. Since they are often visualized by 2-dimensional echocardiography in the long axis, care must be taken to ensure the maximum diameter is recorded to avoid underestimation of dimensions. This is important because the 2-dimensional imaging plane is variable depending on the scan plane. If the aorta and root are assessed in short axis, care must be taken to avoid an oblique imaging plane, which will overestimate the true cross-sectional dimensions. For these reasons, complementary imaging with computed tomography or cardiac magnetic resonance imaging should be strongly considered for a complete assessment of the aorta.

Echocardiography is also limited in its ability to fully assess the entire aorta when trying to understand the exact extent of aortic disease. Transthoracic echocardiography is not able to visualize the distal ascending aorta and much of the descending thoracic aorta. Transesophageal echocardiography also suffers from a blind spot near the distal ascending aorta due to an air shadow from the right mainstem bronchus.

Despite these specific limitations, transthoracic and transesophageal echocardiography remains a primary imaging modality in the assessment for aortic valve and aortic repair evaluation (Figs. 1.18 and 1.19).

1.4.3.3 Magnetic Resonance Imaging

Aortic valve repair has been shown to be an alternative to aortic valve replacement for treatment of aortic valve regurgitation in selected patients [126]. To establish a precise diagnosis, patient selection and risk stratification, imaging, in particular echocardiography, plays a central role. However, the assessment of aortic regurgitation by echocardiography can be difficult and image quality might be limited to the acoustic window and in patients with obesity or lung disease [127].

The pathomechanism of aortic regurgitation includes annular dilatation with central valve leakage due to inadequate cusp apposition, bicuspid valve with retraction and/or prolapse of the conjoint cusp, tricuspid valve with cusp prolapse and cusp perforation in patients with endocarditis [126]. Figure 1.20 is showing a patient with bicuspid aortic valve and severe aortic regurgitation due to leaflet prolapse.

The decision to repair a damaged aortic valve depends on many factures, such as the mechanism of insufficiency, the degree of valve degeneration, left ventricular impairment and associated aortic or coronary disease. MRI has the unique advantage to visualize most of the required informa-

tion [74]. In detail, MRI allows direct quantification of aortic regurgitation by through plane phase-contrast velocity encoding, which provides measurements of the ante- and retrograde flow at the sinotubular junction, thereby allowing accurate quantification of regurgitant volume and regurgitant fraction [24]. Moreover, MRI provides excellent characterisation of different valve morphologies by cine images acquired in a stack of sequential short-axis cine images through the valve and parallel to the valve tips [113, 114]. As gold standard for the assessment of ventricular size, mass and function, MRI is able to add important information on the chronic volume overload with an eccentric hypertrophic response of the left ventricle [27]. In the same investigation magnetic resonance angiography allows to reliable depict aortic dimensions with a high temporal and spatial resolution [128].

Therefore, MRI may allow to add important information for the evaluation of repairability of regurgitant aortic valve. However, there are a few significant limitations which have to be considered. First, MRI has a lower temporal and spatial resolution in comparison to echocardiography [129], thereby exact identification of the underlying pathomechanism of aortic regurgitation might be difficult. Second, valve calcification is very hard to visualize by MRI as calcium is usually present as a signal void [130]. This is of great importance, as the degree of valvular calcification is a central parameter for the decision of repair versus replace. Third, cardiac motion can result in artifact, which might impair correct measurements of the aorta, in particular of the aortic root.

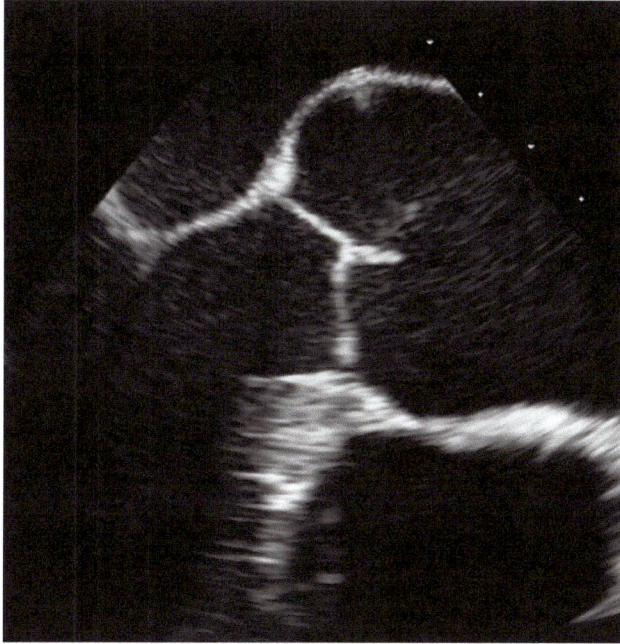

Fig. 1.18 Zoomed long axis view of the aortic valve on transesophageal echocardiography where cusp prolapse, cusp effective height and coaptation length can be measured

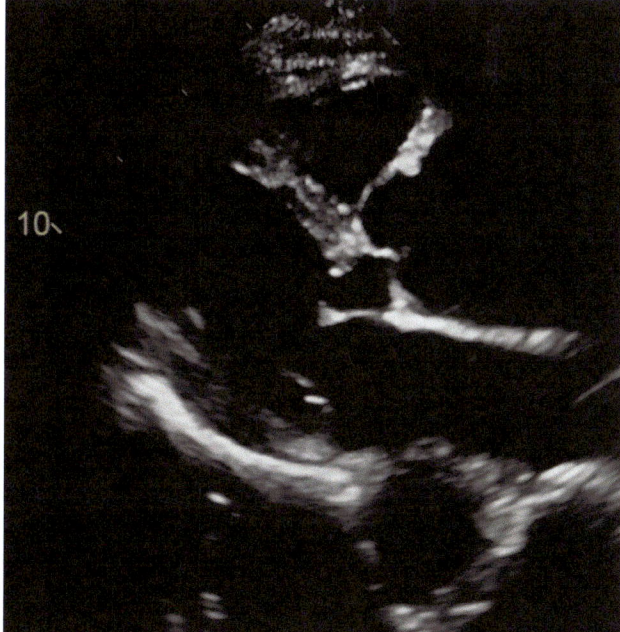

Fig. 1.19 Dilated proximal ascending aorta with effacement of the sinotubuluar junction seen by transthoracic echocardiography on the parasternal long axis view

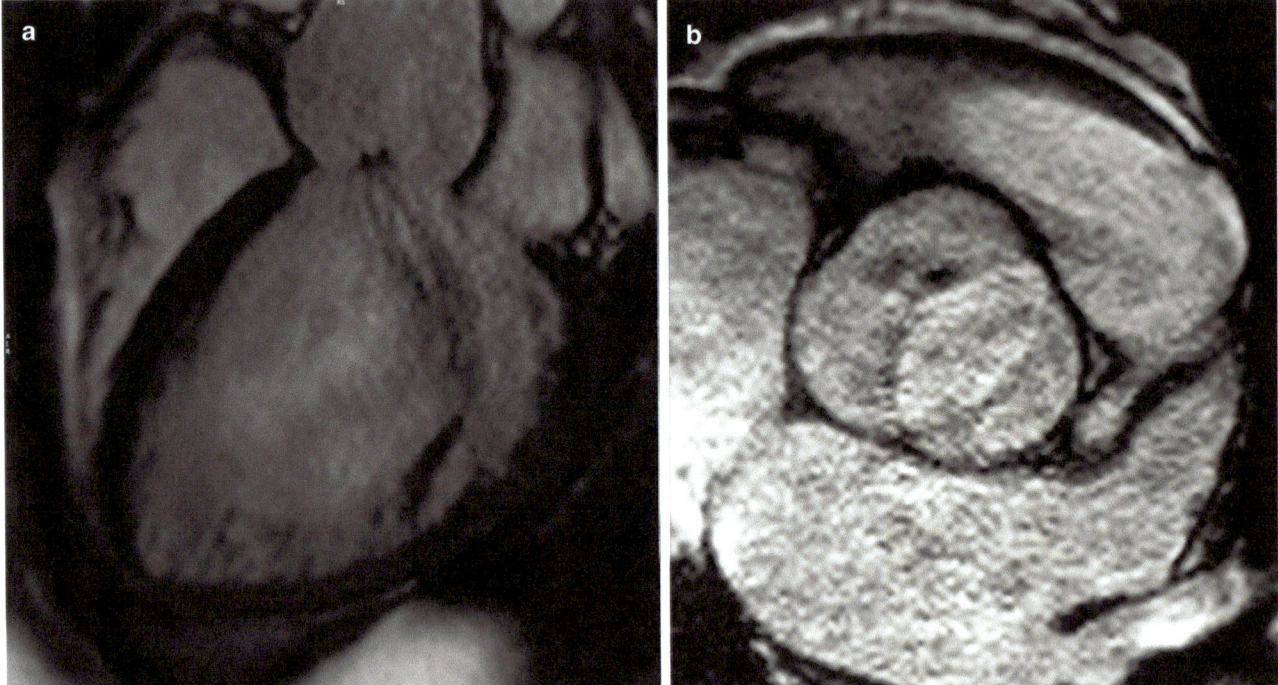

Fig. 1.20 3-chamber (**a**) and short axis cine images (**b**) showing a patient with bicuspid aortic valve with severe regurgitation due to cusp prolapse. Note the severely volume overloaded left ventricle and some calcification on the bicuspid valve presented as signal void

1.4.3.4 Angiography

Direct visualization of the leaflets and the appearance of the tissue of the aortic valve is not possible using angiography. Therefore only the overall anatomical appearance, dimensions of the aortic annulus, sinotubular junction and ascending aorta, and most importantly, the extent of calcifications of the valve and the surrounding tissue can be assessed. 2 orthogonal projections are necessary to evaluate eccentricity. For assessment of calcification, zoomed images with increased X-ray dosage (for better image quality) and inspiration respiration hold are advised. Rotational angiography without contrast helps to identify the exact location of the calcium (Fig. 1.21).

1.4.4 Assessment of Aortic Valve Calcification

1.4.4.1 Introduction

Degenerative changes of the aortic valve often include variable degrees of leaflet calcification. This can further extend into the aortic annulus or the aortic-mitral continuity. An assessment of the degree of pattern of calcification can be useful for both diagnosis and planning an intervention.

For example, it is known that the calcium burden of an aortic valve correlates with the degree of stenosis and is therefore recognized as a supplementary imaging parameter that can be used in determining the severity of aortic stenosis [121]. Additionally, the degree of calcification has been found to be independently associated with clinical outcomes

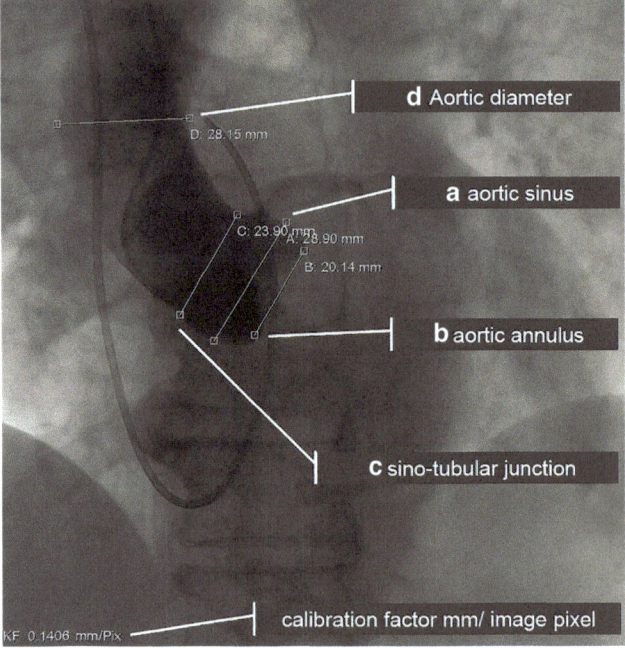

Fig. 1.21 Aortic root injection with measurements of key anatomic landmarks: (**a**) aortic sinus (**b**) aortic annulus (**c**) sino-tubular junction and (**d**) Aortic diameter. Calibration factor is given in mm/pixel of the native image

[95, 101]. Calcification of the aortic annulus may also require more aggressive surgical debulking during a surgical valve replacement. In the setting of transcatheter aortic valve replacement, the pattern of calcification in the aortic root is

very important because it may restrict the expansion of the crimped valve and lead to valve dysfunction or a higher risk of paravalvular regurgitation [131–133]. Some patterns of calcification have also be associated with increased risk of complete heart block requiring a permanent pacemaker [96]. Even more concerning, calcification extending into the left ventricular outflow tract appears to increase the risk of aortic root rupture and overall 2-year mortality [97, 98]. It is also possible that eccentric annular calcification may also increase the risk of complications or paravalvular regurgitation.

Since computed tomography is based on the same radiographic principles as X-ray imaging, it is ideally suited to detect and measure calcification [12, 13, 134]. Additionally, the 3-dimensional dataset can be manipulated using multiplanar reconstruction to specifically localize calcification in the aortic valve leaflets or annulus. Software tools also allow for precise quantification of calcium burden and distribution, but may be subject to differences in scan settings [94].

Echocardiography can also visualize calcification, but ultrasound beams are subject to significant shadowing and blooming artifact by calcification, which limits the utility of this modality for this specific component of valve assessment if detailed quantification is needed. However, an approximation of the burden and distribution of calcium is generally still possible and some researchers have developed scores or proprietary software tools to better standardize the echocardiographic assessment of calcium [99, 100, 135–137]. Magnetic resonance imaging is also able to assess for the presence of aortic valve calcification but is not used regularly to quantify the exact burden. Although calcified leaflets makes valve visualization more difficult, spatial resolution is still excellent, allowing even measurements such as direct planimetry of valve area [63].

Details regarding the role of each modality in detecting aortic valve calcium will be described in this section.

1.4.4.2 Computed Tomography

Echocardiographic diagnosis of low-flow, low-gradient aortic stenosis with preserved ejection fraction remains challenging. Quantification of Aortic valve calcification (AVC) by computed tomography (CT) has gained in importance, especially in patients with paradoxical low-flow, low-gradient aortic stenosis. Quantification of aortic valve calcification on CT is easy to perform and highly reproducible. Quantification of AVC with CT is performed using the method proposed by Agaston requiring the acquisition of a non-enhanced CT scan at 120 kVp. Previously, the European Society of Cardiology recommended cut-off values for the AVC Agaston Score to assess the likelihood of severe aortic stenosis according to AVC load. On contrast-enhanced CT, mathematical formulas may enable the quantification of aortic valve calcification even with variable degree of enhancement of the aortic root. The aortic valve quantification is performed using the same software and the same Hounsfield

Unit threshold as for quantification of coronary calcification (Fig. 1.22).

1.4.4.3 Echocardiography

Transthoracic echocardiography can be used to assess for general aortic valve calcification but is limited by shadowing of ultrasound beams by dense calcium. This may obscure structures or details past the area of calcification. Additionally, because calcium is a strong reflector of ultrasound beams, blooming artifact may occur and cause calcified structures to appear larger than reality by echocardiography. These artifacts are present in both 2-dimensional and 3-dimensional echocardiography.

It is generally otherwise straightforward to detect calcification of the aortic valve leaflets, which will look bulky, echodense and may have restricted mobility. This is first noted on the parasternal long axis view, which can also show whether calcification extends into the aortic annulus, left ventricular outflow tract or aortic-mitral continuity. The parasternal short axis view can reveal if there is asymmetric leaflet calcification, nodular calcification, or if calcification is causing mobility restriction of a specific leaflet or commissure. A modified parasternal short axis view panning into the aortic annulus and left ventricular outflow tract may also reveal calcification pattern in these areas. This assessment can also be performed using biplane imaging, by sweeping from the valve level into the left ventricular outflow tract based on the parasternal long axis view to generate corresponding parasternal short axis views. Other transthoracic views that may be helpful in assessing aortic valve, annular and left ventricular outflow tract calcium include the apical 5 and apical 3 chamber views.

Like transthoracic echocardiography, calcification of the aortic valve can be seen by transesophageal echocardiography. Leaflets are best assessed using the midesophageal long axis and short axis views. The aortic annulus, left ventricular outflow tract and aortic-mitral continuity can be seen either by sliding below the aortic valve in the short axis plane or by using biplane imaging and sweeping from the long axis view. 3-dimensional echocardiography may be of limited use because although leaflets will look bulky, the echodensity of specific areas relative to others is generally not well rendered using current technology and blooming artifact may accentuate areas of calcification. Significant valve calcification may make direct planimetry of the aortic valve area impossible or less accurate [93]. Nonetheless, this can still be a useful strategy to help better understand the degree of stenosis when other parameters are unclear and as part of a comprehensive, integrative assessment of aortic stenosis [15].

Calcium assessment on echocardiography is important because it has been shown to correlate with calcium burden detected by computed tomography and overall valve weight on explanted samples [101, 138]. It is also associated with clinical outcomes including cardiovascular morbidity and

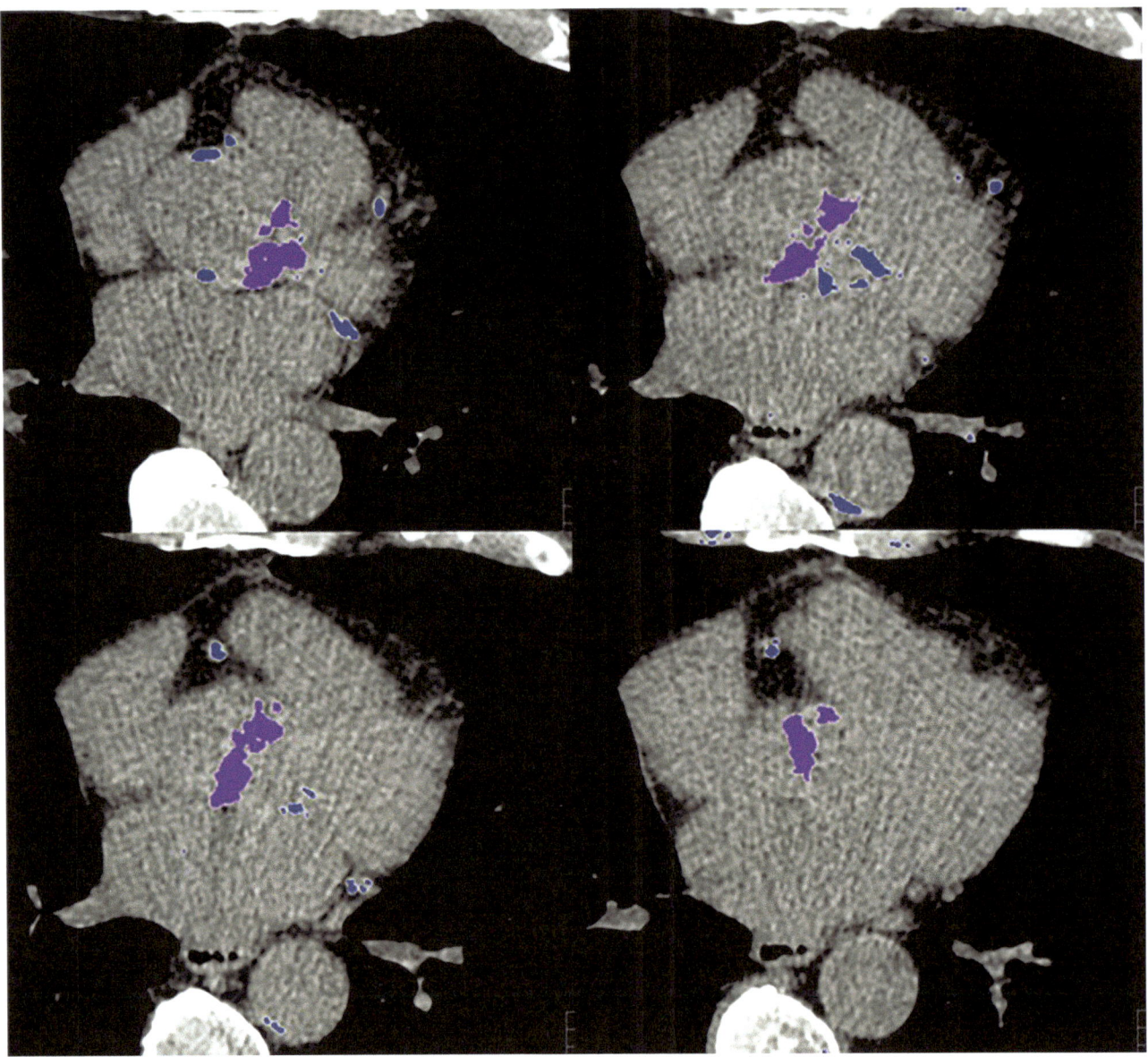

Fig. 1.22 Aortic valve calcification. The Agatston Score of aortic valve calcification is quantified using the same software and the same Hounsfield Unit threshold as for quantification of coronary calcification

all-cause mortality [4]. However, visual estimates of the degree of calcification is subject to significant interobserver variability [136]. Some scores have been proposed in a research setting to attempt to standardize the reporting of calcium by echocardiography, but are not in routine clinical use [100, 137]. Additionally, dedicated software to quantify calcium burden by echocardiography can be developed and has been reported to correlate reasonably well with quantification by computed tomography and valve weight on pathologic inspection [99].

In addition to the degree of calcification, the pattern of calcification is also important to assess during evaluation of the aortic valve. This is usually easily detectable by echocardiography on the short axis view. Both commissural calcification as well overall calcium burden have been shown to be associated with paravalvular regurgitation after transcatheter aortic valve implantation [131, 132]. Additionally, calcium extending into the left ventricular outflow tract by computed tomography has been shown to be associated with an increased risk of annular rupture during these procedures and 2-year survival [97, 98]. Although this has not been validated by echocardiography, this pattern of calcification is readily visible on standard transthoracic or transesophageal echocardiographic studies.

In the setting of a bicuspid aortic valve, the degree of calcification and leaflet mobility restriction are important in the echocardiographic assessment if valve repair is being considered or planned. The presence of significant calcification will often require debridement and is associated with a lower likelihood of successful repair [83, 87, 121] (Fig. 1.23).

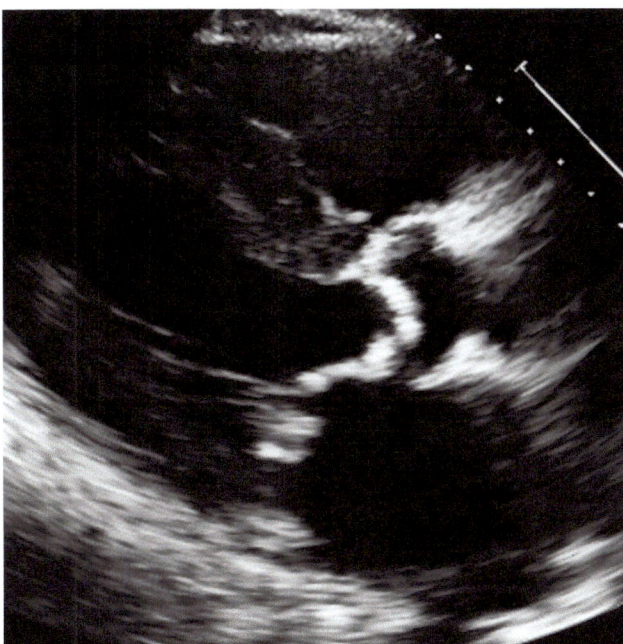

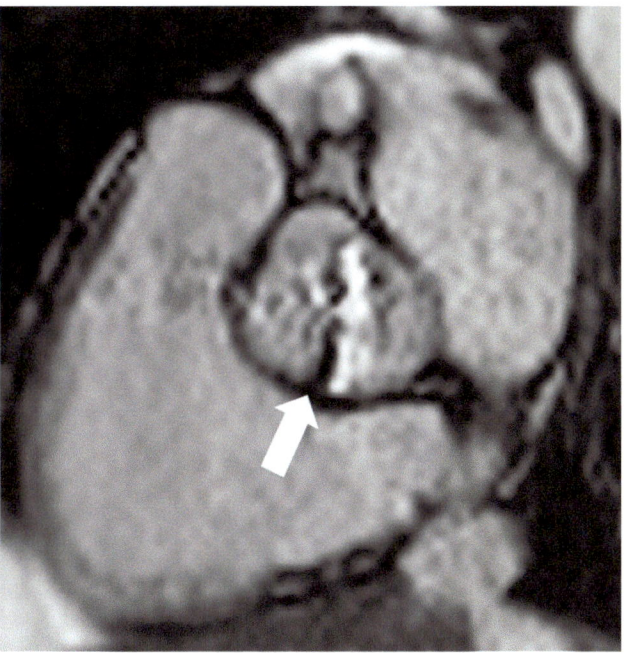

Fig. 1.23 Severe aortic calcification extending into the aortic root, left ventricular outflow tract, aortic-mitral continuity and body of the anterior mitral valve leaflet seen by transthoracic echocardiography on the parasternal long axis view. Posterior mitral annular calcification is also visible

Fig. 1.24 Moderate stenosis in a patient with bicuspid aortic valve. The calcification is present as a signal void (arrow)

1.4.4.4 Magnetic Resonance Imaging

Most aortic valves with severe stenosis and some aortic valves with severe regurgitation are usually severely calcified. Whereas CT is considered the gold standard for the detection of calcification, echocardiography is limited by the acoustic shadow and magnetic resonance imaging (MRI) by the lower proton density with very low signal on both T1 and T2 weighted images as well as the extremely short life-times of the proton signal in water bound to solid-like entities [130]. The latter makes the identification of calcium very difficult and calcium is usually present as signal void (Fig. 1.24). Although in ex-vivo studies or newer techniques, like susceptibility-weighted-magnetic resonance imaging, have been shown to at least partially overcome these limitations and allow detection of calcification in solid soft tissue [139, 140], visualization of calcium in moving structures, such as the aortic valve, remains difficult and is not used in routinely in clinical practice.

1.5   Timing of Intervention and Functional Assessment

1.5.1   Introduction

Once a diagnosis of severe aortic valvular disease is made, the most important clinical decision following this is whether an intervention is indicated. If it is not at the time of initial diagnosis, serial imaging plays an important role to help determine optimal timing for intervention [2, 3, 15].

Generally, there are two primary concerns related to severe valvular disease. The first is symptoms due to a hemodynamic effect of the lesion on cardiac output, pulmonary pressures, myocardial perfusion and wall stress. The second is the consequence to the left ventricle with chronic severe aortic valvular disease.

In the setting of aortic stenosis, the left ventricle becomes pressure overloaded due to the high afterload from the stenosed valve. This increases wall stress, can lead to left ventricular hypertrophy, and in late stages with development of fibrotic changes, dysfunction in left ventricular contractility or relaxation [141, 142].

In aortic regurgitation, the left ventricle is volume overloaded. Chronic remodeling due to this can also result in left ventricular dilation and systolic dysfunction [143, 144]. Therefore, in both cases, the left ventricular size and systolic function need to be carefully followed if symptoms requiring intervention are absent.

Several imaging modalities are able to evaluate the left ventricle in the setting of severe aortic valve disease to assess for either masked underlying symptoms or to detect chronic adverse left ventricular remodeling. These include echocardiography, cardiac magnetic resonance imaging, computed tomography, invasive angiography and nuclear medicine studies. Each has its own advantages and limitations and will be discussed in greater detail in this section. Some methods are able to evaluate both systolic and diastolic function while others are only able to assess systolic function. In addition to studies done at rest, there may also be a role in performing exercise testing in selected asymptomatic individuals [60, 145]. Functional testing may reveal symptoms that are underreported or additional high risk factors suggesting a need for intervention.

1.5.2 Left Ventricular Function, Functional Reserve, Stress Testing, Low Flow Low Gradient Stenosis

1.5.2.1 Introduction

An integrated approach to assessment of the left ventricle in the presence of significant aortic valve disease can be helpful in making management decisions.

Left ventricular size and systolic function are two of the most important imaging parameters to determine. This is because it can determine if chronic valvular disease has caused damage and remodeling to the left ventricle. As remodeling progresses, there is generally myocardial fibrosis that can cause systolic and diastolic dysfunction as well as chamber enlargement. The left ventricular size and volumes can be determined using different imaging modalities and calculation methods. When fewer assumptions about the left ventricular geometry are made, the measurement method tends to be more accurate [6]. However, prognostic clinical data for aortic valve disease may be limited to older methods of ventricular size measurements, such as the 2-dimensional end diastolic or end systolic diameter as measured by echocardiography. This is why treatment guidelines still incorporate these simple and common measurements in treatment algorithms [2, 3, 15].

Left ventricular dimensions, volumes and ejection fraction is most commonly measured by echocardiography but can also be assessed by cardiac magnetic resonance imaging [112], computed tomography, left ventricular angiography and by nuclear medicine techniques.

In addition to understanding the consequence of the valve lesion on the ventricle, the left ventricular systolic function is also important because it provides context in terms of the observed valvular hemodynamics relative to the suspected or known degree of valve disease. For example, a left ventricle with normal size and contractility that generates a normal forward stroke volume will generate higher gradients for the same degree of stenosis compared to either a small ventricle with normal contractility or one with severe impairment in systolic function. In the setting of aortic stenosis, this phenomenon is called low-flow low-gradient aortic stenosis and may cause discrepancy in the measured transvalvular gradient compared to the calculated aortic valve area [146].

Low-flow low-gradient aortic stenosis is an important clinical entity because of the subtypes and associated prognostic differences [146–148]. One subset are those with low gradients due to reduced left ventricular ejection fraction. The other have a preserved left ventricular ejection fraction, but the stroke volume is low due to small overall ventricular size. This second subset is somewhat controversial among clinicians and is also called paradoxical low-flow low-gradient aortic stenosis. Care must be taken in this setting to ensure that measurement errors have not misclassified individuals into this group.

Testing for left ventricular functional reserve and to clarify the true severity of valve stenosis is generally recommended if the etiology of symptoms or need for intervention are unclear. The most common method to evaluate low-flow low-gradient aortic stenosis is with low-dose Dobutamine stress echocardiography [112]. This attempt to augment left ventricular contractility to increase stroke volume provides both information about the left ventricular systolic reserve as well as clarifies whether the degree of aortic stenosis is truly severe. In some situations, the aortic valve may appear to be open poorly due to insufficient stroke volume as opposed to restriction at the valve level [149]. This is often referred to as peudosevere aortic stenosis.

In this section, multimodality imaging assessment of the left ventricular size and systolic function will be reviewed. In addition, methods to assess functional reserve and low-flow low-gradient aortic stenosis will be covered (Fig. 1.25).

1.5.2.2 Assessing Left Ventricular Ejection Fraction and Left Ventricular Dimensions

1.5.2.2.1 Introduction

The basic assessment of the left ventricle by an imaging modality is evaluation of the left ventricular dimensions and estimation of the left ventricular ejection fraction. This can be performed by echocardiography, cardiac magnetic resonance imaging, computed tomography, invasive angiography and nuclear medicine imaging [6, 7].

Population studies with normal patients have established reference values specific to each modality [150]. It is likely most accurate when indexed to body surface area. Reference values are also different between men and women. There are likely also differences by ethnic background but insufficient data exists to allow for guidelines to recommend adjustment of sex-specific reference ranges based on race.

Left ventricular dimensions are measured at both end diastole and end systole. The end diastolic measurement is the more useful measure in determining overall left ventricular size for dilation whereas the end systolic measurement may be more useful as a gross indicator of systolic function. Left ventricular end diastolic volume is likely a better method to define left ventricular dilation than a linear dimension since it accounts for variability in left ventricular geometry and avoids errors introduced by the location of a single linear measurement.

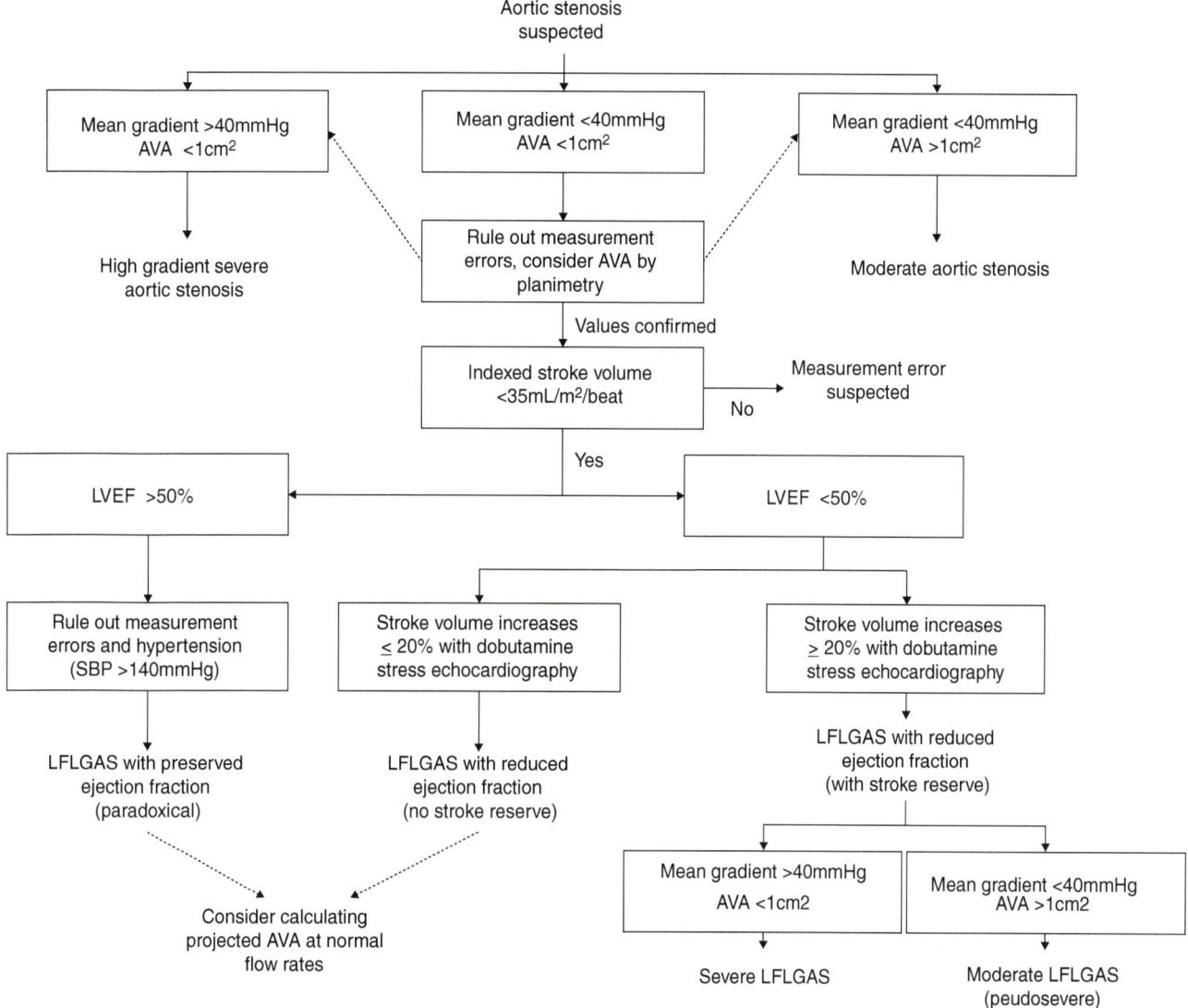

Fig. 1.25 A clinical diagnostic algorithm outlining the possible diagnoses after imaging for suspected aortic stenosis (*AVA* aortic valve area, *LVEF* left ventricular ejection fraction, *SBP* systolic blood pressure, *LFLGAS* low flow low gradient aortic stenosis)

Left ventricular ejection fraction is defined as the percentage or proportion of the left ventricular end diastolic volume ejected from the chamber by end systole. This value is calculated by finding the difference between the end diastolic and end systolic volume of the left ventricle and then dividing by the end diastolic volume. These volumes can be measured in various ways but is most commonly done by the Simpson's method of stacked discs. There are also multiple formulas that can be used to estimate the left ventricular ejection fraction, but because there are assumptions about the left ventricular geometry, accuracy may be limited in the setting of left ventricular remodeling [6]. Accurate measurements of the left ventricular volumes and ejection fraction require good visualization of the endocardium if the method requires tracing or tracking this landmark as the border of the ventricular chamber.

In this section, assessment of left ventricular size and ejection fraction using different imaging modalities will be reviewed.

1.5.2.2.2 Echocardiography

Transthoracic echocardiography is the most commonly used method of evaluating left ventricular dimensions and ejection fraction because it is widely available, relatively inexpensive and does not involve exposure to ionizing radiation.

Left ventricular dimensions can be measured using 2 dimensional imaging. This is usually performed in the parasternal long axis view. End diastolic and end systolic diameters are measured at the mitral valve tips with both points of the cardiac cycle defined by the closure of the mitral and aortic valves, respectively. Previous methods of measuring the left ventricular diameter using m-mode imaging is no longer recommended because depending on the m-mode plane, these dimensions may not be correctly perpendicular to the long axis of the left ventricular cavity.

Left ventricular volumes can also be measured using 2 dimensional imaging [6]. The most common method of performing this measurement is the Simpson's biplane method of stacked discs. The left ventricular cavity is traced at end diastole and end systole in apical 4 and 2 chamber views. Ideally, dedicated zoomed views of the left ventricle paying special attention to avoiding foreshortening should be used. It is also important to perform the tracing along the true endocardial border as defined by the edge of the compacted myocardium.

Left ventricular ejection fraction can then be calculated using the measured volumes by Simpson's biplane method. The end systolic volume is subtracted by the end diastolic volume and then this difference is divided by the end diastolic volume. Other methods of estimating the left ventricular ejection fraction that use only a single linear measurement, such as Teichholz method, may be less accurate because of assumptions regarding the left ventricular geometry.

One limitation of the Simpson's biplane method of stacked discs to measure left ventricular volumes and left ventricular ejection fraction is that measurements are made in the apical 4 and 2 chamber views only. Therefore, if there are significant wall motion abnormalities or an aneurysm affecting only or predominantly the posterior wall or anterior septum of the left ventricle, the effect on volumes and ejection fraction may be underestimated. One method to correct for this is to perform a stacked disc measurement using three planes instead of two. This is done by tracing the endocardial border in apical 4, 3 and 2 chamber views if the software package allows.

Microbubble echocardiographic contrast agents can also be used to assist with left ventricular volume measurement if the endocardial definition on non-contrast imaging is suboptimal [151, 152]. Studies comparing 2 dimensional measurements of left ventricular ejection fraction with and without microbubble contrast suggest that there is less measurement variability when echocardiographic contrast agents are used.

3 dimensional echocardiography is a promising tool to improve the reliability and accuracy of left ventricular volume and ejection fraction measurements [153]. This is performed using a 3 dimensional transthoracic probe. A large volume dataset is obtained that includes the entire left ventricular cavity. Depending on the volume rate of the probe, an electrocardiographic gated multi-beat acquisition may be necessary. If this is done, the patient should perform a breath hold to prevent a stitching artifact from translation of the heart through the imaging volume. Once a dataset with an adequate volume rate is captured, vendor specific software packages allow for semi-automatic endocardial tracking to measure volumes and ejection fraction. This can be verified and adjusted if there are problems with tracking. A significant advantage of using 3 dimensional echocardiography for this purpose is that abnormalities of left ventricular geometry are accounted for, assuming tracking is correct. There is also evidence to suggest that 3 dimensional measurements of left ventricular volumes and ejection fraction shows less variability that 2 dimensional methods [154, 155].

An important consideration of the left ventricular ejection fraction is that this value represents the absolute change in volume of the left ventricle from end diastole to end systole, but does not describe the direction of blood flow. While this is usually almost entirely forward flow that exits the left ventricular outflow tract though the aortic valve into the aorta, the presence of certain cardiac lesions may cause a significant volume of blood to be ejected into another cardiac chamber. With significant mitral regurgitation there is flow into the left atrium, with a ventricular septal defect blood flows into the right ventricle and with a Gerbode defect blood flows into the right atrium. Therefore, ejection fraction should be interpreted in the context of any cardiac lesion that may cause significant blood flow to another location other than the aorta.

Transesophageal echocardiography can also be used to measure left ventricular linear dimensions, volumes and ejection fraction [111]. However, accuracy may be limited due to the greater distance of the left ventricle from the image transducer compared to transthoracic imaging. Left ventricular apical foreshortening may also be significant in transesophageal imaging.

Echocardiography allows for measurement of left ventricular dimensions, volumes and ejection fraction using different techniques. Greater use of 3 dimensional imaging or contrast echocardiography may improve the reliability of these measurements in the future (Figs. 1.26, 1.27, 1.28 and 1.29).

1.5.2.2.3 Magnetic Resonance Imaging

Accurate measurement of left ventricular (LV) mass, volumes and ejection fraction (EF) is crucial, as these variables are important for diagnosis, treatment decisions and prognosis in patients with cardiac diseases. Cardiovascular magnetic resonance imaging (CMR) is the gold standard for assessing LV dimensions and function as it allows more accurate and reproducible measurements compared to other noninvasive imaging techniques such as echocardiography and nuclear imaging [156]. Unlike echocardiography, CMR has the ability to obtain high-resolution tomographic imaging in different planes. Furthermore, CMR is particularly useful for the evaluation of LV function in patients with limited acoustic windows and poor echocardiographic quality. Due to the superior spatial resolution and more precise border definition in CMR compared to echocardiography and nuclear imaging [28], inter- and intra-reader as well as inter-scan variability is low [28, 156]. Acquisition of dimensions and functions of the LV in CMR is noninvasive, involves no exposure to ionizing radiation, can be easily performed without contrast within less than 10 minutes. Typically, during a series

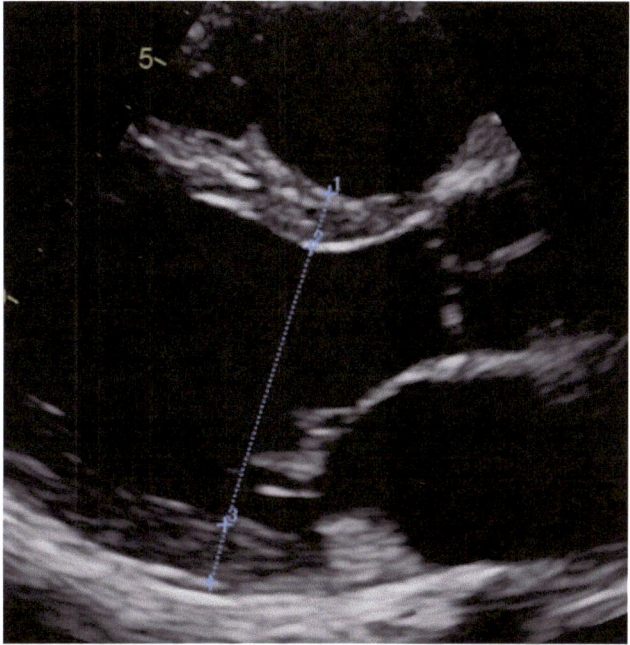

Fig. 1.26 Left ventricular linear end diastolic dimensions measured on the parasternal long axis view of a transthoracic echocardiogram

of short breath-holds, gated cardiac images are acquired over 6- to 10-mm tomographic cine short-axis cross-sections of the heart. The summation of discs method is then applied to determine the myocardial volumes by tracing the endocardial contours in systole and diastole. Furthermore, multiple phases of the cardiac cycle in long axis (e.g. 2 chamber, 3 chamber and 4 chamber) are performed and reconstructed into a "cine" movie (Fig. 1.30). LVEF, represented by the volumetric blood fraction ejected from the LV chamber with each contraction, is calculated using the Simpson's method by dividing the volume of blood pumped from the LV per beat (stroke volume) by the volume of blood collected in the left ventricle at the end of diastolic filling. Further, LV mass can be derived from the short-axis cine-slices stack in the diastolic phase. Normal LV volumes decrease with age and are smaller for women than men, even after adjustment for body size. Therefore, normal LV volumes and function values in CMR are based on age- and sex-specific reference ranges [157–159].

1.5.2.2.4 Computed Tomography

Multidetector computed tomography allows for accurate quantification of left ventricular (LV) function, with a high accuracy as compared to magnetic resonance imaging [160]. Left ventricular end-diastolic volume (EDV), end-systolic volume (ESV) and the ejection fraction (EF) can be calculated (Fig. 1.31). LV function is an important prognostic parameter in valvular disease. In particular in aortic stenosis, the low-flow (LF), low-gradient (LG) type (i.e. stroke volume

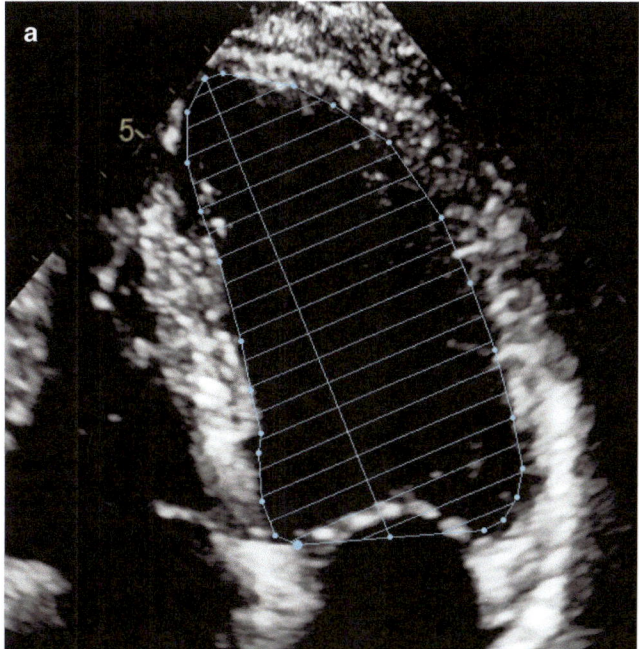

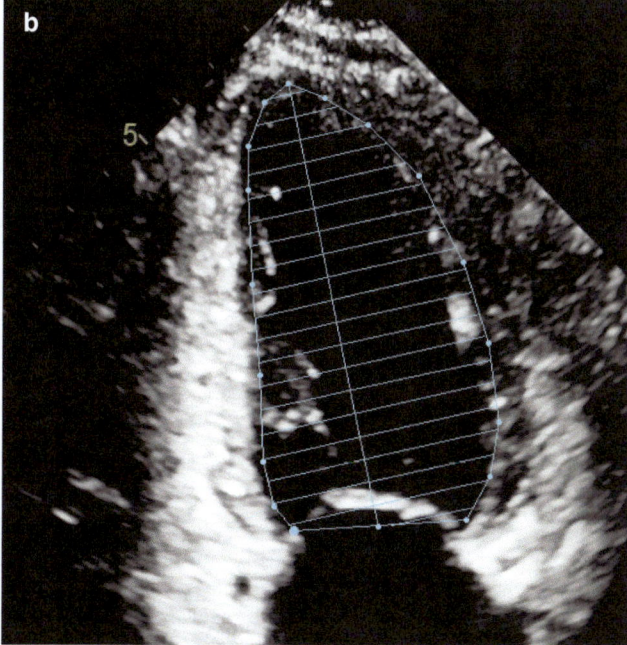

Fig. 1.27 Left ventricular end diastolic volume measured by transthoracic echocardiography using Simpson's biplane method without microbubble contrast in the apical 4 chamber (**a**) and 2 chamber (**b**) views. Measurement of end diastolic and end systolic volumes allows for calculation of left ventricular ejection fraction

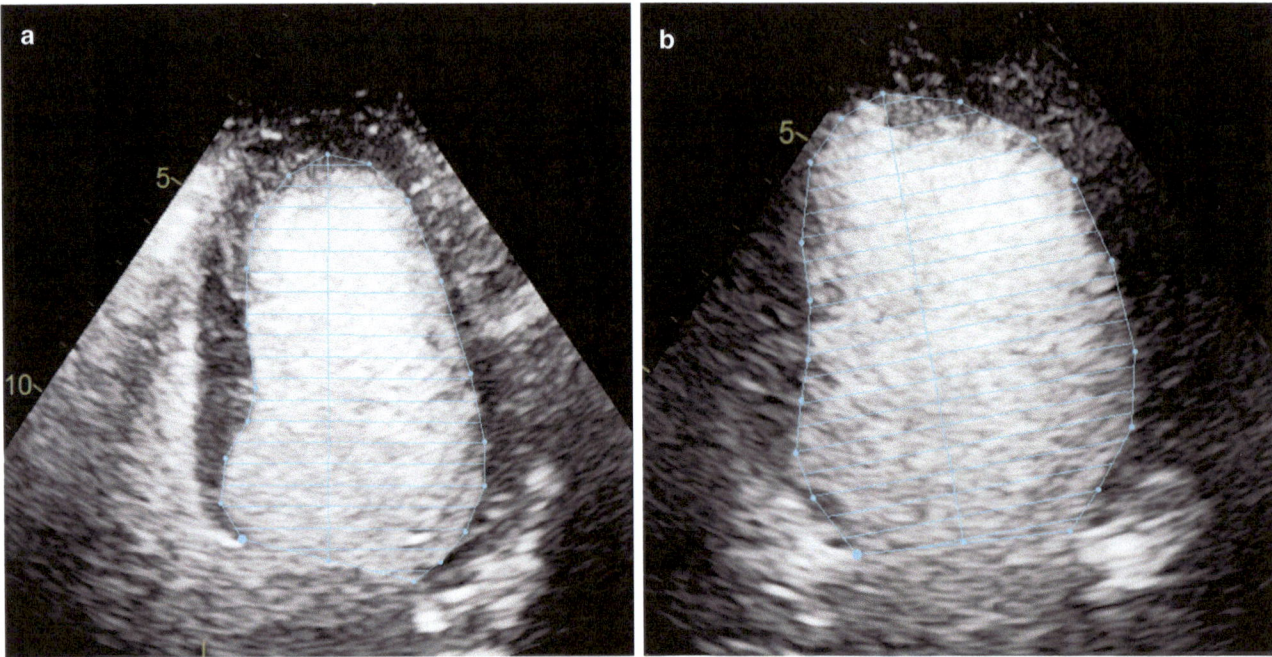

Fig. 1.28 Left ventricular end diastolic volume measured by transthoracic echocardiography using Simpson's biplane method with microbubble contrast in the apical 4 chamber (**a**) and 2 chamber (**b**) views. Measurement of end diastolic and end systolic volumes allows for calculation of left ventricular ejection fraction

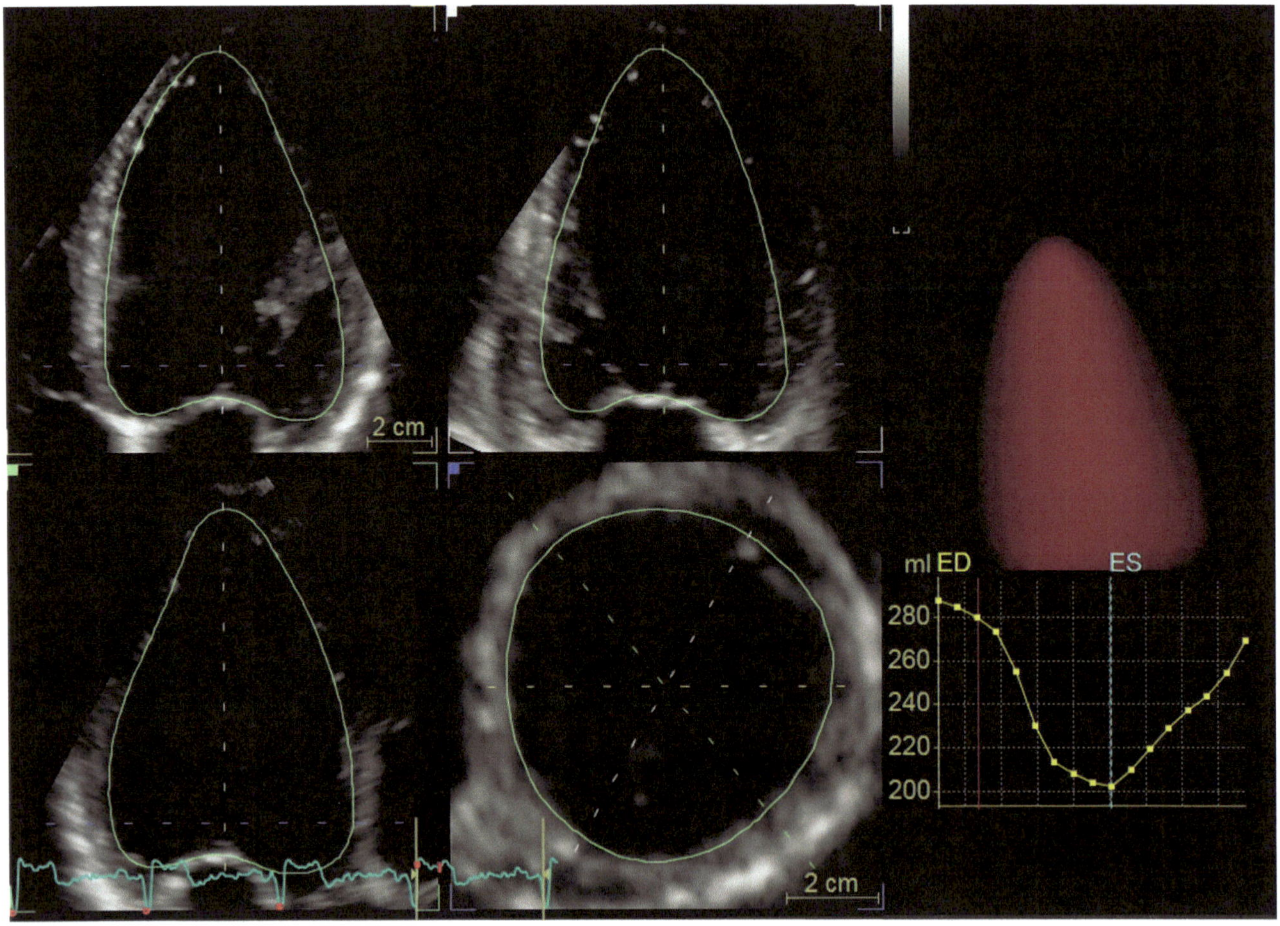

Fig. 1.29 Left ventricular volumes and ejection fraction measured using 3-dimensional transthoracic echocardiography and a semi-automated software algorithm

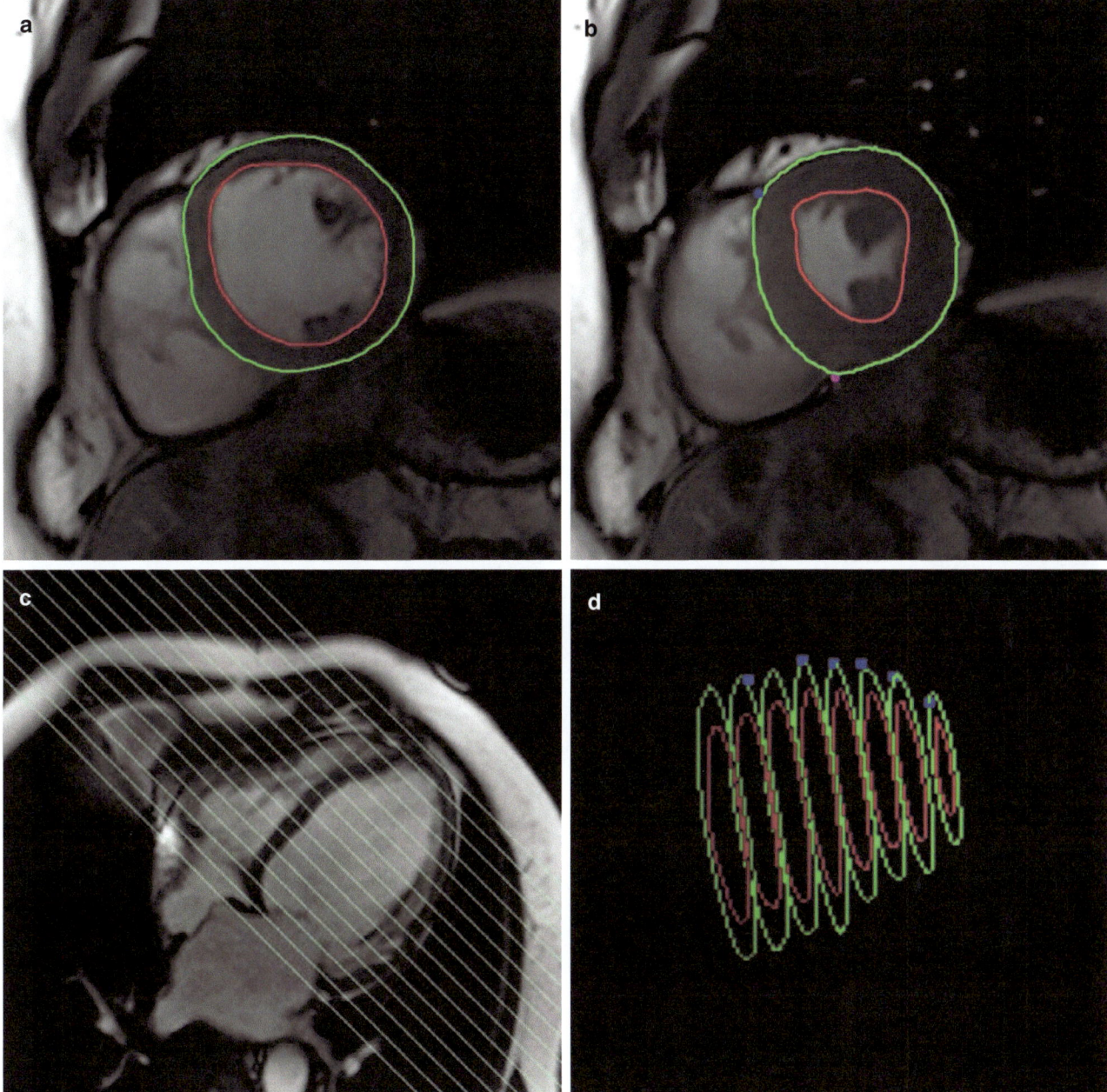

Fig. 1.30 Left ventricular mass is calculated from tracing the endocardium (red) and epicardium (red) in diastole (panel **a**). For left ventricular volume and function assessment, endocardium contours (red) are drawn in short axis slices in diastole (panel **a**) and systole (panel **b**) in a stack of short-axis slices from basal to the apex in order to cover the entire heart as shown in the 4-chamber view on panel **c** and in the three dimensional view on panel **d**

index <35 mL/m^2 and a gradient of <40 mmHg in the absense of hypertension) may occur with depressed or preserved EF (≥50%), the latter being called "paradoxical" LF-LG [161].

Quantification of LV function by CTA is feasible using the same CT datasets acquired for a coronary CT angiography, if multiphase datasets encompassing the entire cardiac cycle are available. The ECG-gating technique of choice is the "retrospective" mode, while certain CT vendors also provide prospective ECG-gating technology covering the entire R-R interval at reduced tube current (mAs) exposure. Image reconstruction of axial datasets at 10% increments (or 5% increments) using thin slices (≤1 mm) in order to ensure high accuracy is recommended. The lowest end-systolic and maximal end-diastolic dataset is usually selected by automated tools and displayed as absolute and indexed values to the body surface area (BSA) (Fig. 1.31, right upper panel).

1.5.2.2.5 Left Ventricular Angiography

Attempts to quantify left ventricular size and function have been done as early as the beginning of the last century

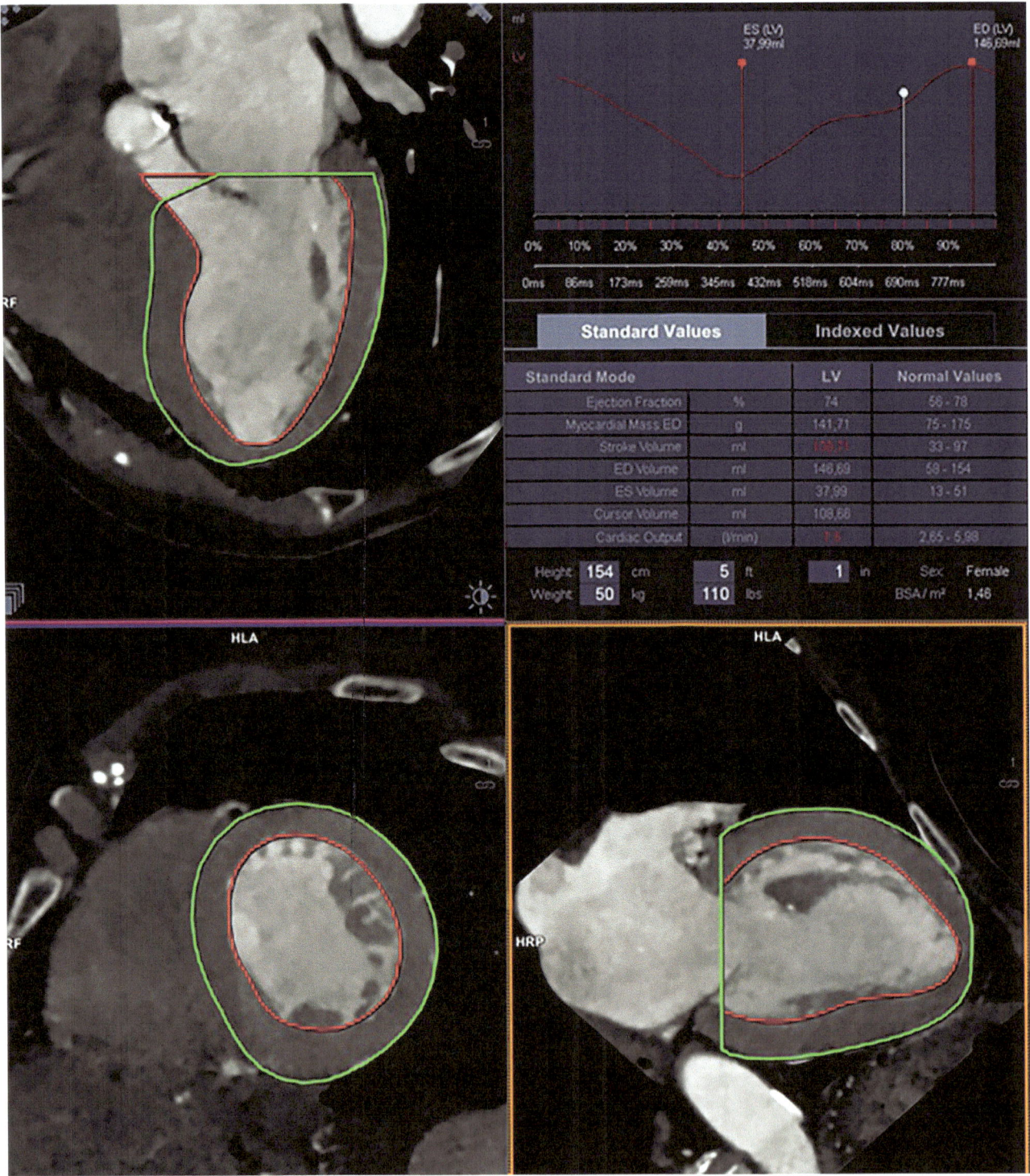

Fig. 1.31 Quantification of left ventricular function and dimensions by computed tomography (CT). The minimal end-systolic (ES) volume (at 45% of R-R interval) and the maximal end-diastolic (ED) volume (at 95% of the R-R interval) were selected for computation of EF and stroke volume in a patient with severe aortic stenosis. Ejection fraction (EF) was 74% (hyperdynamic). Myocardial mass during the ED phase can be segmented and computed automatically

using indirect cine roentgenography to visualize heart movement [162]. Geigel calculated cardiac volumes as a sphere in 1914. Chapman et al. described the use of biplane Cinefluorography for measurement of ventricular volume in 1958 [163]. They calculated LV Volume by a modified Simpson's rule equation which is basically still used today. A sufficient and quick contrast power injection into the left ventricle is necessary. A total of 30 cc with a flow of

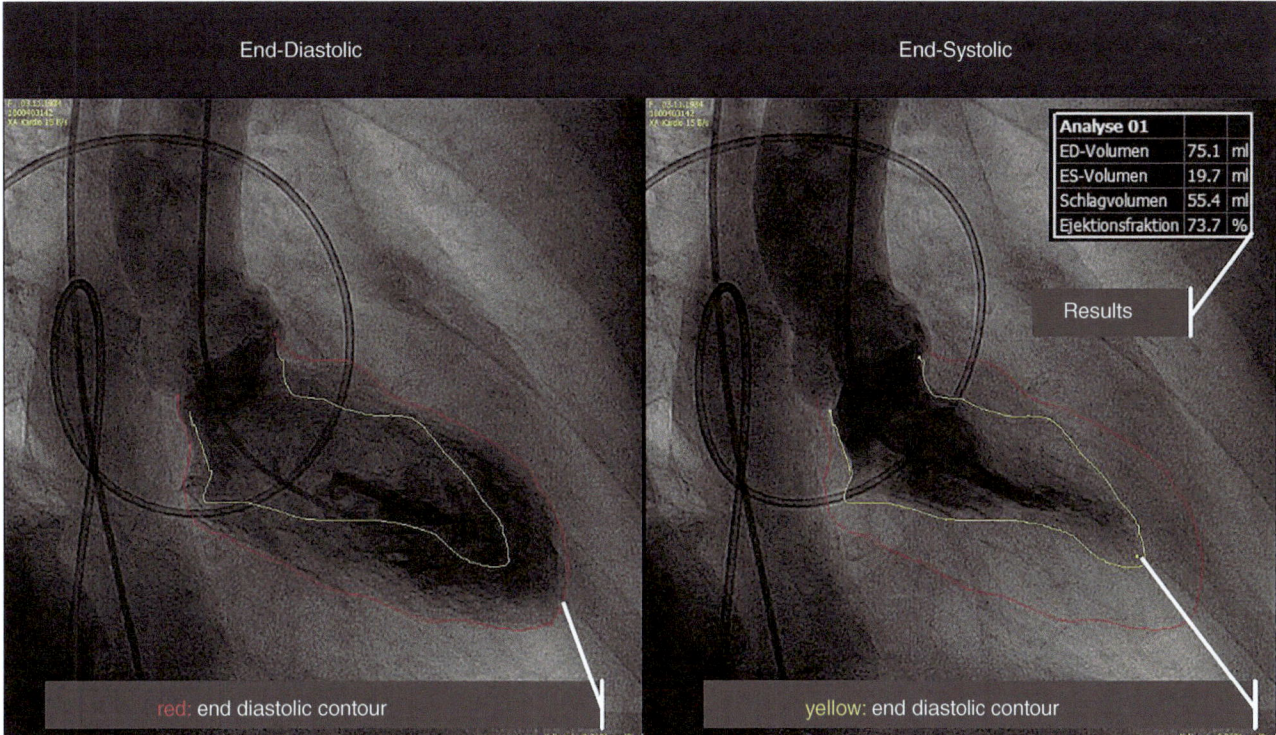

Fig. 1.32 Semi automatic contour detection by dedicated software to perform off-line analysis of left ventricular function from LV-angiography. Results of end diastolic (ED), end sytolic (ES) and stroke volume (Schlagvolumen) are given in millilitres (ml), ejection fraction (Ejektionsfraktion) in %

12–15 cc/s is enough. A biplane technique is preferable to reduce the amount of contrast use. During inspiration and breath hold a scene with at least 25 frames/s is obtained. High frame rate is necessary to identify the still frames with maximal endsystolic (lowest) and enddiastolic (biggest) volume for correct calculation of the ejection fraction. Using the method used by Chapman, exact volumes can also be calculated. Adding the heart rate at timepoint of injection, stroke volume and cardiac output can be obtained. Current software packages included by vendors for X-ray machines or as an add-on for the offline workstations allow automatic methodology to delineate LV contours in the enddiastolic and endsystolic phase with high accuracy and less time effort. Due to the algorithm-based approach, inter- and intra-observer variability is also reduced [164].

The beauty of the angiography method is that it is luminography. Therefore, its sensitivity to detect small fistula, diverticula and recesses is very high, and due to the high spatial resolution, in most cases is still better than non-contrast enhanced echocardiography. This advantage is likely to degrade with ongoing technologic advancementsin echocardiography and nowadays cineventriculography does not play a routine role in daily practices since most patients who enter the cath lab often have had a non-invasive echocardiographic exam before. But if echocardiography is not conclusive, LV angiography enables a quick and powerful solution for assement of local and global LV function (Fig. 1.32).

1.5.2.2.6 Nuclear Medicine

Nuclear cardiology offers a variety of different techniques for assessment of left ventricular (LV) function: first-pass and equilibrium radionuclide ventriculography (RNV), gated myocardial perfusion single-photon-emission-computed-tomography (SPECT), and gated positron emission tomography (PET) [165]. Intravascular tracers, including 99m-Technetium (Tc)-labelled erythrocytes and 99mTc-labelled human serum albumin, can be used for equilibrium radionuclide ventriculography (ERNV) while first-pass radionuclide ventriculography (FPRNV) can be performed with many other 99mTc-labelled radiopharmaceuticals. While ERNV represents a well-validated technique for accurate determination of left ventricular (LV) ejection fraction (EF) and LV volumes, it also offers high reproducibility, rendering it particularly useful for sequential assessments over time. However, it requires particular local expertise due to the need for in-vivo or in-vitro radionuclide-labeling of the erythrocytes or the serum albumin. Acquired using planar scintigraphy or SPECT, data are collected from many cardiac cycles to generate an image set of the heart that is then summed to obtain a single, composite cycle. ERNV may be acquired at rest or during exercise. By contrast, an FPRNV study is obtained from a short sequence of cardiac cycles acquired during the

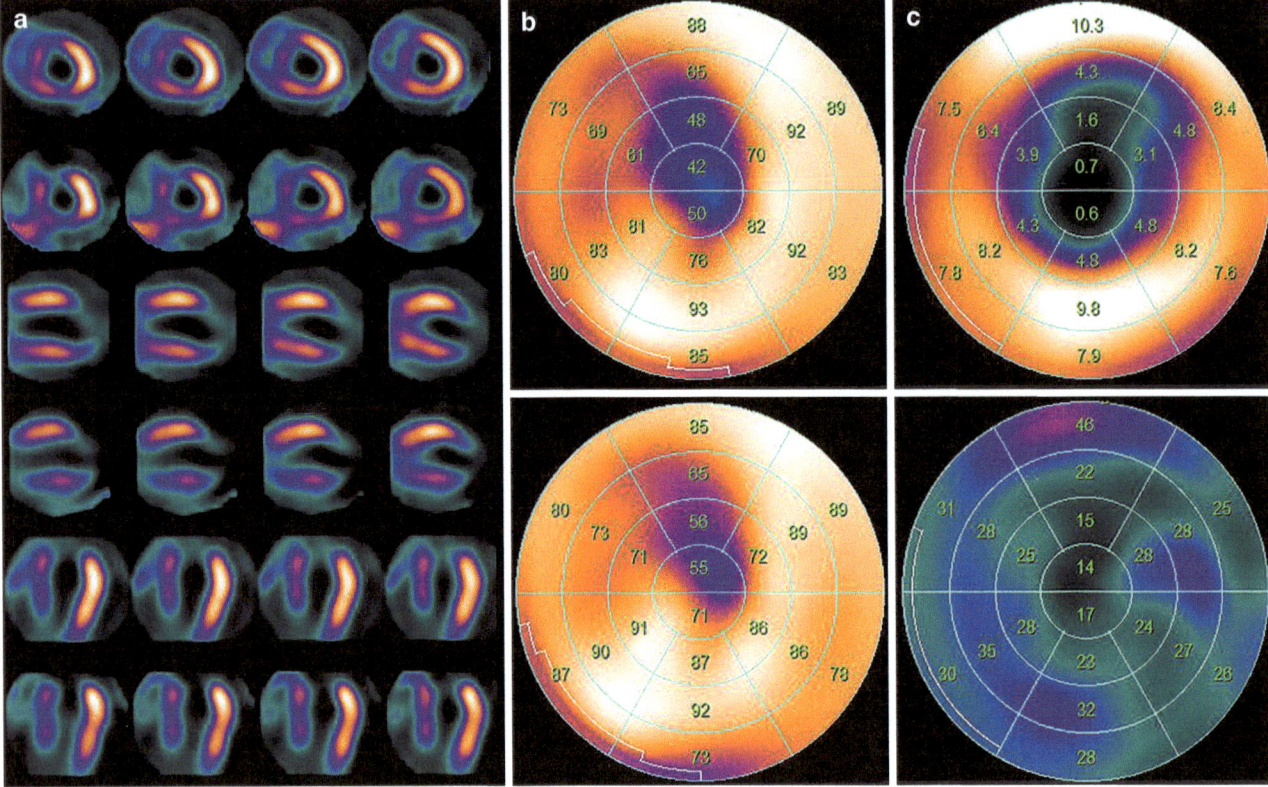

Fig. 1.33 Electrocardiogram-gated myocardial perfusion SPECT imaging of a patient with ischemic heart disease and a history of anterior myocardial infarction. Selected short axis, vertical long axis and horizontal long axis slices at rest (bottom) and during pharmacologically induced stress (top) are depicted (**a**), as well as the corresponding polar plots (**b**). While ischemia can be excluded, SPECT reveals an anterior myocardial scar (green-blue-violet) with corresponding hypokinesia (black-green-blue-violet) in the anterior wall as shown in the analysis of the gated datasets (**c**): The polar plot at the top depicts segmental motion (in mm), and the polar plot at the bottom depicts myocardial thickening (in %) during the cardiac cycle. Global left ventricular ejection fraction was 52%

first-pass transit of a radioactive tracer through the central circulation, cardiac chambers, and the lungs, after intravenous bolus injection. It provides a high target to background ratio, but imaging is possible in only one scintigraphic projection. Finally, myocardial perfusion imaging is now widely available, as it performed in electrocardiogram (ECG) gated mode. After reconstruction and reorientation of the gated SPECT projection data sets, fully automated algorithms may be used to quantify LVEF, LV EDV, and ESV (Fig. 1.33).

A validation study of gated myocardial perfusion SPECT using cardiac magnetic resonance imaging as a standard of reference for LVEF yielded high correlation [166]. While relatively easily obtainable as an adjunct to myocardial perfusion assessment, use of different acquisition and reconstruction parameters can substantially influence LVEF quantification from gated SPECT or PET [167].

1.5.2.3 Assessing Left Ventricular Function and Functional Reserve

1.5.2.3.1 Introduction

Left ventricular mechanics is a complex function and reflected in the myocyte architecture of left ventricular myocardium. The myofibers in the sub-endocardial region of the myocardium are oriented in a right-handed helical structure, while orientation gradually changes into a sub-epicardial left-handed helical arrangement; hence, the longitudinal axis of the myofibers rotates continuously. This architecture results in an almost longitudinal direction of the subendocardial fibers more or less corresponding to the long axis of the left ventricle, while the fibers display a circumferential orientation in the midventricular region and an oblique direction in the apical region. The complex arrangement of myofibers determines left ventricular deformation during systole in that the subendocardial region contributes primarily to longitudinal deformation, while the sub-epicardial region determines the rotational component. Circumferential deformation is more pronounced than longitudinal deformation and thus represents an important component of ventricular systole. Therefore, the left ventricle exhibits a wringing contraction during the cardiac cycle with clock-wise rotation at the base and counter-clockwise rotation at the apex, resulting in a mechanically highly-effective twisting [168].

Left ventricular ejection fraction is a robust parameter associated with extensive prognostic information; however, it does not reflect the complex twisting motion of the ventricle in an appropriate manner. This is particularly important as many pathological alterations of the left ventricle primarily affect the subendocardial region and thereby longitudinal motion and deformation. However, left ventricular longitudinal displacement can be determined by mitral anulus plane systolic excursion using M-mode, longitudinal velocity by tissue Doppler imaging, and ventricular deformation in the longitudinal, circumferential, and rotational direction by strain imaging [168–172].

During early diastole, the potential energy primarily stored in the interstitial connective tissue induces the recoil of left ventricular twist leading to ventricular untwisting and resulting in early diastolic suction. The major part of the untwisting motion occurs during isovolumetric relaxation phase, while the rest is completed during early diastole. In ventricles exhibiting a decreased compliance, there is less untwisting resulting in a disturbed relaxation and finally diastolic dysfunction. With progressive diastolic dysfunction, left ventricular filling pressure increases leading to secondary alterations such as left atrial dilatation and pulmonary hypertension. The assessment of diastolic function is an important component of left ventricular imaging and involves characterization of the filling pattern with analysis of blood flow during early and late diastole both across the mitral valve and in the pulmonary veins, the velocity of myocardial tissue motion in early and late diastole, and the velocity of myocardial deformation in early diastole [168].

A complete and integrative assessment of left ventricular function therefore involves both systolic and diastolic function and applies different methods such as measurement of ventricular dimensions, blood flow velocity, tissue velocity, and tissue deformation [6, 173].

1.5.2.3.2 Echocardiography

Aortic stenosis induces increased afterload on the left ventricle. It usually tolerates this pressure overload for long time periods; however, it adapts by developing myocardial hypertrophy. This allows it to maintain stroke volume but leads to ventricular remodeling with thickening of the myocardial layer, decreased myocardial compliance, reduced longitudinal function, and progressive diastolic dysfunction [173, 174].

The myocardial hypertrophy occurring secondary to aortic stenosis in combination with the elevated ventricular systolic pressure results in increased transmural pressure with subendocardial ischemia and fibrosis. These alterations induce subtle changes in left ventricular longitudinal function, which are observed despite maintained ejection fraction. Decreased longitudinal displacement can be measured with M-mode as reduced mitral anulus plane systolic excursion [172], decreased longitudinal velocity by determining S′ in tissue Doppler imaging [175], and decreased longitudinal deformation by assessing global longitudinal peak systolic strain in speckle tracking imaging [6, 171, 173, 174]. All of these parameters for longitudinal systolic function have been associated with an impaired outcome and should be measured in patients with aortic stenosis [176]. As compared to longitudinal strain imaging, the assessment of radial and circumferential strain is less helpful in clinical practice because these parameters as well as their implications for outcome have been less well studied [171, 177].

If the increased afterload is maintained after this adaptation phase, not only longitudinal systolic function of the left ventricle will suffer, but radial and circumferential function will deteriorate as well. These alterations become evident as a decreased transversal motion resulting in a decreased ejection fraction. If there is an afterload mismatch only, the left ventricle has the potential to recover and the reduced ejection fraction normalizes after aortic valve replacement [178]. In contrast, if the ventricle has started to fail, irreversible morphological and functional damage occurs, and ejection fraction does not improve after intervention or operation [179–181]. In both situations, however, there may also be significant secondary mitral regurgitation due to anular dilatation and papillary muscle displacement. This is particularly important because the presence of mitral regurgitation hampers the assessment of both systolic left ventricular function and aortic stenosis severity. Since forward stroke volume decreases in the presence of a significant mitral regurgitation, both planimetry of the anatomic aortic valve orifice area and calculation of the effective aortic valve orifice area overestimate the severity of aortic stenosis under such conditions [15, 169].

In patients with aortic stenosis, diastolic dysfunction typically occurs prior to a decrease in left ventricular ejection fraction and thus is a form of heart failure with preserved ejection fraction in patients with the respective symptoms and/or signs. Hence, careful assessment of diastolic function is essential in such individuals. Typically, there is delayed relaxation without secondary alterations such as left atrial dilatation and pulmonary hypertension. Only at later stages, when left ventricular hypertrophy is evident and an afterload mismatch is observed, a higher degree diastolic dysfunction with a pseudo-normal or restrictive filling pattern is observed. All the diastolic function parameters available and also early diastolic strain rate can be applied to analyze diastolic function in aortic stenosis patients [15, 173].

1.5.2.3.3 Stress Echocardiography

In patients with aortic stenosis and symptoms and/or a reduced ejection fraction, there is a clear indication for aortic valve replacement, and stress echo is contraindicated under these conditions [2, 182]. However, exercise testing is important for revealing symptoms or an abnormal blood pressure response in patients who claim to be asymptomatic. Patients who are limited by symptoms during exercise testing have a worse outcome and thus an indication for aortic valve replacement. Exercise stress echocardiography should be used instead of electrocardiographic exercise testing, because stress echo displays incremental diagnostic value over exercise testing alone. Exercise stress echocardiography can be performed by means of a treadmill or a supine bicycle; the latter has the advantage that images can be acquired throughout the exercise phase and at true peak workload, while this is only possible before and immediately after exercise with the treadmill. The absence of an increase, or alternatively, a decrease in left ventricular ejection fraction during exercise indicates left ventricular dysfunction. An increase in pulmonary pressure above 60 mmHg during exercise is suggestive of a severe aortic stenosis. Both parameters are associated with a reduced outcome and are in favor of an aortic valve replacement [182].

Another important indication for stress echocardiography in patients with aortic stenosis is a severe aortic stenosis causing left ventricular dysfunction due to afterload mismatch. A patient with reduced left ventricular ejection fraction and mean systolic pressure gradient >40 mmHg and/or peak systolic flow velocity >4 m/s across the aortic valve does not necessarily suffer from reduced left ventricular systolic function; such a ventricle rather displays a normal response to afterload mismatch. However, mean systolic pressure gradient and/or peak systolic flow velocity across the aortic valve may decrease when stroke volume and left ventricular systolic function are severely impaired. This constellation of findings should be differentiated from patients with a moderate aortic stenosis and an impaired left ventricular systolic function due to other reasons. In these patients the severity of the aortic stenosis usually is overestimated because the small stroke volume and low contractility are not sufficient for overcoming the aortic valve tissue resistance and opening the valve to the maximal possible extent. Such patients do not meet the criteria for aortic valve replacement and should receive a state-of-the-art heart failure therapy instead [2, 4, 183]. Dobutamine stress echocardiography is applied in patients with afterload mismatch, because this drug exerts a positive inotropic effect on the left ventricular myocardium and may thus unmask contractile reserve of the ventricle, leading to an increase in the systolic pressure gradient over the aortic valve. Dobutamine is only used at a low dose (5, 10, and 20 µg/kg/m^2) in this situation because at higher doses the predominant effect of dobutamine is chronotropic as opposed to inotropic. True severe aortic stenosis is diagnosed when the mean systolic pressure gradient reaches >30 mmHg and the peak systolic flow velocity ≥4 m/s, while the effective orifice area does not exceed 1 cm^2. The contractile reserve is defined is an increase in stroke volume of at least 20%. The absence of a contractile reserve indicates a poor long-term outcome, although aortic valve replacement may be beneficial in such patients as well [2, 4, 15, 182, 183].

1.5.2.3.4 Magnetic Resonance Imaging

Left ventricular (LV) function can be assessed in CMR by calculating LV ejection fraction (LVEF) (using the stroke volume derived from end diastolic and end systolic LV volume) or by visual regional wall motion grading. Wall motion can be categorized in each segment as being normal, hypokinetic, akinetic and dyskinetic. Myocardial strain analysis is a tool to more accurately assess myocardial deformation and helps to quantitatively assess myocardial function (Fig. 1.34). Myocardial strain analysis can also detect the decline of myocardial function preceding the reduction of LVEF [184] and is therefore increasingly recognized as an important myocardial performance index [185]. Myocardial strain can be assessed using CMR tagging [186]. In this method, specialized radiofrequency pulses are applied prior to the beginning of the cine CMR pulses sequence. These additional pulses result in alteration of the magnetic properties of the heart, typically in a grid stripe pattern [186]. The grids or stripes are dark relative to the remaining myocardium, and the grids are displaced as a result of myocardial motion. CMR tagging has allowed precise quantification of regional heterogeneity in myocardial contraction [187]. Other tissue tracking methods include DENSE (displacement encoding with stimulated echoes in CMR) and HARP (harmonic phase may offer more automated methods for myocardial strain

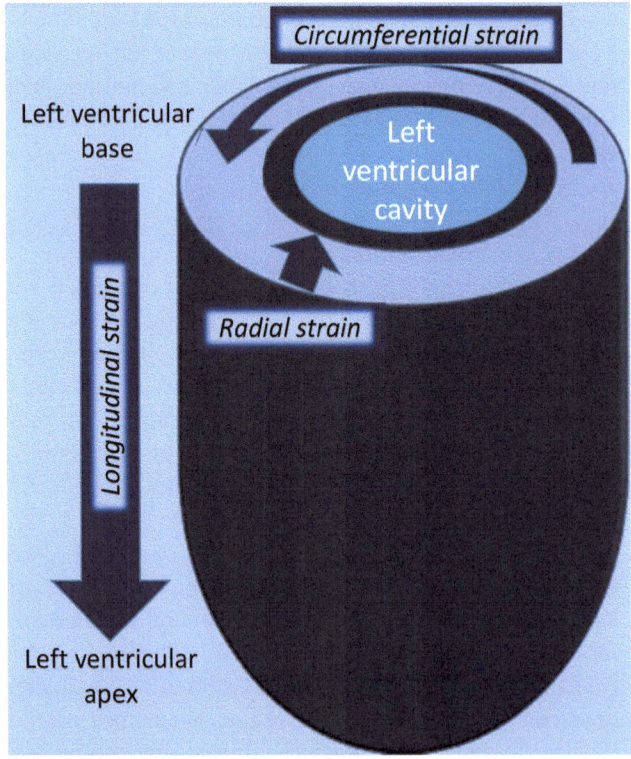

Fig. 1.34 Cardiac magnetic resonance imaging myocardial feature tracking is used to analyze myocardial deformation over time with circumferential strain, radial strain and longitudinal strain

analysis). However, image analysis is mainly performed qualitatively with considerable operator dependency, and as mentioned before, quantitative analysis with myocardial tagging requires the acquisition of additional sequences and involves lengthy post processing [187]. Recently, CMR myocardial feature tracking (FT) has been introduced, which is similar to echocardiographic speckle tracking [171]. This technique tracks tissue voxel motion (strain points) in cine CMR images and allows assessment of the displacement or deformation of the heart muscle over time without the need of additional sequences acquisition (Fig. 1.35). CMR FT provides information on the longitudinal shortening, circumferential shortening and radial thickening of the myocardium. Aside from the peak strain (%), strain rate (the rate of strain changes over the course of time), time to peak strain (ms), peak systolic strain rate (1/s), peak diastolic strain rate (1/s) can be measured. Other parameters include peak displacement (mm), time to peak displacement (ms), peak systolic velocity (mm/s) and peak diastolic velocity (mm/s) which can be all assessed in 2D and 3D as well. Good agreement has been demonstrated between CMR FT and other sequence based tissue tracking sequences [188].

Due to its excellent image quality, in addition to assessment of myocardial function at rest, CMR can also clearly visualize LV endocardial wall motion during low- and high-dose dobutamine challenges for the assessment of myocardial viability and ischemia [189]. The goal of dobutamine stress CMR imaging is to differentiate between normal myocardium, scarred myocardium, viable myocardium and ischemic myocardium. Dobutamine stress CMR is performed following doses and imaging protocols that are comparable to dobutamine stress echocardiography [190]. To assess ischemia, the goal of the dobutamine infusion is to achieve a minimum heart rate of 85% of the predicted maximal heart rate for the patient's age. Accordingly, the dobutamine dose is increased every 3–5 min to doses of 10, 20, and 30, and finally to 40 µg/kg per minute, and if needed, additionally atropine 0.5 or 1 mg (maximum 2 mg). Ischemic myocardial segments become hypo-akinetic or dyskinetic under maximal stress conditions. Viable myocardium shows the typical pattern of a "biphasic response", where a myocardial territory augments its contraction at a low dobutamine dose (low inotrope dose) but later becomes hypokinetic or akinetic at higher dobutamine doses. In non-viable scar segments, dobutamine has no effect on akinetic or dyskinetic segments. CMR can also determine viability with late gadolinium enhancement (LGE) methods [191]. The gadolinium-based contrast agents used for LGE differentiate viable myocardium from scar on the basis of differences in cell membrane integrity in acute myocardial infarction and to changes in extracellular volume fraction in chronic myocardial infarction [192].

1.5.2.3.5 Computed Tomography

In severe aortic stenosis (AS), especially the asymptomatic and low-flow, low-gradient subtypes, prediction of outcome is based on a wide spectrum of clinical and imaging-based parameters. Apart from aortic valve calcification, novel biomarkers (NT-proBNP, hs-troponin) but also left ventricular function are independent and valuable prognostic parameters. While LV-EF is a less specific criterion, quantification

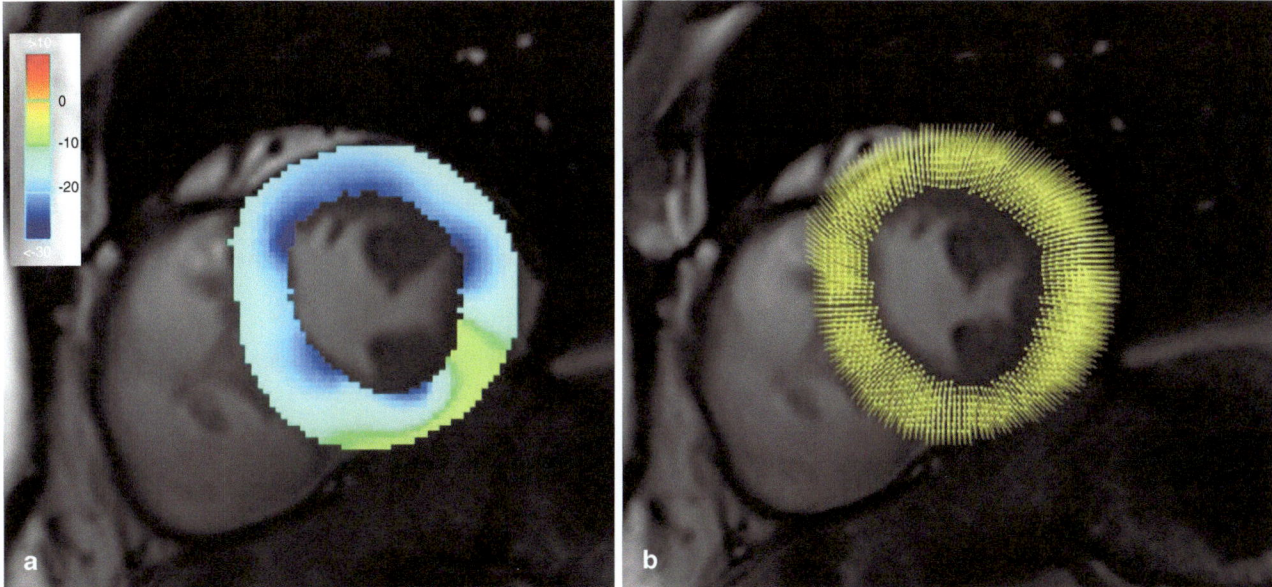

Fig. 1.35 Circumferential strain analysis using cardiac magnetic resonance imaging feature tracking in a short axis midventricular cine slice is depicted in panel **a**. In panel **b** the strain point over time in the cardiac cycle can be followed

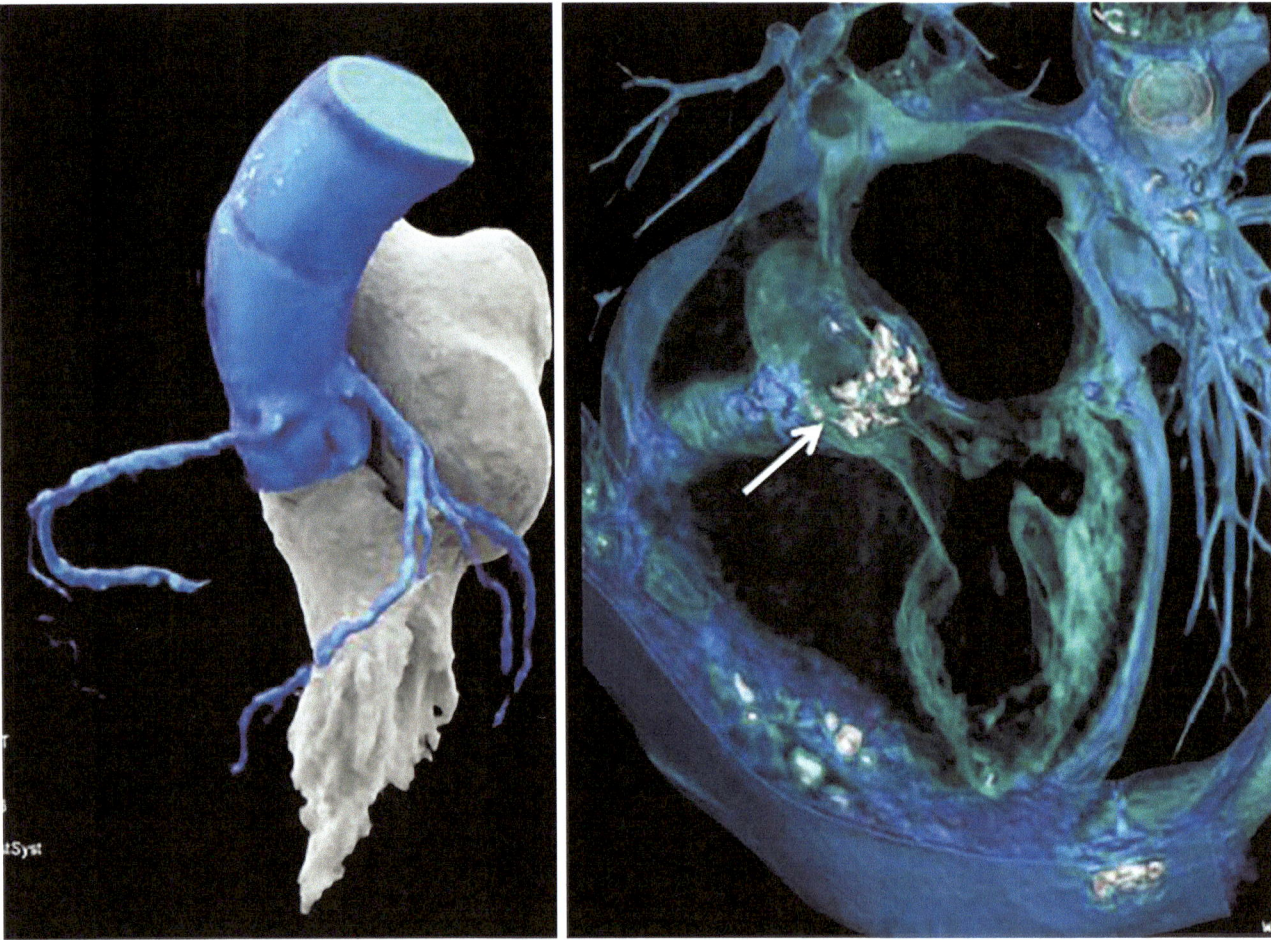

Fig. 1.36 84 year-old female with severe aortic stenosis. Automated 3D segmentation of the left ventricle during end-systolic phase (42% of the R-R interval) **(left)** from a coronary CTA dataset acquired for TAVR planning is shown. LV blood volume is colored white and coronary arteries/aorta blue. End-diastolic phase **(right)** (89% of R-R interval) with a different VRT setting allows for visualization of aortic valve calcification severity (white arrow) and the LV myocardium (green). The LV blood volume is colored black

of longitudinal and global LV strain by echocardiography has emerged as a more sensitive method for defining myocardial contraction and detect early deterioration.

Accordingly, left ventricular strain has emerged as incremental prognostic parameter for predicting adverse outcome [193], especially in those with asymptomatic AS, and low-flow, low-gradient AS, in which timing of surgery is often debated and difficult to decide. LV strain is also predictive of worse outcome in patients with aortic regurgitation [194] and heart failure.

Novel, recently introduced computed tomography (CT) post-processing tools [195] now allow for quantification of CT-derived longitudinal LV strain, as recently shown in 25 patients pre- and post-transcatheter aortic valve replacement (TAVR). In this study, 4 chamber, 3 chamber and 2 chamber views from CT data were rendered and peak global and peak longitudinal strain were computed. CT–derived LV strain showed good interobserver agreement (r = 0.85), but systematic underestimation as compared to echocardiography.

However, CT-based strain improved (p = 0.006) after TAVR, indicating a promising potential for monitoring of procedural success. These post-processing tools require further validation prior to widespread commercial market implementation (Fig. 1.36).

1.5.2.4 Low-Flow-Low-Gradient Aortic Stenosis

1.5.2.4.1 Introduction

In patients with aortic stenosis, one can distinguish between 'normal flow' (stroke volume index >35 mL/m^2) and 'low flow' (stroke volume index <35 mL/m^2); these expressions are widely used, although not technically correct, as they describe stroke volume rather than flow. Similarly, in such patients, one can differentiate between a 'normal gradient' (mean systolic pressure gradient >40 mmHg) and a 'low gradient' (mean systolic pressure gradient <40 mmHg). In a population with severe aortic stenosis diagnosed according to current guidelines, all four constellations of findings will be present [2, 4, 15]. However, the distinction of these four conditions is affected by systematic errors, which are mainly related to calculation of stroke volume, while the determination of the systolic pressure gradient is much more reliable. Stroke volume can be calculated by subtracting the end-systolic from the end-diastolic left ventricular volume, which are both determined in echocardiography by the modified Simpson's biplane method. Alternatively, stroke volume can be derived from the velocity time integral in the left ventricular outflow tract multiplied by the area of the outflow tract. Both methods are known to underestimate stroke volume; the Simpson's biplane method due to foreshortening and tracing errors, and the outflow tract method due to underestimation of its area. Indeed, when calculation of stroke volume is corrected for the true planimetered area of the left ventricular outflow tract, both the low flow—normal gradient and the low flow—low gradient constellations of findings in aortic stenosis are much less often diagnosed [15].

While the low flow—normal gradient constellation is consistent with a severe aortic stenosis and afterload mismatch leading to lower stroke volume, the low flow—low gradient constellation is a diagnostic problem when it is associated with a small effective orifice area. In principle, the finding of a low stroke volume, a low systolic pressure gradient, and a small effective orifice area may occur due to two different situations which should whenever possible be distinguished because of the therapeutic implications associated with this distinction. One possible situation is a patient with severe aortic stenosis and an impaired left ventricular systolic function due to the aortic stenosis alone or in combination with other reasons, the other situation is a patient with a moderate aortic stenosis and an impaired left ventricular systolic function unrelated to the aortic stenosis. The first type of patient should be treated by aortic valve replacement, while the second type should receive an optimal medical and device therapy for heart failure. Hence, the distinction between the two entities is important and is based on clinical assessment as well as advanced imaging [15, 59, 196–198].

1.5.2.4.2 Echocardiography
Low flow low gradient aortic stenosis is defined as mean systolic pressure gradient <40 mmHg, peak systolic flow velocity <4 m/s, effective orifice area <1 cm², and reduced left ventricular ejection fraction (<50%) [2, 4, 15]. A very important aspect of the echocardiographic assessment in patients with low flow low gradient aortic stenosis is ensuring that there are no mistakes related to calculation of stroke volume and, to a lesser extent, measurement of pressure gradients [15, 197, 198]. The diagnosis is indeed much less frequent when the true shape of the left ventricular outflow tract is considered, either using 3-dimensional transoesophageal

echocardiography or computed tomography [197, 198]. Both methods yield similar results regarding the planimetric analysis of left ventricular outflow tract area [15, 42].

In patients exhibiting low flow low gradient aortic stenosis even after correct assessment of left ventricular outflow tract area, the severity of aortic stenosis should be evaluated carefully under consideration of all the parameters recommended for its classification. Assessment of cardiac remodeling including left ventricular hypertrophy, diastolic dysfunction, and pulmonary hypertension is particularly important. In patients with small diameter of the proximal aorta, pressure recovery may be considered, and the energy loss index calculated [15, 197]. Finally, a dobutamine stress echocardiogram should be performed in such patients to improve the differentiation between true severe and pseudo-severe (moderate) aortic stenosis [59, 196].

A particularly challenging problem are patients with so-called "paradoxical" low flow low gradient aortic stenosis [161, 199]. These patients exhibit a small stroke volume with all the associated diagnostic problems, but a normal ejection fraction (>50%). This constellation of findings is possible in patients with small ventricles, myocardial hypertrophy, diastolic dysfunction, and high peripheral resistance. However, it is particularly important to exclude the measurement errors discussed above for low flow low gradient aortic stenosis in these patients. A dobutamine stress echo cannot be recommended for these patients based on the currently available literature [2, 4, 15].

1.5.2.4.3 Stress Echocardiography
Dobutamine stress echocardiography is recommended in patients with low flow low gradient aortic stenosis for the differentiation between patients with true severe from those with pseudo-severe (moderate) aortic stenosis. Such patients exhibit reduced left ventricular ejection fraction (<50%), mean systolic pressure gradient <40 mmHg, peak systolic flow velocity <4 m/s, and an effective orifice area <1 cm². As a rule of thumb, a mean systolic pressure gradient <20 mmHg in combination with an effective orifice area <1 cm² is highly suspicious of underlying moderate aortic stenosis and such patients should be evaluated for measurement errors with particular care [196, 200].

The stress echo is performed at dobutamine doses of 5, 10, and 20 µg/kg/m². The imaging assessment includes left ventricular ejection fraction determined by Simpson's biplane method, left ventricular contractile reserve assessed by increase in stroke volume (>20% compared to baseline), pulsed-wave Doppler over the left ventricular outflow tract, and continuous-wave Doppler across the aortic valve. Due to dobutamine stimulation, stroke volume and heart rate increase leading to enhanced transvalvular flow with an increase in systolic pressure gradient. Typically, true severe aortic stenosis results in a mean systolic pressure gradient

>40 mmHg and a peak systolic flow velocity >4 m/s, while the effective orifice area remains <1 cm².

In about one third of patients, there is no sufficient contractile reserve of the left ventricle, and these individuals are known to exhibit an increased mortality during surgical valve replacement. This observation has lost much of its importance since transcatheter aortic valve replacement has been introduced. Very important is the information that the absence of a contractile reserve does not exclude an improvement of left ventricular ejection fraction after aortic valve replacement. Hence, the major aim for dobutamine stress echocardiographic studies in low flow low gradient aortic stenosis should be to identify cases with moderate aortic stenosis as these patients should receive an optimal medical and device therapy for heart failure instead of valve replacement. In contrast, patients with true severe low flow low gradient aortic stenosis should undergo aortic valve replacement, preferentially by a transcatheter approach. The patients with no sufficient contractile reserve and strong suspicion of a severe symptomatic aortic stenosis should be considered for transcatheter aortic valve replacement as well, because they have the potential for an improvement of left ventricular ejection fraction after valve replacement [2, 4, 15].

If the situation remains unclear after the stress echocardiogram because the systolic pressure gradient has not increased sufficiently or the contractile reserve is not large enough, the concept of the projected aortic valve area at a normal flow rate might be applied. With this concept the effective orifice area is calculated for a projected normal flow rate of, for example, 250 mL/s. The same cut-off of 1 cm² applies for this method as for the conventional approach [15, 196, 200].

1.5.2.4.4 Magnetic Resonance Imaging

Patients with low-flow-low-gradient aortic stenosis represent a highly challenging subset from both a diagnostic and a therapeutic standpoint. A multimodality imaging approach, including comprehensive resting echocardiography, dobutamine stress echocardiography, and multidetector computed tomography, is the key to successful diagnosis and management. In selected cases with poor echocardiographic windows or difficulties in myocardial function evaluation, cardiac magnetic resonance imaging (CMR) is an ideal additional modality to accurately assess left ventricular dimensions and functions [156]. Furthermore, tissue characterization can be performed using Late Gadolinium Enhancement in CMR. The amount of myocardial fibrosis assessed by CMR, may provide incremental information for risk stratification and therapeutic management in low-flow-low-gradient aortic stenosis. In fact, Hermann et al. could show that in patients with aortic stenosis a low gradient is associated with a higher degree of fibrosis, decreased longitudinal function, and poorer clinical outcome despite pre-

served ejection fraction [201]. It is reasonable to hypothesize that patients with extensive fibrosis would be less likely to demonstrate improved left ventricular function after aortic valve replacement. However, additional studies are needed to validate and refine these emerging biomarkers. A newer technique, CMR feature tracking, can accurately detect myocardial deformation. Reduction of longitudinal strain and an impairment of longitudinal velocity could be observed in patients with low-flow-low-gradient aortic stenosis [202], but it is unknown whether these new technique is predictive of reversibility of left ventricular remodeling after aortic valve replacement.

1.5.2.4.5 Nuclear Medicine

There is no established use for nuclear medicine in the setting of low-flow-low-gradient AS.

1.5.3 Left Ventricular Fibrosis and Diastolic Function

1.5.3.1 Introduction

In addition to evaluation of left ventricular systolic function by ejection fraction and using strain analysis, the degree of diastolic dysfunction and myocardial fibrotic changes may also be prognostically significant in individuals with aortic valve disease before and after intervention [203–207]. It is also associated with worse symptoms prior to valve replacement [208, 209].

Diastolic function of the left ventricle refers to myocardial relaxation, which is an active process that requires energy consumption by cardiac myocytes. It determines how the left ventricle fills and potential elevation in the left atrial pressure. Diastolic filling is divided into predominantly three phases: early filling (rapid filling), diastasis (slow filling) and atrial contraction [210]. With normal diastolic function, a majority of blood enters the left ventricle in the early filling phase, followed by much less flow during diastasis and a somewhat smaller volume of blood pushed in during atrial systole.

The early diastolic component of flow is secondary to rapid relaxation of the contracted myocardium, creating a vacuum effect that opens the mitral valve and creates a favorable gradient to promote left atrial to left ventricular blood flow. As the myocardium becomes more stiff and unable to relax rapidly, less blood enters the left ventricle in the early phase of diastole. Increased filling during atrial contraction compensates for this initially, followed by progressively increasing left atrial pressure to push more blood into the left ventricle in early and mid diastole.

The most severe form of diastolic dysfunction is called restrictive filing. This occurs when the myocardial relaxation is so abnormal, diastolic filling is achieved due to a marked elevation in left atrial pressure that forces blood into the left ventricle. Very rapid early filling occurs in this situation with little flow during the remaining parts of diastole [211].

Echocardiography is the primary method of evaluating diastolic function since it is able to assess velocities of the blood pool as well as the myocardium throughout the diastolic filling period. However, it is limited in the ability to detect abnormalities in the myocardial tissue itself such as fibrosis. Cardiac magnetic resonance imaging is more useful for this specific application [180]. In this section the role of multimodality imaging in the evaluation of diastolic function and left ventricular fibrosis will be reviewed [212].

1.5.3.2 Echocardiography

Left ventricular diastolic function assessment by echocardiography is based on the principles of left ventricular filling mechanisms. In the early phase of diastole, flow is usually due to a left atrium to left ventricular gradient created by rapid relaxation of the contracted myocardium. This is called the "E" wave when looking at flow through the mitral valve. In diastasis, a small ongoing gradient causes slow filling. There is usually only very low velocity flow during this period but when it is increased, a prominent "L" wave can be detected. Lastly, atrial systole pushes a further volume of blood into the left ventricle. This is what creates the "A" wave.

All the three components can be assessed by looking at the mitral valve leaflets, mitral valve blood flow and myocardial tissue velocities [210, 211].

The mitral valve leaflets typically open widely in early diastole during early rapid filling (corresponding with the E wave), followed by partial closing in diastasis and then opening widely again during atrial systole (corresponding with the A wave). M-mode echocardiography of the mitral leaflet tips demonstrates this pattern of opening quite clearly. Although this will demonstrate all three phases of diastole, flow is not directly analyzed so it is not generally used to determine if diastolic dysfunction exists.

Flow across the mitral valve is assessed using pulse wave Doppler at the level of the mitral valve tips. This demonstrates the velocity of flow during each phase of diastole. The E and A wave peak velocity should be similar when diastolic function is normal. The E wave usually begins to reduce in velocity relative to the A wave progressively as diastolic dysfunction progresses. In later stages, a prominent L wave in mid diastole may be visible. With late-stage restrictive filling, the E wave becomes much more prominent than the A wave (usually greater than a 2:1 ratio) and the E wave velocity decreases from peak rapidly (deceleration time of under 180 ms, measured by tracing the spectral Doppler profile from the peak E velocity to the end of the E wave) due to rapid equalization of pressure between the left atrium and left ventricle.

Myocardial tissue velocity can be analyzed using specialized tissue Doppler imaging by echocardiography. This mode only detects low velocities in the heart and therefore excludes the blood pool. A colour Doppler overlay can be visualized over the left ventricular myocardium and pulse wave Doppler can be applied to specific locations to track motion velocity. Pulse wave Doppler analysis of the septal and lateral left ventricular base should be done by placing the sample volume at the basal myocardium, taking care not to sample too apically, at the fibrous junction between the ventricle and atrium or in the atrial wall. The spectral Doppler recording follows a similar diastolic pattern seen with the mitral valve leaflets or inflow, with tissue movement away from the transducer during early and late diastole corresponding with the E and A waves. The early diastolic motion is of interest and is labeled E'. Low E' velocities (below 8 cm/s septally and 10 cm/s laterally), especially relative to the peak mitral inflow E velocity, are associated with abnormal myocardial relaxation. Additionally, a high E/E' ratio (above 14 when septal and lateral ratios are averaged) is correlated with elevated left atrial pressure.

Doppler measurements by echocardiography face important limitations. The angulation of motion must be oriented as parallel as possible towards the transducer to avoid underestimation of velocities. The sample volume of pulse wave Doppler recordings must also be placed carefully at the appropriate location. Lastly, the accurate evaluation of all diastolic parameters described above may be limited in the setting of other cardiac diseases that may change transmitral flow and myocardial motion abnormalities. This includes significant mitral valve disease (annular calcification, regurgitation, stenosis, repair, annuloplasty, replacement), arrhythmia (atrial fibrillation or flutter, idioventricular rhythm, heart blocked, paced rhythm, atrioventricular dissociation) and atrial abnormalities (loss of atrial contraction and A wave).

To overcome these limitations, the most recent guidelines by the American Society of Echocardiography and the European Association of Cardiovascular Imaging recommends an integrative approach [1]. This includes evaluation of downstream consequences expected in the setting of diastolic dysfunction. Longstanding increases in left atrial pressure usually result in dilation of this thin-walled structure and transmission of elevated pressures into the pulmonary circulation. Therefore, left atrial dilation and pulmonary hypertension are used as evaluation criteria in the new algorithm. Since neither finding is specific to left ventricular diastolic dysfunction, a combined assessment of 4 features is recommended and in some cases, presence and absence of diastolic dysfunction may still be "indeterminate".

Another limitation in the assessment of diastolic dysfunction is age related change in left ventricular relaxation. Advanced age is associated with worse myocardial relaxation and is seen echocardiographically by lower E and E′ velocities compared to younger individuals. However, this may be common with age and may not be prognostically significant.

Lastly, it is important to note that in the presence of left ventricular systolic dysfunction or myocardial disease, diastolic dysfunction is also always present. In these settings, echocardiography is used primarily to determine the grade of diastolic dysfunction. Grade I refers to impaired myocardial relaxation with no evidence of elevated left atrial pressure. Grade II refers to evidence of moderately elevated left atrial pressure. Grade III refers to a restrictive filling pattern that is consistent with severe impairment of myocardial relaxation and markedly elevated left atrial pressure.

Assessment of myocardial fibrosis by echocardiography is difficult since it cannot characterize tissue quality like other imaging modalities. There is also no direct way to stain and detect fibrotic areas. Transmural injury with subsequent scar formation may appear as a thinned wall segment that is akinetic or dyskinetic and more echogenic than other wall segments. However, non-transmural fibrosis such as injury due to chronic pressure of volume overload from aortic valve disease is not visualized.

Future advancements in the echocardiographic evaluation of left ventricular diastolic function may include novel cardiac strain parameters. For example, left atrial strain has been described as being associated with diastolic dysfunction [213]. Global left ventricular strain rate has also been shown to be closely associated with left ventricular filling pressures and may outperform traditional Doppler parameters [214, 215].

Echocardiography plays an important role in the assessment of left ventricular diastolic function but is limited by concurrent cardiac disease that alters the Doppler parameters being assessed. Additionally, abnormalities in individual parameters are not specific to diastolic dysfunction so an integrated approach should be taken and disease states that reduce accuracy of assessment should be ruled out. Myocardial fibrosis related to valve disease is not readily visualized by echocardiography and alternative imaging modalities should be considered (Fig. 1.37).

1.5.3.3 Magnetic Resonance Imaging

Left ventricular remodeling in patients with aortic stenosis is a consequence of chronic pressure overload. The results are myocyte hypertrophy, increased interstitial left ventricular volume caused initially by reactive fibrosis (increase in collagen volume) and at a later stage by replacement fibrosis (replacement by fibrous tissue) due to myocyte apoptosis (scar). In cardiac magnetic resonance, both reactive fibrosis and replacement fibrosis and can be directly visualized and quantified by sophisticated techniques.

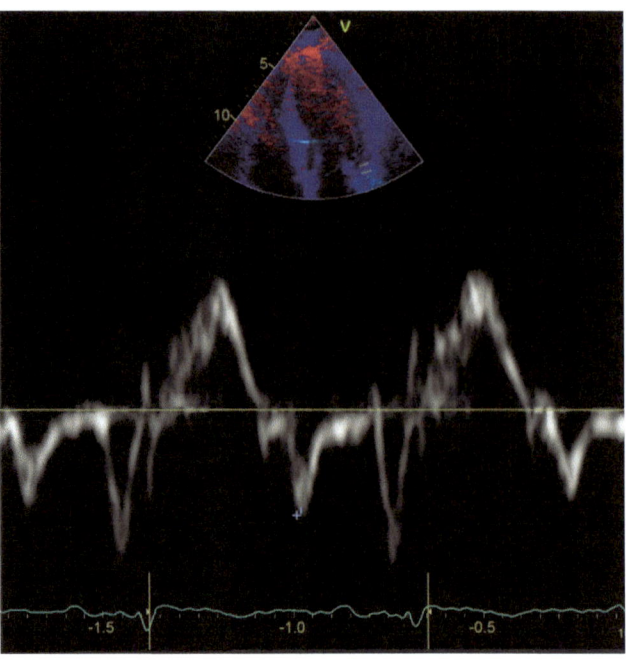

Fig. 1.37 Tissue Doppler imaging by transthoracic echocardiography of the lateral mitral annulus

T1-mapping techniques allow quantification of the longitudinal magnetization relaxation time of a given tissue (T1 time) [216]. T1 maps in cardiac magnetic resonance tomography give the myocardial T1 time, which represents a mixture of the native signal of myocytes and the interstitium [217]. Increasing extent of fibrosis leads to prolonged native T1 mapping values. In addition to native T1 maps, those maps can be acquired post injection of gadolinium based contrast agents. Due to the contrast kinetics and the T1 shortening effect of gadolinium based contrast agents, the post contrast T1 mapping values become shorter with an increase of interstitial fibrosis. Putting both the pre- and post-contrast T1 myocardial mapping values and the hematocrit of the patient into a formula, the extracellular left ventricular fraction can be calculated, which is mainly an expression of collagen I in absence of amyloid deposition or edema [218]. In summary, cardiac magnetic resonance T1 mapping techniques pre- and post-contrast media injections allow one to quantify extracellular (interstitial) myocardial tissue and thus fibrosis quantitatively. Compared to late gadolinium contrast enhanced cardiac magnetic resonance, T1 mapping offers the advantage to detect and to quantify diffuse interstitial fibrosis which is particularly important in patients with aortic stenosis as the left ventricular remodeling in those patients is typically caused by reactive fibrosis (increase in collagen volume) and not by replacement fibrosis, assuming there is no coexisting cardiac diseases such as coronary artery disease with myocardial infarction. The clinical implication of myocardial fibrosis assessed by T1 mapping techniques in patients with aortic stenosis has been demonstrated in several studies. Increased T1 mapping values and extracellular volume have been shown to correlate with the severity of aortic stenosis [219] as well as with poor prognostic markers such as symptoms [180], cardiac decompensation [180], ventricular dysfunction [220] and increased cardiac biomarkers [221]. Importantly, mortality has been shown to be significantly higher in patients with aortic stenosis and increased extracellular volume assessed by T1 mapping techniques [180].

Late gadolinium contrast enhanced cardiac magnetic resonance offers the possibility to visualize and quantify myocardial replacement fibrosis and myocardial scar. Due to the delayed washout of gadolinium based contrast agents in fibrotic tissue compared to the rapid washout of the contrast media in normal myocardium, fibrosis appears bright in late enhanced images. In these images, inversion time is chosen to null the myocardium, so the healthy myocardium looks black [222]. According to the pattern and distribution of myocardial fibrosis, underlying pathologies can be distinguished. The ischemic pattern is typically described as subendocardial in the territory of a coronary artery. In contrast, multiple non-ischemic patterns (midwall, epicardial, or patchy) have been reported (Fig. 1.38) [223]. Late gadolinium enhancement is common in patients with severe aortic

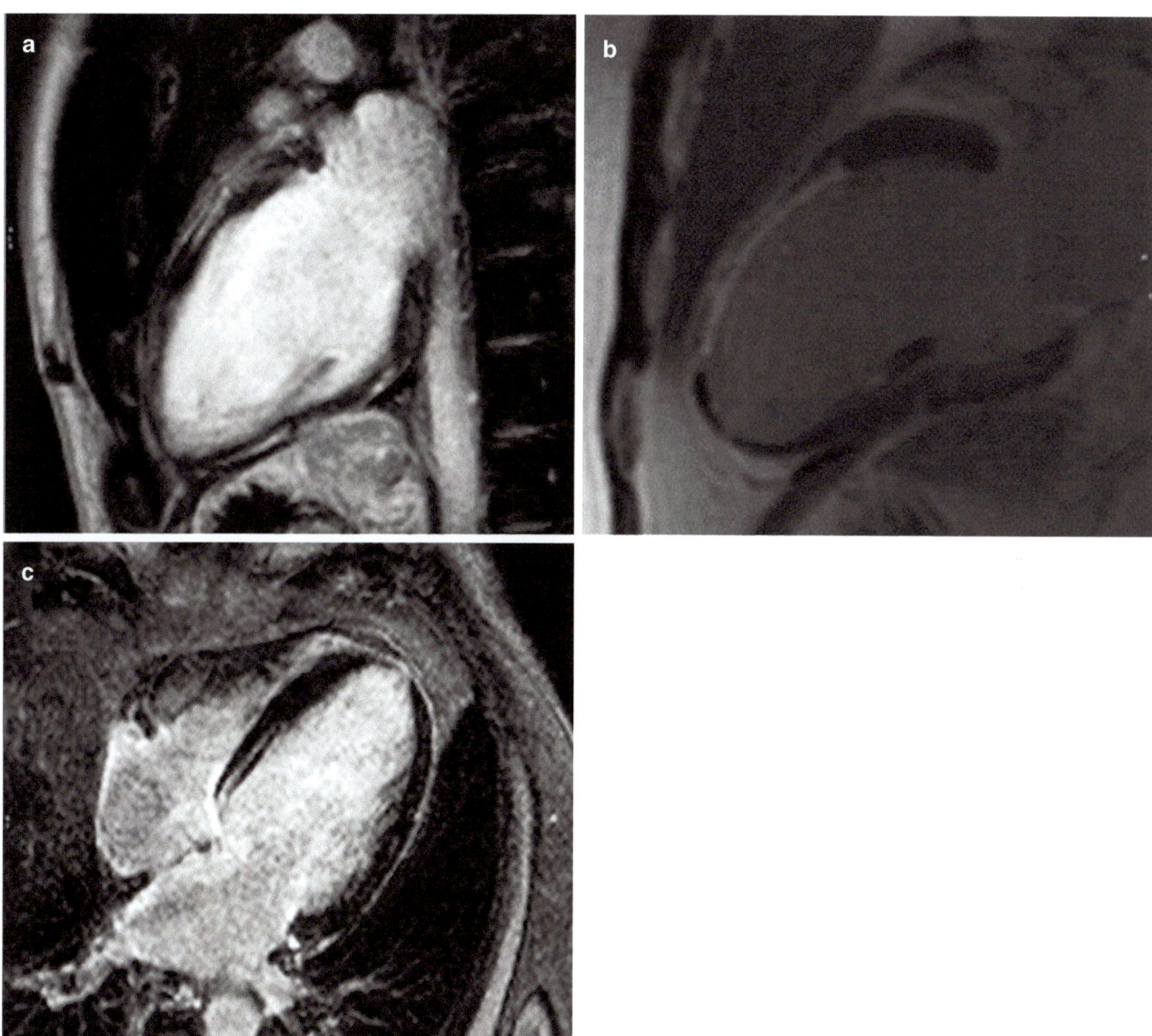

Fig. 1.38 Late gadolinium enhanced images of three different patients illustrating different patterns. (**a**) Epicardial and patchy late enhancement in a patient with myocarditis. (**b**) Subendocardial late enhancement in the territory of the left anterior descending coronary due to myocardial infarction. (**c**) Septal midwall late enhancement in a patient with severe aortic stenosis

stenosis and is associated with increased left ventricular mass, poor left ventricular function and increased cardiac biomarkers [221, 224]. Furthermore, fibrosis assessed by late gadolinium enhancement serves as an independent predictor of mortality in patients with moderate and severe aortic stenosis [225]. This is important as late gadolinium enhancement is an irreversible morphological substrate and a marker of postoperative clinical outcomes in patients with severe aortic stenosis [172]. Higher degrees of myocardial replacement fibrosis accumulation were associated with worse long term survival in patients with severe aortic valve disease. Specifically, patients with midwall fibrosis had the worst prognosis [29].

Tagging and feature tracking are novel techniques which allow assessment of the function of the left ventricle in patients with aortic stenosis, especially with respect to stiffness and diastolic impairment, which are consequences of the left ventricular remodeling process consisting of myocyte hypertrophy and fibrosis. Both techniques allow quantification of radial, circumferential and longitudinal strain by acquisition of special sequences (tagging) or via post processing of cine images (feature tracking). Strain values and extent of fibrosis correlate inversely with outcome, and impaired longitudinal strain is significantly lower in patients with significant symptomatic severe aortic stenosis compared to asymptomatic patients [226]. Furthermore, impaired pre-operative circumferential strain is associated with post-operative mortality [227].

As stated in the current 2017 ESC/EACTS Guidelines for the management of valvular heart disease, cardiac magnetic resonance is classified as a useful modality for the detection and quantification of myocardial fibrosis. It provides additional prognostic information regardless of the presence of coronary artery disease as the extent of fibrosis has been shown to be an important risk marker in patients with aortic stenosis [228].

Novel promising techniques such as molecular magnetic resonance imaging with dedicated contrast agents might allow more specific detection of fibrosis in the future; however, those are not yet implemented in routine clinical practice since they are investigational at this time.

1.6 Special Conditions and Other Problems

1.6.1 Endocarditis

1.6.1.1 Introduction

Infective endocarditis (IE) occurs mostly on the cardiac valves but it may involve any surface of the endocardium, including the chordae of the atrioventricular valves and the endocardial walls of the cardiac chambers, congenital defects, and prosthetic tissue or cardiac devices. The clinical diagnosis is made according to a combination of clinical, echocardiographic, and laboratory findings as defined in the modified Duke criteria. The prevalence of IE reported in different observational studies is about 2.7–2.5 per 100,000 persons-years and is potentially fatal, with a 1-year mortality rate after completion of treatment of 10–20% [229–231]. Several risk factors predispose to the development IE such any type of prosthetic valve, previous episode of IE, and any type of cyanotic congenital heart disease. Other patient related risk factors are older age (>60 years), male sex, injection drug use, or poor dental hygiene. The clinical manifestations are variable depending on the presence of an acute, subacute, or chronic onset. Fever and new cardiac murmurs are the most common symptom and sign, respectively, while cutaneous manifestations like petechiae or splinter hemorrhages, Janeway lesions, Osler nodes, and Roth spots are more uncommon, but highly suggestive of IE [232]. Echocardiography should be performed in all patients with suspected IE as it is the technique of choice for detection of valvular vegetation or complications of an IE with identification of vegetations representing one of two major diagnostic criteria for IE.

The pathogenesis of endocarditis varies depending on the infecting organism. The first step in the formation of a vegetation is endocardial injury followed by a secondarily infected platelet-fibrin nidus. The endocardial injury is associated with high velocity jets where blood travels from a high pressure chamber through a narrow orifice into a low-pressure chamber [231]. Vegetations are usually located on the ventricular side of incompetent semilunar valves or the atrial side of incompetent atrioventricular valves. If aortic regurgitation is present, vegetations may also adhere to the chordae tendineae of the anterior leaflet of the mitral valve and, in case of mitral regurgitation, may also develop on the left atrial wall. Such so-called jet lesions may also develop on all other locations of endocarditis; for example, in cases of ventricular septal defect, vegetations may develop on the right ventricular side of the defect and secondarily on right sided heart valves [233].

The differential diagnosis for endocarditis is wide and two clinical categories should be distinguished. Patients with bacteremia in the absence of vegetation and patients with valvular vegetation in absence of bacteremia. In the first case, alternative causes of bacteremia (e.g. infection of intravascular catheter, cardiac device, skin and soft tissue, osteomyelitis, prosthetic joint) should be evaluated. In the second case, non-bacterial thrombotic endocarditis (e.g. marantic, Libman-Sacks, or verrucous endocarditis) should be considered. It is particularly important to distinguish between true non-bacterial thrombotic endocarditis and patients with negative blood cultures due to previous antibiotic therapy or organisms that are difficult to incubate and require extended cultures.

1.6.1.2 Echocardiography

The role of echocardiography, either transthoracic (TTE) or transoesophagial (TOE), is crucial in the diagnosis and evaluation of infective endocarditis. The common approach is to begin with a TTE. However, in special occasions such as patients with one or more prosthetic valves or known poor image quality in TTE, TOE may be used as first-line diagnostic tool. TOE should also be performed in patients with positive TTE to rule out local complications as well as in case of negative TTE if the clinical suspicion for endocarditis is high. TOE should not be performed if it is unlikely to acquire additional diagnostic information, if the clinical risk factors are prohibitive, and if the findings will implicate no change in the clinical management of the patient. When a TTE has moderate or good ultrasound quality, normal anatomy, less than mild valvular regurgitation, no valvular stenoses or scleroses, no significant pericardial effusion, no catheter or pacemaker leads, and no evidence of vegetations, the negative predictive value is about 97% [234]. The sensitivity of TTE for endocarditis in native and prosthetic valves is 70% and 50%, respectively, and that of TOE is 96% and 92%, respectively; the specificity for both methods is about 90%. TTE underestimates the size and complexity of large vegetations and may be non-diagnostic in small vegetations (<3 mm), redundant leaflet tissue, and shadowing because of severe calcification or prosthetic valves.

It may be difficult to differentiate vegetations from thrombi, tumors such as fibroelastoma, degenerative lesions such as Lambl's excrescences, and sterile vegetations as in Libman-sacks endocarditis and marantic endocarditis. In those cases, pre-test probability according to clinical presentation, laboratory findings, and likelihood of endocarditis should be taken into consideration. False positive findings may occur because of small degenerative processes such as strands, which are mostly seen on the aortic and mitral valves, representing a normal degenerative process. Amputated chordae after valve surgery, redundant or aberrant chordae or false tendons in the left ventricle, the Chiari network in the right atrium, or annular calcifications may be confused with a vegetation as well. The echocardiographic characteristics typical of infective endocarditis are (1) an oscillating mass on a valve, supporting tissue or intravascular device, (2) an abscess typically seen as thickend, non-homogeneous, echodense or echolucent perivalvular area, (3) a pseudoaneurysm, indentified as a pulsatile perivalvular echo-free space with color-Doppler flow, (4) a perforation, depicted as interruption of endocardial tissue continuity, (5) a fistula, seen as a communication between two neighbouring cavities, (6) a valve aneurysm and (7) dehiscence of a prosthetic valve [229]. Vegetations characteristically prolapse into the upstream chamber and have a lobulated and amorphous appearance unlike the hair-like and shorter strands. Characteristics which are associated with higher risk of embolism are larger size, highly mobile, less dense and greater extension of the vegetation [235].

Prosthetic valve endocarditis should always be considered in case of dehiscence on the prosthetic valve, as it may be the only manifestation of IE. A dehiscence may be seen as a rocking motion of the prosthesis or even as new paravalvular regurgitation. If there are no previous examinations for comparison, greater than mild paravalvular regurgitation should always raise the suspicion of prosthetic endocarditis.

A TTE and/or TEE should be repeated within 5–7 days if the first examination is negative, but the clinical probability remains high. Follow-up echocardiograms should be considered in uncomplicated endocarditis in order not to overlook new silent complications and monitor vegetations. After completion of antibiotic therapy, a TTE should be performed again in order to analyze valve morphology and function as well as the ventricular function [229].

1.6.1.3 Positron Emission Tomography-Computed Tomography

Two nuclear imaging modalities are currently available that have been shown to offer added value over echocardiography for the diagnosis of endocarditis: radiolabeled leukocyte scintigraphy [236] and, more recently, 18F-fluorodeoxyglucose (FDG) positron emission tomography/computed tomography (PET/CT) [237]. While the former offers high specificity for detection of infection, it requires specialized equipment and expertise, including direct handling of blood products, rendering this technique cumbersome and time-consuming. Scintigraphy and SPECT/CT acquisitions use commonly performed 4 and 24 h after the injection of radiolabelled leucocytes. Sensitivity, specificity, positive predictive value, negative predictive value, and accuracy for the diagnosis of prosthetic valve endocarditis has been reported as 64%, 100%, 100%, 81%, and 86%, respectively [238].

On the other hand, 18F-FDG PET/CT has the advantage of short acquisition times and wide-spread availability without the need for cumbersome labeling-procedures, thus overcoming the major limitations of leukocyte scintigraphy while yielding an extremely high sensitivity for the detection of tissue with high metabolic activity. FDG, an analogue of glucose, is metabolized similarly to glucose. FDG is transported across cell membranes by glucose transporters and is enzymatically phosphorylated to FDG-6-phosphate which cannot further undergo glycolysis and becomes metabolically trapped intracellularly. Therefore, 18F-FDG can be used to identify cells with high metabolic activity, such as inflammatory cells. Of note, however, 18F-FDG PET/CT does not allow for discrimination between infection and sterile inflammation. The latter may be particularly problematic within the first weeks after the surgery or intervention due to sterile inflammatory reactions after implantation of foreign material. Therefore, 18F-FDG PET/CT should not be used for the diagnosis of prosthetic valve infection within three months of implantation [228]. Finally, special patient preparation consisting of a strict carbohydrate-free diet before 18F-FDG injection is mandatory to ensure suppression of physiological glucose uptake in the myocardium adjacent to the valve. If physiological uptake can be suppressed successfully 18F-FDG PET/CT has 91% sensitivity, 91% specificity, and 93% positive and 88% negative predictive values for the diagnosis of prosthetic valve infective endocarditis [239]. In this setting, the addition of 18F-FDG PET/CT to the modified Duke criteria has been shown to substantially increase sensitivity from 52–70% to >90%. In contrast, in the setting of native valve endocarditis, the sensitivity of 18F-FDG PET/CT for diagnosis is inadequate and ranges below 15% [239]. This is mainly due to the limited temporal resolution of PET/CT, rendering detection of small and mobile (e.g., in the case of isolated vegetations on native valves) difficult, if not impossible. Exceptions where 18F-FDG PET/CT offers added diagnostic value over echocardiography and other imaging modalities in the setting of native valve endocarditis are suspected abscess and differentiation between pseudoaneurysm and abscess.

In conclusion, current guidelines recommend the use of 18F-FDG PET/CT or radiolabeled leukocyte SPECT/CT as a second-line imaging modality after transthoracic and transoesophageal echocardiography if infective endocarditis of a prosthetic valve remains possible according to the modified Duke criteria. Abnormal radionuclide accumulation around the site of implantation currently constitutes a major imaging criterion for the diagnosis of infective endocarditis (Fig. 1.39) [228].

The choice of nuclear modality must, of course, be based on local expertise and availability. If both are available, 18F-FDG PET/CT should be considered the first choice because of its high sensitivity. However, radiolabeled leukocyte SPECT/CT seems particularly interesting for the assessment of patients with suspected prosthetic valve infection in the first months after valve implantation of in cases of inconclusive 18F-FDG PET/CT results due to its higher specificity.

1.6.1.4 Angiography and Catheterization

Echocardiography is accurate and reproducible in patients with good image quality for chamber quantification, morphology and grading valvular heart disease severity. It is also possible to assess the hemodynamic status in terms of estimation of right sided blood pressures by using transvalvular gradients. But we must recognize that it is limited in accuracy with respect to systematic under- and overestimation [240]. Therefore the ESC Guidelines for Diagnosis and Treatment of Pulmonary Hypertension recommend to express not the exact diagnosis or severity of pulmonary hypertension but to use the term of "unlikely", "possible" or "very likely" [240]. It should also be noted that the RV/RA gradient is severely underestimated in patients with relevant tricuspid regurgitation. To overcome this limitation, it is necessary and recommended to perform invasive measurements. In patients with severe aortic stenosis, the presence of pulmonary hypertension (PHT) is common, different in mechanism and associated with bad outcomes depending on whether it is precapillary, postcapillary or combined [241].

Therefore, a complete hemodynamic assessment by performing left and right-heart catherization is recommended in all patients with dyspnea as clinical symptoms, signs of pulmonary hypertension, left atrial enlargement, enlarged right ventricle, depressed right ventricular function and additional valvular heart disease.

Catheterization can be easily done using a femoral approach, or even easier in our experience, from brachial access when radial access for coronary angiography is used. Coming from the superior vena cava, it is almost always a straightforward process to enter into the RV and pulmonary artery with less need for X-ray use as it is done in the intensive care unit for monitoring purposes. If pulmonary wedge position is achieved, position of the ballon can be confirmed using fluoroscopy. This is especially relevant in patients with pulmonary hypertension, as it can be difficult (and even in some cases impossible) to achive a stable position of the ballon.

Some rare but relevant pathologies like subvalvular stenosis or the entity of a double chambered right ventricle cannot be overseen in preoperative workup.

Cardiac output can be measured using thermodilution or Ficks principle. For the latter, the exact Oxygen demand of the resting body has to be determined. In clinical practice, we use standard tables in a comfortable resting situation for the patient. External oxygen supply has to be discontinued for 10 minutes before taking blood samples (Fig. 1.40).

1.6.1.5 Scintigraphy

Nuclear imaging is useful for the assessment of right ventricular volume and function through radionuclide ventriculography (see Sect. 1.5.2.2.6).

Furthermore, ventilation-perfusion scintigraphy plays an essential role in the diagnosis of chronic thromboembolic pulmonary hypertension (CTEPH) which constitutes a differential diagnosis in pulmonary hypertension. Patients with pulmonary arterial hypertension (PAH) usually demonstrate regular or heterogeneous perfusion, while a ventilation-perfusion scan with multiple mismatched segmental or larger perfusion defects indicates a high probability of CTEPH. By contrast, a normal or low probability scan excludes CTEPH with a sensitivity and a specificity of 90% to 100% and 94% to 100%, respectively. As a ventilation-

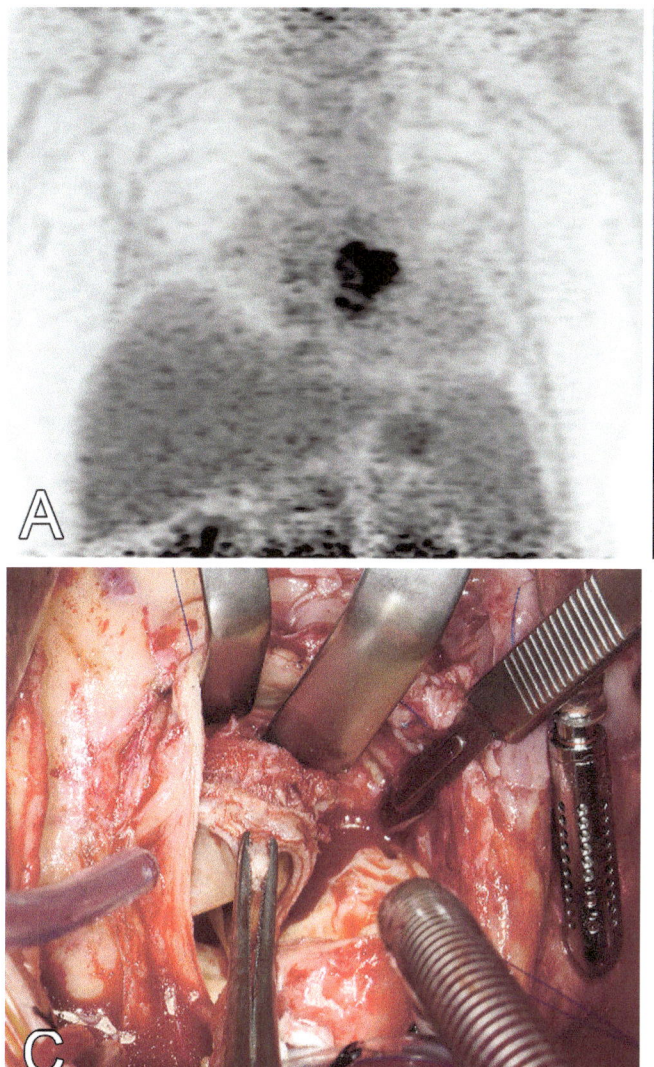

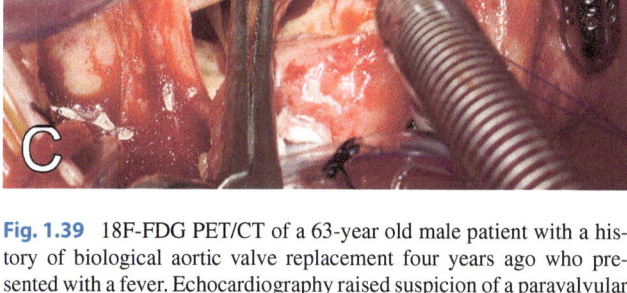

Fig. 1.39 18F-FDG PET/CT of a 63-year old male patient with a history of biological aortic valve replacement four years ago who presented with a fever. Echocardiography raised suspicion of a paravalvular abscess. PET maximum intensity projection (MIP, **a**) depicts strong focal FDG accumulation in the area of the aortic root. Fused PET/CT reformatted in a sagittal view (**b**) allows clear localization of the increased metabolic activity. Surgery (**c**) confirmed a large posterior abscess and a homograft was implanted

perfusion scan provides higher sensitivity than CT pulmonary angiography, it is recommended as the screening test of choice [242].

Finally, while myocardial perfusion imaging (see Sect. 1.2.2.6) is often used to rule out ischemic heart disease as a potential cause for pulmonary hypertension, it may also be able to detect the presence of right ventricular pressure overload by assessing the structure and radionuclide uptake of the right ventricle. Some studies found that the right ventricular wall thickness as assessed during myocardial SPECT was associated with electrocardiographic evidence of right ventricular hypertrophy and that tracer uptake was increased in patients with chronic obstructive pulmonary disease (COPD) [243]. Flattening of the interventricular septum (D-shaping) in addition to increased right ventricular tracer uptake and volume on gated SPECT studies strongly correlated with right ventricular overload [244] (Fig. 1.41).

1.6.1.6 Magnetic Resonance Imaging

Marfan syndrome is a connective tissue disease affecting a mutation in the fibrillin 1 gene in most of the cases with an incidence of 1:5000 [245]. The cardiovascular, ocular and skeletal systems are mainly involved in this disease. Cardiovascular manifestations of the disease affect the aorta, the myocardium, the valves and the pulmonary arteries. As aortic dissection is the most common cause of death in patients with Marfan syndrome, particular attention has to be paid regarding the imaging of the entire aorta. According to the guidelines of the European Society of

Cardiology, these patients need an assessment of the entire aorta at the time point of diagnosis and a follow-up by advanced imaging every one to five years (depending on the aortic root dimensions) in addition to transthoracic echocardiography [246]. Both cardiac magnetic resonance or computed tomography can be used to assess the whole aorta with both advantages and disadvantages of each technique. It is essential to report measurements of the aortic annulus, the sinus of valsalva, the sinutubular junction, and

the ascending and descending aorta. The entire aorta can be visualized by cardiac magnetic resonance as well as complications including aneurysm formation, dissection, and complications of previous surgery. Additionally, biophysical properties such as the aortic distensibility can be assessed [247]. Due to its diversity, different sequences can be used to assess the aorta. Steady-state free precession cine images and T2 black blood sequences are most commonly used. Furthermore, ECG-gated contrast-enhanced 3D sequences can also be acquired. However, contrast media injection is needed for the latter sequence. One advantage of cardiac magnetic resonance tomography is that biventricular function, valves and extra-cardiac manifestations like dural ectasia can be simultaneously assessed in addition to aortic measurement. Of course, the assessment of the aorta plays also an important role in patients with collagen diseases such as Ehlers-Danlos syndrome type IV, in which disease manly arteries of large and medium diameter are affected [248].

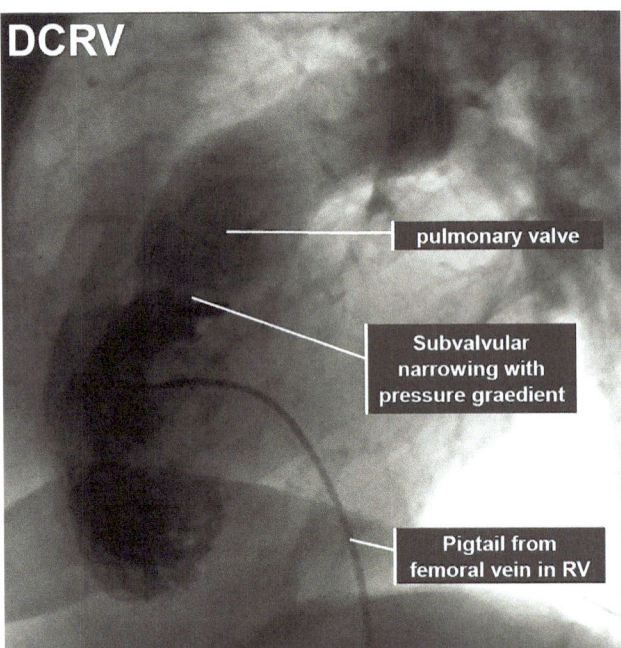

Fig. 1.40 Double chambered right ventricle (DCRV) from almost 90° left lateral oblique position. Pigtail comes from the femoral vein into the right ventricle with elevated pressures. Cranial to this, the intraventricular constriction is visible forming a subvalvular normal pressure chamber. No pressure gradient is measured across the anatomically normal pulmonary valve

Although, in most cases bicuspid aortic valve is an isolated cardiac disease, coexistence with other congenital cardiovascular malformations is common such as coarctation of the aorta, Turner syndrome, patent ductus arteriosus, and supravalvular aortic stenosis. Additionally, patients with bicuspid aortic valves are at an increased risk for aortic valve stenosis, regurgitation, aortic dilatation, aneurysm and dissection [249, 250]. Cardiac magnetic resonance allows the assessment of the valve morphology, function, and complications. Through visualization of the cusps in steady-state free precession cine images in long and short axis views perpendicular to the valve, the morphology including fusion of cusps can be assessed. Unfortunately, valvular calcifications cannot be directly visualized, since calcium appears black regardless of the sequence used. In addition to the morphology, the function of the bicuspid valve can be quantified by

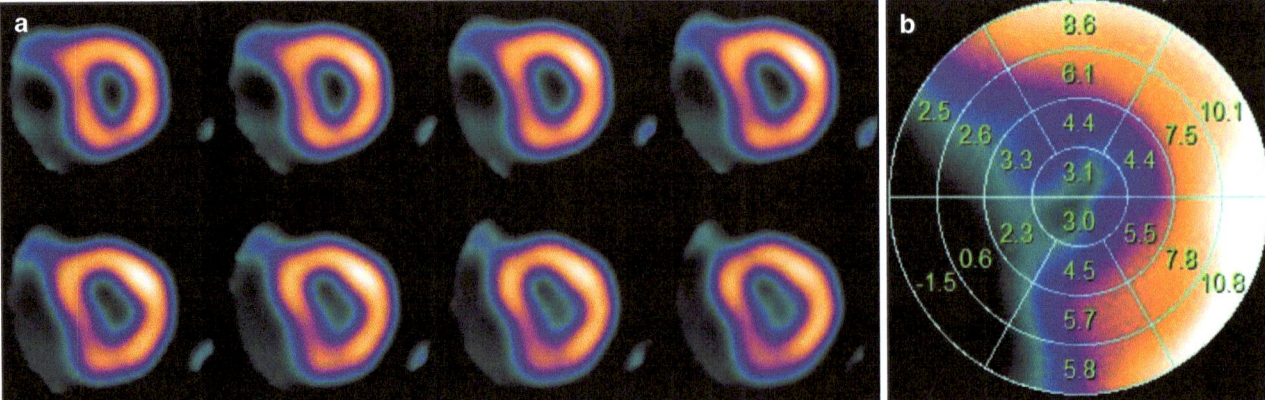

Fig. 1.41 Electrocardiogram-gated myocardial perfusion SPECT imaging of a patient with known severe chronic obstructive pulmonary disease. Short axis slices at rest (**a**) depict clearly a flattening of the interventricular septum, resulting in the typical D-shaped pattern. Analysis of the gated dataset depicted as absolute motion (in mm) in a polar plot (**b**), reveals marked septal dyssynchrony

calculation of blood flow and velocity through the aortic valve with phase contrast imaging. This sequence uses the differences in the phase of moving blood compared to static tissue to quantify forward flow and backward flow as well as maximum velocity over the aortic valve [24]. However, compared to transthoracic doppler echocardiography, which offers very high temporal resolution, maximal velocity in cardiac magnetic resonance can be underestimated due to the lower temporal resolution [251]. Planimetry of the aortic valve is another method to quantify aortic valve area, which however might result in a degree of inaccuracy. One caveat using this method is that the directly calculated orifice area representing the maximal instantaneous valve area in systole is lower compared to the continuity equation, which represents the mean area in systole. Recently, studies have shown that the left ventricular outflow tract area, which is estimated in transthoracic echocardiography, is not a circular but an oval structure. Of course, the left ventricular outflow tract can be visualized by cardiac magnetic resonance [252]. According to the guidelines of the European Society of Cardiology, in every patient with diagnosis of a bicuspid aortic valve, the aortic root and the ascending aorta should be visualized with transthoracic echocardiography alone or in association with another imaging modality, preferably cardiac magnetic resonance at the time of diagnosis. Additionally, magnetic resonance tomography or computed tomography is indicated if there is an increase in diameter >3 mm/year or a diameter >45 mm [246]. Recently, time resolved three-dimensional phase-contrast cardiac magnetic resonance (4D-Flow) has demonstrated different flow patterns in patients with bicuspid aortic valve which might explain different aortic dilatation morphologies [253]. Shear stress can be also be calculated from the latter acquisitions [254]. To assess the benefits and clinical impact of these novel techniques on patient treatment and risk classification, further studies are needed (Fig. 1.42).

1.6.1.7 Angiography

Contrast Power injection into the aortic root using a pigtail catheter visualizes very well the coronary sinuses, the annulus, the sinutubular junction and the ascending aorta. Standard settings are comparable with Settings for Aortic regurgitation. Care has to be taken not to interfere with the aortic valve and the aortic wall. Therefore the pigtail should be placed 1–2 cm above the sino-tubular-junction (STJ). The diameter can be taken by calibrating the system in comparison with the size of the catheter used or using a geometric calibration with the known geometry of the X-ray system with a good reproducibility. Due to the fact that measurements are based off of a 2D transparent image, the true diameter of a tubular structure can be missed. Biplane imaging using a perpendicular view can overcome

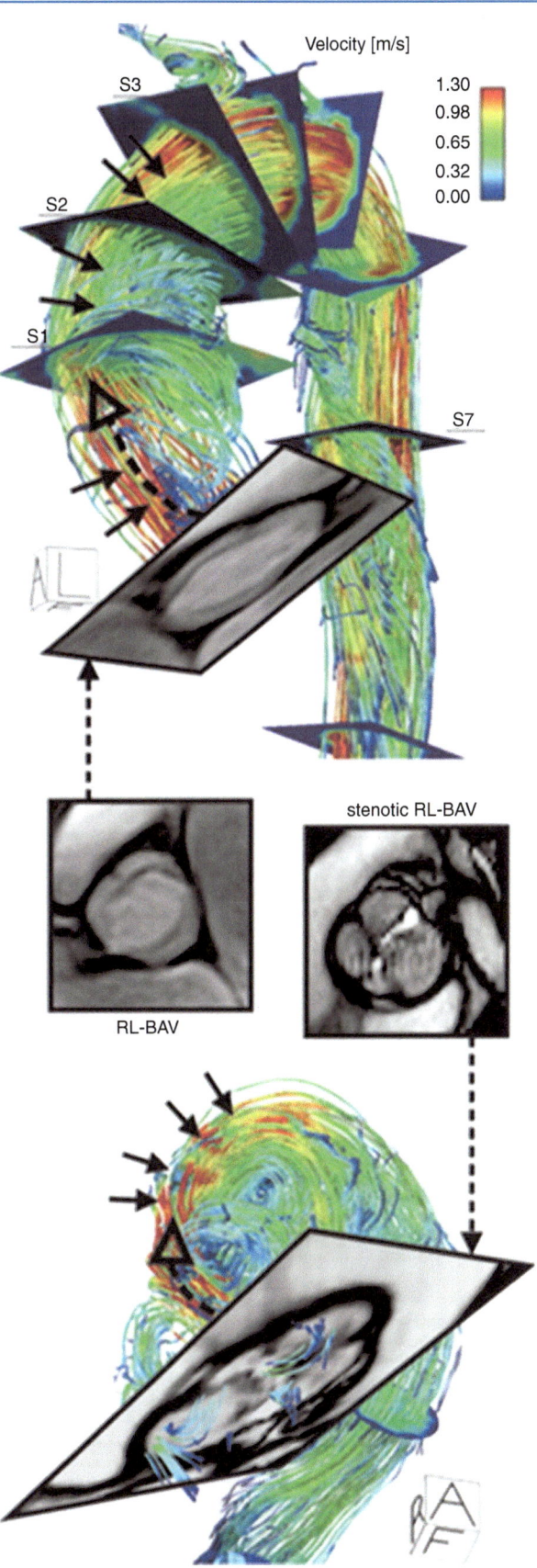

Fig. 1.42 Velocity and systolic wall shear stress measurements in a patient with nonstenotic (upper panel) and stenotic (lower panel) bicuspid aortic valve. (Reprinted with permission from Alex J. Barker et al.)

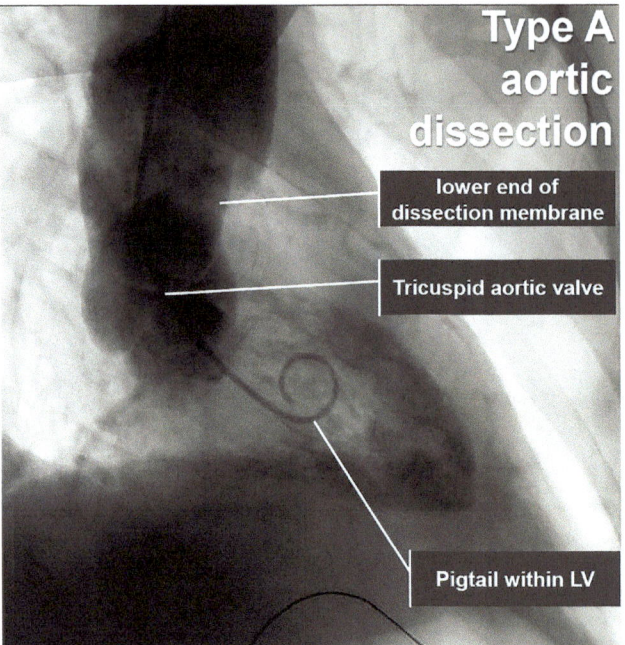

Fig. 1.43 Type A aortic dissection picked up during LV angiogram in a patient with acute chest pain and ST segment changes but normal coronary arteries. Dissection was not picked up during fast screening cardiac ultrasound at the emergency room

this limitation at the price of higher X-ray exposure and contrast use if monoplane equipment is used. Today, this method is rarely used due to the widespread availability of CT-Angiography which offers more information with less contrast. Still, in emergency settings like missed aortic dissections as the reason for coronary angiography, or during percutaneous intervention without transesophageal echo monitoring, it is still very useful (Fig. 1.43).

1.6.2 Aortic Valve Tumors

1.6.2.1 Introduction
Primary cardiac tumors are much rarer than metastatic disease, and tumors on the cardiac valves are even rarer. However, there are important pathologies that may be seen on the aortic valve [255]. They are clinically relevant because they may embolize from the highly mobile leaflets and cause a stroke [256].

The most common aortic valvular tumor described is a papillary fibroelastoma. These are frond-like masses that are often attached by a stalk [257]. Histologically, they are avascular and contain fibroelastic tissue within a shell of endocardium [258]. They can be highly mobile and while historically were noted incidentally on autopsy, have been

reported more frequently now due to improvements in cardiac imaging. The largest observational case series of papillary fibroelastomas noted that they were most frequently found on the aortic valve. This series also found that surgical excision was associated with a lower rate of stroke and all-cause mortality [259].

Other tumors can also be seen on the aortic valve, including myxomas or myofibroblastic tumors [260, 261]. It is important to differentiate a neoplastic valvular lesion from other causes for valve masses or benign degenerative findings. Thrombus or vegetation (infectious or non-infectious) can also be causes of valvular masses. Degenerative elements can sometimes be seen on the valve such as Lambl's excrescences [262]. These are thin, filamentous strands seen originating from the valve cusp edges. Nodules of Arantius can also be seen at the center of the valve cusps where they meet at the central coaptation point. This finding is generally considered normal with no clinical consequence although hypertrophy causing regurgitation has been described [263].

Although valve masses can be seen by different imaging modalities, they are best visualized when both temporal and spatial resolution are high [264]. This is because they are highly mobile with the cardiac cycle. In this section, the use and appearance of aortic tumors by different imaging modalities will be described.

1.6.2.2 Echocardiography
Aortic valve tumors are well assessed by echocardiography because they may be highly mobile. The high temporal resolution of this modality allows for adequate sensitivity in visualizing a valve tumor [264]. It should be noted that overall, primary cardiac tumors are rare, and those involving the valves are even rarer.

Papillary fibroelastomas are the most commonly seen aortic valve tumor and typically appear as a discrete round, oval or irregular well-demarcated echodensity on the valve leaflets. They may be highly mobile and are usually seen on the aortic side of the valve. Interference with valve leaflet coaptation causing regurgitation can occur, but this is rare [265].

Standard transthoracic or transesophageal echocardiographic short- and long-axis views of the aortic valve with 2 dimensional or 3 dimensional imaging may be able to visualize the mass, but sometimes modified imaging planes or sweeping the plane through the valve leaflets is needed [5, 111]. Additionally, using biplane imaging can help localize masses that may not be visible on standard views. Of course, colour and spectral Doppler assessment of the valve for functional effects such as regurgitation should also be assessed [7, 8].

The location and attachment point of this type of tumor is important to note because papillary fibroelastomas typically shrink when not in an aqueous environment, making them difficult to visualize in the operating room once the valve is being inspected directly while the heart is on cardiopulmonary bypass. The indication for surgical management in these cases is typically due to the embolic risk associated with papillary fibroelastomas. [266]

Other rare tumors that may be seen on the aortic valve include myxomas or inflammatory myofibroblastic tumors [260, 261, 267]. There may also be benign valvular masses or mass-like thickening seen by echocardiography including Lambl's excrescences, degenerative strands or hypertrophy of the Nodules of Arantius [262, 268] (Fig. 1.44).

1.6.2.3 Magnetic Resonance Imaging

Cardiac magnetic resonance (CMR) provides uniquely a non-invasive tissue characterization based on a multiparametric imaging approach. Typically used sequences for tissue differentiation of cardiac masses are T1- and T2-weighted sequences followed by fat suppression triple inversion recovery images. Perfusion images and late enhanced images provide further information about the tissue morphology. Steady state free precession sequences through the cardiac cycle provide functional information.

Cardiac valve tumors are rare. Papillary fibroelastomas are the most common primary tumor of the cardiac valves [269]. As papillary fibroelastomas are small and highly mobile structures, they are usually diagnosed by echocardiography, which provides very high temporal resolution. However, in atypical cases cardiac magnetic resonance can provide further information due to its tissue characterization ability. On steady state free precession cine images papillary fibroelastomas appear as small highly mobile structures with low signal typically located on the aortic surface of the aortic valve or on the atrial side of the mitral valve. On T1- weighted images fibroelastomas appear with intermediate—hyperintense signal and hyperintense on T2-weighted images [270]. After injection of contrast media there is homogenous late gadolinium enhancement [271]. Most important differential diagnoses are vegetations due to endocarditis or thrombi, which can be differentiated within the clinical context and tissue characterization by CMR. The signal of a thrombus depends on its age. A thrombus typically does not show any late enhancement and provides high signal intensity in T1- and T2-weighted images in the acute phase; however in subacute and chronic phase the signal intensity in T2 weighted images gets lower [270] (Fig. 1.45).

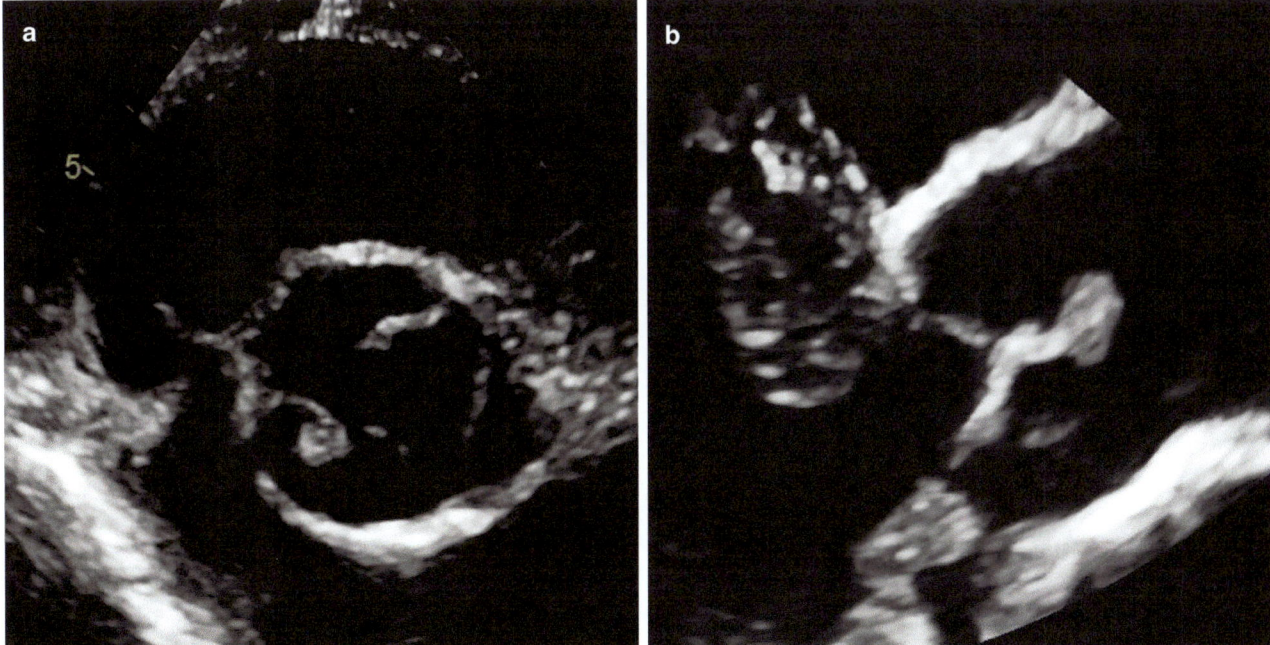

Fig. 1.44 A papillary fibroelastoma of the aortic valve seen on transesophageal echocardiography in a modified short axis (**a**) and long axis (**b**) views of the aortic valve

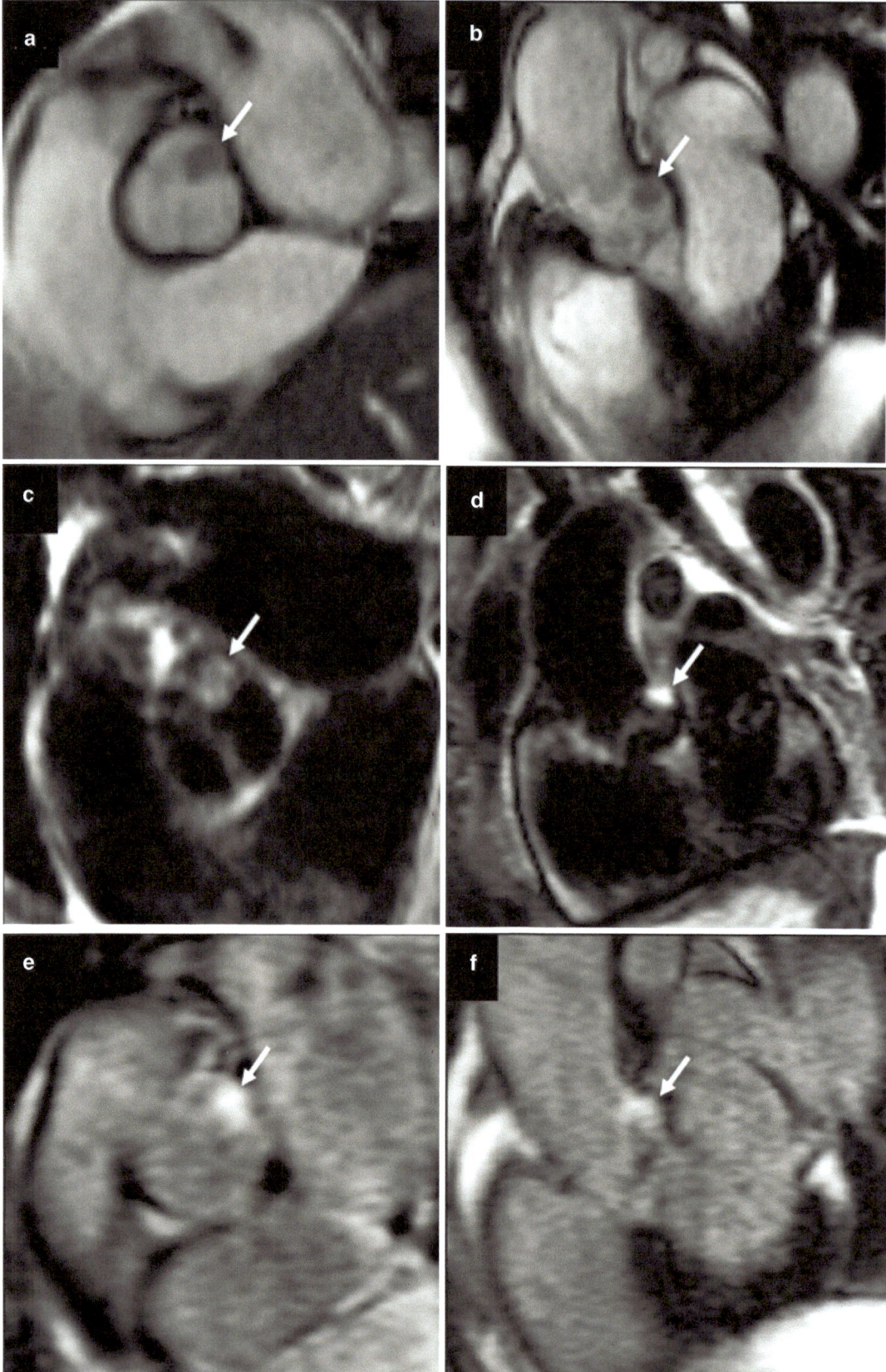

Fig. 1.45 Cardiovascular magnetic resonance images of an aortic papillary fibroelastoma on steady state free percession images (**a**, **b**) with intermediate signal intensity on T1 weighted spin-echo sequences (**c**) high signal intensity on T2 weighted sequences (**d**) and homogenous late enhancement (**e**, **f**). Reprinted with permission from Carpenter JP et al.

References

1. Nkomo VT, Gardin JM, Skelton TN, Gottdiener JS, Scott CG, Enriquez-Sarano M. Burden of valvular heart diseases: a population-based study. Lancet. 2006;368(9540):1005–11.
2. Nishimura RA, Otto CM, Bonow RO, Carabello BA, Erwin JP 3rd, Fleisher LA, Jneid H, Mack MJ, McLeod CJ, O'Gara PT, Rigolin VH, Sundt TM 3rd, Thompson A. 2017 AHA/ACC Focused Update of the 2014 AHA/ACC Guideline for the Management of Patients With Valvular Heart Disease: a report of the American College of Cardiology/American Heart Association Task Force on Clinical Practice Guidelines. Circulation. 2017;135(25):e1159–95.
3. Nishimura RA, Otto CM, Bonow RO, Carabello BA, Erwin JP 3rd, Guyton RA, O'Gara PT, Ruiz CE, Skubas NJ, Sorajja P, Sundt TM 3rd, Thomas JD. 2014 AHA/ACC guideline for the management of patients with valvular heart disease: a report of the American College of Cardiology/American Heart Association Task Force on Practice Guidelines. J Am Coll Cardiol. 2014;63(22):e57–185.
4. Baumgartner H, Falk V, Bax JJ, De Bonis M, Hamm C, Holm PJ, Iung B, Lancellotti P, Lansac E, Rodriguez Munoz D, Rosenhek R, Sjogren J, Tornos Mas P, Vahanian A, Walther T, Wendler O, Windecker S, Zamorano JL. 2017 ESC/EACTS Guidelines for the management of valvular heart disease. Eur Heart J. 2017;38(36):2739–91.
5. Mitchell C, Rahko PS, Blauwet LA, Canaday B, Finstuen JA, Foster MC, Horton K, Ogunyankin KO, Palma RA, Velazquez EJ. Guidelines for Performing a Comprehensive Transthoracic Echocardiographic Examination in Adults: recommendations from the American Society of Echocardiography. J Am Soc Echocardiogr. 2019;32(1):1–64.
6. Lang RM, Badano LP, Mor-Avi V, Afilalo J, Armstrong A, Ernande L, Flachskampf FA, Foster E, Goldstein SA, Kuznetsova T, Lancellotti P, Muraru D, Picard MH, Rietzschel ER, Rudski L, Spencer KT, Tsang W, Voigt JU. Recommendations for cardiac chamber quantification by echocardiography in adults: an update from the American Society of Echocardiography and the European Association of Cardiovascular Imaging. Eur Heart J Cardiovasc Imaging. 2015;16(3):233–70.
7. Zoghbi WA, Adams D, Bonow RO, Enriquez-Sarano M, Foster E, Grayburn PA, Hahn RT, Han Y, Hung J, Lang RM, Little SH, Shah DJ, Shernan S, Thavendiranathan P, Thomas JD, Weissman NJ. Recommendations for Noninvasive Evaluation of Native Valvular Regurgitation: a report from the American Society of Echocardiography Developed in Collaboration with the Society for Cardiovascular Magnetic Resonance. J Am Soc Echocardiogr. 2017;30(4):303–71.
8. Lancellotti P, Tribouilloy C, Hagendorff A, Popescu BA, Edvardsen T, Pierard LA, Badano L, Zamorano JL. Recommendations for the echocardiographic assessment of native valvular regurgitation: an executive summary from the European Association of Cardiovascular Imaging. Eur Heart J Cardiovasc Imaging. 2013;14(7):611–44.
9. Baumgartner H, Hung J, Bermejo J, Chambers JB, Evangelista A, Griffin BP, Iung B, Otto CM, Pellikka PA, Quinones M. Echocardiographic assessment of valve stenosis: EAE/ASE recommendations for clinical practice. J Am Soc Echocardiogr. 2009;22(1):1–23; quiz 101-2.
10. Feuchtner GM, Dichtl W, Friedrich GJ, Frick M, Alber H, Schachner T, Bonatti J, Mallouhi A, Frede T, Pachinger O, zur Nedden D, Muller S. Multislice computed tomography for detection of patients with aortic valve stenosis and quantification of severity. J Am Coll Cardiol. 2006;47(7):1410–7.
11. Pawade TA, Newby DE, Dweck MR. Calcification in aortic stenosis: the skeleton key. J Am Coll Cardiol. 2015;66(5):561–77.
12. Ko SM, Song MG, Hwang HK. Evaluation of the aortic and mitral valves with cardiac computed tomography and cardiac magnetic resonance imaging. Int J Cardiovasc Imaging. 2012;28(Suppl 2):109–27.
13. Achenbach S, Delgado V, Hausleiter J, Schoenhagen P, Min JK, Leipsic JA. SCCT expert consensus document on computed tomography imaging before transcatheter aortic valve implantation (TAVI)/transcatheter aortic valve replacement (TAVR). J Cardiovasc Comput Tomogr. 2012;6(6):366–80.
14. Iung B, Baron G, Butchart EG, Delahaye F, Gohlke-Barwolf C, Levang OW, Tornos P, Vanoverschelde JL, Vermeer F, Boersma E, Ravaud P, Vahanian A. A prospective survey of patients with valvular heart disease in Europe: the Euro Heart Survey on Valvular Heart Disease. Eur Heart J. 2003;24(13):1231–43.
15. Baumgartner HC, Hung JC-C, Bermejo J, Chambers JB, Edvardsen T, Goldstein S, Lancellotti P, LeFevre M, Miller F Jr, Otto CM. Recommendations on the echocardiographic assessment of aortic valve stenosis: a focused update from the European Association of Cardiovascular Imaging and the American Society of Echocardiography. Eur Heart J Cardiovasc Imaging. 2017;18(3):254–75.
16. Currie PJ, Seward JB, Reeder GS, Vlietstra RE, Bresnahan DR, Bresnahan JF, Smith HC, Hagler DJ, Tajik AJ. Continuous-wave Doppler echocardiographic assessment of severity of calcific aortic stenosis: a simultaneous Doppler-catheter correlative study in 100 adult patients. Circulation. 1985;71(6):1162–9.
17. Smith MD, Kwan OL, DeMaria AN. Value and limitations of continuous-wave Doppler echocardiography in estimating severity of valvular stenosis. JAMA. 1986;255(22):3145–51.
18. Burwash IG, Forbes AD, Sadahiro M, Verrier ED, Pearlman AS, Thomas R, Kraft C, Otto CM. Echocardiographic volume flow and stenosis severity measures with changing flow rate in aortic stenosis. Am J Phys. 1993;265(5 Pt 2):H1734–43.
19. Baumgartner H, Stefenelli T, Niederberger J, Schima H, Maurer G. "Overestimation" of catheter gradients by Doppler ultrasound in patients with aortic stenosis: a predictable manifestation of pressure recovery. J Am Coll Cardiol. 1999;33(6):1655–61.
20. Quinones MA, Otto CM, Stoddard M, Waggoner A, Zoghbi WA. Recommendations for quantification of Doppler echocardiography: a report from the Doppler Quantification Task Force of the Nomenclature and Standards Committee of the American Society of Echocardiography. J Am Soc Echocardiogr. 2002;15(2):167–84.
21. Lancellotti P, Tribouilloy C, Hagendorff A, Moura L, Popescu BA, Agricola E, Monin JL, Pierard LA, Badano L, Zamorano JL. European Association of Echocardiography recommendations for the assessment of valvular regurgitation. Part 1: aortic and pulmonary regurgitation (native valve disease). Eur J Echocardiogr. 2010;11(3):223–44.
22. Niederberger J, Schima H, Maurer G, Baumgartner H. Importance of pressure recovery for the assessment of aortic stenosis by Doppler ultrasound. Role of aortic size, aortic valve area, and direction of the stenotic jet in vitro. Circulation. 1996;94(8):1934–40.
23. Schlosser T, Malyar N, Jochims M, Breuckmann F, Hunold P, Bruder O, Erbel R, Barkhausen J. Quantification of aortic valve stenosis in MRI-comparison of steady-state free precession and fast low-angle shot sequences. Eur Radiol. 2007;17(5):1284–90.
24. Myerson SG. Heart valve disease: investigation by cardiovascular magnetic resonance. J Cardiovasc Magn Reson. 2012;14:7.
25. Gatehouse PD, Keegan J, Crowe LA, Masood S, Mohiaddin RH, Kreitner KF, Firmin DN. Applications of phase-contrast flow and velocity imaging in cardiovascular MRI. Eur Radiol. 2005;15(10):2172–84.
26. Cawley PJ, Maki JH, Otto CM. Cardiovascular magnetic resonance imaging for valvular heart disease: technique and validation. Circulation. 2009;119(3):468–78.

27. Bellenger NG, Burgess MI, Ray SG, Lahiri A, Coats AJ, Cleland JG, Pennell DJ. Comparison of left ventricular ejection fraction and volumes in heart failure by echocardiography, radionuclide ventriculography and cardiovascular magnetic resonance; are they interchangeable? Eur Heart J. 2000;21(16):1387–96.

28. Grothues F, Smith GC, Moon JC, Bellenger NG, Collins P, Klein HU, Pennell DJ. Comparison of interstudy reproducibility of cardiovascular magnetic resonance with two-dimensional echocardiography in normal subjects and in patients with heart failure or left ventricular hypertrophy. Am J Cardiol. 2002;90(1):29–34.

29. Dweck MR, Joshi S, Murigu T, Alpendurada F, Jabbour A, Melina G, Banya W, Gulati A, Roussin I, Raza S, Prasad NA, Wage R, Quarto C, Angeloni E, Refice S, Sheppard M, Cook SA, Kilner PJ, Pennell DJ, Newby DE, Mohiaddin RH, Pepper J, Prasad SK. Midwall fibrosis is an independent predictor of mortality in patients with aortic stenosis. J Am Coll Cardiol. 2011;58(12):1271–9.

30. Nigri M, Azevedo CF, Rochitte CE, Schraibman V, Tarasoutchi F, Pommerantzeff PM, Brandao CM, Sampaio RO, Parga JR, Avila LF, Spina GS, Grinberg M. Contrast-enhanced magnetic resonance imaging identifies focal regions of intramyocardial fibrosis in patients with severe aortic valve disease: Correlation with quantitative histopathology. Am Heart J. 2009;157(2):361–8.

31. Stankovic Z, Allen BD, Garcia J, Jarvis KB, Markl M. 4D flow imaging with MRI. Cardiovasc Diagn Ther. 2014;4(2):173–92.

32. Markl M, Wallis W, Harloff A. Reproducibility of flow and wall shear stress analysis using flow-sensitive four-dimensional MRI. J Magn Reson Imaging. 2011;33(4):988–94.

33. Bock J, Frydrychowicz A, Lorenz R, Hirtler D, Barker AJ, Johnson KM, Arnold R, Burkhardt H, Hennig J, Markl M. In vivo noninvasive 4D pressure difference mapping in the human aorta: phantom comparison and application in healthy volunteers and patients. Magn Reson Med. 2011;66(4):1079–88.

34. Dyverfeldt P, Gardhagen R, Sigfridsson A, Karlsson M, Ebbers T. On MRI turbulence quantification. Magn Reson Imaging. 2009;27(7):913–22.

35. Mahadevia R, Barker AJ, Schnell S, Entezari P, Kansal P, Fedak PW, Malaisrie SC, McCarthy P, Collins J, Carr J, Markl M. Bicuspid aortic cusp fusion morphology alters aortic three-dimensional outflow patterns, wall shear stress, and expression of aortopathy. Circulation. 2014;129(6):673–82.

36. Omran H, Schmidt H, Hackenbroch M, Illien S, Bernhardt P, von der Recke G, Fimmers R, Flacke S, Layer G, Pohl C, Luderitz B, Schild H, Sommer T. Silent and apparent cerebral embolism after retrograde catheterisation of the aortic valve in valvular stenosis: a prospective, randomised study. Lancet. 2003;361(9365):1241–6.

37. Oh JK, Taliercio CP, Holmes DR Jr, Reeder GS, Bailey KR, Seward JB, Tajik AJ. Prediction of the severity of aortic stenosis by Doppler aortic valve area determination: prospective Doppler-catheterization correlation in 100 patients. J Am Coll Cardiol. 1988;11(6):1227–34.

38. Otto CM, Pearlman AS, Comess KA, Reamer RP, Janko CL, Huntsman LL. Determination of the stenotic aortic valve area in adults using Doppler echocardiography. J Am Coll Cardiol. 1986;7(3):509–17.

39. Zoghbi WA, Farmer KL, Soto JG, Nelson JG, Quinones MA. Accurate noninvasive quantification of stenotic aortic valve area by Doppler echocardiography. Circulation. 1986;73(3):452–9.

40. Evangelista A, Garcia-Dorado D, Garcia del Castillo H, Gonzalez-Alujas T, Soler-Soler J. Cardiac index quantification by Doppler ultrasound in patients without left ventricular outflow tract abnormalities. J Am Coll Cardiol. 1995;25(3):710–6.

41. Pibarot P, Clavel MA. Left ventricular outflow tract geometry and dynamics in aortic stenosis: implications for the echocardiographic assessment of aortic valve area. J Am Soc Echocardiogr. 2015;28(11):1267–9.

42. Michelena HI, Margaryan E, Miller FA, Eleid M, Maalouf J, Suri R, Messika-Zeitoun D, Pellikka PA, Enriquez-Sarano M. Inconsistent echocardiographic grading of aortic stenosis: is the left ventricular outflow tract important? Heart. 2013;99(13):921–31.

43. LaBounty TM, Miyasaka R, Chetcuti S, Grossman PM, Deeb GM, Patel HJ, Booher A, Patel S, Bach DS. Annulus instead of LVOT diameter improves agreement between echocardiography effective orifice area and invasive aortic valve area. JACC Cardiovasc Imaging. 2014;7(10):1065–6.

44. Mehrotra P, Flynn AW, Jansen K, Tan TC, Mak G, Julien HM, Zeng X, Picard MH, Passeri JJ, Hung J. Differential left ventricular outflow tract remodeling and dynamics in aortic stenosis. J Am Soc Echocardiogr. 2015;28(11):1259–66.

45. Caballero L, Saura D, Oliva-Sandoval MJ, Gonzalez-Carrillo J, Espinosa MD, Garcia-Navarro M, Valdes M, Lancellotti P, de la Morena G. Three-dimensional morphology of the left ventricular outflow tract: impact on grading aortic stenosis severity. J Am Soc Echocardiogr. 2017;30(1):28–35.

46. Hahn RT, Pibarot P. Accurate measurement of left ventricular outflow tract diameter: comment on the updated recommendations for the echocardiographic assessment of aortic valve stenosis. J Am Soc Echocardiogr. 2017;30(10):1038–41.

47. Saitoh T, Shiota M, Izumo M, Gurudevan SV, Tolstrup K, Siegel RJ, Shiota T. Comparison of left ventricular outflow geometry and aortic valve area in patients with aortic stenosis by 2-dimensional versus 3-dimensional echocardiography. Am J Cardiol. 2012;109(11):1626–31.

48. Rosenhek R, Binder T, Porenta G, Lang I, Christ G, Schemper M, Maurer G, Baumgartner H. Predictors of outcome in severe, asymptomatic aortic stenosis. N Engl J Med. 2000;343(9):611–7.

49. Otto CM, Burwash IG, Legget ME, Munt BI, Fujioka M, Healy NL, Kraft CD, Miyake-Hull CY, Schwaegler RG. Prospective study of asymptomatic valvular aortic stenosis. Clinical, echocardiographic, and exercise predictors of outcome. Circulation. 1997;95(9):2262–70.

50. Kim CJ, Berglund H, Nishioka T, Luo H, Siegel RJ. Correspondence of aortic valve area determination from transesophageal echocardiography, transthoracic echocardiography, and cardiac catheterization. Am Heart J. 1996;132(6):1163–72.

51. Lancellotti P, Lebois F, Simon M, Tombeux C, Chauvel C, Pierard LA. Prognostic importance of quantitative exercise Doppler echocardiography in asymptomatic valvular aortic stenosis. Circulation. 2005;112(9 Suppl):I377–82.

52. Okura H, Yoshida K, Hozumi T, Akasaka T, Yoshikawa J. Planimetry and transthoracic two-dimensional echocardiography in noninvasive assessment of aortic valve area in patients with valvular aortic stenosis. J Am Coll Cardiol. 1997;30(3):753–9.

53. Cormier B, Iung B, Porte JM, Barbant S, Vahanian A. Value of multiplane transesophageal echocardiography in determining aortic valve area in aortic stenosis. Am J Cardiol. 1996;77(10):882–5.

54. Stoddard MF, Arce J, Liddell NE, Peters G, Dillon S, Kupersmith J. Two-dimensional transesophageal echocardiographic determination of aortic valve area in adults with aortic stenosis. Am Heart J. 1991;122(5):1415–22.

55. Pontone G, Andreini D, Bartorelli AL, Bertella E, Cortinovis S, Mushtaq S, Annoni A, Formenti A, Baggiano A, Conte E, Tamborini G, Muratori M, Gripari P, Bovis F, Veglia F, Foti C, Alamanni F, Ballerini G, Fiorentini C, Pepi M. Aortic annulus area assessment by multidetector computed tomography for predicting paravalvular regurgitation in patients undergoing balloon-expandable transcatheter aortic valve implantation: a comparison with transthoracic and transesophageal echocardiography. Am Heart J. 2012;164(4):576–84.

56. Nguyen G, Leipsic J. Cardiac computed tomography and computed tomography angiography in the evaluation of patients prior

to transcatheter aortic valve implantation. Curr Opin Cardiol. 2013;28(5):497–504.

57. Blais C, Burwash IG, Mundigler G, Dumesnil JG, Loho N, Rader F, Baumgartner H, Beanlands RS, Chayer B, Kadem L, Garcia D, Durand LG, Pibarot P. Projected valve area at normal flow rate improves the assessment of stenosis severity in patients with low-flow, low-gradient aortic stenosis: the multicenter TOPAS (Truly or Pseudo-Severe Aortic Stenosis) study. Circulation. 2006;113(5):711–21.

58. Monin JL, Monchi M, Gest V, Duval-Moulin AM, Dubois-Rande JL, Gueret P. Aortic stenosis with severe left ventricular dysfunction and low transvalvular pressure gradients: risk stratification by low-dose dobutamine echocardiography. J Am Coll Cardiol. 2001;37(8):2101–7.

59. Monin JL, Quere JP, Monchi M, Petit H, Baleynaud S, Chauvel C, Pop C, Ohlmann P, Lelguen C, Dehant P, Tribouilloy C, Gueret P. Low-gradient aortic stenosis: operative risk stratification and predictors for long-term outcome: a multicenter study using dobutamine stress hemodynamics. Circulation. 2003;108(3):319–24.

60. Lancellotti P, Pellikka PA, Budts W, Chaudhry FA, Donal E, Dulgheru R, Edvardsen T, Garbi M, Ha JW, Kane GC, Kreeger J, Mertens L, Pibarot P, Picano E, Ryan T, Tsutsui JM, Varga A. The clinical use of stress echocardiography in non-ischaemic heart disease: recommendations from the European Association of Cardiovascular Imaging and the American Society of Echocardiography. Eur Heart J Cardiovasc Imaging. 2016;17(11):1191–229.

61. Barkhausen J, Ruehm SG, Goyen M, Buck T, Laub G, Debatin JF. MR evaluation of ventricular function: true fast imaging with steady-state precession versus fast low-angle shot cine MR imaging: feasibility study. Radiology. 2001;219(1):264–9.

62. Sommer THM KR, Axel L,. Evaluation of aortic stenosis by direct planimetric assessment of the aortic valve area using steady-state free precession sequences (balanced FFE). J Cardiovasc Magn Reson. 2002;4.

63. Kupfahl C, Honold M, Meinhardt G, Vogelsberg H, Wagner A, Mahrholdt H, Sechtem U. Evaluation of aortic stenosis by cardiovascular magnetic resonance imaging: comparison with established routine clinical techniques. Heart. 2004;90(8):893–901.

64. Debl K, Djavidani B, Seitz J, Nitz W, Schmid FX, Muders F, Buchner S, Feuerbach S, Riegger G, Luchner A. Planimetry of aortic valve area in aortic stenosis by magnetic resonance imaging. Investig Radiol. 2005;40(10):631–6.

65. Buchner S, Debl K, Schmid FX, Luchner A, Djavidani B. Cardiovascular magnetic resonance assessment of the aortic valve stenosis: an in vivo and ex vivo study. BMC Med Imaging. 2015;15:34.

66. Alkadhi H, Wildermuth S, Plass A, Bettex D, Baumert B, Leschka S, Desbiolles LM, Marincek B, Boehm T. Aortic stenosis: comparative evaluation of 16-detector row CT and echocardiography. Radiology. 2006;240(1):47–55.

67. Shah RG, Novaro GM, Blandon RJ, Whiteman MS, Asher CR, Kirsch J. Aortic valve area: meta-analysis of diagnostic performance of multi-detector computed tomography for aortic valve area measurements as compared to transthoracic echocardiography. Int J Cardiovasc Imaging. 2009;25(6):601–9.

68. Hillis LD, Firth BG, Winniford MD. Analysis of factors affecting the variability of Fick versus indicator dilution measurements of cardiac output. Am J Cardiol. 1985;56(12):764–8.

69. Gorlin R, Gorlin SG. Hydraulic formula for calculation of the area of the stenotic mitral valve, other cardiac valves, and central circulatory shunts. Am Heart J. 1951;41(1):1–29.

70. Cannon SR, Richards KL, Crawford M. Hydraulic estimation of stenotic orifice area: a correction of the Gorlin formula. Circulation. 1985;71(6):1170–8.

71. Goldstein SA, Evangelista A, Abbara S, Arai A, Asch FM, Badano LP, Bolen MA, Connolly HM, Cuellar-Calabria H, Czerny M, Devereux RB, Erbel RA, Fattori R, Isselbacher EM, Lindsay JM, McCulloch M, Michelena HI, Nienaber CA, Oh JK, Pepi M, Taylor AJ, Weinsaft JW, Zamorano JL, Dietz H, Eagle K, Elefteriades J, Jondeau G, Rousseau H, Schepens M. Multimodality imaging of diseases of the thoracic aorta in adults: from the American Society of Echocardiography and the European Association of Cardiovascular Imaging: endorsed by the Society of Cardiovascular Computed Tomography and Society for Cardiovascular Magnetic Resonance. J Am Soc Echocardiogr. 2015;28(2):119–82.

72. Chatzimavroudis GP, Oshinski JN, Franch RH, Pettigrew RI, Walker PG, Yoganathan AP. Quantification of the aortic regurgitant volume with magnetic resonance phase velocity mapping: a clinical investigation of the importance of imaging slice location. J Heart Valve Dis. 1998;7(1):94–101.

73. Lotz J, Meier C, Leppert A, Galanski M. Cardiovascular flow measurement with phase-contrast MR imaging: basic facts and implementation. Radiographics. 2002;22(3):651–71.

74. Nishimura RA, Otto CM, Bonow RO, Carabello BA, Erwin JP 3rd, Guyton RA, O'Gara PT, Ruiz CE, Skubas NJ, Sorajja P, Sundt TM 3rd, Thomas JD. 2014 AHA/ACC guideline for the management of patients with valvular heart disease: executive summary: a report of the American College of Cardiology/American Heart Association Task Force on Practice Guidelines. J Am Coll Cardiol. 2014;63(22):2438–88.

75. Lee JKT, Franzone A, Lanz J, Siontis GCM, Stortecky S, Grani C, Roost E, Windecker S, Pilgrim T. Early detection of subclinical myocardial damage in chronic aortic regurgitation and strategies for timely treatment of asymptomatic patients. Circulation. 2018;137(2):184–96.

76. Myerson SG, d'Arcy J, Mohiaddin R, Greenwood JP, Karamitsos TD, Francis JM, Banning AP, Christiansen JP, Neubauer S. Aortic regurgitation quantification using cardiovascular magnetic resonance: association with clinical outcome. Circulation. 2012;126(12):1452–60.

77. Kammerlander AA, Wiesinger M, Duca F, Aschauer S, Binder C, Zotter Tufaro C, Nitsche C, Badre-Eslam R, Schonbauer R, Bartko P, Beitzke D, Loewe C, Hengstenberg C, Bonderman D, Mascherbauer J. Diagnostic and prognostic utility of cardiac magnetic resonance imaging in aortic regurgitation. JACC Cardiovasc Imaging. 2018.

78. Sellers RD, Levy MJ, Amplatz K, Lillehei CW. Left retrograde cardioangiography in acquired cardiac disease: technic, indications and interpretations in 700 cases. Am J Cardiol. 1964;14:437–47.

79. Schultz CJ, Slots TL, Yong G, Aben JP, Van Mieghem N, Swaans M, Rahhab Z, El Faquir N, van Geuns R, Mast G, Zijlstra F, de Jaegere PP. An objective and reproducible method for quantification of aortic regurgitation after TAVI. EuroIntervention. 2014;10(3):355–63.

80. Pascarelli EF, Bertrand CA. Comparison of arm and leg blood-pressures in aortic insufficiency: an appraisal of Hill's sign. Br Med J. 1965;2(5453):73–5.

81. Sinning JM, Hammerstingl C, Vasa-Nicotera M, Adenauer V, Lema Cachiguango SJ, Scheer AC, Hausen S, Sedaghat A, Ghanem A, Muller C, Grube E, Nickenig G, Werner N. Aortic regurgitation index defines severity of peri-prosthetic regurgitation and predicts outcome in patients after transcatheter aortic valve implantation. J Am Coll Cardiol. 2012;59(13):1134–41.

82. El Khoury G, Vanoverschelde JL, Glineur D, Pierard F, Verhelst RR, Rubay J, Funken JC, Watremez C, Astarci P, Lacroix V, Poncelet A, Noirhomme P. Repair of bicuspid aortic valves in patients with aortic regurgitation. Circulation. 2006;114(1 Suppl):I610–6.

83. Ridley CH, Vallabhajosyula P, Bavaria JE, Patel PA, Gutsche JT, Shah R, Feinman JW, Weiss SJ, Augoustides JG. The Sievers classification of the bicuspid aortic valve for the perioperative echocardiographer: the importance of valve phenotype for aortic valve repair in the era of the functional aortic annulus. J Cardiothorac Vasc Anesth. 2016;30(4):1142–51.

84. Prodromo J, D'Ancona G, Amaducci A, Pilato M. Aortic valve repair for aortic insufficiency: a review. J Cardiothorac Vasc Anesth. 2012;26(5):923–32.

85. Aicher D, Kunihara T, Abou Issa O, Brittner B, Graber S, Schafers HJ. Valve configuration determines long-term results after repair of the bicuspid aortic valve. Circulation. 2011;123(2):178–85.

86. Pettersson GB, Crucean AC, Savage R, Halley CM, Grimm RA, Svensson LG, Naficy S, Gillinov AM, Feng J, Blackstone EH. Toward predictable repair of regurgitant aortic valves: a systematic morphology-directed approach to bicommissural repair. J Am Coll Cardiol. 2008;52(1):40–9.

87. Nash PJ, Vitvitsky E, Li J, Cosgrove DM 3rd, Pettersson G, Grimm RA. Feasibility of valve repair for regurgitant bicuspid aortic valves—an echocardiographic study. Ann Thorac Surg. 2005;79(5):1473–9.

88. Perlman GY, Blanke P, Webb JG. Transcatheter aortic valve implantation in bicuspid aortic valve stenosis. EuroIntervention. 2016;12(Y):Y42–5.

89. Bauer T, Linke A, Sievert H, Kahlert P, Hambrecht R, Nickenig G, Hauptmann KE, Sack S, Gerckens U, Schneider S, Zeymer U, Zahn R. Comparison of the effectiveness of transcatheter aortic valve implantation in patients with stenotic bicuspid versus tricuspid aortic valves (from the German TAVI Registry). Am J Cardiol. 2014;113(3):518–21.

90. Jilaihawi H, Chen M, Webb J, Himbert D, Ruiz CE, Rodes-Cabau J, Pache G, Colombo A, Nickenig G, Lee M, Tamburino C, Sievert H, Abramowitz Y, Tarantini G, Alqoofi F, Chakravarty T, Kashif M, Takahashi N, Kazuno Y, Maeno Y, Kawamori H, Chieffo A, Blanke P, Dvir D, Ribeiro HB, Feng Y, Zhao ZG, Sinning JM, Kliger C, Giustino G, Pajerski B, Imme S, Grube E, Leipsic J, Vahanian A, Michev I, Jelnin V, Latib A, Cheng W, Makkar R. A bicuspid aortic valve imaging classification for the TAVR era. JACC Cardiovasc Imaging. 2016;9(10):1145–58.

91. Makkar R, Chakravarty T, Jilaihawi H. Transcatheter aortic valve replacement for bicuspid aortic stenosis: are we ready for the challenge? J Am Coll Cardiol. 2016;68(11):1206–8.

92. Phan K, Wong S, Phan S, Ha H, Qian P, Yan TD. Transcatheter aortic valve implantation (TAVI) in patients with bicuspid aortic valve stenosis—systematic review and meta-analysis. Heart Lung Circ. 2015;24(7):649–59.

93. Saura D, de la Morena G, Flores-Blanco PJ, Oliva MJ, Caballero L, Gonzalez-Carrillo J, Espinosa MD, Lopez-Ruiz M, Garcia-Navarro M, Valdes M. Aortic valve stenosis planimetry by means of three-dimensional transesophageal echocardiography in the real clinical setting: feasibility, reliability and systematic deviations. Echocardiography. 2015;32(3):508–15.

94. Boulif J, Gerber B, Slimani A, Lazam S, de Meester C, Pierard S, Pasquet A, Pouleur AC, Vancraeynest D, El Khoury G, de Kerchove L, Noirhomme P, Vanoverschelde JL. Assessment of aortic valve calcium load by multidetector computed tomography. Anatomical validation, impact of scanner settings and incremental diagnostic value. J Cardiovasc Comput Tomogr. 2017;11(5):360–6.

95. Clavel MA, Pibarot P, Messika-Zeitoun D, Capoulade R, Malouf J, Aggarval S, Araoz PA, Michelena HI, Cueff C, Larose E, Miller JD, Vahanian A, Enriquez-Sarano M. Impact of aortic valve calcification, as measured by MDCT, on survival in patients with aortic stenosis: results of an international registry study. J Am Coll Cardiol. 2014;64(12):1202–13.

96. Fujita B, Kutting M, Seiffert M, Scholtz S, Egron S, Prashovikj E, Borgermann J, Schafer T, Scholtz W, Preuss R, Gummert J,

Steinseifer U, Ensminger SM. Calcium distribution patterns of the aortic valve as a risk factor for the need of permanent pacemaker implantation after transcatheter aortic valve implantation. Eur Heart J Cardiovasc Imaging. 2016;17(12):1385–93.

97. Maeno Y, Abramowitz Y, Yoon SH, Israr S, Jilaihawi H, Watanabe Y, Sharma R, Kawamori H, Miyasaka M, Kazuno Y, Takahashi N, Hariri B, Mangat G, Kashif M, Chakravarty T, Nakamura M, Cheng W, Makkar RR. Relation between left ventricular outflow tract calcium and mortality following transcatheter aortic valve implantation. Am J Cardiol. 2017;120(11):2017–24.

98. Barbanti M, Yang TH, Rodes Cabau J, Tamburino C, Wood DA, Jilaihawi H, Blanke P, Makkar RR, Latib A, Colombo A, Tarantini G, Raju R, Binder RK, Nguyen G, Freeman M, Ribeiro HB, Kapadia S, Min J, Feuchtner G, Gurtvich R, Alqoofi F, Pelletier M, Ussia GP, Napodano M, de Brito FS Jr, Kodali S, Norgaard BL, Hansson NC, Pache G, Canovas SJ, Zhang H, Leon MB, Webb JG, Leipsic J. Anatomical and procedural features associated with aortic root rupture during balloon-expandable transcatheter aortic valve replacement. Circulation. 2013;128(3):244–53.

99. d'Humieres T, Faivre L, Chammous E, Deux JF, Bergoend E, Fiore A, Radu C, Couetil JP, Benhaiem N, Derumeaux G, Dubois-Rande JL, Ternacle J, Fard D, Lim P. A new three-dimensional echocardiography method to quantify aortic valve calcification. J Am Soc Echocardiogr. 2018;31(10):1073–9.

100. Pressman GS, Crudu V, Parameswaran-Chandrika A, Romero-Corral A, Purushottam B, Figueredo VM. Can total cardiac calcium predict the coronary calcium score? Int J Cardiol. 2011;146(2):202–6.

101. Thomassen HK, Cioffi G, Gerdts E, Einarsen E, Midtbo HB, Mancusi C, Cramariuc D. Echocardiographic aortic valve calcification and outcomes in women and men with aortic stenosis. Heart. 2017;103(20):1619–24.

102. Michelena HI, Della Corte A, Prakash SK, Milewicz DM, Evangelista A, Enriquez-Sarano M. Bicuspid aortic valve aortopathy in adults: Incidence, etiology, and clinical significance. Int J Cardiol. 2015;201:400–7.

103. Schaefer BM, Lewin MB, Stout KK, Gill E, Prueitt A, Byers PH, Otto CM. The bicuspid aortic valve: an integrated phenotypic classification of leaflet morphology and aortic root shape. Heart. 2008;94(12):1634–8.

104. Sievers HH, Schmidtke C. A classification system for the bicuspid aortic valve from 304 surgical specimens. J Thorac Cardiovasc Surg. 2007;133(5):1226–33.

105. Krepp JM, Roman MJ, Devereux RB, Bruce A, Prakash SK, Morris SA, Milewicz DM, Holmes KW, Ravekes W, Shohet RV, Pyeritz RE, Maslen CL, Kroner BL, Eagle KA, Preiss L, Asch FM. Bicuspid and unicuspid aortic valves: different phenotypes of the same disease? Insight from the GenTAC Registry. Congenit Heart Dis. 2017;12(6):740–5.

106. Mookadam F, Thota VR, Garcia-Lopez AM, Emani UR, Alharthi MS, Zamorano J, Khandheria BK. Unicuspid aortic valve in adults: a systematic review. J Heart Valve Dis. 2010;19(1):79–85.

107. Tsang MY, Abudiab MM, Ammash NM, Naqvi TZ, Edwards WD, Nkomo VT, Pellikka PA. Quadricuspid aortic valve: characteristics, associated structural cardiovascular abnormalities, and clinical outcomes. Circulation. 2016;133(3):312–9.

108. Hayakawa M, Asai T, Kinoshita T, Suzuki T. Quadricuspid aortic valve: a report on a 10-year case series and literature review. Ann Thorac Cardiovasc Surg. 2014;20(Suppl):941–4.

109. Yuan SM. Quadricuspid aortic valve: a comprehensive review. Braz J Cardiovasc Surg. 2016;31(6):454–60.

110. Michelena HI, Prakash SK, Della Corte A, Bissell MM, Anavekar N, Mathieu P, Bosse Y, Limongelli G, Bossone E, Benson DW, Lancellotti P, Isselbacher EM, Enriquez-Sarano M, Sundt TM 3rd, Pibarot P, Evangelista A, Milewicz DM, Body SC. Bicuspid aortic valve: identifying knowledge gaps and rising to the

challenge from the International Bicuspid Aortic Valve Consortium (BAVCon). Circulation. 2014;129(25):2691–704.

111. Hahn RT, Abraham T, Adams MS, Bruce CJ, Glas KE, Lang RM, Reeves ST, Shanewise JS, Siu SC, Stewart W, Picard MH. Guidelines for performing a comprehensive transesophageal echocardiographic examination: recommendations from the American Society of Echocardiography and the Society of Cardiovascular Anesthesiologists. Anesth Analg. 2014;118(1):21–68.

112. Doherty JU, Kort S, Mehran R, Schoenhagen P, Soman P. ACC/AATS/AHA/ASE/ASNC/HRS/SCAI/SCCT/SCMR/STS 2017 appropriate use criteria for multimodality imaging in valvular heart disease: a report of the American College of Cardiology Appropriate Use Criteria Task Force, American Association for Thoracic Surgery, American Heart Association, American Society of Echocardiography, American Society of Nuclear Cardiology, Heart Rhythm Society, Society for Cardiovascular Angiography and Interventions, Society of Cardiovascular Computed Tomography, Society for Cardiovascular Magnetic Resonance, and Society of Thoracic Surgeons. J Nucl Cardiol. 2017;24(6):2043–63.

113. Buchner S, Hulsmann M, Poschenrieder F, Hamer OW, Fellner C, Kobuch R, Feuerbach S, Riegger GA, Djavidani B, Luchner A, Debl K. Variable phenotypes of bicuspid aortic valve disease: classification by cardiovascular magnetic resonance. Heart. 2010;96(15):1233–40.

114. Wassmuth R, von Knobelsdorff-Brenkenhoff F, Gruettner H, Utz W, Schulz-Menger J. Cardiac magnetic resonance imaging of congenital bicuspid aortic valves and associated aortic pathologies in adults. Eur Heart J Cardiovasc Imaging. 2014;15(6):673–9.

115. Schulz-Menger J, Abdel-Aty H, Busjahn A, Wassmuth R, Pilz B, Dietz R, Friedrich MG. Left ventricular outflow tract planimetry by cardiovascular magnetic resonance differentiates obstructive from non-obstructive hypertrophic cardiomyopathy. J Cardiovasc Magn Reson. 2006;8(5):741–6.

116. Vogel-Claussen J, Santaularia Tomas M, Newatia A, Boyce D, Pinheiro A, Abraham R, Abraham T, Bluemke DA. Cardiac MRI evaluation of hypertrophic cardiomyopathy: left ventricular outflow tract/aortic valve diameter ratio predicts severity of LVOT obstruction. J Magn Reson Imaging. 2012;36(3):598–603.

117. Lim WY, Lloyd G, Bhattacharyya S. Mechanical and surgical bioprosthetic valve thrombosis. Heart. 2017;103(24):1934–41.

118. Mankad S. Management of prosthetic heart valve complications. Curr Treat Options Cardiovasc Med. 2012;14(6):608–21.

119. Yanagawa B, Whitlock RP, Verma S, Gersh BJ. Anticoagulation for prosthetic heart valves: unresolved questions requiring answers. Curr Opin Cardiol. 2016;31(2):176–82.

120. Rodriguez-Gabella T, Voisine P, Puri R, Pibarot P, Rodes-Cabau J. Aortic bioprosthetic valve durability: incidence, mechanisms, predictors, and management of surgical and transcatheter valve degeneration. J Am Coll Cardiol. 2017;70(8):1013–28.

121. Cherry SV, Jain P, Rodriguez-Blanco YF, Fabbro M 2nd. Noninvasive evaluation of native valvular regurgitation: a review of the 2017 American Society of Echocardiography Guidelines for the Perioperative Echocardiographer. J Cardiothorac Vasc Anesth. 2018;32(2):811–22.

122. Ridley C, Sohmer B, Vallabhajosyula P, Augoustides JGT. Aortic leaflet billowing as a risk factor for repair failure after aortic valve repair. J Cardiothorac Vasc Anesth. 2017;31(3):1001–6.

123. Szymanski T, Maslow A, Mahmood F, Singh A. Three-dimensional echocardiographic assessment of coaptation after aortic valve repair. J Cardiothorac Vasc Anesth. 2017;31(3):993–1000.

124. Habertheuer A, Milewski RK, Bavaria JE, Siki M, Freas M, Desai N, Szeto W, Ram C, Hu R, Vallabhajosyula P. Predictors of recurrent aortic insufficiency in type i bicuspid aortic valve repair. Ann Thorac Surg. 2018;106(5):1316–24.

125. de Kerchove L, Mastrobuoni S, Boodhwani M, Astarci P, Rubay J, Poncelet A, Vanoverschelde JL, Noirhomme P, El Khoury G. The role of annular dimension and annuloplasty in tricuspid aortic valve repair. Eur J Cardiothorac Surg. 2016;49(2):428–37; discussion 437-8.

126. Minakata K, Schaff HV, Zehr KJ, Dearani JA, Daly RC, Orszulak TA, Puga FJ, Danielson GK. Is repair of aortic valve regurgitation a safe alternative to valve replacement? J Thorac Cardiovasc Surg. 2004;127(3):645–53.

127. Everett RJ, Newby DE, Jabbour A, Fayad ZA, Dweck MR. The role of imaging in aortic valve disease. Curr Cardiovasc Imaging Rep. 2016;9:21.

128. Baliyan V, Verdini D, Meyersohn NM. Noninvasive aortic imaging. Cardiovasc Diagn Ther. 2018;8(Suppl 1):S3–s18.

129. Gulsin GS, Singh A, McCann GP. Cardiovascular magnetic resonance in the evaluation of heart valve disease. BMC Med Imaging. 2017;17(1):67.

130. Wehrli FW. Magnetic resonance of calcified tissues. J Magn Reson. 2013;229:35–48.

131. Colli A, D'Amico R, Kempfert J, Borger MA, Mohr FW, Walther T. Transesophageal echocardiographic scoring for transcatheter aortic valve implantation: impact of aortic cusp calcification on postoperative aortic regurgitation. J Thorac Cardiovasc Surg. 2011;142(5):1229–35.

132. Gripari P, Ewe SH, Fusini L, Muratori M, Ng AC, Cefalu C, Delgado V, Schalij MJ, Bax JJ, Marsan NA, Tamborini G, Pepi M. Intraoperative 2D and 3D transoesophageal echocardiographic predictors of aortic regurgitation after transcatheter aortic valve implantation. Heart. 2012;98(16):1229–36.

133. Mihara H, Shibayama K, Berdejo J, Harada K, Itabashi Y, Siegel RJ, Kashif M, Jilaihawi H, Makkar RR, Shiota T. Impact of device landing zone calcification on paravalvular regurgitation after transcatheter aortic valve replacement: a real-time three-dimensional transesophageal echocardiographic study. J Am Soc Echocardiogr. 2015;28(4):404–14.

134. Pawade T, Clavel MA, Tribouilloy C, Dreyfus J, Mathieu T, Tastet L, Renard C, Gun M, Jenkins WSA, Macron L, Sechrist JW, Lacomis JM, Nguyen V, Galian Gay L, Cuellar Calabria H, Ntalas I, Cartlidge TRG, Prendergast B, Rajani R, Evangelista A, Cavalcante JL, Newby DE, Pibarot P, Messika Zeitoun D, Dweck MR. Computed tomography aortic valve calcium scoring in patients with aortic stenosis. Circ Cardiovasc Imaging. 2018;11(3):e007146.

135. Koos R, Kuhl HP, Muhlenbruch G, Wildberger JE, Gunther RW, Mahnken AH. Prevalence and clinical importance of aortic valve calcification detected incidentally on CT scans: comparison with echocardiography. Radiology. 2006;241(1):76–82.

136. Quader N, Wilansky S, Click RL, Katayama M, Chaliki HP. Visual estimation of the severity of aortic stenosis and the calcium burden by 2-dimensional echocardiography: is it reliable? J Ultrasound Med. 2015;34(10):1711–7.

137. Sheng SP, Howell LA, Caughey MC, Yeung M, Vavalle JP. Relation of an echocardiographic-based cardiac calcium score to mitral stenosis severity and coronary artery disease in patients with severe aortic stenosis. Am J Cardiol. 2018;121(2):249–55.

138. Thaden JJ, Nkomo VT, Suri RM, Maleszewski JJ, Soderberg DJ, Clavel MA, Pislaru SV, Malouf JF, Foley TA, Oh JK, Miller JD, Edwards WD, Enriquez-Sarano M. Sex-related differences in calcific aortic stenosis: correlating clinical and echocardiographic characteristics and computed tomography aortic valve calcium score to excised aortic valve weight. Eur Heart J. 2016;37(8):693–9.

139. Le Ven F, Tizon-Marcos H, Fuchs C, Mathieu P, Pibarot P, Larose E. Valve tissue characterization by magnetic resonance imaging in calcific aortic valve disease. Can J Cardiol. 2014;30(12):1676–83.

140. Adams LC, Bressem K, Boker SM, Bender YY, Norenberg D, Hamm B, Makowski MR. Diagnostic performance of susceptibility-weighted magnetic resonance imaging for the detection of calcifications: a systematic review and meta-analysis. Sci Rep. 2017;7(1):15506.

141. Rader F, Sachdev E, Arsanjani R, Siegel RJ. Left ventricular hypertrophy in valvular aortic stenosis: mechanisms and clinical implications. Am J Med. 2015;128(4):344–52.

142. Everett RJ, Clavel MA, Pibarot P, Dweck MR. Timing of intervention in aortic stenosis: a review of current and future strategies. Heart. 2018;104(24):2067–76.

143. Hiendlmayr B, Nakda J, Elsaid O, Wang X, Flynn A. Timing of surgical intervention for aortic regurgitation. Curr Treat Options Cardiovasc Med. 2016;18(11):63.

144. Nadeau-Routhier C, Marsit O, Beaudoin J. Current management of patients with severe aortic regurgitation. Curr Treat Options Cardiovasc Med. 2017;19(2):9.

145. Magne J, Lancellotti P, Pierard LA. Exercise testing in asymptomatic severe aortic stenosis. JACC Cardiovasc Imaging. 2014;7(2):188–99.

146. Clavel MA, Magne J, Pibarot P. Low-gradient aortic stenosis. Eur Heart J. 2016;37(34):2645–57.

147. Tribouilloy C, Rusinaru D, Marechaux S, Castel AL, Debry N, Maizel J, Mentaverri R, Kamel S, Slama M, Levy F. Low-gradient, low-flow severe aortic stenosis with preserved left ventricular ejection fraction: characteristics, outcome, and implications for surgery. J Am Coll Cardiol. 2015;65(1):55–66.

148. Vogelgesang A, Hasenfuss G, Jacobshagen C. Low-flow/low-gradient aortic stenosis-Still a diagnostic and therapeutic challenge. Clin Cardiol. 2017;40(9):654–9.

149. Clavel MA, Burwash IG, Pibarot P. Cardiac imaging for assessing low-gradient severe aortic stenosis. JACC Cardiovasc Imaging. 2017;10(2):185–202.

150. Galderisi M, Cosyns B, Edvardsen T, Cardim N, Delgado V, Di Salvo G, Donal E, Sade LE, Ernande L, Garbi M, Grapsa J, Hagendorff A, Kamp O, Magne J, Santoro C, Stefanidis A, Lancellotti P, Popescu B, Habib G. Standardization of adult transthoracic echocardiography reporting in agreement with recent chamber quantification, diastolic function, and heart valve disease recommendations: an expert consensus document of the European Association of Cardiovascular Imaging. Eur Heart J Cardiovasc Imaging. 2017;18(12):1301–10.

151. Porter TR, Mulvagh SL, Abdelmoneim SS, Becher H, Belcik JT, Bierig M, Choy J, Gaibazzi N, Gillam LD, Janardhanan R, Kutty S, Leong-Poi H, Lindner JR, Main ML, Mathias W Jr, Park MM, Senior R, Villanueva F. Clinical applications of ultrasonic enhancing agents in echocardiography: 2018 American Society of Echocardiography Guidelines update. J Am Soc Echocardiogr. 2018;31(3):241–74.

152. Mulvagh SL, Rakowski H, Vannan MA, Abdelmoneim SS, Becher H, Bierig SM, Burns PN, Castello R, Coon PD, Hagen ME, Jollis JG, Kimball TR, Kitzman DW, Kronzon I, Labovitz AJ, Lang RM, Mathew J, Moir WS, Nagueh SF, Pearlman AS, Perez JE, Porter TR, Rosenbloom J, Strachan GM, Thanigaraj S, Wei K, Woo A, Yu EH, Zoghbi WA. American Society of Echocardiography consensus statement on the clinical applications of ultrasonic contrast agents in echocardiography. J Am Soc Echocardiogr. 2008;21(11):1179–201; quiz 1281.

153. Bhave NM, Lang RM. Evaluation of left ventricular structure and function by three-dimensional echocardiography. Curr Opin Crit Care. 2013;19(5):387–96.

154. Dorosz JL, Lezotte DC, Weitzenkamp DA, Allen LA, Salcedo EE. Performance of 3-dimensional echocardiography in measuring left ventricular volumes and ejection fraction: a systematic review and meta-analysis. J Am Coll Cardiol. 2012;59(20):1799–808.

155. Caiani EG, Corsi C, Zamorano J, Sugeng L, MacEneaney P, Weinert L, Battani R, Gutierrez-Chico JL, Koch R, Perez de Isla L, Mor-Avi V, Lang RM. Improved semiautomated quantification of left ventricular volumes and ejection fraction using 3-dimensional echocardiography with a full matrix-array transducer: comparison with magnetic resonance imaging. J Am Soc Echocardiogr. 2005;18(8):779–88.

156. Hundley WG, Bluemke DA, Finn JP, Flamm SD, Fogel MA, Friedrich MG, Ho VB, Jerosch-Herold M, Kramer CM, Manning WJ, Patel M, Pohost GM, Stillman AE, White RD, Woodard PK. ACCF/ACR/AHA/NASCI/SCMR 2010 expert consensus document on cardiovascular magnetic resonance: a report of the American College of Cardiology Foundation Task Force on Expert Consensus Documents. J Am Coll Cardiol. 2010;55(23):2614–62.

157. Petersen SE, Aung N, Sanghvi MM, Zemrak F, Fung K, Paiva JM, Francis JM, Khanji MY, Lukaschuk E, Lee AM, Carapella V, Kim YJ, Leeson P, Piechnik SK, Neubauer S. Reference ranges for cardiac structure and function using cardiovascular magnetic resonance (CMR) in Caucasians from the UK Biobank population cohort. J Cardiovasc Magn Reson. 2017;19(1):18.

158. Chuang ML, Gona P, Hautvast GL, Salton CJ, Breeuwer M, O'Donnell CJ, Manning WJ. CMR reference values for left ventricular volumes, mass, and ejection fraction using computer-aided analysis: the Framingham Heart Study. J Magn Reson Imaging. 2014;39(4):895–900.

159. Aquaro GD, Camastra G, Monti L, Lombardi M, Pepe A, Castelletti S, Maestrini V, Todiere G, Masci P, di Giovine G, Barison A, Dellegrottaglie S, Perazzolo Marra M, Pontone G, Di Bella G. Reference values of cardiac volumes, dimensions, and new functional parameters by MR: a multicenter, multivendor study. J Magn Reson Imaging. 2017;45(4):1055–67.

160. Maffei E, Messalli G, Martini C, Nieman K, Catalano O, Rossi A, Seitun S, Guaricci AI, Tedeschi C, Mollet NR, Cademartiri F. Left and right ventricle assessment with Cardiac CT: validation study vs Cardiac MR. Eur Radiol. 2012;22(5):1041–9.

161. Pibarot P, Dumesnil JG. Low-flow, low-gradient aortic stenosis with normal and depressed left ventricular ejection fraction. J Am Coll Cardiol. 2012;60(19):1845–53.

162. Lomon A, Comandon J. La Radiocinematographie par la photographie des ecrans renforsateurs. Bull. et miiein. Soc. radiol. med. de Paris 1911;3;127.

163. Chapman CB, Baker O, Reynolds J, Bonte FJ. Use of biplane cine-fluorography for measurement of ventricular volume. Circulation. 1958;18(6):1105–17.

164. Oost E, Oemrawsingh P, Reiber JH, Lelieveldt B. Automated left ventricular delineation in X-ray angiograms: a validation study. Catheter Cardiovasc Interv. 2009;73(2):231–40.

165. Hesse B, Lindhardt TB, Acampa W, Anagnostopoulos C, Ballinger J, Bax JJ, Edenbrandt L, Flotats A, Germano G, Stopar TG, Franken P, Kelion A, Kjaer A, Le Guludec D, Ljungberg M, Maenhout AF, Marcassa C, Marving J, McKiddie F, Schaefer WM, Stegger L, Underwood R. EANM/ESC guidelines for radionuclide imaging of cardiac function. Eur J Nucl Med Mol Imaging. 2008;35(4):851–85.

166. Schaefer WM, Lipke CS, Standke D, Kuhl HP, Nowak B, Kaiser HJ, Koch KC, Buell U. Quantification of left ventricular volumes and ejection fraction from gated 99mTc-MIBI SPECT: MRI validation and comparison of the Emory Cardiac Tool Box with QGS and 4D-MSPECT. J Nucl Med. 2005;46(8):1256–63.

167. Kubo N, Mabuchi M, Katoh C, Morita K, Tsukamoto E, Morita Y, Tamaki N. Accuracy and reproducibility of left ventricular function from quantitative, gated, single photon emission computed tomography using dynamic myocardial phantoms: effect of pre-reconstruction filters. Nucl Med Commun. 2002;23(6):529–36.

168. Sengupta PP, Tajik AJ, Chandrasekaran K, Khandheria BK. Twist mechanics of the left ventricle: principles and application. JACC Cardiovasc Imaging. 2008;1(3):366–76.

169. Chengode S. Left ventricular global systolic function assessment by echocardiography. Ann Card Anaesth. 2016;19(Supplement):S26–s34.

170. Dunlay SM, Roger VL, Weston SA, Jiang R, Redfield MM. Longitudinal changes in ejection fraction in heart failure patients with preserved and reduced ejection fraction. Circ Heart Fail. 2012;5(6):720–6.

171. Aurich M, Keller M, Greiner S, Steen H, Aus dem Siepen F, Riffel J, Katus HA, Buss SJ, Mereles D. Left ventricular mechanics assessed by two-dimensional echocardiography and cardiac magnetic resonance imaging: comparison of high-resolution speckle tracking and feature tracking. Eur Heart J Cardiovasc Imaging. 2016;17(12):1370–8.

172. Weidemann F, Herrmann S, Stork S, Niemann M, Frantz S, Lange V, Beer M, Gattenlohner S, Voelker W, Ertl G, Strotmann JM. Impact of myocardial fibrosis in patients with symptomatic severe aortic stenosis. Circulation. 2009;120(7):577–84.

173. Nagueh SF, Smiseth OA, Appleton CP, Byrd BF 3rd, Dokainish H, Edvardsen T, Flachskampf FA, Gillebert TC, Klein AL, Lancellotti P, Marino P, Oh JK, Popescu BA, Waggoner AD. Recommendations for the evaluation of left ventricular diastolic function by echocardiography: an update from the American Society of Echocardiography and the European Association of Cardiovascular Imaging. J Am Soc Echocardiogr. 2016;29(4):277–314.

174. Ozkan A, Kapadia S, Tuzcu M, Marwick TH. Assessment of left ventricular function in aortic stenosis. Nat Rev Cardiol. 2011;8(9):494–501.

175. Chahal NS, Lim TK, Jain P, Chambers JC, Kooner JS, Senior R. Normative reference values for the tissue Doppler imaging parameters of left ventricular function: a population-based study. Eur J Echocardiogr. 2010;11(1):51–6.

176. Capoulade R, Le Ven F, Clavel MA, Dumesnil JG, Dahou A, Thebault C, Arsenault M, O'Connor K, Bedard E, Beaudoin J, Senechal M, Bernier M, Pibarot P. Echocardiographic predictors of outcomes in adults with aortic stenosis. Heart. 2016;102(12):934–42.

177. Smiseth OA, Torp H, Opdahl A, Haugaa KH, Urheim S. Myocardial strain imaging: how useful is it in clinical decision making? Eur Heart J. 2016;37(15):1196–207.

178. Quere JP, Monin JL, Levy F, Petit H, Baleynaud S, Chauvel C, Pop C, Ohlmann P, Lelguen C, Dehant P, Gueret P, Tribouilloy C. Influence of preoperative left ventricular contractile reserve on postoperative ejection fraction in low-gradient aortic stenosis. Circulation. 2006;113(14):1738–44.

179. Dweck MR, Boon NA, Newby DE. Calcific aortic stenosis: a disease of the valve and the myocardium. J Am Coll Cardiol. 2012;60(19):1854–63.

180. Chin CWL, Everett RJ, Kwiecinski J, Vesey AT, Yeung E, Esson G, Jenkins W, Koo M, Mirsadraee S, White AC, Japp AG, Prasad SK, Semple S, Newby DE, Dweck MR. Myocardial fibrosis and cardiac decompensation in aortic stenosis. JACC Cardiovasc Imaging. 2017;10(11):1320–33.

181. Hein S, Arnon E, Kostin S, Schonburg M, Elsasser A, Polyakova V, Bauer EP, Klovekorn WP, Schaper J. Progression from compensated hypertrophy to failure in the pressure-overloaded human heart: structural deterioration and compensatory mechanisms. Circulation. 2003;107(7):984–91.

182. Lancellotti P, Pellikka PA, Budts W, Chaudhry FA, Donal E, Dulgheru R, Edvardsen T, Garbi M, Ha JW, Kane GC, Kreeger J, Mertens L, Pibarot P, Picano E, Ryan T, Tsutsui JM, Varga A. The clinical use of stress echocardiography in non-ischaemic heart disease: recommendations from the European Association of Cardiovascular Imaging and the American Society of Echocardiography. J Am Soc Echocardiogr. 2017;30(2):101–38.

183. Henri C, Pierard LA, Lancellotti P, Mongeon FP, Pibarot P, Basmadjian AJ. Exercise testing and stress imaging in valvular heart disease. Can J Cardiol. 2014;30(9):1012–26.

184. Thavendiranathan P, Poulin F, Lim KD, Plana JC, Woo A, Marwick TH. Use of myocardial strain imaging by echocardiography for the early detection of cardiotoxicity in patients during and after cancer chemotherapy: a systematic review. J Am Coll Cardiol. 2014;63(25 Pt A):2751–68.

185. Schuster A, Paul M, Bettencourt N, Morton G, Chiribiri A, Ishida M, Hussain S, Jogiya R, Kutty S, Bigalke B, Perera D, Nagel E. Cardiovascular magnetic resonance myocardial feature tracking for quantitative viability assessment in ischemic cardiomyopathy. Int J Cardiol. 2013;166(2):413–20.

186. Zerhouni EA, Parish DM, Rogers WJ, Yang A, Shapiro EP. Human heart: tagging with MR imaging—a method for noninvasive assessment of myocardial motion. Radiology. 1988;169(1):59–63.

187. Cao JJ, Ngai N, Duncanson L, Cheng J, Gliganic K, Chen Q. A comparison of both DENSE and feature tracking techniques with tagging for the cardiovascular magnetic resonance assessment of myocardial strain. J Cardiovasc Magn Reson. 2018;20(1):26.

188. Hor KN, Gottliebson WM, Carson C, Wash E, Cnota J, Fleck R, Wansapura J, Klimeczek P, Al-Khalidi HR, Chung ES, Benson DW, Mazur W. Comparison of magnetic resonance feature tracking for strain calculation with harmonic phase imaging analysis. JACC Cardiovasc Imaging. 2010;3(2):144–51.

189. Nagel E, Lehmkuhl HB, Bocksch W, Klein C, Vogel U, Frantz E, Ellmer A, Dreysse S, Fleck E. Noninvasive diagnosis of ischemia-induced wall motion abnormalities with the use of high-dose dobutamine stress MRI: comparison with dobutamine stress echocardiography. Circulation. 1999;99(6):763–70.

190. Afridi I, Kleiman NS, Raizner AE, Zoghbi WA. Dobutamine echocardiography in myocardial hibernation. Optimal dose and accuracy in predicting recovery of ventricular function after coronary angioplasty. Circulation. 1995;91(3):663–70.

191. Kim RJ, Wu E, Rafael A, Chen EL, Parker MA, Simonetti O, Klocke FJ, Bonow RO, Judd RM. The use of contrast-enhanced magnetic resonance imaging to identify reversible myocardial dysfunction. N Engl J Med. 2000;343(20):1445–53.

192. Arai AE. The cardiac magnetic resonance (CMR) approach to assessing myocardial viability. J Nucl Cardiol. 2011;18(6):1095–102.

193. Vollema EM, Sugimoto T, Shen M, Tastet L, Ng ACT, Abou R, Marsan NA, Mertens B, Dulgheru R, Lancellotti P, Clavel MA, Pibarot P, Genereux P, Leon MB, Delgado V, Bax JJ. Association of left ventricular global longitudinal strain with asymptomatic severe aortic stenosis: natural course and prognostic value. JAMA Cardiol. 2018;3(9):839–47.

194. Alashi A, Mentias A, Abdallah A, Feng K, Gillinov AM, Rodriguez LL, Johnston DR, Svensson LG, Popovic ZB, Griffin BP, Desai MY. Incremental prognostic utility of left ventricular global longitudinal strain in asymptomatic patients with significant chronic aortic regurgitation and preserved left ventricular ejection fraction. JACC Cardiovasc Imaging. 2018;11(5):673–82.

195. Marwan M, Ammon F, Bittner D, Rother J, Mekkhala N, Hell M, Schuhbaeck A, Gitsioudis G, Feyrer R, Schlundt C, Achenbach S, Arnold M. CT-derived left ventricular global strain in aortic valve stenosis patients: A comparative analysis pre and post transcatheter aortic valve implantation. J Cardiovasc Comput Tomogr. 2018;12(3):240–4.

196. Nishimura RA, Grantham JA, Connolly HM, Schaff HV, Higano ST, Holmes DR Jr. Low-output, low-gradient aortic stenosis in

patients with depressed left ventricular systolic function: the clinical utility of the dobutamine challenge in the catheterization laboratory. Circulation. 2002;106(7):809–13.

197. Stahli BE, Abouelnour A, Nguyen TD, Vecchiati A, Maier W, Luscher TF, Frauenfelder T, Tanner FC. Impact of three-dimensional imaging and pressure recovery on echocardiographic evaluation of severe aortic stenosis: a pilot study. Echocardiography. 2014;31(8):1006–16.

198. Stahli BE, Stadler T, Holy EW, Nguyen-Kim TDL, Hoffelner L, Erhart L, Obeid S, Niemann M, Jenni R, Hamada S, Manka R, Luscher TF, Maisano F, Nietlispach F, Frauenfelder T, Tanner FC. Impact of stroke volume assessment by integrating multidetector computed tomography and Doppler data on the classification of aortic stenosis. Int J Cardiol. 2017;246:80–6.

199. Hachicha Z, Dumesnil JG, Bogaty P, Pibarot P. Paradoxical low-flow, low-gradient severe aortic stenosis despite preserved ejection fraction is associated with higher afterload and reduced survival. Circulation. 2007;115(22):2856–64.

200. Clavel MA, Ennezat PV, Marechaux S, Dumesnil JG, Capoulade R, Hachicha Z, Mathieu P, Bellouin A, Bergeron S, Meimoun P, Arsenault M, Le Tourneau T, Pasquet A, Couture C, Pibarot P. Stress echocardiography to assess stenosis severity and predict outcome in patients with paradoxical low-flow, low-gradient aortic stenosis and preserved LVEF. JACC Cardiovasc Imaging. 2013;6(2):175–83.

201. Herrmann S, Stork S, Niemann M, Lange V, Strotmann JM, Frantz S, Beer M, Gattenlohner S, Voelker W, Ertl G, Weidemann F. Low-gradient aortic valve stenosis myocardial fibrosis and its influence on function and outcome. J Am Coll Cardiol. 2011;58(4):402–12.

202. Buckert D, Cieslik M, Tibi R, Radermacher M, Rasche V, Bernhardt P, Hombach V, Rottbauer W, Wohrle J. Longitudinal strain assessed by cardiac magnetic resonance correlates to hemodynamic findings in patients with severe aortic stenosis and predicts positive remodeling after transcatheter aortic valve replacement. Clin Res Cardiol. 2018;107(1):20–9.

203. Kampaktsis PN, Kokkinidis DG, Wong SC, Vavuranakis M, Skubas NJ, Devereux RB. The role and clinical implications of diastolic dysfunction in aortic stenosis. Heart. 2017;103(19):1481–7.

204. Yarbrough WM, Mukherjee R, Ikonomidis JS, Zile MR, Spinale FG. Myocardial remodeling with aortic stenosis and after aortic valve replacement: mechanisms and future prognostic implications. J Thorac Cardiovasc Surg. 2012;143(3):656–64.

205. Obasare E, Bhalla V, Gajanana D, Rodriguez Ziccardi M, Codolosa JN, Figueredo VM, Morris DL, Pressman GS. Natural history of severe aortic stenosis: diastolic wall strain as a novel prognostic marker. Echocardiography. 2017;34(4):484–90.

206. Blair JEA, Atri P, Friedman JL, Thomas JD, Brummel K, Sweis RN, Mikati I, Malaisrie SC, Davidson CJ, Flaherty JD. Diastolic function and transcatheter aortic valve replacement. J Am Soc Echocardiogr. 2017;30(6):541–51.

207. Dahl JS, Barros-Gomes S, Videbaek L, Poulsen MK, Issa IF, Carter-Storch R, Christensen NL, Kumme A, Pellikka PA, Moller JE. Early diastolic strain rate in relation to systolic and diastolic function and prognosis in aortic stenosis. JACC Cardiovasc Imaging. 2016;9(5):519–28.

208. Dahl JS, Christensen NL, Videbaek L, Poulsen MK, Carter-Storch R, Hey TM, Pellikka PA, Steffensen FH, Moller JE. Left ventricular diastolic function is associated with symptom status in severe aortic valve stenosis. Circ Cardiovasc Imaging. 2014;7(1):142–8.

209. Kamimura D, Suzuki T, Fox ER, Skelton TN, Winniford MD, Hall ME. Increased left ventricular diastolic stiffness is associated with heart failure symptoms in aortic stenosis patients with preserved ejection fraction. J Card Fail. 2017;23(8):581–8.

210. Nagueh SF, Appleton CP, Gillebert TC, Marino PN, Oh JK, Smiseth OA, Waggoner AD, Flachskampf FA, Pellikka PA, Evangelisa A. Recommendations for the evaluation of left ventricular diastolic function by echocardiography. Eur J Echocardiogr. 2009;10(2):165–93.

211. Nagueh SF, Smiseth OA, Appleton CP, Byrd BF 3rd, Dokainish H, Edvardsen T, Flachskampf FA, Gillebert TC, Klein AL, Lancellotti P, Marino P, Oh JK, Alexandru Popescu B, Waggoner AD. Recommendations for the evaluation of left ventricular diastolic function by echocardiography: an update from the American Society of Echocardiography and the European Association of Cardiovascular Imaging. Eur Heart J Cardiovasc Imaging. 2016;17(12):1321–60.

212. Kinno M, Nagpal P, Horgan S, Waller AH. Comparison of echocardiography, cardiac magnetic resonance, and computed tomographic imaging for the evaluation of left ventricular myocardial function: part 2 (diastolic and regional assessment). Curr Cardiol Rep. 2017;19(1):6.

213. Singh A, Addetia K, Maffessanti F, Mor-Avi V, Lang RM. LA strain for categorization of LV diastolic dysfunction. JACC Cardiovasc Imaging. 2017;10(7):735–43.

214. Wang J, Khoury DS, Thohan V, Torre-Amione G, Nagueh SF. Global diastolic strain rate for the assessment of left ventricular relaxation and filling pressures. Circulation. 2007;115(11):1376–83.

215. Dokainish H, Sengupta R, Pillai M, Bobek J, Lakkis N. Usefulness of new diastolic strain and strain rate indexes for the estimation of left ventricular filling pressure. Am J Cardiol. 2008;101(10):1504–9.

216. Haaf P, Garg P, Messroghli DR, Broadbent DA, Greenwood JP, Plein S. Cardiac T1 mapping and extracellular volume (ECV) in clinical practice: a comprehensive review. J Cardiovasc Magn Reson. 2016;18(1):89.

217. Coelho-Filho OR, Shah RV, Mitchell R, Neilan TG, Moreno H Jr, Simonson B, Kwong R, Rosenzweig A, Das S, Jerosch-Herold M. Quantification of cardiomyocyte hypertrophy by cardiac magnetic resonance: implications for early cardiac remodeling. Circulation. 2013;128(11):1225–33.

218. Miller CA, Naish JH, Bishop P, Coutts G, Clark D, Zhao S, Ray SG, Yonan N, Williams SG, Flett AS, Moon JC, Greiser A, Parker GJ, Schmitt M. Comprehensive validation of cardiovascular magnetic resonance techniques for the assessment of myocardial extracellular volume. Circ Cardiovasc Imaging. 2013;6(3):373–83.

219. Bull S, White SK, Piechnik SK, Flett AS, Ferreira VM, Loudon M, Francis JM, Karamitsos TD, Prendergast BD, Robson MD, Neubauer S, Moon JC, Myerson SG. Human non-contrast T1 values and correlation with histology in diffuse fibrosis. Heart. 2013;99(13):932–7.

220. Dusenbery SM, Jerosch-Herold M, Rickers C, Colan SD, Geva T, Newburger JW, Powell AJ. Myocardial extracellular remodeling is associated with ventricular diastolic dysfunction in children and young adults with congenital aortic stenosis. J Am Coll Cardiol. 2014;63(17):1778–85.

221. Chin CW, Shah AS, McAllister DA, Joanna Cowell S, Alam S, Langrish JP, Strachan FE, Hunter AL, Maria Choy A, Lang CC, Walker S, Boon NA, Newby DE, Mills NL, Dweck MR. High-sensitivity troponin I concentrations are a marker of an advanced hypertrophic response and adverse outcomes in patients with aortic stenosis. Eur Heart J. 2014;35(34):2312–21.

222. Croisille P, Revel D, Saeed M. Contrast agents and cardiac MR imaging of myocardial ischemia: from bench to bedside. Eur Radiol. 2006;16(9):1951–63.

223. Mahrholdt H, Wagner A, Judd RM, Sechtem U, Kim RJ. Delayed enhancement cardiovascular magnetic resonance assessment of non-ischaemic cardiomyopathies. Eur Heart J. 2005;26(15):1461–74.

224. Rudolph A, Abdel-Aty H, Bohl S, Boye P, Zagrosek A, Dietz R, Schulz-Menger J. Noninvasive detection of fibrosis applying

contrast-enhanced cardiac magnetic resonance in different forms of left ventricular hypertrophy relation to remodeling. J Am Coll Cardiol. 2009;53(3):284–91.

225. Barone-Rochette G, Pierard S, De Meester de Ravenstein C, Seldrum S, Melchior J, Maes F, Pouleur AC, Vancraeynest D, Pasquet A, Vanoverschelde JL, Gerber BL. Prognostic significance of LGE by CMR in aortic stenosis patients undergoing valve replacement. J Am Coll Cardiol. 2014;64(2):144–54.

226. Al Musa T, Uddin A, Swoboda PP, Garg P, Fairbairn TA, Dobson LE, Steadman CD, Singh A, Erhayiem B, Plein S, McCann GP, Greenwood JP. Myocardial strain and symptom severity in severe aortic stenosis: insights from cardiovascular magnetic resonance. Quant Imaging Med Surg. 2017;7(1):38–47.

227. Musa TA, Uddin A, Swoboda PP, Fairbairn TA, Dobson LE, Singh A, Garg P, Steadman CD, Erhayiem B, Kidambi A, Ripley DP, McDiarmid AK, Haaf P, Blackman DJ, Plein S, McCann GP, Greenwood JP. Cardiovascular magnetic resonance evaluation of symptomatic severe aortic stenosis: association of circumferential myocardial strain and mortality. J Cardiovasc Magn Reson. 2017;19(1):13.

228. Baumgartner H, Falk V, Bax JJ, De Bonis M, Hamm C, Holm PJ, Iung B, Lancellotti P, Lansac E, Rodriguez Munoz D, Rosenhek R, Sjogren J, Tornos Mas P, Vahanian A, Walther T, Wendler O, Windecker S, Zamorano JL, Group ESCSD. 2017 ESC/EACTS Guidelines for the management of valvular heart disease. Eur Heart J. 2017;38(36):2739–91.

229. Habib G, Lancellotti P, Antunes MJ, Bongiorni MG, Casalta JP, Del Zotti F, Dulgheru R, El Khoury G, Erba PA, Iung B, Miro JM, Mulder BJ, Plonska-Gosciniak E, Price S, Roos-Hesselink J, Snygg-Martin U, Thuny F, Tornos Mas P, Vilacosta I, Zamorano JL, Group ESCSD. 2015 ESC Guidelines for the management of infective endocarditis: The Task Force for the Management of Infective Endocarditis of the European Society of Cardiology (ESC). Endorsed by: European Association for Cardio-Thoracic Surgery (EACTS), the European Association of Nuclear Medicine (EANM). Eur Heart J. 2015;36(44):3075–128.

230. Olmos C, Vilacosta I, Fernandez-Perez C, Bernal JL, Ferrera C, Garcia-Arribas D, Perez-Garcia CN, San Roman JA, Maroto L, Macaya C, Elola FJ. The evolving nature of infective endocarditis in Spain: a population-based study (2003 to 2014). J Am Coll Cardiol. 2017;70(22):2795–804.

231. Rodbard S. Blood velocity and endocarditis. Circulation. 1963;27:18–28.

232. Cahill TJ, Prendergast BD. Infective endocarditis. Lancet. 2016;387(10021):882–93.

233. Bansal RC. Infective endocarditis. Med Clin North Am. 1995;79(5):1205–40.

234. Sivak JA, Vora AN, Navar AM, Schulte PJ, Crowley AL, Kisslo J, Corey GR, Liao L, Wang A, Velazquez EJ, Samad Z. An approach to improve the negative predictive value and clinical utility of transthoracic echocardiography in suspected native valve infective endocarditis. J Am Soc Echocardiogr. 2016;29(4):315–22.

235. Sanfilippo AJ, Picard MH, Newell JB, Rosas E, Davidoff R, Thomas JD, Weyman AE. Echocardiographic assessment of patients with infectious endocarditis: prediction of risk for complications. J Am Coll Cardiol. 1991;18(5):1191–9.

236. Hyafil F, Rouzet F, Lepage L, Benali K, Raffoul R, Duval X, Hvass U, Iung B, Nataf P, Lebtahi R, Vahanian A, Le Guludec D. Role of radiolabelled leucocyte scintigraphy in patients with a suspicion of prosthetic valve endocarditis and inconclusive echocardiography. Eur Heart J Cardiovasc Imaging. 2013;14(6):586–94.

237. Saby L, Laas O, Habib G, Cammilleri S, Mancini J, Tessonnier L, Casalta JP, Gouriet F, Riberi A, Avierinos JF, Collart F, Mundler O, Raoult D, Thuny F. Positron emission tomography/computed tomography for diagnosis of prosthetic valve endocarditis:

increased valvular 18F-fluorodeoxyglucose uptake as a novel major criterion. J Am Coll Cardiol. 2013;61(23):2374–82.

238. Rouzet F, Chequer R, Benali K, Lepage L, Ghodbane W, Duval X, Iung B, Vahanian A, Le Guludec D, Hyafil F. Respective performance of 18F-FDG PET and radiolabeled leukocyte scintigraphy for the diagnosis of prosthetic valve endocarditis. J Nucl Med. 2014;55(12):1980–5.

239. Gomes A, Glaudemans A, Touw DJ, van Melle JP, Willems TP, Maass AH, Natour E, Prakken NHJ, Borra RJH, van Geel PP, Slart R, van Assen S, Sinha B. Diagnostic value of imaging in infective endocarditis: a systematic review. Lancet Infect Dis. 2017;17(1):e1–e14.

240. Fisher MR, Forfia PR, Chamera E, Housten-Harris T, Champion HC, Girgis RE, Corretti MC, Hassoun PM. Accuracy of Doppler echocardiography in the hemodynamic assessment of pulmonary hypertension. Am J Respir Crit Care Med. 2009;179(7):615–21.

241. Weber L, Rickli H, Haager PK, Joerg L, Weilenmann D, Brenner R, Taramasso M, Baier P, Maisano F, Maeder MT. Haemodynamic mechanisms and long-term prognostic impact of pulmonary hypertension in patients with severe aortic stenosis undergoing valve replacement. Eur J Heart Fail. 2019;21(2):172–81.

242. Galie N, Humbert M, Vachiery JL, Gibbs S, Lang I, Torbicki A, Simonneau G, Peacock A, Vonk Noordegraaf A, Beghetti M, Ghofrani A, Gomez Sanchez MA, Hansmann G, Klepetko W, Lancellotti P, Matucci M, McDonagh T, Pierard LA, Trindade PT, Zompatori M, Hoeper M, Group ESCSD. 2015 ESC/ERS Guidelines for the diagnosis and treatment of pulmonary hypertension: The Joint Task Force for the Diagnosis and Treatment of Pulmonary Hypertension of the European Society of Cardiology (ESC) and the European Respiratory Society (ERS): Endorsed by: Association for European Paediatric and Congenital Cardiology (AEPC), International Society for Heart and Lung Transplantation (ISHLT). Eur Heart J. 2016;37(1):67–119.

243. Cohen HA, Baird MG, Rouleau JR, Fuhrmann CF, Bailey IK, Summer WR, Strauss HW, Pitt B. Thallium 201 myocardial imaging in patients with pulmonary hypertension. Circulation. 1976;54(5):790–5.

244. Movahed MR, Hepner A, Lizotte P, Milne N. Flattening of the interventricular septum (D-shaped left ventricle) in addition to high right ventricular tracer uptake and increased right ventricular volume found on gated SPECT studies strongly correlates with right ventricular overload. J Nucl Cardiol. 2005;12(4):428–34.

245. Ho NC, Tran JR, Bektas A. Marfan's syndrome. Lancet. 2005;366(9501):1978–81.

246. Baumgartner H, Bonhoeffer P, De Groot NM, de Haan F, Deanfield JE, Galie N, Gatzoulis MA, Gohlke-Baerwolf C, Kaemmerer H, Kilner P, Meijboom F, Mulder BJ, Oechslin E, Oliver JM, Serraf A, Szatmari A, Thaulow E, Vouhe PR, Walma E, Task Force on the Management of Grown-up Congenital Heart Disease of the European Society of C, Association for European Paediatric C, Guidelines ESCCfP. ESC Guidelines for the management of grown-up congenital heart disease (new version 2010). Eur Heart J. 2010;31(23):2915–57.

247. Mohiaddin RH, Underwood SR, Bogren HG, Firmin DN, Klipstein RH, Rees RS, Longmore DB. Regional aortic compliance studied by magnetic resonance imaging: the effects of age, training, and coronary artery disease. Br Heart J. 1989;62(2):90–6.

248. Kerwin W, Pepin M, Mitsumori L, Yarnykh V, Schwarze U, Byers P. MRI of great vessel morphology and function in Ehlers-Danlos syndrome type IV. Int J Cardiovasc Imaging. 2008;24(5):519–28.

249. Ferencik M, Pape LA. Changes in size of ascending aorta and aortic valve function with time in patients with congenitally bicuspid aortic valves. Am J Cardiol. 2003;92(1):43–6.

250. Guntheroth WG. A critical review of the American College of Cardiology/American Heart Association practice guidelines on

bicuspid aortic valve with dilated ascending aorta. Am J Cardiol. 2008;102(1):107–10.

251. O'Brien KR, Cowan BR, Jain M, Stewart RA, Kerr AJ, Young AA. MRI phase contrast velocity and flow errors in turbulent stenotic jets. J Magn Reson Imaging. 2008;28(1):210–8.

252. Chin CW, Khaw HJ, Luo E, Tan S, White AC, Newby DE, Dweck MR. Echocardiography underestimates stroke volume and aortic valve area: implications for patients with small-area low-gradient aortic stenosis. Can J Cardiol. 2014;30(9):1064–72.

253. Weigang E, Kari FA, Beyersdorf F, Luehr M, Etz CD, Frydrychowicz A, Harloff A, Markl M. Flow-sensitive four-dimensional magnetic resonance imaging: flow patterns in ascending aortic aneurysms. Eur J Cardiothorac Surg. 2008;34(1):11–6.

254. Barker AJ, Markl M, Burk J, Lorenz R, Bock J, Bauer S, Schulz-Menger J, von Knobelsdorff-Brenkenhoff F. Bicuspid aortic valve is associated with altered wall shear stress in the ascending aorta. Circ Cardiovasc Imaging. 2012;5(4):457–66.

255. Edwards FH, Hale D, Cohen A, Thompson L, Pezzella AT, Virmani R. Primary cardiac valve tumors. Ann Thorac Surg. 1991;52(5):1127–31.

256. Kumar V, Soni P, Hashmi A, Moskovits M. Aortic valve fibroelastoma: a rare cause of stroke. BMJ Case Rep. 2016;2016.

257. Fleischmann KE, Schiller NB. Papillary fibroelastoma: move over myxoma. J Am Coll Cardiol. 2015;65(22):2430–2.

258. Klarich KW, Enriquez-Sarano M, Gura GM, Edwards WD, Tajik AJ, Seward JB. Papillary fibroelastoma: echocardiographic characteristics for diagnosis and pathologic correlation. J Am Coll Cardiol. 1997;30(3):784–90.

259. Tamin SS, Maleszewski JJ, Scott CG, Khan SK, Edwards WD, Bruce CJ, Oh JK, Pellikka PA, Klarich KW. Prognostic and bio-epidemiologic implications of papillary fibroelastomas. J Am Coll Cardiol. 2015;65(22):2420–9.

260. Laguna G, Carrascal Y, Arce N, Martinez G. Incidental aortic valve myxoma: tumour excision and aortic valve repair. Eur J Cardiothorac Surg. 2015;48(3):510–1.

261. Butany J, Dixit V, Leong SW, Daniel LB, Mezody M, David TE. Inflammatory myofibroblastic tumor with valvular involvement: a case report and review of the literature. Cardiovasc Pathol. 2007;16(6):359–64.

262. Aziz F, Baciewicz FA Jr. Lambl's excrescences: review and recommendations. Tex Heart Inst J. 2007;34(3):366–8.

263. Shapira N, Fernandez J, McNicholas KW, Serra AJ, Hirschfeld K, Spagna PM, Lemole GM. Hypertrophy of nodules of Arantius and aortic insufficiency: pathophysiology and repair. Ann Thorac Surg. 1991;51(6):969–72.

264. Peters PJ, Reinhardt S. The echocardiographic evaluation of intracardiac masses: a review. J Am Soc Echocardiogr. 2006;19(2):230–40.

265. Saric M, Armour AC, Arnaout MS, Chaudhry FA, Grimm RA, Kronzon I, Landeck BF, Maganti K, Michelena HI, Tolstrup K. Guidelines for the use of echocardiography in the evaluation of a cardiac source of embolism. J Am Soc Echocardiogr. 2016;29(1):1–42.

266. Sun JP, Asher CR, Yang XS, Cheng GG, Scalia GM, Massed AG, Griffin BP, Ratliff NB, Stewart WJ, Thomas JD. Clinical and echocardiographic characteristics of papillary fibroelastomas: a retrospective and prospective study in 162 patients. Circulation. 2001;103(22):2687–93.

267. Luo W, Teng P, Ni Y. A rare cardiac inflammatory myofibroblastic tumor involving aortic valve. J Cardiothorac Surg. 2017;12(1):13.

268. Dumaswala B, Dumaswala K, Hsiung MC, Quiroz LD, Sungur A, Escanuela MG, Mehta K, Oz TK, Bhagatwala K, Karia NM, Nanda NC. Incremental value of three-dimensional transesophageal echocardiography over two-dimensional transesophageal echocardiography in the assessment of Lambl's excrescences and nodules of Arantius on the aortic valve. Echocardiography. 2013;30(8):967–75.

269. Baikoussis NG, Dedeilias P, Argiriou M, Argiriou O, Vourlakou C, Prapa E, Charitos C. Cardiac papillary fibroelastoma; when, how, why? Ann Card Anaesth. 2016;19(1):162–5.

270. Motwani M, Kidambi A, Herzog BA, Uddin A, Greenwood JP, Plein S. MR imaging of cardiac tumors and masses: a review of methods and clinical applications. Radiology. 2013;268(1):26–43.

271. Palaskas N, Thompson K, Gladish G, Agha AM, Hassan S, Iliescu C, Kim P, Durand JB, Lopez-Mattei JC. Evaluation and management of cardiac tumors. Curr Treat Options Cardiovasc Med. 2018;20(4):29.

Patient Screening

2

Buechel Ronny, Gräni Christoph, Edwin Ho, Mizuki Miura,
Alberto Pozzoli, Michael Gagesch, Gregor Freystätter,
Heike A. Bischoff-Ferrari, Philipp Haager, Hans Rickli,
Gudrun Feuchtner, Thomas Senoner, Michel Zuber,
Francesco Maisano, Hatem Alkadhi, and
Philipp Kaufmann

2.1 Introduction

2.1.1 Intro

Beside the assessment of the severity of aortic valve stenosis or regurgitation, valve morphology, access routes and annular sizing, screening of concomitant cardiac and non-cardiac pathologies is crucial for the management of aortic patients. Pre-interventional multimodalty imaging in screening aortic patients plays an important role and includes possible concomitant coronary artery disease, evaluation of other valve involvement and extra cardiac pathologies. For the assessment of coronary artery disease, depending on the pre-test likelihood different imaging modalities including invasive coronary angiography, computed tomography angiography (CTA), stress perfusion magnetic resonance imaging or nuclear perfusion imaging are at choice [1]. For the decision of the treatment of concomitant valve disease, a multimodality approach is indicated. Echocardiography, and in patients with impaired acoustic window magnetic resonance imaging and assessment of calcification using CTA (i.e. mitral annulus calcification visualization in mitral stenosis or regurgitation) are additionally performed. Beyond the intended comprehensive cardiac work-up of aortic patients, pre-interventional CTA of transcatheter aortic valve replacement (TAVR) frequently reveals potentially benign and malignant incidental findings. These incidental findings may provoke additional downstream testing [2]. The presence of potentially malignant incidental findings on CTA is an independent predictor of long-term all-cause and noncardiovascular mortality [3] and has to be therefore integrated in the decision making regarding management of the aortic disease. Other important co-factors of aortic patients include lung function screening, as preoperative pulmonary function tests predict mortality after aortic valve replacement [4] and frailty. Frailty is a risk factor for death and disability following aortic replacement [5].

Based on the screened concomitant pathologies, the treating team finally decides which approach is most

B. Ronny · G. Christoph · P. Kaufmann (✉)
Department of Nuclear Medicine, Cardiac Imaging,
Zurich University Hospital, Zurich, Switzerland
e-mail: ronny.buechel@usz.ch; christoph.graeni@insel.ch;
pak@usz.ch

E. Ho · M. Miura · A. Pozzoli · F. Maisano
University Heart Center, Zurich University Hospital,
Zurich, Switzerland
e-mail: edwin.ho@usz.ch; mizuki.miura@usz.ch;
alberto.pozzoli@usz.ch; francesco.maisano@usz.ch

M. Gagesch · G. Freystätter · H. A. Bischoff-Ferrari
Department of Geriatrics, Zurich University Hospital,
Zurich, Switzerland

Centre on Aging and Mobility, Zurich University Hospital, Waid
City Hospital and University of Zurich, Zurich, Switzerland
e-mail: Michael.gagesch@usz.ch; gregor.freystatter@usz.ch;
heike.Bischoff-Ferrari@usz.ch

P. Haager · H. Rickli
Cardiology Unit, Kantonsspital St. Gallen, St. Gallen, Switzerland
e-mail: philipp.haager@usz.ch; hans.rickli@kssg.ch

G. Feuchtner · T. Senoner
Radiology Unit, Innsbruck University Hospital, Innsbruck, Austria
e-mail: gudrun.feuchtner@i-med.ac.at;
thomas.senoner@i-med.ac.at

M. Zuber
Department of Cardiology, Zurich University Hospital,
Zurich, Switzerland
e-mail: michel.zuber@usz.ch

H. Alkadhi
Institute of Diagnostic and Interventional Radiology, Zurich
University Hospital, Zurich, Switzerland
e-mail: hatem.alkadhi@usz.ch

© Springer Nature Switzerland AG 2020
F. Maisano et al. (eds.), *Multimodality Imaging for Cardiac Valvular Interventions, Volume 1 Aortic Valve*,
https://doi.org/10.1007/978-3-030-27584-6_2

successful. The recently published European guidelines on the treatment of valvular heart disease have placed the "Heart Team", a multidisciplinary team of cardiologists, cardiac surgeons, anaesthetists, care of the elderly physicians and non-medical cardiac care specialists, at the centre of the decision process to select the most appropriate therapy for individual patients [6]. Different established comprehensive risk scores (e.g. Society of Thoracic Surgeons (STS), EuroSCORE, logistic EuroSCORE), including a broad set of parameters like baseline characteristics, laboratory tests, imaging results from concomitant valve disease and other cardiac disorders, co-morbidities etc. are used in the individual decision for the optimal treatment. For example in patients with severe aortic stenosis, surgical aortic valve repair (SAVR) is preferred in younger patients (<70 years old) with a low risk score. Furthermore, SAVR is indicated in the situation where the need for a coronary artery bypass grafting intervention is given with concomitant severe coronary artery disease or suspicion of endocarditis, unfavorable access routes (stenotic and heavily calcified femoral arteries), short distance between the coronary ostia and aortic valve annulus and very large or very narrow aortic valve annulus. In addition, in cases with bicuspid valve morphology, severe primary mitral valve disease, severe tricuspid valve disease, aneurysm of the ascending aorta or septal hypertrophy requiring myomectomy SAVR is the preferred approach. On the contrary, TAVR is preferred in older, frail patients (>70 years) with a higher risk score or when severe concomitant comorbidities are present. Further, TAVR is the indicated procedure when a patient underwent previous cardiac surgery, has restricted mobility and conditions that may affect the rehabilitation process after procedure. The sequelae of chest radiation, porcelain aorta, pre-expected patients-prosthesis mismatch or severe chest deformation/scoliosis also directs the cardiologist and surgeons towards TAVR. To conclude, an adequate assessment before aortic treatment is paramount and indispensable for the treating physicians. Aside from important demographic information, a diagnostic armamentarium of the highest quality should be provided and include multimodality assessment of aortic calve, concomitant cardiac diseases and comprehensive non-cardiac screening.

2.2 Assessment of Concomitant Cardiac Pathologies

2.2.1 Intro

In order to fully understand the clinical impact of aortic valve disease as well as the need for and risk of intervention, a careful assessment of concomitant cardiac pathology is

essential. This includes evaluation for coronary artery disease, multivalvular disease and any other abnormalities that may influence a surgical or transcatheter intervention.

Coronary artery disease is a common cardiac pathology that often accompanies degenerative valve disease [7]. It is important to evaluate because significant coronary artery disease may be the primary driver for symptoms in situations where the valve disease is not severe. Additionally, if a procedure is planned to repair or replace the valve, revascularization may also need to occur.

If surgical valve replacement or repair is planned and significant coronary artery disease coexists, then a single operation including coronary bypass grafting is generally recommended in worldwide guidelines [6, 8, 9]. In the setting of transcatheter aortic valve replacement, it is not clear whether pre-procedure revascularization has a large impact on procedural risk or prognosis relative to the additional risk from treating the coronary artery disease [10–12]. It is also important to consider that some transcatheter valve device designs and implant technique may increase the difficulty of future angioplasty procedures due to strut location relative to the coronary ostia [13].

Identifying coronary artery disease in the setting of significant aortic valve disease is more challenging due to the valvular hemodynamic contribution to myocardial ischemia with exertion. This is a potential pitfall of physiologic testing for ischemia, in addition to baseline patient functional limitations and the underlying potential risk of an exercise study with severe valvular disease. Direct anatomic assessment of the coronary arteries is therefore generally regarded as the best strategy. This is commonly done using invasive coronary angiography. In younger patients at low risk for obstructive coronary disease, a CTA can be considered to avoid the risks associated with invasive angiography [9]. Significant coronary calcification, which is common in older patients treated with transcatheter devices, may make CTA difficult to interpret [14].

Multivalvular disease is becoming more and more common in developed countries due to an aging population [15]. This is especially true for calcific aortic stenosis. In this setting, valvular degeneration and calcification is often not isolated to the aortic valve and significant concomitant mitral or tricuspid valve disease may be seen. The most common accompanying valve disease is mitral regurgitation. Similar to coronary artery disease, multivalvular disease may influence symptoms and an intervention plan.

If a surgical approach is recommended for aortic valve disease, the typical recommendation is to also correct any other hemodynamically significant valve disease at the same time. In the setting of transcatheter valve replacement, novel transcatheter mitral and tricuspid devices have opened up the ability to plan for a staged strategy. This approach is reasonable since it has been described that about half of patients who undergo transcatheter aortic valve replacement will have improvement in pre-existing significant mitral regurgitation due to a reduction in left ventricular afterload [16]. Unfortunately, significant mitral regurgitation, both pre-existing and post-procedure, is also associated with worse prognosis in patients undergoing transcatheter aortic valve replacement [17].

The presence or risk of dynamic left ventricular outflow tract obstruction should also be assessed if valve intervention is being considered for severe aortic stenosis. A small, hypertrophied left ventricle may be at risk of this. Dynamic obstruction may be unmasked or worsened after the valvular afterload on the left ventricle is reduced with valve replacement. Although little data exists on exact parameters that are most predictive of this so-called "suicide left ventricle", it has been described after some cases of transcatheter aortic valve replacement and has been treated by alcohol septal ablation in some cases [18, 19].

In this section, the strategies to assess concomitant coronary artery disease and multivalvular disease will be reviewed. All imaging modalities may play a role, including invasive angiography, computed tomography, echocardiography, nuclear imaging and cardiac magnetic resonance imaging.

2.2.2 Assessment of CAD

2.2.2.1 Intro

The presence of coronary artery disease (CAD) increases morbidity and mortality in patients with valvular heart disease (VHD). In addition, it raises the risk for specific procedures, especially within the surgical theater. Respecting the invasive character of open heart surgery, it is obvious that relevant CAD has to be ruled out so as not to miss the chance to profit from a left internal mammary bypass in case of a proximal LAD or left main stenosis and to rule out ischemic problems during or after the procedure. Therefore it has been common practice that all patients undergo invasive evaluation using standard coronary angiography to rule out relevant CAD.

Nowadays, with the evolution of multislice computed tomography (MSCT) and percutaneous treatment of CAD and valvular heart disease a more differential strategy is possible and necessary.

2.2.2.2 Coronary Angiography and Functional Assessment

Current guidelines on valvular heart disease point out, that all male patients >40 years of age and postmenopausal women undergoing cardiac surgery for valvular heart disease should still undergo invasive coronary angiography to rule out relevant CAD as first diagnostic strategy (Class I, Level C). Also patients with suspected ischemia, history of CAD, left ventricular systolic dysfunction or with one or more cardiovascular risk factors should primarily undergo selective coronary angiography [6].

In patients with a low probability of CAD, CTA can be a good alternative to invasive angiography. This is becoming more and more an extra value for the patient, as CT based procedure planning is now very common practice in an increasing number of centers. Besides traditional risc factors, CT offers additional value to evaluate further cardiac and non-cardiac structures like calcifications, vessel sizes, tumors or also high risk features like endoluminal thrombus.

The indication for myocardial revascularization depends on the extent of the coronary artery disease, the planned type of heart surgery or the structural intervention. Percutaneous therapies now offer the value of staged procedures to address only relevant disease. To better distinguish between non-significant and significant lesions with ischemia, non-invasive stress tests are helpful.

If not performed and an intermediate lesion is detected, invasive functional diagnostic measures are highly recommended. The concept of fractional flow reserve (FFR) was introduced to assess intermediate lesions. A 0.014-inch guidewire with a pressure sensor on its tip is advanced beyond the coronary stenosis. Using a hyperemic stimulus (most often adenosine i.v. or i.c.), the pressure drop behind the stenosis is a marker of hemodynamic severity. Several trials have pointed out, that a cut-off value of 0.8 is considered relevant [20]. On the other hand, if the lesion is not functionally relevant, it is safe to skip the percutaneous or even surgical procedure.

Recently, resting gradients alone have been examined (iFR). The advantage as compared to FFR is the possibility to omit pharmacological vasodilation. On the other hand, the measured differences are smaller and opens up the possibilities for technical errors.

The decision whether or not a revasularisation procedure is required should be discussed together with all other findings within a heart team. In a surgical procedure with indication for aortic valve replacement and severe CAD, a combined procedure with revascularization using the left mammarial artery for a significant proximal complex LAD stenosis is recommended. On the other hand, a non-significant lesion may be left untreated if not relevant and therefore ease up the surgical procedure.

Vice versae, not every moderate aortic stenosis needs to be treated nowadays with valve surgery in a patient receiving bypass grafting. Additional investigations using a "TAVI-CT" has a big value to determine the valvular size, vascular access and other comorbidities. With these additional information, the heart team is able to decide whether or not a patient is still a surgical candidate, whether or not a later percutaneous treatment of the aortic valve is easily feasible, or if the patient would profit from a surgical strategy due to an dilated annulus or aortic aneurysm which needs to be addressed.

2.2.2.3 CT

Coronary computed tomography angiography (CCTA) [21, 22] is a non-invasive imaging modality for the evaluation of CAD, with a high accuracy for stenosis detection >50%, and an excellent performance to "rule out" disease [21–23]. CTA data sets nowadays even allow for 3D computational fluid modelling (CFD) and noninvasive calculation of the FFR [24, 25]. FFR_{CT} improves accuracy of CTA with 93% sensitivity and 82% specificity for detection of lesion-based ischemia [24, 25]. However, noninvasive FFR_{CT} is currently only validated for patients with low calcium scores <800 AU, and caution is warranted in elderly patients with a trend to high coronary calcium load.

Furthermore, CTA allows for atherosclerotic plaque characterization [26–29]: Non-calcified plaque (<200 HU) indicates fibrofatty atheroma [29], and can be distinguished from calcified plaque. Additionally, a very low attenuation plaque (LAP) <30 Hounsfield Units (HU) correlates well with lipid-necrotic core plaque, a criterion for plaque "vulnerability" and a marker for adverse outcome [26] as well as a predictor for ischemia [27], even in the absence of high grade >70% stenosis.

Apart from LAP <30 HU, 3 additional major high-risk plaque (HRP) criteria according to CADRADS [30] classification can be distinguished: Napkin-Ring Sign (NRS), defined as having a hyperdense rim with ≤200 HU and an inner hypodense core [28], remodeling index (RI) >1.1 and spotty calcification <3 mm. High-risk plaque criteria indicate advanced complex atherosclerotic lesions, plaque vulnerablity [31] and higher risk for cardiac events [26].

Examination techniques: Non-contrast CT. An unenhanced ECG-gated coronary calcium score with standardized scan parameters (detector collimation 64 × 1.5 mm; 120 kV) allows for both coronary and simultaneous aortic valve calcium scoring [32] with a good inter-platform performance. The Agatston Score (Agatston units, AU), Mass and Volume Score can be calculated.

Coronary CTA prior to valvular interventions should be performed with ≥64-slice CT technology with a thin detector collimation of ≥0.6 mm and fast rotation times. Prospective ECG-triggering can be applied in regular heart rates <65 bpm (diastolic padding, 70% of RR-interval), while in higher and in particular irregular heart rates, retrospective ECG-gating should be used, which allows for "ECG-editing" and hence the correction of artifacts resulting from arrhythmia. If systolic image reconstruction is required for comprehensive evaluation of valve morphology, multiphase datasets are needed by covering image acquisition over the entire cardiac cycle, as commonly available for retrospective ECG-gating, or novel other algorithms.

An iodine contrast agent has to be injected intravenously (flow rate 4–6 mL/s + 40 cc saline chaser), triggered into arterial phase (bolus tracking or test bolus methods). The contrast volume (65–110 cc) should be adjusted according to the patient's body weight and scan time using standardized recommendations and kept as low as possible. CT scanners with high temporal resolution (<75 ms), such as achieved by dual source technology (e.g. 2nd or 3rd generation dual source 128-slice CT), are a great advantage in patients with aortic stenosis and arrhythmic, fast heart rates.

There are three major challenges in patients with severe aortic stenosis: First, due to their increased age >70 years, comorbidities such as kidney dysfunction are common. Hence, contrast volume should be kept as low as possible, e.g. by applying spectral low-kVp imaging, or ultrafast scan times (e.g. by high–pitch CTA).

Second, the high prevalence of arrhythmia such as atrial fibrillation or multiple ectopic beats may hamper image quality and requires ECG-editing to correct for missaligned image artifacts. Third, high calcium scores, if >400 AU, increase the risk of overestimation of stenosis due to artifacts. Especially in male patients with severe aortic stenosis, advanced age >75 years, and those with a high coronary artery disease risk profile, the probability of high calcium scores is high, and the diagnostic accuracy of coronary CTA for exact stenosis quantification limited. Other tests (e.g. invasive coronary angiography (ICA), myocardial perfusion by MRI, SPECT or PET) are mainly used to confirm the diagnosis of CAD.

Despite advanced age, the calcium scores are usually highly variable among patients with valvular disease, depending on the coronary risk profile, gender and the type of valve disease. Especially in females, calcium scores are in general remarkably lower than in males, and despite of high age, mostly of adequate image quality.

Several studies have investigated the accuracy of CTA in patients prior to cardiac surgery. In the first landmark study, Bettencourt et al. showed in 454 patients undergoing all types of cardiac surgery [33], a safe rule out of >50% stenosis (NPV 99% and sensitivity 95%), but only a moderate-to-low specifity (89%) and a low PPV of 38–66% (per patient and per vessel).

In patients with severe aortic stenosis prior to transcatheter aortic valve replacement (TAVR), several single center studies [14] showed similar results, and a meta-analysis [34] pooling 7 studies with a cumulative sample size of 1275 patients showed a patient-based pooled sensitivity, specificity, PPV and NPV of 95%, 65%, 71% and 94%, respectively. Moderate specificity of 65% is explained by high calcium scores and image quality limitations in patients with severe arrythmia. The meta-analysis [34] had a low risk of bias. In conclusion, for 50% diameter stenosis, CCTA provides acceptable diagnostic accuracy for the exclusion of coronary artery disease in patients referred for TAVR [34], hence CCTA serves as a reliable gatekeeper for invasive coronary angiography and could decrease additional coronary angiographies by 37%, from the same CT datasets performed for procedure planning [34].

CTA image analysis: Coronary stenosis severity should be scored visually as: minimal <25%, mild ≤25–49%; intermediate 50–69% or severe ≥70% according to CADRADS [30]. Then, each coronary segment should be evaluated for plaque morphology and defined as "non-calcified" (hypoattenuating <200 HU), mixed or "calcified" [29]. Next, the presence of "high-risk plaque" criteria [26–28] should be assesed and a patient labeled as "vulnerable" if 2 out of 4 criteria are present [30]. High-risk plaque criteria indicate higher risk for adverse outcomes. Ischemia is more often found in LAP, even if stenosis is less than 50% [27] and may explain chest pain symptoms (ANOCA = angina in the absence of obstructive coronary artery disease).

In conclusions, CCTA is a valuable tool for non-invasive rule out of significant CAD, defined as stenosis greater than 50%. Caution is advised in patients with high calcium scores in terms of overestimation of the degree of stenosis, as well as in renal dysfunction, with regards to iodine contrast exposure. Furthermore, arrhythmias in patients with valvular disease represent a challenge: advanced technology undoubtedly is of benefit and should be preferred in patients prior to cardiac valve intervention, to ensure optimal image quality and minimal contrast and radiation exposure. Notably, coronary CTA datasets are usually available from any cardiac CT

study performed for purpose of valvular intervention planning, without added iodine or contrast agent exposure (Fig. 2.1).

Translational outlook. Currently, machine learning algorithms [35], including radiomics, are being investigated for improved accuracy of CCTA. These are promising tools for overcoming current shortcomings.

2.2.2.4 Stress Test

The most common way to evaluate for the presence of significant CAD is by the use of stress testing. This is recommended by various international guidelines based on pre-test probability and symptoms [36, 37].

A typical stress test would involve some form of myocardial stressor, typically exercise on a treadmill or bicycle according to standardized protocols, in combination with a tracer for ischemia. Exercise induces myocardial ischemia by increasing oxygen demand due to augmentation in heart rate, contractility and blood pressure. The target heart rate for a maximal exercise stress study is 85% of the age-predicted maximum value. The adequacy of peak demand on the myocardium is often reported as the rate pressure product, which is calculated by multiplying the peak heart rate and peak systolic blood pressure. Other stressors can include Dobutamine or vasodilators such as dipyridamole or adenosine [3]. Dobutamine can simulate some of the effects of exercise on the heart by stimulating beta adrenergic receptors to increase inotropy and chronotropy. The systolic blood pressure, however, may not increase with a Dobutamine infusion to the same degree as with true exercise, which can result in a lower peak rate pressure product. Vasodilator stressors

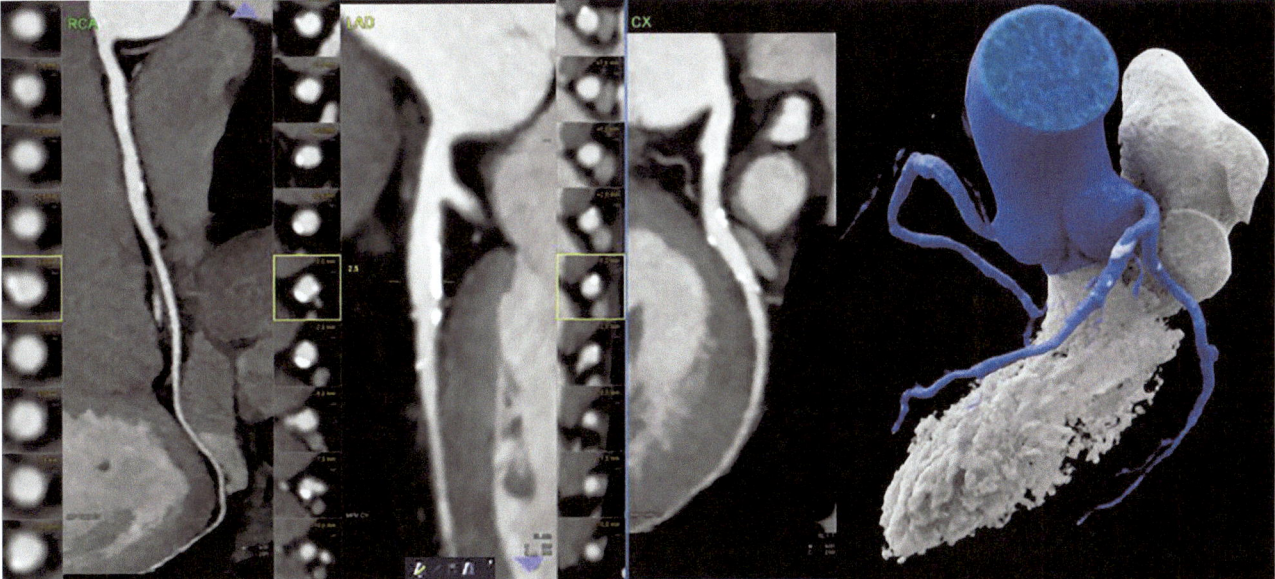

Fig. 2.1 Coronary CTA provides a reliable rule out of significant stenosis. Calcified plaque with less than 50% stenosis in the LAD, CX and RCA shown by multiplanar reformations (mMRP) (upper panel) and 3D VRT (lower panel)

work by exhausting the vasodilatory reserve of diseased coronary artery segments, changing relative perfusion patterns as well as potentially inducing a local steal phenomenon, causing true ischemia.

The most commonly used indicator of ischemia is the continuous 12 lead ECG, but can also include wall motion by echocardiography or perfusion by nuclear imaging, CTA or CMR [4]. Diagnostic ECG changes for ischemia are defined as greater than or equal to 1 mm of horizontal or downsloping ST depression, measured at 60–80 ms after the J point. The PQ segment is used as the baseline. Isolated J point depression with an upsloping ST segment is considered a negative ECG response unless it is marked (greater than 1 mm), which is then defined as an equivocal response because it may be representative of ischemia in some individuals (Fig. 2.2).

Stress echocardiography adds wall motion analysis of all wall segments defined by a 16 or 17 segment model. Nuclear perfusion imaging utilizes a nuclear tracer that distributes proportionately with blood flow and is measured at rest and stress to determine if there are relative perfusion defects that exist only during stress, indicating ischemia, or are present at both rest and stress, indicating an infarct or artifact. Perfusion analysis by computed tomography and magnetic resonance imaging can be achieved using intravenous contrast and a gated acquisition protocol to evaluate myocardial perfusion at stress.

Although investigational, perfusion by echocardiography can also be performed using microbubble contrast agents [5].

Important prognostic data that can be derived from stress tests include total exercise time, peak exercise capacity, the Duke Treadmill Score, wall motion score index by echocardiography as well as the hemodynamic blood pressure and heart rate response to exercise. Some high risk features that can be seen on stress tests include significant ST depression at low workloads, exercise induced ST elevation, exercise induced ventricular arrhythmia, markedly blunted blood pressure response to exercise, severe stress induced left ventricular dysfunction, stress perfusion abnormalities greater than 10% of the myocardium or covering multiple vascular territories, inducible wall motion abnormalities involving more than 2 segments or multiple coronary artery beds and wall motion abnormalities at low workloads [37].

Unfortunately, in the setting of significant valvular heart disease, traditional stress testing may not be a reliable method to detect significant coronary artery disease. Patients may have significant functional limitations that prevent them from reaching the target heart rate needed for a diagnostic study for ischemia. More importantly, there are hemodynamic risks to maximal exercise testing and it is absolutely contraindicated in those with symptomatic severe aortic stenosis [38]. Pharmacologic agents should also be used with caution if not avoided in the presence of significant valvular

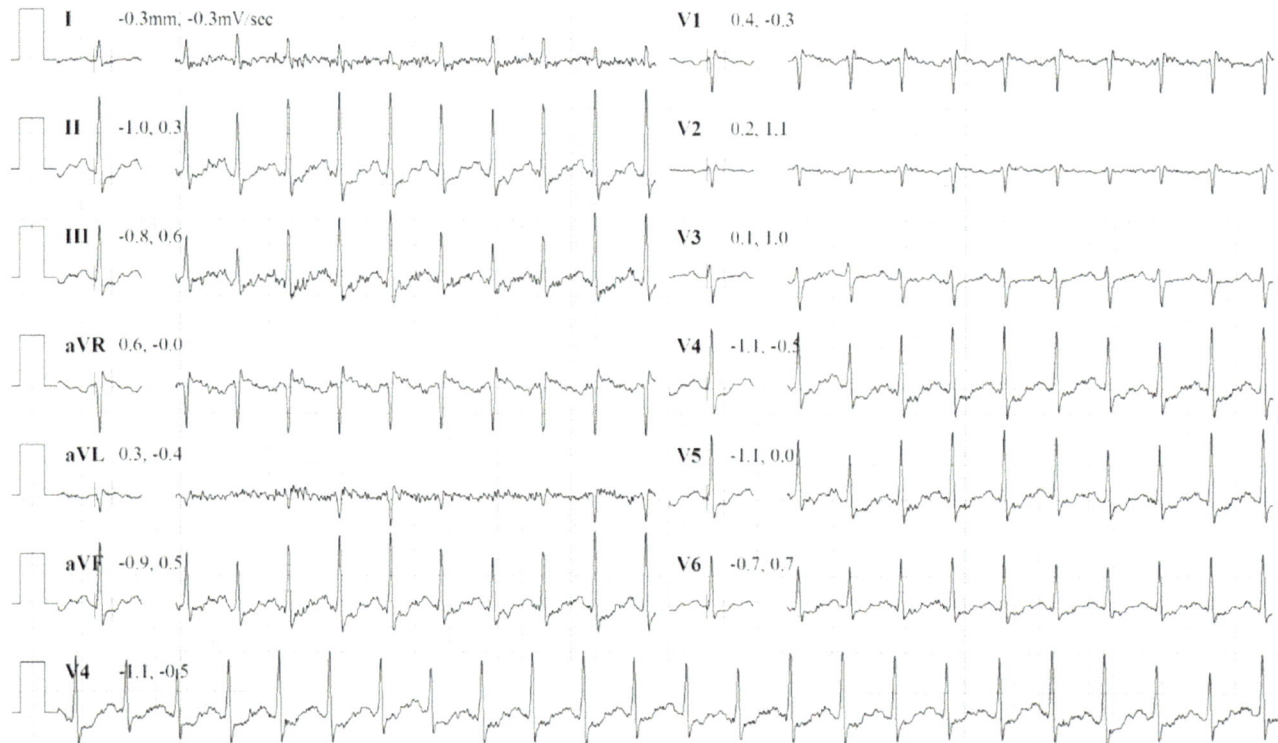

Fig. 2.2 Peak heart rate electrocardiogram of a treadmill stress test demonstrating ST segment depression in leads II, III, aVF, V4, V5 and V6, which may be consistent with ischemia

disease. This is especially true in aortic stenosis. Lastly, increased left ventricular wall strain, left ventricular hypertrophy, effects on the coronary flow reserve and potential changes to myocardial perfusion pressure likely reduce the specificity of traditional markers of ischemia by stress testing. In general, although ischemia can certainly be detected, exercise testing in valvular heart disease is performed to determine the hemodynamic effect of the valve lesion [39].

In light of these limitations, anatomic tests are generally recommended to evaluate for coronary artery disease in the setting of aortic valve disease. This most often occurs in the form of invasive angiography, but in some individuals where the pre-test probability of coronary artery disease is low, computed tomography coronary angiography is considered a reasonable alternative [9, 40]. Some centres will also use invasive functional assessment, such as fractional flow reserve, to assist with evaluating the functional significance of stenotic lesions found through anatomic testing [41].

2.2.2.5 Echo

The echocardiographic assessment for coronary artery disease is focused on the systolic and diastolic function of the left ventricle [42]. Overall left ventricular systolic function including the left ventricular ejection fraction provides significant prognostic information in the presence of coronary artery disease. Regional wall motion abnormalities can be seen if there has been infarction or there is ischemia in a coronary territory. If multivessel disease is present, it is also possible to see global left ventricular systolic dysfunction.

In addition to evaluating systolic regional function by visual inspection of contractility, strain imaging can also identify abnormalities in regional myocardial contractility. Strain is defined as the regional deformation of a myocardial wall segment relative to its baseline length and can be measured longitudinally, circumferentially or radially. It is analyzed using semi-automatic software speckle tracking algorithms. When performed correctly, strain analysis is typically more sensitive in detecting subtle abnormalities in myocardial contractility and thus may have additional benefit in the evaluation of wall motion for suspected coronary artery disease [43–46].

Left ventricular diastolic function is also important to evaluate in the setting of known or suspected coronary artery disease. In the myocardial ischemic cascade, it is known that diastolic dysfunction actually precedes systolic dysfunction [36]. This can be assessed as per the guideline recommendations for diastolic assessment using Doppler parameters and left atrial size [47]. Left ventricular global strain rate or left atrial strain may also be useful markers of diastolic dysfunction but are still investigational [48–50].

Since abnormalities in rest imaging are generally indicative of infarction or significant resting ischemia, such as during an acute coronary syndrome, there is an additional role for stress echocardiography to assess for inducible ischemia

due to coronary artery disease. This is typically performed using treadmill or bicycle exercise stress according to standardized protocols [38]. Resting left ventricular wall motion images are obtained to fully evaluate baseline wall motion according to a 16 or 17 segment model. Peak images should be obtained within 1 (at most 2) minutes after exercise termination and ideally while the heart rate is still at or near the target peak heart rate for the exercise study. This is because wall motion abnormalities may normalize quickly as the heart rate drops back to baseline in recovery. Stress echocardiography can also be performed using pharmacologic agents. Dobutamine is a beta adrenergic agonist that will increase inotropy at lower doses and chronotropy at higher doses, increasing myocardial oxygen demand and potentially inducing ischemia to reveal underlying coronary artery disease. Vasodilators have also been used for stress echocardiography, although wall motion abnormalities will only be seen if a steal phenomenon causes regional ischemia [39]. Perfusion analysis can also be done using microbubble contrast injections and specialized imaging protocols [51].

Unfortunately, in the setting of severe valve disease, the ability to safely perform stress echocardiography may be limited. They may provide useful information about the hemodynamic effect of the valve disease itself but coronary artery disease assessment is mostly limited to resting echocardiography and other imaging modalities (Figs. 2.3 and 2.4).

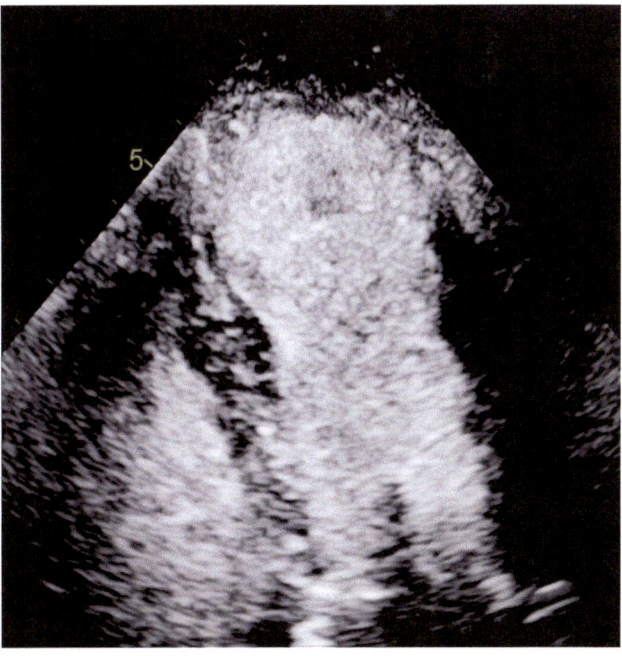

Fig. 2.3 Left ventricular apical aneurysm due to prior infarction seen at end systole on an apical 4 chamber view of a transthoracic echocardiogram with microbubble contrast

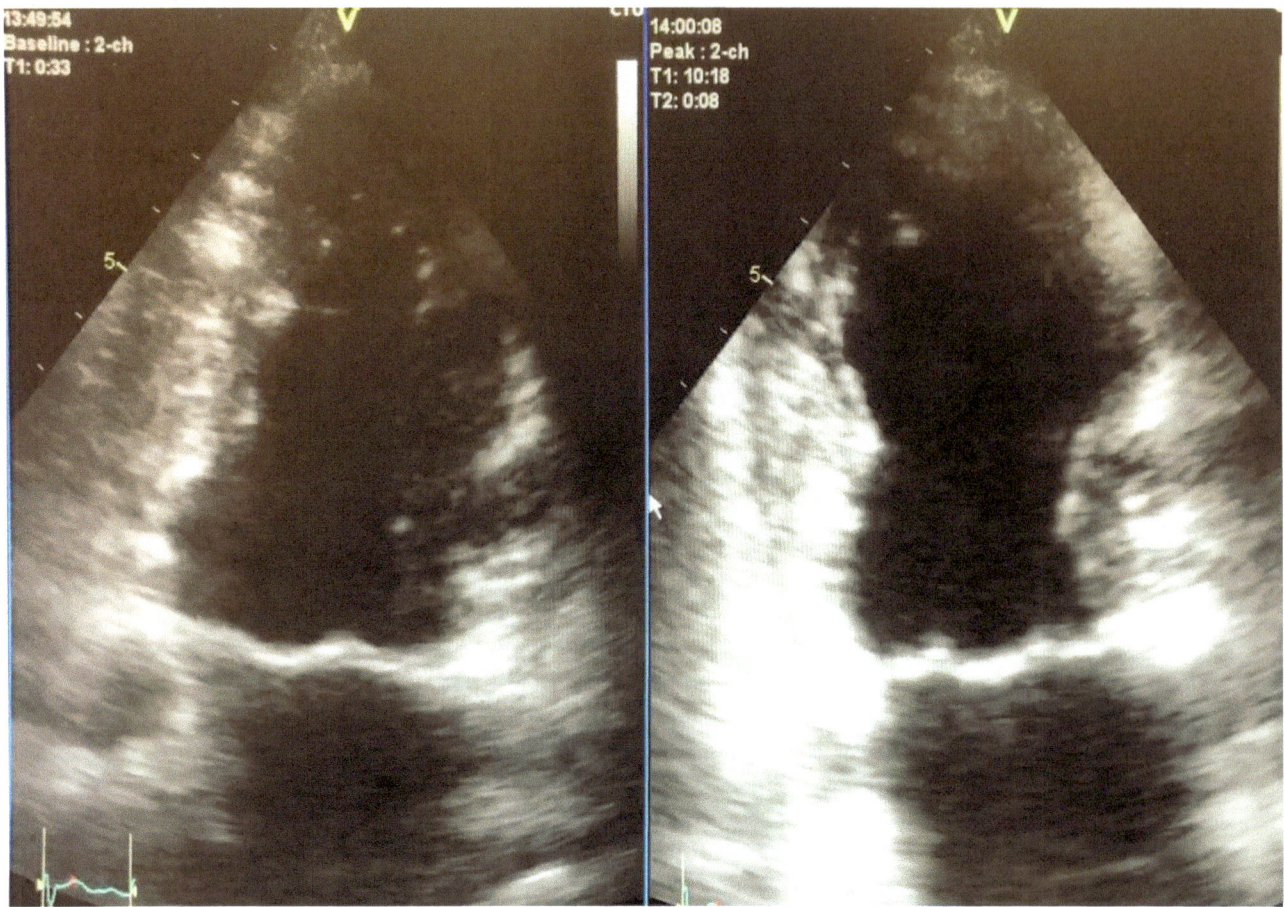

Fig. 2.4 Stress echocardiographic comparison of the end systolic apical 2 chamber view at rest (left) and at peak heart rate (right), demonstrating a peak workload shape deformity due to akinesis of the mid to distal anterior wall extending to the apex, suggesting the presence of inducible ischemia in the LAD territory

2.2.2.6 Nuclear Scan

Nuclear imaging has a pivotal and long-standing role in the assessment of patients with suspected or known coronary artery disease.

Myocardial perfusion SPECT imaging relies on the basic principle of perfusion-dependent tracer uptake into viable myocytes and subsequent detection and imaging of the photon emission resulting from gamma decay. Current radiotracers for SPECT perfusion imaging include 99m-Technetium and 201-Thallium. 99m-Technetium-based tracers should be preferred for their shorter half-life and higher photon energy leading to higher count rates and better image quality at a lower radiation exposure. On the other hand, 201-Thallium exhibits less liver uptake and redistributes into viable hypoperfused myocardium, thereby enabling delayed viability imaging.

Depending on the patient's characteristics, cardiac stress may be achieved through physical exercise or pharmacological agents using intravenous dobutamine or vasodilator infusion. Stress-induced perfusion abnormalities are used to detect obstructive CAD, and its high diagnostic accuracy has been documented in a vast number of studies. By use of concomitant electrocardiogram gating, functional parameters such as left ventricular volumes and contractility become available, thus providing an additional important layer of information for the interpreting physician. Unlike any other modality, SPECT possesses long-term follow-up information in many ten-thousands of patients which firmly establish the critical role of SPECT for risk stratification of CAD patients [52, 53].

As with SPECT, the basic principle of PET is based on the detection of photons originating from radionuclide decay. However, both modalities differ fundamentally concerning some technical characteristics: PET radionuclides exhibit β+-decay and a relatively short half-live which mandates an on-site cyclotron for rapid production (except for 82-Rubidium which can be produced with a generator). Furthermore, PET spatial resolution is significantly better than that of SPECT (Fig. 2.5) and attenuation correction is more robust. These advantages of PET over other functional imaging modalities result in higher diagnostic accuracy for the detection of

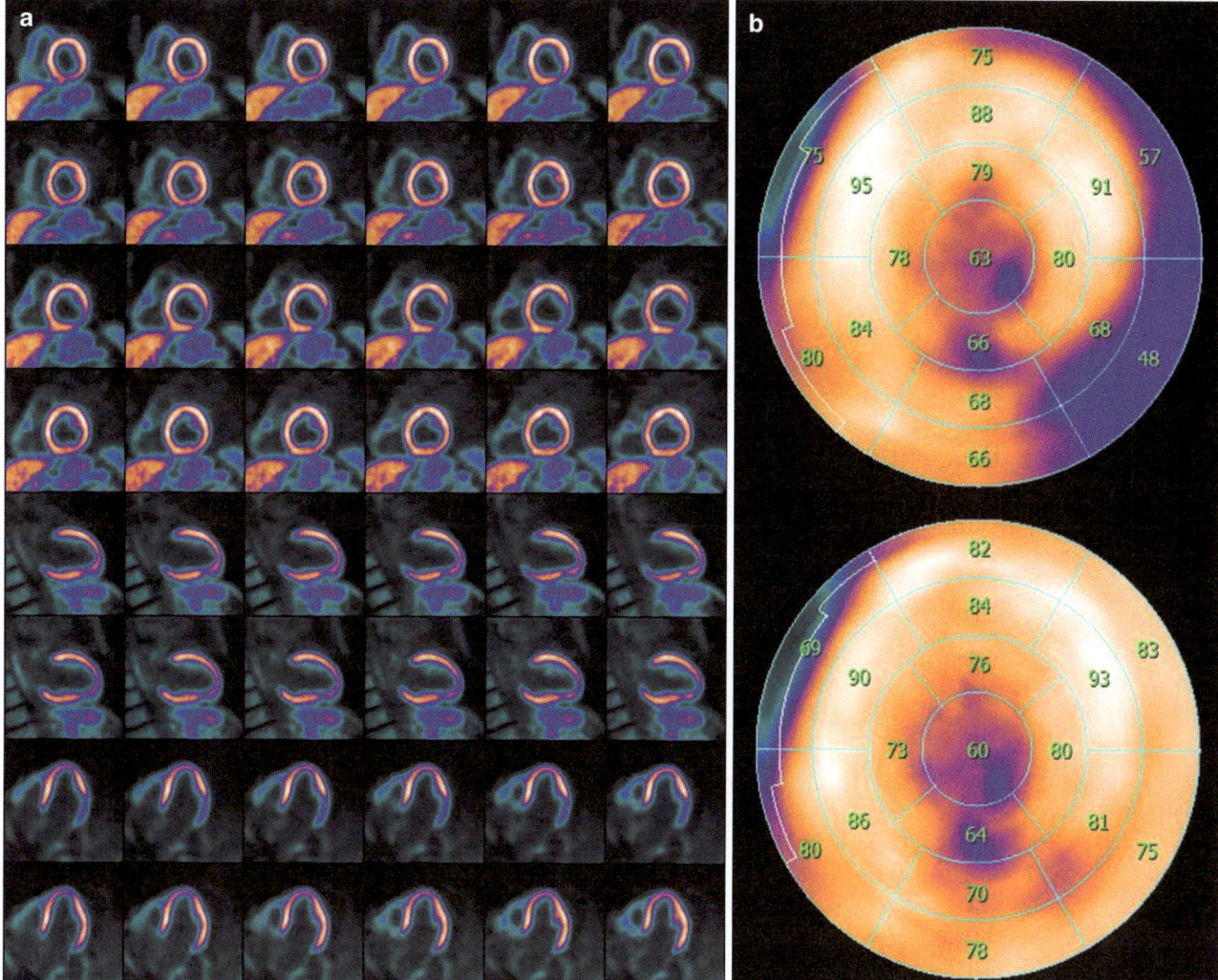

Fig. 2.5 13N-ammonia PET myocardial perfusion imaging of a 67-year old female patient with typical chest pain. Selected short axis, vertical long axis and horizontal long axis slices at rest (bottom) and during pharmacologically induced stress (top) are depicted (**a**), as well as the corresponding polar plots (**b**), revealing a very small inferoapical scar and an inferolaterobasal/laterobasal ischemia

coronary artery disease [54]. Furthermore, PET allows absolute quantification of myocardial blood flow in mL/min/g which may improve detection of balanced ischemia in coronary three-vessel disease or in case of microvascular dysfunction. The prognostic value of PET myocardial perfusion has been demonstrated in several large studies [55].

2.2.3 Assessment of Other Valve Involvement

2.2.3.1 Intro

The presence of multiple valve disease is not uncommon and represents a diagnostic and therapeutic challenge to clinicians because of the heterogeneity between patients and their valve lesions. The most common combination of valve disease in surgical and transcatheter series is aortic and mitral valve disease. The concurrent presence of significant tricuspid valve disease is also significant [56].

One example of a commonly occurring combination of valve lesions is aortic stenosis and mitral regurgitation. Longstanding pressure overload of the left ventricle can cause left ventricular dilation and systolic function. This can cause functional mitral regurgitation due to annular dilation and leaflet tethering. Concomitant coronary artery disease with wall motion abnormalities may also contribute to the secondary mitral regurgitation. This lesion then changes the flow state across the stenosed aortic valve, which can result in a low transvalvular gradient despite significant stenosis. Diagnostically, this may be challenging if the first evaluation is done when both valves are already significantly dysfunctional.

Another example of a diagnostic challenge due to mixed valve disease is the presence of mitral stenosis with aortic stenosis. This is rare outside of the setting of rheumatic valve disease, but severe mitral annular calcification can cause some degree of stenosis. If mitral stenosis is severe, flow rates can be reduced across both mitral and aortic valves, causing an underestimation of transvalvular gradients and stenosis severity.

Mitral stenosis or regurgitation in combination with aortic regurgitation also demonstrates interacting valve hemodynamics. When there is mitral stenosis, the left ventricle is relatively underfilled from the left atrium and therefore the high stroke volume usually observed with severe aortic regurgitation may be absent. Mitral regurgitation on the other hand, may have an additive effect with severe aortic regurgitation due to the absence of a physical barrier between the aortic regurgitant flow and the left atrium, leading to more significant symptoms.

In addition to the diagnostic challenges caused by the presence of multiple significant valve lesions, treatment decisions also become more complex. In the past, surgical treatment of multiple valves was associated with increased procedural risk. Transcatheter treatment options has overcome some of this limitation, but many devices are still investigational and also suffer from their own limitations. This has increased the need for multidisciplinary Heart Valve Teams with access to multiple device categories and treatment options, including conventional surgery. In the end, an individualized recommendation should be made on the basis of a global assessment of the impact of the valve lesions separately and in combination, patient specific variables including risk profile, preference and functional status, local expertise and the risk associated with an intervention on one or multiple valves [57, 58].

Multimodality imaging plays a crucial role in the evaluation of multiple valve disease and in complex decision making in the setting of a multidisciplinary Heart Valve Team [6, 9, 59]. This section will review how different imaging modalities can assess the presence and severity of multiple valve lesions.

2.2.3.2 Echo

Resting transthoracic echocardiography is the primary imaging modality of choice to evaluate for multiple valve disease in the setting of aortic valve disease, since a complete transthoracic echocardiogram protocol provides detailed anatomic and functional assessment of all the cardiac valves [60]. Valvular regurgitation, or rarely, stenosis, can be evaluated based on the guidelines published by international imaging societies [40, 61, 62]. The interpretation and management is best assessed by an experienced multidisciplinary Heart Valve Team if multiple valve lesions exist, since management may be more complex [6, 8, 9].

Mitral valve disease is commonly seen in association with aortic valve disease and may require special attention. For example, calcific degeneration seem in aortic stenosis may also affect the mitral valve and cause regurgitation due to calcific leaflet changes or torn chordae with prolapse or flail. Alternatively, there may be functional mitral regurgitation due to left ventricular systolic dysfunction caused by severe aortic valve disease. Or, there may be mitral regurgitation due to more than one etiology. This information is important for a Heart Valve Team because there may be implications on the expected clinical benefit, procedural risk or overall plan of aortic valve intervention. Less commonly, there may also be a mitral inflow gradient due to significant mitral annular calcification. The degree of functional stenosis and contribution to symptoms is important to consider for this difficult to treat entity.

Transesophageal echocardiography may also have additional utility in clarifying additional valve disease in the setting of aortic valve disease if transthoracic imaging is unclear. The closer proximity of the transducer probe to the cardiac valves provides improved spatial resolution in both 2-dimensional and 3-dimensional echocardiographic imaging. Complete transesophageal echocardiographic imaging protocols have been published including those specific for evaluation prior to transcatheter valve intervention [63–65].

An integrative approach to the evaluation of valve disease may include both transthoracic and transesophageal echocardiography in addition to other cardiac imaging modalities [61, 66]. This may be especially helpful in the setting of multiple valve disease (Figs. 2.6 and 2.7).

2.2.3.3 Stress Echocardiography

Stress echocardiography may play an important role in the evaluation of multiple valve disease in addition to transthoracic and transesophageal evaluation of each individual valve [40, 60, 61, 63, 64]. It is especially helpful when symptoms and resting valvular hemodynamics appear to be discordant [39]. Stress echocardiography allows each individual valve lesion to be assessed systematically using colour flow imaging and Doppler analysis during exercise. This may reveal which lesion is contribution most to a patient's symptoms.

Since a detailed evaluation of multiple valves requires time, supine bicycle stress testing is preferred over treadmill testing. This allows all the valves to be evaluated during exertion as opposed to in recovery. The assessment strategy should also be based on data from the resting echocardiographic study. The suspected dominant lesion should be assessed first and in its entirety, followed by the other valves in sequence based on their interest to the clinician evaluating the patient. Exercise stages may need to be held for longer periods of time to complete the assessment. Valve assessment at early stages of exercise can also be considered.

Specific scenarios highlighted in the guidelines included rheumatic mitral valve disease due to the potential presence

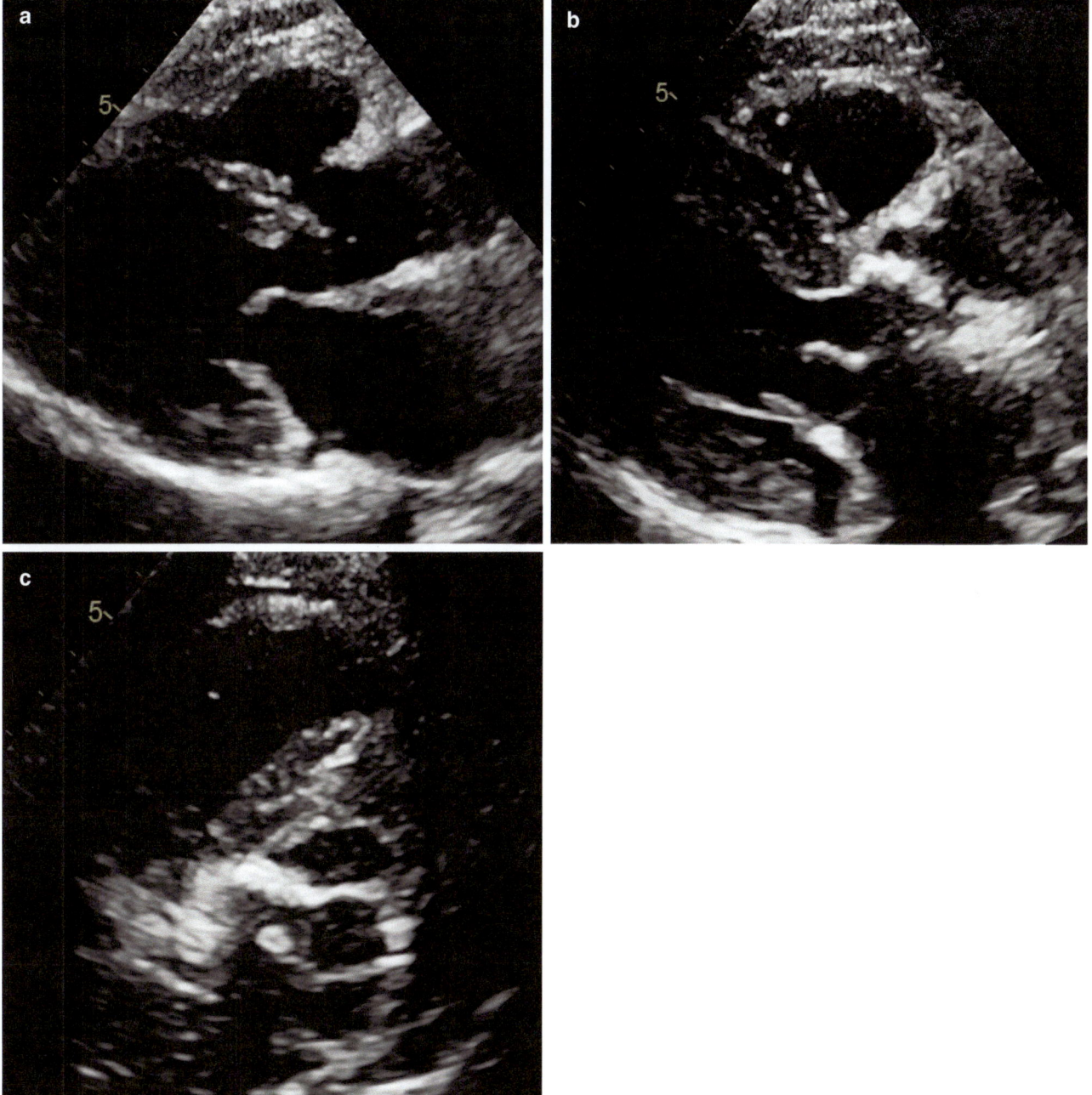

Fig. 2.6 Concomitant mitral stenosis and aortic valve disease due to rheumatic valve disease (**a**) as well as mitral annular calcification (**b**) due to nearly circumferential mitral annular calcification (**c**)

of both stenosis and regurgitation. The hemodynamic significance of each may vary with exercise compared to rest and this should be noted in a stress echocardiography study to help guide management [67]. Mixed aortic valve disease may also demonstrate dynamic changes with exercise and hemodynamic effects may be additive.

In addition to understanding how valve hemodynamics behave with exercise, functional testing allows the clinician to evaluate the true exercise capacity when patients report no apparent symptoms. Valve disease often progresses slowly, leading patients to adapt their lifestyle to their functional limitations (Fig. 2.8).

2.2.3.4 Catheterism

Normally, no invasive technique is necessary to rule out any other relevant valvular disease if a comprehensive echocardiographic examination was performed before. Before transesophageal echo was available, left- and right heart

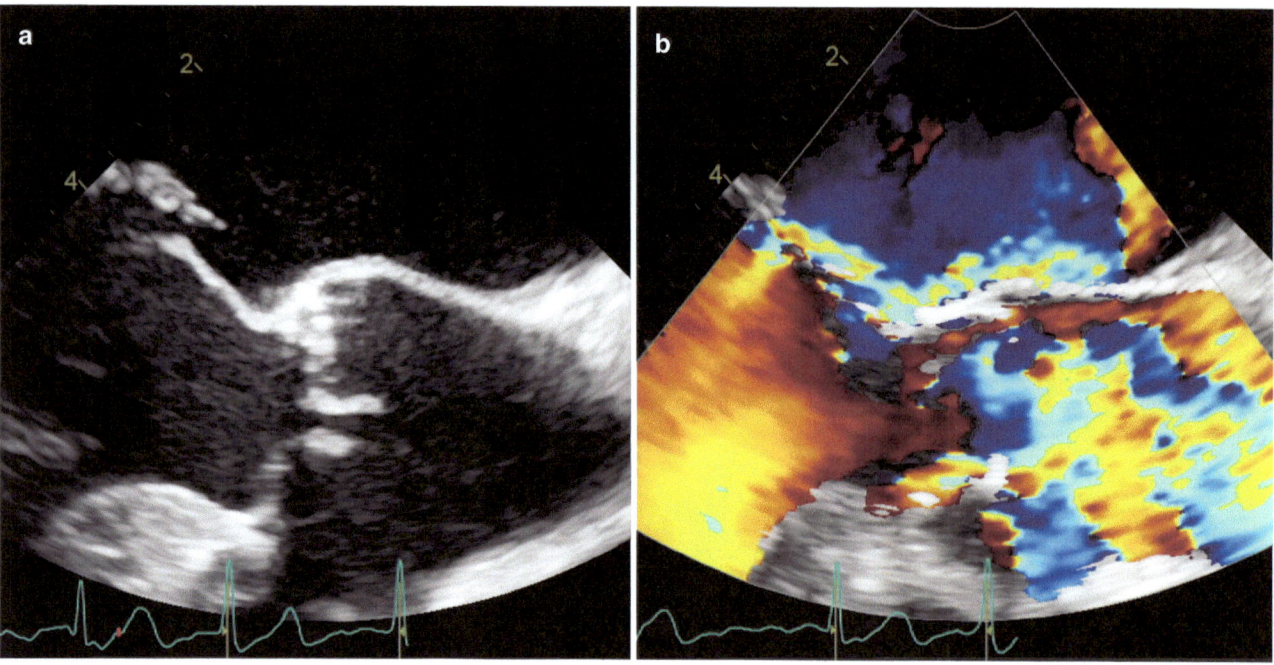

Fig. 2.7 Concomitant mitral regurgitation due to posterior leaflet flail and severe aortic stenosis seen on transesophageal echocardiography in mid-systole seen on 2-dimensional imaging (**a**) and with colour Doppler (**b**)

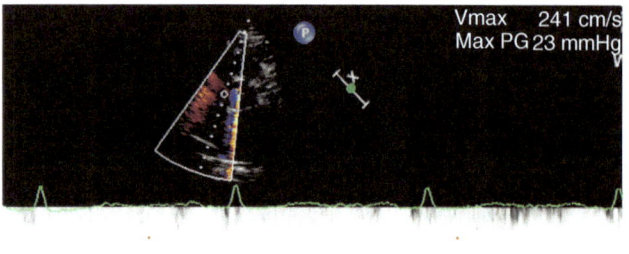

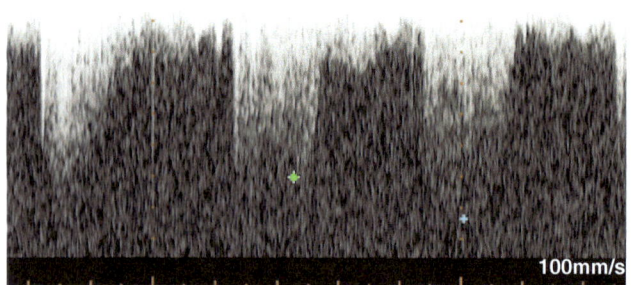

Fig. 2.8 Measurement of peak tricuspid regurgitation jet velocity using continuous wave spectral Doppler during stress echocardiography to assess for a significant increase in pulmonary pressures with exertion in the setting of left sided valvular heart disease

catheterization was performed to quantify stenotic and regurgitant valve disease. If in doubt, additional invasive tests can still be carried out today. Left ventriculography is easily done and yields additional hemodynamic information with measurements of systolic and enddiastolic left ventricular pressure, regional and global wall motion and mitral

regurgitation. The latter is quantified using the semiquantitative method of Seller.

Using aortography, aortic valve regurgitation can be assessed, also a semiquantitative measure as proposed by Seller. Evaluation of right sided heart disease using invasive technique is relatively rare. The peak-to peak gradient of pulmonary stenosis can be obtained easily. Angiography was thought not to have a role for tricuspid regurgitation due to the misleading artefact by the catheter itself. In a small series J. Tunon et al showed in 1994 that there is indeed no influence on the measurement [68] (Fig. 2.9).

2.3   Assessment of Non Cardiac Copathologies

2.3.1   Tumors (Incidental Findings)

2.3.1.1   Intro

CMR is the modality of choice for characterization of cardiac masses. Valvular masses, however, are often small and mobile. In these circumstances, due to its higher spatial resolution, CT is superior to CMR.

2.3.1.2   CT

The advantage of cardiac CT over CMR comprises higher spatial resolution while maintaining high temporal resolution of ≥ 75 ms. Further, CT offers improved visualization of small and mobile masses of less than 1 cm, and an improved

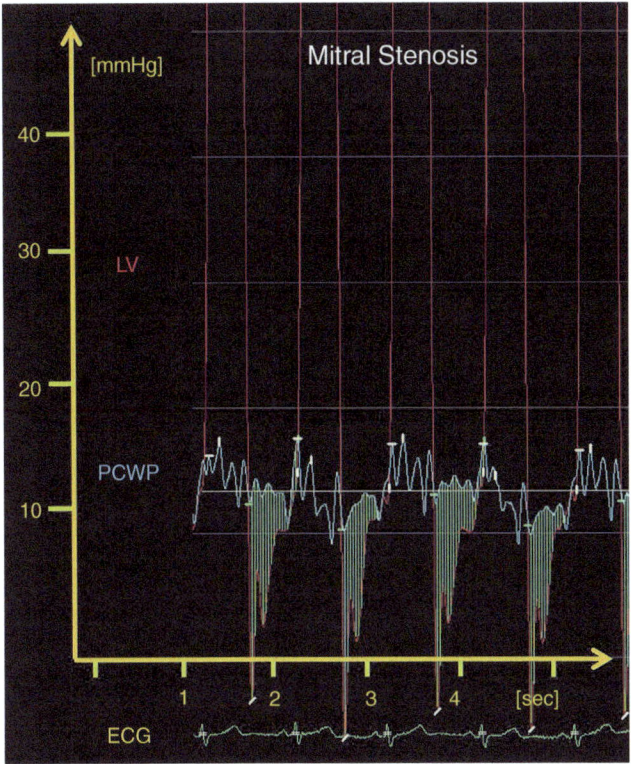

Fig. 2.9 Example of invasive hemodynamics of mitral stenosis. Red LV Pressure curves, blue pulmonary capillary wedge pressure. Green hatched area demonstrates the diastolic pressure gradient above the stenotic valve. Concordant ECG curves are given below

differentiation of soft tissue from calcified mass components.

The most common tumor affecting valves is the papillary fibroelastoma (PFE) (Fig. 2.10). Myxomas, representing the second most common tumor, may arise from valvular endocardium.

PFE are generally benign and composed of collagen (fibro-elastic tissue), avascular papillae, and covered by endothelium. They usually cause no symptoms. However, symptoms may be related to either valvular dysfunction, or embolization into the systemic circulation.

Furthermore, they may cause syncope or other neurological symptoms related to embolism, such as stroke. On CT, PFEs are characterized as hypodense, round shaped masses, with an often irregular surface ("*sea anemone*"—like). Enhancement may be subtle (30–80 HU) or absent. Size typically ranges from 2 mm to 1 cm, and a larger growth is rare. Calcifications are absent. If PFEs are symptomatic, surgery is indicated. PFE typically arise from "downside" endothelium of the valve, hence they are either floating towards the LVOT (if affecting the aortic valve) or the left atrium (if affecting the mitral valve) (Fig. 2.10c, d). The differentiation between PFE and myxoma is very difficult, almost

impossible by CT, and can only reliably be made by pathohistologic examination.

Rarely, thombi attached to native valves may occur. Further, vegetations in the context of infective endocarditis have similar imaging characteristics, but only occur in the presence of inflammatory disease. Calcified masses found on cardiac valves are usually the result of a formerly formed thrombus, vegetation, or chronic rheumatic or degenerative valve disease. Calcified masses appear hyperdense, with CT-attenuation values of >160–200 HU.

Among all cardiac tumors, myxoma represents the most common benign mass. Differential diagnoses are lipomas, which usually occur in the cardiac chambers, and malignant tumors, such as sarcoma, liposarcoma, angiomyolipoma, and lymphoma. Cardiac metastases are rare, and more commonly found in the pericardium and in advanced stages of malignant diseases, such as from melanoma. Notably, cardic masses may be found incidentally on cardiac CT performed for any other indications such as TAVR planning or cororonary artery disease screening.

2.3.1.3 PET

PET has a unique ability to assess the functional and biochemical processes of tissues, which are already altered in the very earliest stages of virtually all diseases. PET allows for detection of these changes usually before anatomical or structural changes occur and become evident on anatomical imaging modalities such as computed tomography or magnetic resonance imaging. Tumor cells maintain a very high glycolytic rate even under aerobic conditions. This constitutes the basis for detection of cancer by FDG-PET, as FDG is an analogon and is metabolized similarly to glucose. FDG is applied in almost all types of cancer diagnosis, staging, restaging, and in monitoring response to cancer treatment with exceptionally high sensitivity. In addition to cancer cells, normal cells such as brain and heart cells or inflammatory cells physiologically metabolize large amounts of glucose due to their high metabolic demand, constituting a potential source of false-positive 18F-FDG PET/CT findings. This may be particularly true in a setting of incidental findings for example during 18F-FDG PET/CT for assessment of infective endocarditis. Therefore, synopsis of all available clinical and imaging information seems mandatory to guide further diagnostic management in these situations.

2.3.2 Frailty Assessment

2.3.2.1 Intro

Frailty is an age related medical syndrome that significantly increases the vulnerability of older adults for negative health outcomes, even when exposed to just minor stressors [69, 70]. Over the past two decades, frailty has been recognized

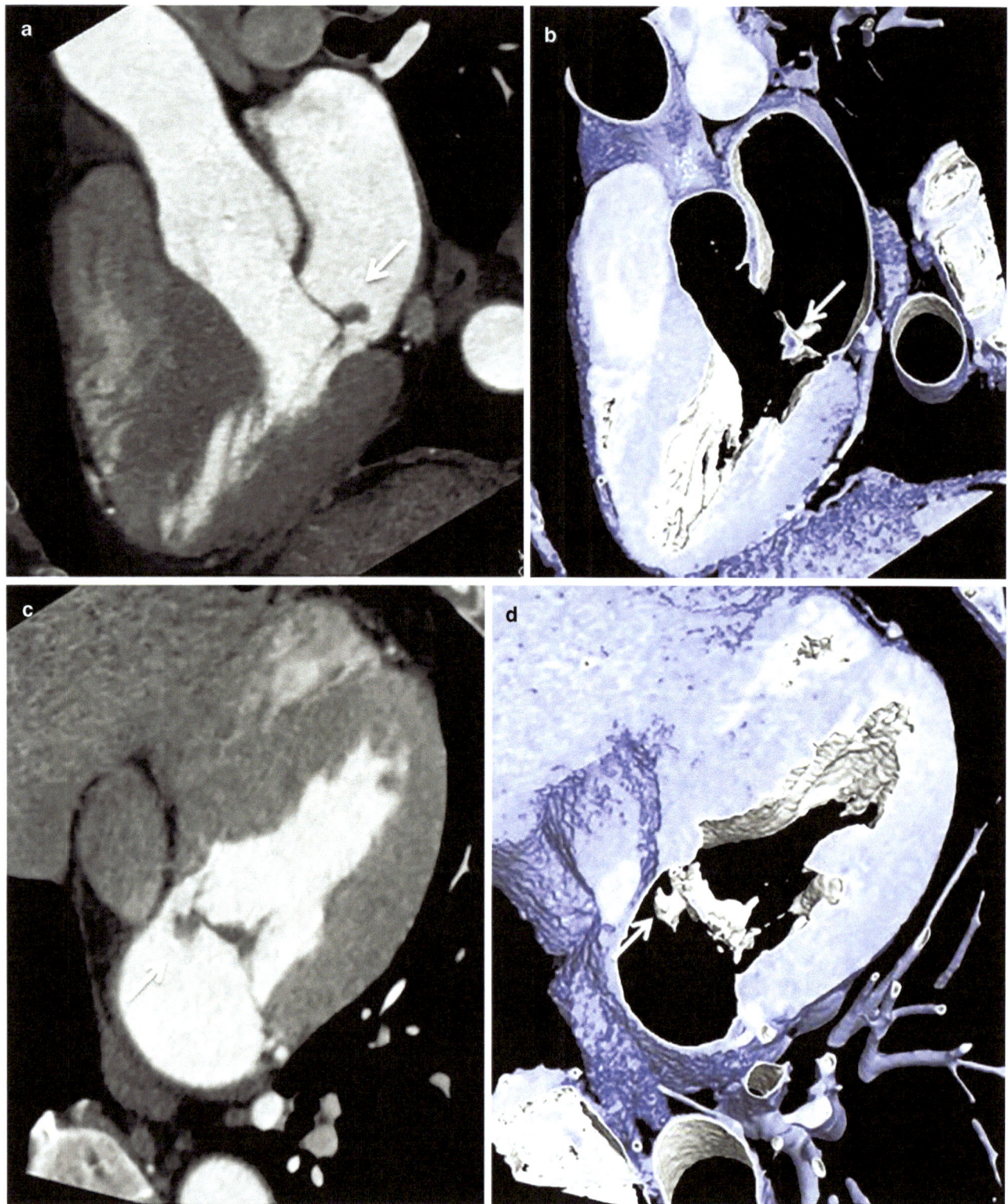

Fig. 2.10 Papillary fibroelastoma (PFE) of the mitral valve: Hypodense mass with irregular surface attached to the anterior cusp, floating into the left atrium on 3-chamber view (**a**. MPR and **b**. corresponding 3-D volume rendering) and thin slice 4-chamber view (**c**., MPR and **d**, volume rendering)

more and more as a state of diminished physiologic resilience [71]. Frailty leads to an increased risk of acute decompensation of health status in multiple situations, from simple urinary tract infections to heart surgery [72, 73]. Today,

advances in medical knowledge and medical technology made formerly invasive surgery procedures, including heart valve replacements within consideration even for frail older adults [6]. In this light, a thorough assessment including frailty status is more important than considering chronological age alone [74]. The current European Society of Cardiology's guidelines acknowledge this development with the recommendation of a structured frailty assessment for the evaluation of older adults with valvular heart disease, since conventional risk prediction scores do not take into account frailty status [6, 73].

In study environments, the frailty phenotype by Fried et al. is the most extensively investigated frailty operationalization together with eight other highly cited instruments [75]. The frailty phenotype is characterized by five signs or symptoms: fatigue, weight loss, weakness, slowness and low activity level. However, no agreement on a reference standard as clinical screening tool has been achieved so far [69, 70]. On the contrary, more than 80 different screening instruments have been published so far for different settings and populations [75]. Notably, the significance of clinically relevant weakness as a core frailty criterion connects frailty with skeletal muscle sarcopenia, characterized by an accelerated decline in muscle-mass and function, and considered a condition preceding frailty [76, 77]. Additionally, and likely closely related to skeletal muscle sarcopenia, there is an evolving concept of age-related cardiac muscle sacropenia [78], which needs further exploration at the human level. Based on animal studies, it has been suggested that cardiac sarcopenia is the age-related involuntary decline in cardiac myocyte numbers and myocardial function [78], very similar to the underlying pathophysiology of skeletal muscle sarcopenia [79–84]. Further, several studies have found an increased risk of skeletal muscle sarcopenia in older adults with chronic heart failure (CHF), the purported clinical picture of cardiac muscle sarcopenia [78, 85–87].

In consequence, a future perspective might be to utilize biomarkers for the detection of sarcopenia obtained from clinical and imaging procedures as a link to frailty status and CHF in older adults [88, 89]. Therefore, the inclusion of geriatric medicine expertise in contemporary heart teams may contribute important risk profiling and treatment of frailty and thereby improve outcomes for older adults evaluated for valvular heart surgery [90, 91].

2.3.2.2 CT

In stable TAVI candidates without acute medical illness, trained nursing staff or medical assistants can conduct a clinical frailty assessment in as little as 15–20 min. For the clinical assessment, weakness is usually evaluated by measuring hand-grip strength with a certified device called dynamometer (in kilograms) or vigorimeter (in kiloPascal) using population-based clinically relevant cut points (lowest 20% or −2 (−2.5) standard deviations below the populations' mean as a threshold [92]. Gait speed, as a robust and convenient marker of physical performance is usually assessed using a standardized 4 m walking test, e.g. from a well validated instrument (Short Physical Performance

Battery) [93]. The low activity criterion is often depicted in different ways. While some authors use an adapted activity questionnaire [94], others simply use reported frequency of going out (i.e. running errands, doing gardening etc.) per week [95] or just classify patients as being "active" or "inactive" [96]. Finally, fatigue is frequently operationalized by items from validated depression screening tools [97] or the presence of tiredness [98]. A score of zero positive items rates a candidate as robust, 1–2 positive items define the at-risk state of "pe-frailty" and ≥3 positive items define present frailty. However, the overall results of the assessment need to be interpreted by a geriatrician and appropriate interventions should be implemented according to the identified risk profile (Fig. 2.11) [99].

Sarcopenia is the age-associated accelerated loss of muscle mass and function [100] and muscle weakness and impaired physical performance are as well core characteristic of physical frailty [101]. Nine different sarcopenia definitions have been published so far, all including lean muscle mass as a biomarker +/− the presence of low muscle strength or low physical performance [83]. Moreover, several working groups have published consensus statements for the diagnosis and treatment of sarcopenia in different settings [76, 88, 102]. Among those, the European Working Group on Sarcopenia in Older People (EWGSOP) published an update of their 2010 clinical definition and consensus diagnostic criteria for sarcopenia in 2018 (EWGSOP2), based on the presence of low muscle mass and either low muscular strength or low physical performance [100]. Of note, the authors highlight the recognition of sarcopenia as an age-related muscle disease ("muscle failure") with its own ICD-10 code (M62.5). Moreover, they state that this should include a perspective change towards focusing more on low muscle strength instead of low muscle mass as the principle determinant for sarcopenia alone in order to expedite the identification of sarcopenia in clinical practice, where the assessment of muscle mass is not always available.

So far, several studies have also investigated CT, MRI, Ultrasonography (US), Dual-energy X-Ray Absorptiometry (DXA) and Bioelectrical Impedance Analysis with promising results for the quantitative and qualitative assessment of muscle mass (examples given in Table 2.1). MRI studies can provide highly reliable information on muscle quality and quantity. However, MRI scans are still not universally available in all health care settings, and are time-consuming and rather expensive. CT scans can be considered to be of almost equal reliability as MRI studies and are a widely available imaging technique in the evaluation of body composition [103]. With CT scans, though, radiation exposition needs to be considered and can limit widespread and repetitive use. DXA represents the most widely used method in assessing appendicular muscle mass (arms and legs) and has the advantage of lower radiation exposure and relatively short duration. Based on DXA, a gold standard

USZ Universitäts Spital Zürich

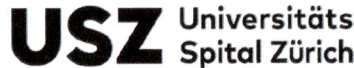

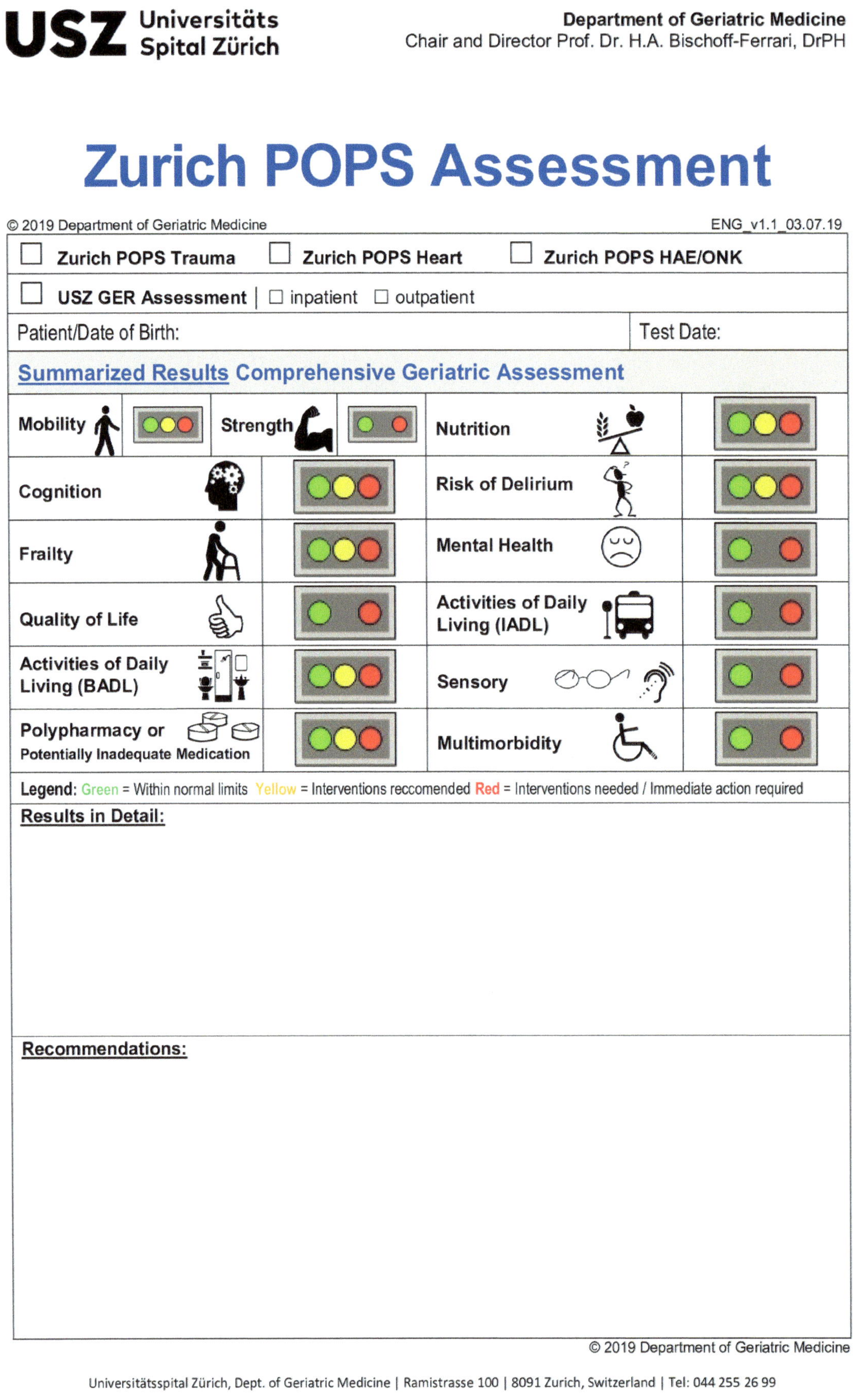

Department of Geriatric Medicine
Chair and Director Prof. Dr. H.A. Bischoff-Ferrari, DrPH

Zurich POPS Assessment

© 2019 Department of Geriatric Medicine — ENG_v1.1_03.07.19

☐ **Zurich POPS Trauma** ☐ **Zurich POPS Heart** ☐ **Zurich POPS HAE/ONK**

☐ **USZ GER Assessment** | ☐ inpatient ☐ outpatient

Patient/Date of Birth: | Test Date:

Summarized Results Comprehensive Geriatric Assessment

Mobility	Strength
Nutrition	
Cognition	Risk of Delirium
Frailty	Mental Health
Quality of Life	Activities of Daily Living (IADL)
Activities of Daily Living (BADL)	Sensory
Polypharmacy or Potentially Inadequate Medication	Multimorbidity

Legend: Green = Within normal limits Yellow = Interventions reccomended Red = Interventions needed / Immediate action required

Results in Detail:

Recommendations:

© 2019 Department of Geriatric Medicine

Universitätsspital Zürich, Dept. of Geriatric Medicine | Ramistrasse 100 | 8091 Zurich, Switzerland | Tel: 044 255 26 99

Fig. 2.11 Overview of the geriatric assessment form as used in the Zurich POPS (Perioperative Care Project for Seniors) project for the evaluation of TAVI candidates)

Table 2.1 Examples of imaging studies for frailty and sarcopenia biomarkers

Study	Measurement	Modality	Setting	Outcome
Wagner (2015) [14] Kleczynski (2018) [22]	Psoas muscle area (PSA/TPA) and Psoas muscle volume (PSV/TPV)	CT	n = 518 patients 65+ scheduled for abdominal surgery n = 153 patients after TAVR	PSA and PSV predicted all-cause mortality at 12 months
Kaplan (2017) [45]	Total muscle cross sectional volume at L3 level. Skeletal muscle index (SMI) thresholds of 52.4 cm^2/m^2 for men and 38.5 cm^2/m^2 for women	CT	n = 450 participants retrospective cohort study from a state trauma registry (USA)	After adjustment, HR was 10.3 (95%CI, 1.3–78.8; P = 0.03) for sarcopenia
Dahya (2016) [43]	Skeletal Muscle Index (SMI, skeletal muscle mass cross-sectional area [cm^2] at L3/height^2)	CT	n = 104 TAVR patients	SMI correlated with age, gender, BMI, handgrip strength, and previous coronary artery bypass graft surgery, but not major complications
Hida (2018) [46]	Thigh muscle thickness (TMT)	US/BIA* *correlation coefficient of 0.38, ($P < 0.001$)	n = 201 participants from Yakumo Study 2014 annual visit, mean age, 66.2 years	Cutoff value, sensitivity, and specificity of TMT in diagnosis of muscle loss were 36 mm, 72.0%, and 73.9%, respectively, for male participants, and 34 mm, 72.2%, and 72.4% for female participants
Melville (2016) [47]	Quadriceps muscle on axial T2 images, and measurement of fractional anisotropy (FA)	MRI	n = 16 participants from Arizona Frailty cohort study (non-frail, pre-frail/ frail) and n = 10 community sample controls	Mean FA values demonstrated significant differences ($P = 0.0030$) between the control and prefrail/frail and non-frail and pre-frail/ frail groups. Significant difference in mean T2 ($P < 0.0001$) and lipid content ($P < 0.0001$) among all three groups in the total quadriceps muscle group
Baumgartner (1998) [37]	Appendicular Skeletal Muscle mass—ASM (Sarcopenia defined as ASM (kg/height^2 (m^2) below 2 SD of mean of a young reference group: ≤ 7.26 kg/m^2 in men, and ≤ 5.45 kg/m^2 in women	DXA	n = 883 community dwelling older adults from New Mexico, USA	Sarcopenia significantly associated with self-reported physical disability

BIA bioelectrical impedance analysis, *CT* computed tomography, *DXA* dual-energy X-Ray absorptiometry, *MRI* magnetic resonance imaging, *US* ultrasonography, *TAVR* trans-catheter aortic valve replacement

method is to calculate the relative skeletal muscle index (RSMI) by Baumgartner et al. with muscle mass (kg) divided by height (m) squared (kg/m^2). Low muscle mass, based on the Baumgartner definition, is defined at values less than 2 SD below a gender specific mean (healthy, younger person) of 7.26 in men, and less than 5.45 in women [104]. This operationalization has shown a high validity in the prediction of falls, a clinical hallmark of frailty and sarcopenia [83]. Current research efforts are in search of alternative biomarkers of frailty, and may extend to other organ systems such as cardiac muscle sarcopenia [78] or cerebral grey matter volume [105].

2.3.2.2.1 Case Finding in a University Geriatric Outpatient Clinic

An 88 year old man with coronary artery disease and recent hospitalization due to heart failure presented to the Geriatric Outpatient Clinic for a follow-up visit after hospital discharge. He complained of nausea and reduced appetite. He reported a loss of 2.5 kg of body weight over the last 6 weeks due to reduced food intake. Geriatric assessment revealed frailty with weight loss, low grip strength, slow gait speed and

low activity level present (4 of 5 Fried criteria positive). Body composition assessment with DXA confirmed low muscle mass with a reduced RSMI of 6.75 kg/m^2 (RSMI ≤ 7.26 kg/m^2 in men is indicative of sarcopenia, Fig. 2.12). We adjusted his medications and started a strength exercise program and protein supplements. In the follow up visit, his appetite and strength improved and he was able to travel again.

In conclusion, A comprehensive frailty assessment in the evaluation of potential heart surgery candidates seems promising as a novel personalized risk evaluation approach in older adults. Clinical frailty imaging in this context provides surgeons with a profound basis for decision-making. As new data gathers, first results seem encouraging to adapt this approach also to other fields of surgery [106, 107].

In summary, we recommend the use of a validated clinical frailty-screening tool in older adults evaluated as candidates for trans-catheter aortic valve replacement. So far, the evidence for imaging techniques including CT, MRI and US have yielded promising results in the detection of sarcopenia, but not frailty so far. To date, there is not enough evidence available to advice for the use of radiologic imaging in clinical routine, as more studies are needed that compare imaging modalities at the

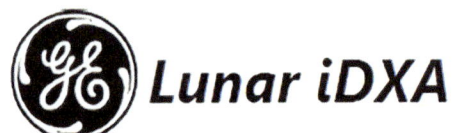

USZ Zurich
Geriatrie RAE B03
CH-8091 Zurich
Phone:

Client	Sex	Ethnicity	Birth Date	Height	Weight	Measured
██████████████	Male	White	01.03.1927	164.0 cm	63.0 kg	23.02.2016

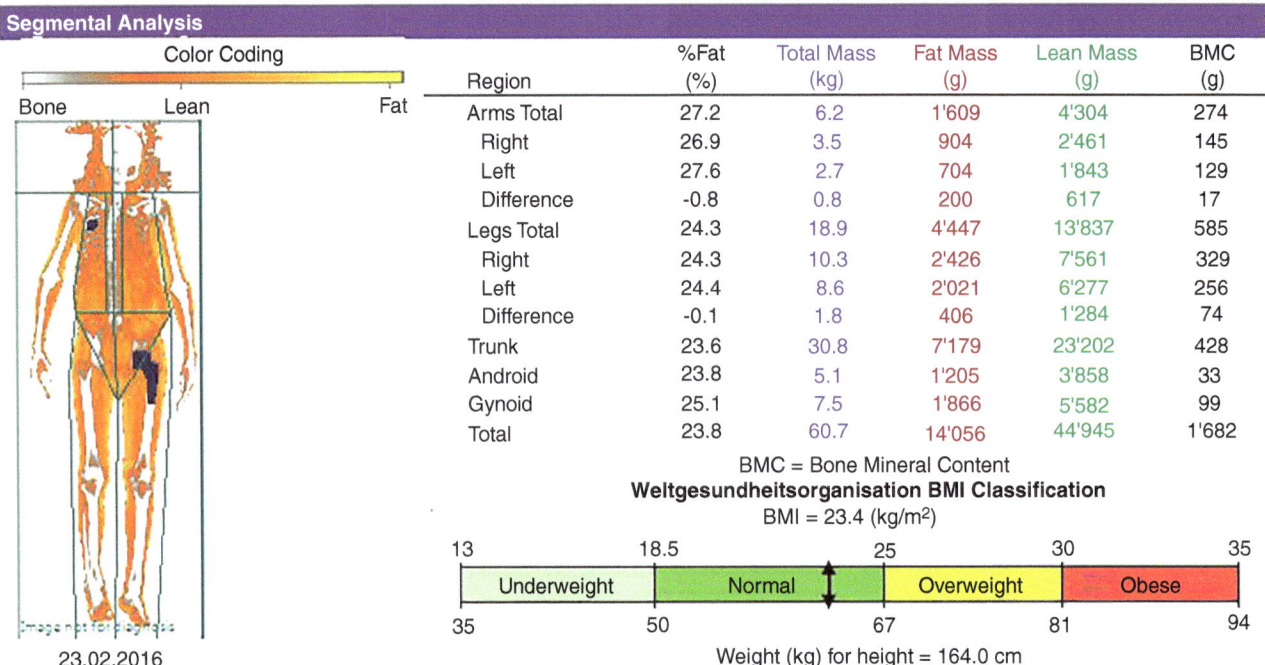

Segmental Analysis						
Region	%Fat (%)	Total Mass (kg)	Fat Mass (g)	Lean Mass (g)	BMC (g)
Arms Total	27.2	6.2	1'609	4'304	274
Right	26.9	3.5	904	2'461	145
Left	27.6	2.7	704	1'843	129
Difference	-0.8	0.8	200	617	17
Legs Total	24.3	18.9	4'447	13'837	585
Right	24.3	10.3	2'426	7'561	329
Left	24.4	8.6	2'021	6'277	256
Difference	-0.1	1.8	406	1'284	74
Trunk	23.6	30.8	7'179	23'202	428
Android	23.8	5.1	1'205	3'858	33
Gynoid	25.1	7.5	1'866	5'582	99
Total	23.8	60.7	14'056	44'945	1'682

BMC = Bone Mineral Content

Weltgesundheitsorganisation BMI Classification

BMI = 23.4 (kg/m²)

23.02.2016

Weight (kg) for height = 164.0 cm

Fig. 2.12 Body composition as measured by iDXA indicating total mass, fat mass and lean mass. Calculated Relative Skeletal Muscle Index (RSMI) was low (6.75 kg/m²) indicating Sarcopenia (cut points ≤7.26 kg/m² in men, and ≤5.45 kg/m² in women)

same time in the same patient group. Therefore, it seems rather unlikely that a comprehensive clinical evaluation of frailty can be substituted by a single imaging technique measurement in the near future. At the same time, novel methods and biomarkers should be incorporated in future research studies on the operationalization of frailty [108].

2.4 Valvular Disease as Result of Chronic Medical Disorders

2.4.1 Amyloidosis

Amyloidosis represents a heterogeneous group of acquired or hereditary pathologies, localized or systemic, that share a characteristic: the extracellular deposition of insoluble fibrillary proteins that determines a disorganization of the structure of the tissues involved with consequent organ - dysfunction. In general, the heart is one of the "target" organs in which amyloid is most frequently deposited [109, 110].

Amyloid can infiltrate any cardiovascular structure, infiltration of the conduction system may lead to branch blocks or even atrioventricular blocks and sinoatrial blocks. The results of myocardial infiltration are instead represented by a progressive increase in the thickness of the walls of the left and right ventricle and the interatrial septum. In fact, cardiac amyloidosis is often described as a cardiac disease with a "hypertrophic phenotype" and restrictive physiology leading to diastolic heart failure. Heart valve involvement is frequent and generally accompanied by a variable (usually mild) degree of valvular regurgitation.

2.4.1.1 Echocardiography

Echocardiography is the main instrumental examination for the non-invasive diagnosis of cardiac amyloidosis. As in other etiologies, *Transthyretin* (TTR)-related amyloidosis is characterized by thickening of the ventricular walls with a typical "granular sparkling" appearance in the absence of dilation of the left ventricle. Further indications for infiltrative heart disease include thickening of the free wall of the right ventricle and interatrial septum, bi-atrial dilatation, diffuse thickening of the atrioventricular valves and mild pericardial effusion. The ejection fraction of the left ventricle is often normal, but the speed of movement of the ventricular

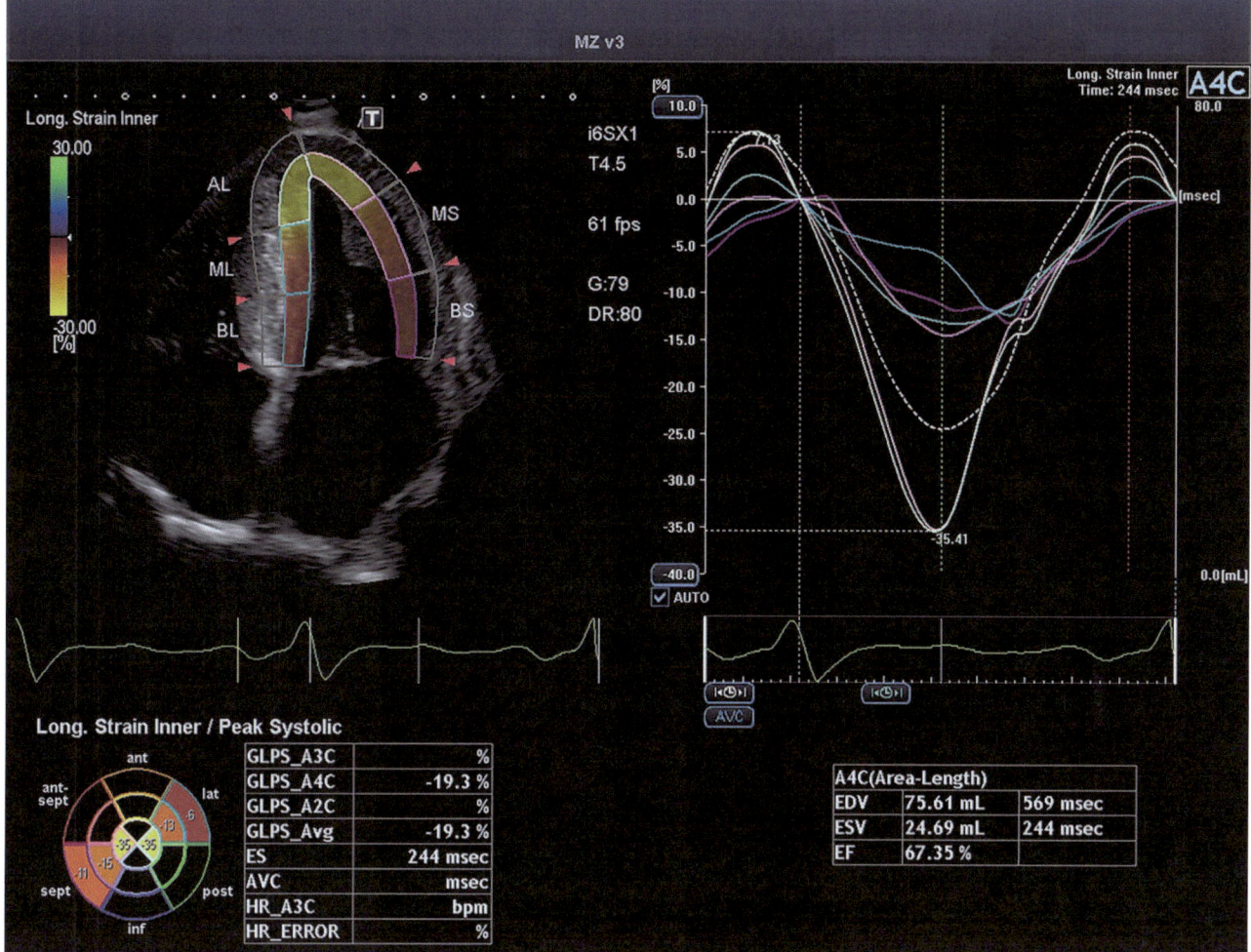

Fig. 2.13 Four-chamber view of ventricular depressed global longitudinal strain in a patient affected by Amyloidosis

walls and both the degree of deformation ("strain") and the rate of deformation over time ("strain rate") of the ventricular myocardium are frequently depressed (Fig. 2.13) [111].

Alterations in the longitudinal contractility of the left ventricle (detectable with tissue Doppler and speckle tracking images) are frequent and appear in the early stages of the disease, when the shortening function is still preserved. The longitudinal "strain" also has a typical pattern that differentiates it from other cardiomyopathies: severe reduction of the deformation values at the base of the left ventricle and saving of the apex. The combined analysis of the transmitral Doppler and the tissue Doppler frequently suggests a high telediastolic pressure and/or a restrictive filling pattern.

2.4.1.2 Scintigraphy

Scintigraphy using bone tracers, in particular 99mTc-3,3-diphosphone-1,2-propane-carboxylic acid (99mTc-DPD) has been documented to bind to TTR deposits but not to conventional (AL) deposits. The method has been shown to be highly sensitive for the detection of cardiac ATTR amyloidosis and,

within certain limits, allows for the differential diagnosis between the two etiological forms [112, 113]. It is important to underline the sensitivity of this technique, which is capable of identifying early myocardial infiltration even before the appearance of echocardiographic abnormalities (Fig. 2.14).

2.5 Special Precautions for Imaging in Patients Subsets

2.5.1 Pregnancy Echo, MRI, CT, PET, Nuclear

Fortunately, cardiac imaging offers a diversity of modalities with each technique providing advantages and disadvantages. Due to the availability of all those modalities, it is important to select the best one for each patient, especially in a vulnerable population such as pregnant women. The American College of Obstetricians and Gynecologists published guidelines for diagnostic imaging during pregnancy and lactation [114] and amended a committee opinion in 2017 [115].

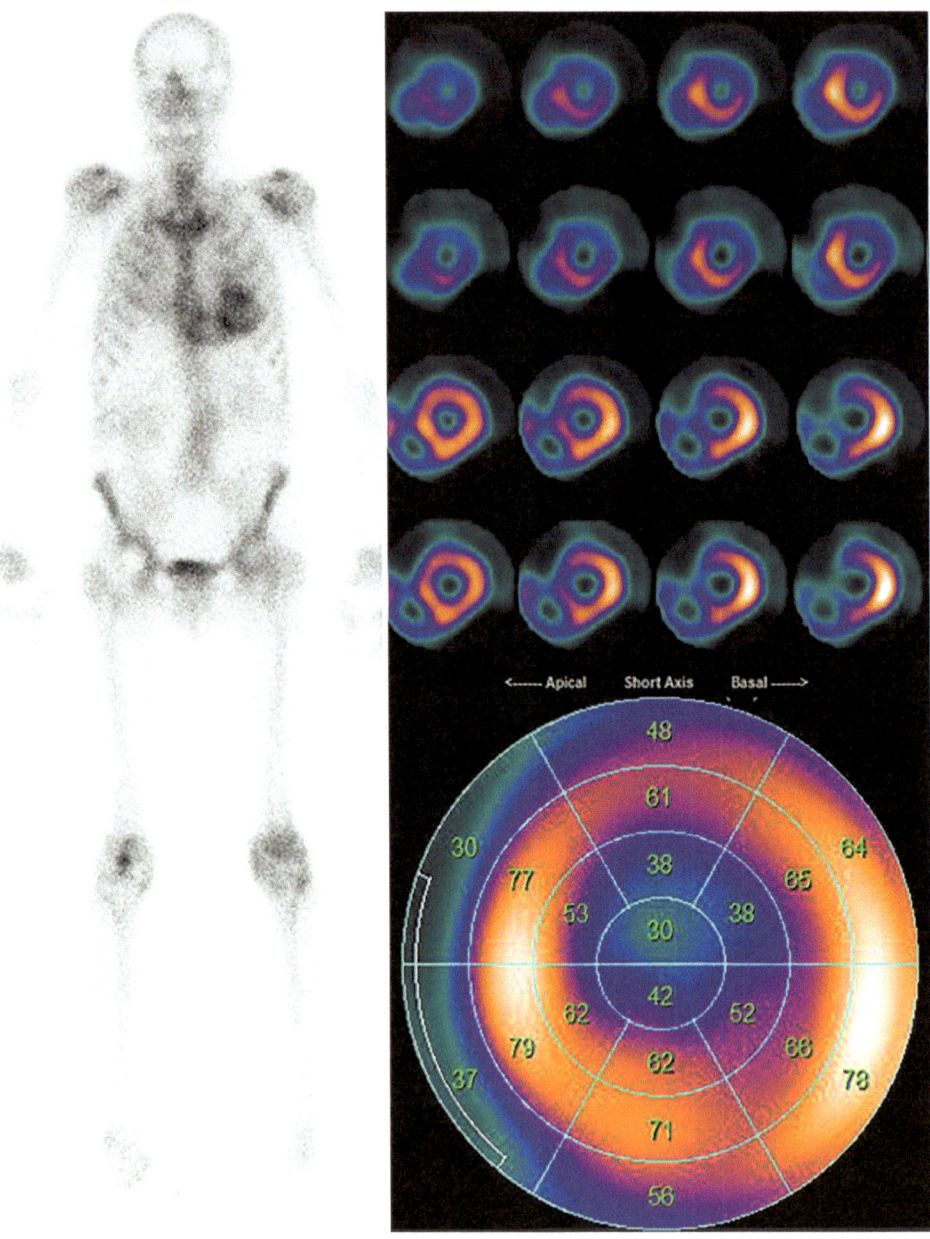

Fig. 2.14 99mTc-DPD whole-body scintigraphy (left) and single-photon-emission-computed-tomography (SPECT, right) reveals significant tracer accumulation in the heart with apical sparing, typical for cardiac ATTR-Amyloidosis in the absence of evidence for AL-Amyloidosis

Ultrasound waves can increase temperature of the fetus >2°C if transducers with high spatial peak temporal average intensity (>720 ms/cm²) are used. If machines are used that are configured correctly, ultrasound does not pose a risk to the fetus [115].

CMR uses electromagnetic radio waves. Direct biologic effects of magnetic resonance imaging (heating) and acoustic damage from high intense noise might play a role in pregnant women undergoing CMR. However, heating of the fetus has been proposed to be negligible during magnetic resonance imaging [116] and no acoustic injuries to the fetus have been reported [117]. Based on this evidence, the American College of Radiology recommended no special consideration for the first (versus any other) trimester in pregnancy [118]. Beside the magnetic resonance itself, the injection of gadolinium-based contrast agents has to be discussed, as this is often necessary for further tissue-characterization in MRI and for perfusion images. Gadolinium-based contrast agents cross the placenta and are excreted by the fetus into the amniotic fluid [118]. Recently, the use of linear gadolinium based contrast agents has been restricted as gadolinium brain deposits were found. Based on current findings the use of gadolinium based contrast agents should be limited to situations in which the benefits clearly outweigh the possible risk [115].

In contrast to CMR, CTA is based on ionizing radiation. The risk of ionizing radiation to harm the fetus depends on two factors: the effective radiation dose and the age of the fetus. Growth restriction, microcephaly, and intellectual disability are adverse effects from high-dose radiation exposure within the most vulnerable period (8–15 weeks of gestation) and an estimated threshold dose of 60–310 mGy, which increases to 250–280 mGy between 16 and 25 weeks of gestation [115, 119]. Whether in-utero exposure of ionizing radiation results in risk of carcinogenesis is unclear. A 10–20 mGy fetal exposures may increase the risk of leukemia by a factor of 1.5–2 [120]. It is important to know that modern ECG-triggered computed tomography of the heart is possible with less than 0.5 mSv. According to the American College of Obstetricians and Gynecologists committee, the use of CT should not be withheld if clinically indicated [115]. If available in a timely manner, MRI should be considered as an alternative to CT during pregnancy if both modalities are equivalent for diagnosis. Although iodinated contrast media can cross the placenta, animal studies have reported no teratogenic or mutagenic effects [121]. Despite this lack of known harm, it is recommended that contrast media should only be used if absolutely required to obtain additional diagnostic information that will affect the care of the fetus or woman during pregnancy [115].

During pregnancy, the fetal exposure during nuclear medicine studies depends on the properties of the radioisotope. Technetium 99m is one of the most commonly used isotope for the cardiovascular system. In general, these procedures result in a fetal exposure of less than 5 mGy which is considered a safe dose in pregnancy [115]. However, other radioisotopes such as iodine 131—which is not used for the cardiovascular system—cannot be used safely during pregnancy. Of note PET myocardial perfusion studies require an even lower radiation exposure in the range of 1–3 mSv.

2.5.2 Renal Failure Echo, MRI, CT, PET, Nuclear

Echocardiography: Image quality in echocardiography may be impaired in obese patients or in patients with lung disease. In such cases an ultrasonic contrast medium based on microbubbles can be injected. These microbubbles have a substantial persistence in the blood stream and are small enough to pass through the microcirculation and finally increase left ventricular opacification and enhancement of the endocardial border. The contrast medium is rapidly eliminated from the blood by means of the lungs in the expired air. Relative to renal function, there is no evidence of any adverse effect [122].

MRI: A substantial number of MRI sequences are depending on the use of intravenous injection of a Gadolinium (Gd) based contrast agend (GBCA) to improve diagnostic power. Because free Gd ions are highly toxic to the body, they have to be tightly bound within the GBCA. Depending on the chemical structure GBCAs can be divided into cyclic versus linear, respectively ionic versus non-ionic compound.

Recently, there have been two major health issues described with GBCAs, i.e. nephrogenic systemic fibrosis (NSF) and the deposition of Gd in the brain tissue [123, 124]. The risk of these conditions is partly related to their molecular structure and particular NSF is specific to certain patient groups, such as renal failure [123–125].

NSF is a rare, progressive, life-threatening condition with fibrosis of multiple organs after GBCA injection in patients with severe renal insufficiency. Based on their chemical properties GBCAs have been categorised to NSF risk. Fortunately, NSF could be vastly decreased by following safety precautions, such as abandonment of non-ionic linear GBCAs, limiting GBCA to a maximum dose, and dialyzing patients with severe chronic insufficiency rapidly following GBCA use [126].

The extend of Gd deposits in the brain varies between different agents. Linear GBCA appear to cause greater signal changes than cyclic compounds. So far, no adverse clinical effects could be observed. However, more data is needed to evaluate the relevance of the described Gd deposition [126].

CT: One of the most important side effects of diagnostic CT contrast agents is contrast-induced acute kidney injury (CI-AKI). CI-AKI is defined as a sudden decrease in renal function within a few days after injection of CT contrast agent that cannot be attributed to other causes. It is well accepted that there is no risk of CI-AKI in patients with normal renal function, however in subjects with pre-existing renal failure, particular with an eGFR <30 mL/min/1.73 m^2, CI-AKI might be a serious complication [127]. In these patients it is important to lower the risk of CI-AKI by reduction of contrast medium and intravenous hydration once there is a lack of alternatives to contrast-enhanced CT [128].

Nuclear cardiology: Single Emission Computed Tomography (SPECT) and Positron Emission Tomography (PET) are both nuclear imaging techniques using radioactive imaging agents designed to visualize myocardial perfusion. SPECT requires a gamma- (i.e. 99m-Technetium Tetrofosmin), PET a beta-emitting radionuclide (i.e. 13N-ammonia). The administration of radioactive substances to humans for diagnostic purposes is a well established and individual organ doses as well as total body effective doses are given for these specified examinations [129].

2.5.3 Patient with Permanent PM Echo, MRI, CT, PET, Nuclear

Echocardiography can be used safely in patients with pacemaker. During echocardiography, there is a typical wall motion appearance in patients with pacemaker due to pacemaker induced left bundle branch block and described as septal flash and apical rocking.

Cardiac magnetic resonance consists of the static and the gradient magnetic field and the radiofrequency energy.

The combination of those fields or one field alone are able to interact with metallic objects and potentially harm the patient due to magnetic field-induced forces (generator movement) [130], currents in conductive wires (myocardial capture) [131], heating (thermal damage) [132], effects on reed switch activity [133], electrical reset [134], inappropriate function ant therapy [135]. Additionally pacemaker systems can cause various types of artefacts. In 2017 an expert consensus statement on magnetic resonance imaging and radiation exposure in patients with cardiovascular implantable electronic devices was published by the Heart Rhythm Society [136]. Based on the consensus statement, magnetic resonance conditional systems are distinguished from non-conditional systems. For conditional systems, a specified magnetic resonance environment with specified conditions of use does not pose a known hazard. It is important that the whole pacemaker system has to be checked, e.g. generator and leads. In the past few years, due to advances in engineering and manufacturing, a variety of pacemakers and defibrillators have been approved as magnetic resonance conditional. However, a magnetic resonance conditional device is only conditional if product leveling is adhered to. This includes programming of the device to an appropriate magnetic resonance mode and scanning with the prerequisites specific for the device.

Computed tomography is considered safe for patients with cardiac implantable electronic devices and it is therefore recommended that patients with a cardiac implantable electronic device undergo clinical diagnostic computed tomography without any additional device interrogation, programming or monitoring [136]. However, imaging artefacts such as beam hardening may reduce image quality. Novel techniques such as 640-slice computed tomography [137] or single energy metal artifact reduction technique have drastically reduced such artefacts [138].

There is no direct interference between diagnostic nuclear studies and pacemakers. This provides an unique advantage over other modalities as there are no imaging artefacts due to the pacemaker leads. During diagnostic procedures radiation exposure is too low to cause harm, however as much higher doses are used during radiation therapy, this can result in a damage of the device. Cumulative dose damage formed the basis of the recommendations in the American Association of Physicists in Medicine (AAPM) 1994 report, which set 2 Gy as a threshold dose above which the device could be at an elevated risk of damage [139].

References

1. Montalescot G, Sechtem U, Achenbach S, Andreotti F, Arden C, Budaj A, Bugiardini R, Crea F, Cuisset T, Di Mario C, Ferreira JR, Gersh BJ, Gitt AK, Hulot JS, Marx N, Opie LH, Pfisterer M, Prescott E, Ruschitzka F, Sabate M, Senior R, Taggart DP, van der Wall EE, Vrints CJ, Zamorano JL, Achenbach S, Baumgartner H, Bax JJ, Bueno H, Dean V, Deaton C, Erol C, Fagard R, Ferrari R, Hasdai D, Hoes AW, Kirchhof P, Knuuti J, Kolh P, Lancellotti P, Linhart A, Nihoyannopoulos P, Piepoli MF, Ponikowski P, Sirnes PA, Tamargo JL, Tendera M, Torbicki A, Wijns W, Windecker S, Knuuti J, Valgimigli M, Bueno H, Claeys MJ, Donner-Banzhoff N, Erol C, Frank H, Funck-Brentano C, Gaemperli O, Gonzalez-Juanatey JR, Hamilos M, Hasdai D, Husted S, James SK, Kervinen K, Kolh P, Kristensen SD, Lancellotti P, Maggioni AP, Piepoli MF, Pries AR, Romeo F, Ryden L, Simoons ML, Sirnes PA, Steg PG, Timmis A, Wijns W, Windecker S, Yildirir A, Zamorano JL. 2013 ESC guidelines on the management of stable coronary artery disease: the Task Force on the management of stable coronary artery disease of the European Society of Cardiology. Eur Heart J. 2013;34(38):2949–3003.

2. Lindsay AC, Sriharan M, Lazoura O, Sau A, Roughton M, Jabbour RJ, Di Mario C, Davies SW, Moat NE, Padley SP, Rubens MB, Nicol ED. Clinical and economic consequences of non-cardiac incidental findings detected on cardiovascular computed tomography performed prior to transcatheter aortic valve implantation (TAVI). Int J Cardiovasc Imaging. 2015;31(7):1435–46.

3. van Kesteren F, Wiegerinck EMA, van Mourik MS, Vis MM, Koch KT, Piek JJ, Stoker J, Tijssen JG, Baan J Jr, Planken RN. Impact of potentially malignant incidental findings by computed tomographic angiography on long-term survival after transcatheter aortic valve implantation. Am J Cardiol. 2017;120(6):994–1001.

4. Henn MC, Zajarias A, Lindman BR, Greenberg JW, Melby SJ, Quader N, Vatterott AM, Lawler C, Damiano MS, Novak E, Lasala JM, Moon MR, Lawton JS, Damiano RJ Jr, Maniar HS. Preoperative pulmonary function tests predict mortality after surgical or transcatheter aortic valve replacement. J Thorac Cardiovasc Surg. 2016;151(2):578–85, 586.e1-2.

5. Afilalo J, Lauck S, Kim DH, Lefevre T, Piazza N, Lachapelle K, Martucci G, Lamy A, Labinaz M, Peterson MD, Arora RC, Noiseux N, Rassi A, Palacios IF, Genereux P, Lindman BR, Asgar AW, Kim CA, Trnkus A, Morais JA, Langlois Y, Rudski LG, Morin JF, Popma JJ, Webb JG, Perrault LP. Frailty in older adults undergoing aortic valve replacement: the FRAILTY-AVR Study. J Am Coll Cardiol. 2017;70(6):689–700.

6. Baumgartner H, Falk V, Bax JJ, De Bonis M, Hamm C, Holm PJ, Iung B, Lancellotti P, Lansac E, Rodriguez Munoz D, Rosenhek R, Sjogren J, Tornos Mas P, Vahanian A, Walther T, Wendler O, Windecker S, Zamorano JL. 2017 ESC/EACTS Guidelines for the management of valvular heart disease. Eur Heart J. 2017;38(36):2739–91.

7. Paradis JM, Fried J, Nazif T, Kirtane A, Harjai K, Khalique O, Grubb K, George I, Hahn R, Williams M, Leon MB, Kodali S. Aortic stenosis and coronary artery disease: what do we know? What don't we know? A comprehensive review of the literature with proposed treatment algorithms. Eur Heart J. 2014;35(31):2069–82.

8. Nishimura RA, Otto CM, Bonow RO, Carabello BA, Erwin JP 3rd, Fleisher LA, Jneid H, Mack MJ, McLeod CJ, O'Gara PT, Rigolin VH, Sundt TM 3rd, Thompson A. 2017 AHA/ACC focused update of the 2014 AHA/ACC guideline for the management of patients with valvular heart disease: a report of the American College of Cardiology/American Heart Association Task Force on Clinical Practice Guidelines. Circulation. 2017;135(25):e1159–95.

9. Nishimura RA, Otto CM, Bonow RO, Carabello BA, Erwin JP 3rd, Guyton RA, O'Gara PT, Ruiz CE, Skubas NJ, Sorajja P, Sundt TM 3rd, Thomas JD. 2014 AHA/ACC guideline for the management of patients with valvular heart disease: a report of the American College of Cardiology/American Heart Association Task Force on Practice Guidelines. J Am Coll Cardiol. 2014;63(22):e57–185.

10. Kotronias RA, Kwok CS, George S, Capodanno D, Ludman PF, Townend JN, Doshi SN, Khogali SS, Genereux P, Herrmann HC, Mamas MA, Bagur R. Transcatheter aortic valve implantation with or without percutaneous coronary artery revascularization strategy: a systematic review and meta-analysis. J Am Heart Assoc. 2017;6(6):e005960.

11. Huczek Z, Zbronski K, Grodecki K, Scislo P, Rymuza B, Kochman J, Dabrowski M, Witkowski A, Wojakowski W, Parma R, Ochala A, Grygier M, Olasinska-Wisniewska A, Araszkiewicz A, Jagielak D, Ciecwierz D, Puchta D, Paczwa K, Filipiak KJ, Wilimski R, Zembala M, Opolski G. Concomitant coronary artery disease and its management in patients referred to transcatheter aortic valve implantation: Insights from the POL-TAVI Registry. Catheter Cardiovasc Interv. 2018;91(1):115–23.

12. Sankaramangalam K, Banerjee K, Kandregula K, Mohananey D, Parashar A, Jones BM, Jobanputra Y, Mick S, Krishnaswamy A, Svensson LG, Kapadia SR. Impact of coronary artery disease on 30-day and 1-year mortality in patients undergoing transcatheter aortic valve replacement: a meta-analysis. J Am Heart Assoc. 2017;6(10):e006092.

13. Zivelonghi C, Pesarini G, Scarsini R, Lunardi M, Piccoli A, Ferrero V, Gottin L, Vassanelli C, Ribichini F. Coronary catheterization and percutaneous interventions after transcatheter aortic valve implantation. Am J Cardiol. 2017;120(4):625–31.

14. Rossi A, De Cecco CN, Kennon SRO, Zou L, Meinel FG, Toscano W, Segreto S, Achenbach S, Hausleiter J, Schoepf UJ, Pugliese F. CT angiography to evaluate coronary artery disease and revascularization requirement before trans-catheter aortic valve replacement. J Cardiovasc Comput Tomogr. 2017;11(5):338–46.

15. Nkomo VT, Gardin JM, Skelton TN, Gottdiener JS, Scott CG, Enriquez-Sarano M. Burden of valvular heart diseases: a population-based study. Lancet. 2006;368(9540):1005–11.

16. Cortes C, Amat-Santos IJ, Nombela-Franco L, Munoz-Garcia AJ, Gutierrez-Ibanes E, De La Torre Hernandez JM, Cordoba-Soriano JG, Jimenez-Quevedo P, Hernandez-Garcia JM, Gonzalez-Mansilla A, Ruano J, Jimenez-Mazuecos J, Castrodeza J, Tobar J, Islas F, Revilla A, Puri R, Puerto A, Gomez I, Rodes-Cabau J, San Roman JA. Mitral regurgitation after transcatheter aortic valve replacement: prognosis, imaging predictors, and potential management. JACC Cardiovasc Interv. 2016;9(15):1603–14.

17. Chakravarty T, Van Belle E, Jilaihawi H, Noheria A, Testa L, Bedogni F, Ruck A, Barbanti M, Toggweiler S, Thomas M, Khawaja MZ, Hutter A, Abramowitz Y, Siegel RJ, Cheng W, Webb J, Leon MB, Makkar RR. Meta-analysis of the impact of mitral regurgitation on outcomes after transcatheter aortic valve implantation. Am J Cardiol. 2015;115(7):942–9.

18. Suh WM, Witzke CF, Palacios IF. Suicide left ventricle following transcatheter aortic valve implantation. Catheter Cardiovasc Interv. 2010;76(4):616–20.

19. Sorajja P, Booker JD, Rihal CS. Alcohol septal ablation after transaortic valve implantation: the dynamic nature of left outflow tract obstruction. Catheter Cardiovasc Interv. 2013;81(2):387–91.

20. Neumann FJ, Sousa-Uva M, Ahlsson A, Alfonso F, Banning AP, Benedetto U, Byrne RA, Collet JP, Falk V, Head SJ, Juni P, Kastrati A, Koller A, Kristensen SD, Niebauer J, Richter DJ, Seferovic PM, Sibbing D, Stefanini GG, Windecker S, Yadav R, Zembala MO. 2018 ESC/EACTS Guidelines on myocardial revascularization. Eur Heart J. 2019;40(2):87–165.

21. Douglas PS, Hoffmann U. Anatomical versus functional testing for coronary artery disease. N Engl J Med. 2015;373(1):91.

22. Budoff MJ, Dowe D, Jollis JG, Gitter M, Sutherland J, Halamert E, Scherer M, Bellinger R, Martin A, Benton R, Delago A, Min JK. Diagnostic performance of 64-multidetector row coronary computed tomographic angiography for evaluation of coronary artery stenosis in individuals without known coronary artery disease: results from the prospective multicenter ACCURACY (Assessment by Coronary Computed Tomographic Angiography of Individuals Undergoing Invasive Coronary Angiography) trial. J Am Coll Cardiol. 2008;52(21):1724–32.

23. Nakazato R, Arsanjani R, Achenbach S, Gransar H, Cheng VY, Dunning A, Lin FY, Al-Mallah M, Budoff MJ, Callister TQ, Chang HJ, Cademartiri F, Chinnaiyan K, Chow BJ, Delago A, Hadamitzky M, Hausleiter J, Kaufmann P, Raff G, Shaw LJ, Villines T, Cury RC, Feuchtner G, Kim YJ, Leipsic J, Berman DS, Min JK. Age-related risk of major adverse cardiac event risk and coronary artery disease extent and severity by coronary CT angiography: results from 15 187 patients from the International Multisite CONFIRM Study. Eur Heart J Cardiovasc Imaging. 2014;15(5):586–94.

24. Leipsic J, Yang TH, Thompson A, Koo BK, Mancini GB, Taylor C, Budoff MJ, Park HB, Berman DS, Min JK. CT angiography (CTA) and diagnostic performance of noninvasive fractional flow reserve: results from the Determination of Fractional Flow Reserve by Anatomic CTA (DeFACTO) study. Am J Roentgenol. 2014;202(5):989–94.

25. Hlatky MA, De Bruyne B, Pontone G, Patel MR, Norgaard BL, Byrne RA, Curzen N, Purcell I, Gutberlet M, Rioufol G, Hink U, Schuchlenz HW, Feuchtner G, Gilard M, Andreini D, Jensen JM, Hadamitzky M, Wilk A, Wang F, Rogers C, Douglas PS. Quality-of-life and economic outcomes of assessing fractional flow reserve with computed tomography angiography: PLATFORM. J Am Coll Cardiol. 2015;66(21):2315–23.

26. Thomsen C, Abdulla J. Characteristics of high-risk coronary plaques identified by computed tomographic angiography and associated prognosis: a systematic review and meta-analysis. Eur Heart J Cardiovasc Imaging. 2016;17(2):120–9.

27. Ahmadi A, Leipsic J, Ovrehus KA, Gaur S, Bagiella E, Ko B, Dey D, LaRocca G, Jensen JM, Botker HE, Achenbach S, De Bruyne B, Norgaard BL, Narula J. Lesion-specific and vessel-related determinants of fractional flow reserve beyond coronary artery stenosis. JACC Cardiovasc Imaging. 2018;11(4):521–30.

28. Maurovich-Horvat P, Schlett CL, Alkadhi H, Nakano M, Otsuka F, Stolzmann P, Scheffel H, Ferencik M, Kriegel MF, Seifarth H, Virmani R, Hoffmann U. The napkin-ring sign indicates advanced atherosclerotic lesions in coronary CT angiography. JACC Cardiovasc Imaging. 2012;5(12):1243–52.

29. Leber AW, Knez A, Becker A, Becker C, von Ziegler F, Nikolaou K, Rist C, Reiser M, White C, Steinbeck G, Boekstegers P. Accuracy of multidetector spiral computed tomography in identifying and differentiating the composition of coronary atherosclerotic plaques: a comparative study with intracoronary ultrasound. J Am Coll Cardiol. 2004;43(7):1241–7.

30. Cury RC, Abbara S, Achenbach S, Agatston A, Berman DS, Budoff MJ, Dill KE, Jacobs JE, Maroules CD, Rubin GD, Rybicki FJ, Schoepf UJ, Shaw LJ, Stillman AE, White CS, Woodard PK, Leipsic JA. CAD-RADS (TM) Coronary Artery Disease—Reporting and Data System. An expert consensus document of the Society of Cardiovascular Computed Tomography (SCCT), the American College of Radiology (ACR) and the North American Society for Cardiovascular Imaging (NASCI). Endorsed by the American College of Cardiology. J Cardiovasc Comput Tomogr. 2016;10(4):269–81.

31. Nakazato R, Otake H, Konishi A, Iwasaki M, Koo BK, Fukuya H, Shinke T, Hirata K, Leipsic J, Berman DS, Min JK. Atherosclerotic plaque characterization by CT angiography for identification of high-risk coronary artery lesions: a comparison to optical coherence tomography. Eur Heart J Cardiovasc Imaging. 2015;16(4):373–9.

32. Eberhard M, Hinzpeter R, Polacin M, Morsbach F, Maisano F, Nietlispach F, Nguyen-Kim TDL, Tanner FC, Alkadhi H. Reproducibility of aortic valve calcification scoring with com-

puted tomography–an interplatform analysis. J Cardiovasc Comput Tomogr. 2019;13(2):92–8.

33. Bettencourt N, Rocha J, Carvalho M, Leite D, Toschke AM, Melica B, Santos L, Rodrigues A, Goncalves M, Braga P, Teixeira M, Simoes L, Rajagopalan S, Gama V. Multislice computed tomography in the exclusion of coronary artery disease in patients with pre-surgical valve disease. Circ Cardiovasc Imaging. 2009;2(4):306–13.

34. van den Boogert TPW, Vendrik J, Claessen B, Baan J, Beijk MA, Limpens J, Boekholdt SAM, Hoek R, Planken RN, Henriques JP. CTCA for detection of significant coronary artery disease in routine TAVI work-up: a systematic review and meta-analysis. Neth Heart J. 2018;26(12):591–9.

35. Singh G, Al'Aref SJ, Van Assen M, Kim TS, van Rosendael A, Kolli KK, Dwivedi A, Maliakal G, Pandey M, Wang J, Do V, Gummalla M, De Cecco CN, Min JK. Machine learning in cardiac CT: Basic concepts and contemporary data. J Cardiovasc Comput Tomogr. 2018;12(3):192–201.

36. Fihn SD, Gardin JM, Abrams J, Berra K, Blankenship JC, Dallas AP, Douglas PS, Foody JM, Gerber TC, Hinderliter AL, King SB 3rd, Kligfield PD, Krumholz HM, Kwong RY, Lim MJ, Linderbaum JA, Mack MJ, Munger MA, Prager RL, Sabik JF, Shaw LJ, Sikkema JD, Smith CR Jr, Smith SC Jr, Spertus JA, Williams SV, Anderson JL. 2012 ACCF/AHA/ACP/AATS/PCNA/SCAI/STS guideline for the diagnosis and management of patients with stable ischemic heart disease: a report of the American College of Cardiology Foundation/American Heart Association task force on practice guidelines, and the American College of Physicians, American Association for Thoracic Surgery, Preventive Cardiovascular Nurses Association, Society for Cardiovascular Angiography and Interventions, and Society of Thoracic Surgeons. Circulation. 2012;126(25):e354–471.

37. Mancini GB, Gosselin G, Chow B, Kostuk W, Stone J, Yvorchuk KJ, Abramson BL, Cartier R, Huckell V, Tardif JC, Connelly K, Ducas J, Farkouh ME, Gupta M, Juneau M, O'Neill B, Raggi P, Teo K, Verma S, Zimmermann R. Canadian Cardiovascular Society guidelines for the diagnosis and management of stable ischemic heart disease. Can J Cardiol. 2014;30(8):837–49.

38. Fletcher GF, Ades PA, Kligfield P, Arena R, Balady GJ, Bittner VA, Coke LA, Fleg JL, Forman DE, Gerber TC, Gulati M, Madan K, Rhodes J, Thompson PD, Williams MA. Exercise standards for testing and training: a scientific statement from the American Heart Association. Circulation. 2013;128(8):873–934.

39. Lancellotti P, Pellikka PA, Budts W, Chaudhry FA, Donal E, Dulgheru R, Edvardsen T, Garbi M, Ha JW, Kane GC, Kreeger J, Mertens L, Pibarot P, Picano E, Ryan T, Tsutsui JM, Varga A. The clinical use of stress echocardiography in non-ischaemic heart disease: recommendations from the European Association of Cardiovascular Imaging and the American Society of Echocardiography. Eur Heart J Cardiovasc Imaging. 2016;17(11):1191–229.

40. Baumgartner HC, Hung JC-C, Bermejo J, Chambers JB, Edvardsen T, Goldstein S, Lancellotti P, LeFevre M, Miller F Jr, Otto CM. Recommendations on the echocardiographic assessment of aortic valve stenosis: a focused update from the European Association of Cardiovascular Imaging and the American Society of Echocardiography. Eur Heart J Cardiovasc Imaging. 2017;18(3):254–75.

41. Pesarini G, Scarsini R, Zivelonghi C, Piccoli A, Gambaro A, Gottin L, Rossi A, Ferrero V, Vassanelli C, Ribichini F. Functional assessment of coronary artery disease in patients undergoing transcatheter aortic valve implantation: influence of pressure overload on the evaluation of lesions severity. Circ Cardiovasc Interv. 2016;9(11):e004088.

42. Lang RM, Badano LP, Mor-Avi V, Afilalo J, Armstrong A, Ernande L, Flachskampf FA, Foster E, Goldstein SA, Kuznetsova T, Lancellotti P, Muraru D, Picard MH, Rietzschel ER, Rudski L, Spencer KT, Tsang W, Voigt JU. Recommendations for car-diac chamber quantification by echocardiography in adults: an update from the American Society of Echocardiography and the European Association of Cardiovascular Imaging. Eur Heart J Cardiovasc Imaging. 2015;16(3):233–70.

43. Norum IB, Ruddox V, Edvardsen T, Otterstad JE. Diagnostic accuracy of left ventricular longitudinal function by speckle tracking echocardiography to predict significant coronary artery stenosis. A systematic review. BMC Med Imaging. 2015;15:25.

44. Liou K, Negishi K, Ho S, Russell EA, Cranney G, Ooi SY. Detection of obstructive coronary artery disease using peak systolic global longitudinal strain derived by two-dimensional speckle-tracking: a systematic review and meta-analysis. J Am Soc Echocardiogr. 2016;29(8):724–735.e4.

45. Caspar T, Samet H, Ohana M, Germain P, El Ghannudi S, Talha S, Morel O, Ohlmann P. Longitudinal 2D strain can help diagnose coronary artery disease in patients with suspected non-ST-elevation acute coronary syndrome but apparent normal global and segmental systolic function. Int J Cardiol. 2017;236:91–4.

46. Zuo HJ, Yang XT, Liu QG, Zhang Y, Zeng HS, Yan JT, Wang DW, Wang H. Global longitudinal strain at rest for detection of coronary artery disease in patients without diabetes mellitus. Curr Med Sci. 2018;38(3):413–21.

47. Nagueh SF, Smiseth OA, Appleton CP, Byrd BF 3rd, Dokainish H, Edvardsen T, Flachskampf FA, Gillebert TC, Klein AL, Lancellotti P, Marino P, Oh JK, Alexandru Popescu B, Waggoner AD. Recommendations for the evaluation of left ventricular diastolic function by echocardiography: an update from the American Society of Echocardiography and the European Association of Cardiovascular Imaging. Eur Heart J Cardiovasc Imaging. 2016;17(12):1321–60.

48. Wang J, Khoury DS, Thohan V, Torre-Amione G, Nagueh SF. Global diastolic strain rate for the assessment of left ventricular relaxation and filling pressures. Circulation. 2007;115(11):1376–83.

49. Dokainish H, Sengupta R, Pillai M, Bobek J, Lakkis N. Usefulness of new diastolic strain and strain rate indexes for the estimation of left ventricular filling pressure. Am J Cardiol. 2008;101(10):1504–9.

50. Singh A, Addetia K, Maffessanti F, Mor-Avi V, Lang RM. LA strain for categorization of LV diastolic dysfunction. JACC Cardiovasc Imaging. 2017;10(7):735–43.

51. Porter TR, Mulvagh SL, Abdelmoneim SS, Becher H, Belcik JT, Bierig M, Choy J, Gaibazzi N, Gillam LD, Janardhanan R, Kutty S, Leong-Poi H, Lindner JR, Main ML, Mathias W Jr, Park MM, Senior R, Villanueva F. Clinical applications of ultrasonic enhancing agents in echocardiography: 2018 American Society of Echocardiography guidelines update. J Am Soc Echocardiogr. 2018;31(3):241–74.

52. Hachamovitch R, Rozanski A, Shaw LJ, Stone GW, Thomson LE, Friedman JD, Hayes SW, Cohen I, Germano G, Berman DS. Impact of ischaemia and scar on the therapeutic benefit derived from myocardial revascularization vs. medical therapy among patients undergoing stress-rest myocardial perfusion scintigraphy. Eur Heart J. 2011;32(8):1012–24.

53. Shaw LJ, Iskandrian AE. Prognostic value of gated myocardial perfusion SPECT. J Nucl Cardiol. 2004;11(2):171–85.

54. Danad I, Raijmakers PG, Driessen RS, Leipsic J, Raju R, Naoum C, Knuuti J, Maki M, Underwood RS, Min JK, Elmore K, Stuijfzand WJ, van Royen N, Tulevski II, Somsen AG, Huisman MC, van Lingen AA, Heymans MW, van de Ven PM, van Kuijk C, Lammertsma AA, van Rossum AC, Knaapen P. Comparison of coronary CT angiography, SPECT, PET, and hybrid imaging for diagnosis of ischemic heart disease determined by fractional flow reserve. JAMA Cardiol. 2017;2(10):1100–7.

55. Juarez-Orozco LE, Tio RA, Alexanderson E, Dweck M, Vliegenthart R, El Moumni M, Prakken N, Gonzalez-Godinez I, Slart R. Quantitative myocardial perfusion evaluation with

positron emission tomography and the risk of cardiovascular events in patients with coronary artery disease: a systematic review of prognostic studies. Eur Heart J Cardiovasc Imaging. 2018;19(10):1179–87.

56. Unger P, Rosenhek R, Dedobbeleer C, Berrebi A, Lancellotti P. Management of multiple valve disease. Heart. 2011;97(4):272–7.

57. Unger P, Clavel MA, Lindman BR, Mathieu P, Pibarot P. Pathophysiology and management of multivalvular disease. Nat Rev Cardiol. 2016;13(7):429–40.

58. Vahanian A, Himbert D, Brochet E. Multiple valve disease—assessment, strategy and intervention. EuroIntervention. 2015;11(Suppl W):W14–6.

59. Grimaldi A, Vermi AC, Pappalardo F, Benussi S, Fumero A, Maisano F, Colombo A, La Canna G, Alfieri O. The pivotal role of echocardiography in the assessment of multivalvular heart disease. Minerva Cardioangiol. 2013;61(2):229–42.

60. Mitchell C, Rahko PS, Blauwet LA, Canaday B, Finstuen JA, Foster MC, Horton K, Ogunyankin KO, Palma RA, Velazquez EJ. Guidelines for performing a comprehensive transthoracic echocardiographic examination in adults: recommendations from the American Society of Echocardiography. J Am Soc Echocardiogr. 2019;32(1):1–64.

61. Zoghbi WA, Adams D, Bonow RO, Enriquez-Sarano M, Foster E, Grayburn PA, Hahn RT, Han Y, Hung J, Lang RM, Little SH, Shah DJ, Shernan S, Thavendiranathan P, Thomas JD, Weissman NJ. Recommendations for noninvasive evaluation of native valvular regurgitation: a report from the American Society of Echocardiography developed in collaboration with the Society for Cardiovascular Magnetic Resonance. J Am Soc Echocardiogr. 2017;30(4):303–71.

62. Lancellotti P, Tribouilloy C, Hagendorff A, Popescu BA, Edvardsen T, Pierard LA, Badano L, Zamorano JL. Recommendations for the echocardiographic assessment of native valvular regurgitation: an executive summary from the European Association of Cardiovascular Imaging. Eur Heart J Cardiovasc Imaging. 2013;14(7):611–44.

63. Hahn RT, Abraham T, Adams MS, Bruce CJ, Glas KE, Lang RM, Reeves ST, Shanewise JS, Siu SC, Stewart W, Picard MH. Guidelines for performing a comprehensive transesophageal echocardiographic examination: recommendations from the American Society of Echocardiography and the Society of Cardiovascular Anesthesiologists. Anesth Analg. 2014;118(1):21–68.

64. Flachskampf FA, Wouters PF, Edvardsen T, Evangelista A, Habib G, Hoffman P, Hoffmann R, Lancellotti P, Pepi M. Recommendations for transoesophageal echocardiography: EACVI update 2014. Eur Heart J Cardiovasc Imaging. 2014;15(4):353–65.

65. Zamorano JL, Badano LP, Bruce C, Chan KL, Goncalves A, Hahn RT, Keane MG, La Canna G, Monaghan MJ, Nihoyannopoulos P, Silvestry FE, Vanoverschelde JL, Gillam LD. EAE/ASE recommendations for the use of echocardiography in new transcatheter interventions for valvular heart disease. Eur Heart J. 2011;32(17):2189–214.

66. Doherty JU, Kort S, Mehran R, Schoenhagen P, Soman P. ACC/AATS/AHA/ASE/ASNC/HRS/SCAI/SCCT/SCMR/STS 2017 Appropriate Use Criteria for Multimodality Imaging in Valvular Heart Disease: A Report of the American College of Cardiology Appropriate Use Criteria Task Force, American Association for Thoracic Surgery, American Heart Association, American Society of Echocardiography, American Society of Nuclear Cardiology, Heart Rhythm Society, Society for Cardiovascular Angiography and Interventions, Society of Cardiovascular Computed Tomography, Society for Cardiovascular Magnetic Resonance, and Society of Thoracic Surgeons. J Nucl Cardiol. 2017;24(6):2043–63.

67. Tischler MD, Battle RW, Saha M, Niggel J, LeWinter MM. Observations suggesting a high incidence of exercise-induced severe mitral regurgitation in patients with mild rheumatic mitral valve disease at rest. J Am Coll Cardiol. 1995;25(1):128–33.

68. Tunon J, Cordoba M, Rey M, Almeida P, Rabago R, Sanchez-Cascos A, Rabago P. Assessment of chronic tricuspid regurgitation by colour Doppler echocardiography: a comparison with angiography in the catheterization room. Eur Heart J. 1994;15(8):1074–84.

69. Morley JE, Vellas B, van Kan GA, Anker SD, Bauer JM, Bernabei R, Cesari M, Chumlea WC, Doehner W, Evans J, Fried LP, Guralnik JM, Katz PR, Malmstrom TK, McCarter RJ, Gutierrez Robledo LM, Rockwood K, von Haehling S, Vandewoude MF, Walston J. Frailty consensus: a call to action. J Am Med Dir Assoc. 2013;14(6):392–7.

70. Rodriguez-Manas L, Feart C, Mann G, Vina J, Chatterji S, Chodzko-Zajko W, Gonzalez-Colaco Harmand M, Bergman H, Carcaillon L, Nicholson C, Scuteri A, Sinclair A, Pelaez M, Van der Cammen T, Beland F, Bickenbach J, Delamarche P, Ferrucci L, Fried LP, Gutierrez-Robledo LM, Rockwood K, Rodriguez Artalejo F, Serviddio G, Vega E. Searching for an operational definition of frailty: a Delphi method based consensus statement: the frailty operative definition-consensus conference project. J Gerontol A Biol Sci Med Sci. 2013;68(1):62–7.

71. Dent E, Kowal P, Hoogendijk EO. Frailty measurement in research and clinical practice: a review. Eur J Intern Med. 2016;31:3–10.

72. Clegg A, Young J, Iliffe S, Rikkert MO, Rockwood K. Frailty in elderly people. Lancet. 2013;381(9868):752–62.

73. Taramasso M, Pozzoli A, Buzzatti N, Alfieri O. Assessing operative risk and benefit in elderly patients with heart valve disease. Eur Heart J. 2013;34(36):2788–91.

74. Rockwood K, Mogilner A, Mitnitski A. Changes with age in the distribution of a frailty index. Mech Ageing Dev. 2004;125(7):517–9.

75. Buta BJ, Walston JD, Godino JG, Park M, Kalyani RR, Xue QL, Bandeen-Roche K, Varadhan R. Frailty assessment instruments: systematic characterization of the uses and contexts of highly-cited instruments. Ageing Res Rev. 2016;26:53–61.

76. Cruz-Jentoft AJ, Baeyens JP, Bauer JM, Boirie Y, Cederholm T, Landi F, Martin FC, Michel JP, Rolland Y, Schneider SM, Topinkova E, Vandewoude M, Zamboni M, European Working Group on Sarcopenia in Older People. Sarcopenia: European consensus on definition and diagnosis: report of the European Working Group on Sarcopenia in Older People. Age Ageing. 2010;39(4):412–23.

77. Cesari M, Landi F, Vellas B, Bernabei R, Marzetti E. Sarcopenia and physical frailty: two sides of the same coin. Front Aging Neurosci. 2014;6:192.

78. Lin J, Lopez EF, Jin Y, Van Remmen H, Bauch T, Han HC, Lindsey ML. Age-related cardiac muscle sarcopenia: combining experimental and mathematical modeling to identify mechanisms. Exp Gerontol. 2008;43(4):296–306.

79. Sayer AA. Sarcopenia. BMJ. 2010;341:c4097.

80. Abellan van Kan G, Andre E, Bischoff Ferrari HA, Boirie Y, Onder G, Pahor M, Ritz P, Rolland Y, Sampaio C, Studenski S, Visser M, Vellas B. Carla Task Force on Sarcopenia: propositions for clinical trials. J Nutr Health Aging. 2009;13(8):700–7.

81. Cruz-Jentoft AJ, Baeyens JP, Bauer JM, Boirie Y, Cederholm T, Landi F, Martin FC, Michel JP, Rolland Y, Schneider SM, Topinkova E, Vandewoude M, Zamboni M. Sarcopenia: European consensus on definition and diagnosis: report of the European Working Group on Sarcopenia in Older People. Age Ageing. 2010;39(4):412–23.

82. Visser M. Towards a definition of sarcopenia—results from epidemiologic studies. J Nutr Health Aging. 2009;13(8):713–6.

83. Bischoff-Ferrari HA, Orav JE, Kanis JA, Rizzoli R, Schlogl M, Staehelin HB, Willett WC, Dawson-Hughes B. Comparative performance of current definitions of sarcopenia against the prospective incidence of falls among community-dwelling seniors age 65 and older. Osteoporos Int. 2015;26(12):2793–802.

84. Dawson-Hughes B, Bischoff-Ferrari H. Considerations concerning the definition of sarcopenia: response to comments. Osteoporos Int. 2016;27(11):3147–8.

85. Springer J, Springer JI, Anker SD. Muscle wasting and sarcopenia in heart failure and beyond: update 2017. ESC Heart Fail. 2017;4(4):492–8.

86. Bekfani T, Pellicori P, Morris DA, Ebner N, Valentova M, Steinbeck L, Wachter R, Elsner S, Sliziuk V, Schefold JC, Sandek A, Doehner W, Cleland JG, Lainscak M, Anker SD, von Haehling S. Sarcopenia in patients with heart failure with preserved ejection fraction: impact on muscle strength, exercise capacity and quality of life. Int J Cardiol. 2016;222:41–6.

87. Saitoh M, Ebner N, von Haehling S, Anker SD, Springer J. Therapeutic considerations of sarcopenia in heart failure patients. Expert Rev Cardiovasc Ther. 2018;16(2):133–42.

88. Studenski SA, Peters KW, Alley DE, Cawthon PM, McLean RR, Harris TB, Ferrucci L, Guralnik JM, Fragala MS, Kenny AM, Kiel DP, Kritchevsky SB, Shardell MD, Dam TT, Vassileva MT. The FNIH sarcopenia project: rationale, study description, conference recommendations, and final estimates. J Gerontol A Biol Sci Med Sci. 2014;69(5):547–58.

89. Kleczynski P, Tokarek T, Dziewierz A, Sorysz D, Bagienski M, Rzeszutko L, Dudek D. Usefulness of Psoas muscle area and volume and frailty scoring to predict outcomes after transcatheter aortic valve implantation. Am J Cardiol. 2018;122(1):135–40.

90. Adams HS, Ashokkumar S, Newcomb A, MacIsaac AI, Whitbourn RJ, Palmer S. A contemporary review of severe aortic stenosis. Intern Med J. 2019;49(3):297–305.

91. Pulignano G, Gulizia MM, Baldasseroni S, Bedogni F, Cioffi G, Indolfi C, Romeo F, Murrone A, Musumeci F, Parolari A, Patane L, Pino PG, Mongiardo A, Spaccarotella C, Di Bartolomeo R, Musumeci G. ANMCO/SIC/SICI-GISE/SICCH Executive Summary of Consensus Document on Risk Stratification in elderly patients with aortic stenosis before surgery or transcatheter aortic valve replacement. Eur Heart J Suppl. 2017;19(Suppl D):D354–d369.

92. Sipers WM, Verdijk LB, Sipers SJ, Schols JM, van Loon LJ. The Martin Vigorimeter represents a reliable and more practical tool than the Jamar dynamometer to assess handgrip strength in the geriatric patient. J Am Med Dir Assoc. 2016;17(5):466.e1–7.

93. Guralnik JM, Ferrucci L, Pieper CF, Leveille SG, Markides KS, Ostir GV, Studenski S, Berkman LF, Wallace RB. Lower extremity function and subsequent disability: consistency across studies, predictive models, and value of gait speed alone compared with the short physical performance battery. J Gerontol A Biol Sci Med Sci. 2000;55(4):M221–31.

94. Saum KU, Muller H, Stegmaier C, Hauer K, Raum E, Brenner H. Development and evaluation of a modification of the Fried frailty criteria using population-independent cutpoints. J Am Geriatr Soc. 2012;60(11):2110–5.

95. Santos-Eggimann B, Cuenoud P, Spagnoli J, Junod J. Prevalence of frailty in middle-aged and older community-dwelling Europeans living in 10 countries. J Gerontol A Biol Sci Med Sci. 2009;64(6):675–81.

96. Joseph SM, Manghelli JL, Vader JM, Keeney T, Novak EL, Felius J, Martinez SC, Nassif ME, Lima B, Silvestry SC, Rich MW. Prospective assessment of frailty using the fried criteria in patients undergoing left ventricular assist device therapy. Am J Cardiol. 2017;120(8):1349–54.

97. Ensrud KE, Blackwell TL, Redline S, Ancoli-Israel S, Paudel ML, Cawthon PM, Dam TT, Barrett-Connor E, Leung PC, Stone KL. Sleep disturbances and frailty status in older community-dwelling men. J Am Geriatr Soc. 2009;57(11):2085–93.

98. Rockwood K, Andrew M, Mitnitski A. A comparison of two approaches to measuring frailty in elderly people. J Gerontol A Biol Sci Med Sci. 2007;62(7):738–43.

99. Cesari M, Marzetti E, Thiem U, Perez-Zepeda MU, Abellan Van Kan G, Landi F, Petrovic M, Cherubini A, Bernabei R. The geriatric management of frailty as paradigm of "The end of the disease era". Eur J Intern Med. 2016;31:11–4.

100. Cruz-Jentoft AJ, Bahat G, Bauer J, Boirie Y, Bruyère O, Cederholm T, Cooper C, Landi F, Rolland Y, Sayer AA, Schneider SM, Sieber CC, Topinkova E, Vandewoude M, Visser M, Zamboni M, Writing Group for the European Working Group on Sarcopenia in Older People, the Extended Group for E. Sarcopenia: revised European consensus on definition and diagnosis. Age Ageing. 2019;48:16–31.

101. Fried LP, Tangen CM, Walston J, Newman AB, Hirsch C, Gottdiener J, Seeman T, Tracy R, Kop WJ, Burke G, McBurnie MA, Cardiovascular Health Study Collaborative Research Group. Frailty in older adults: evidence for a phenotype. J Gerontol A Biol Sci Med Sci. 2001;56(3):M146–56.

102. Chumlea WC, Cesari M, Evans WJ, Ferrucci L, Fielding RA, Pahor M, Studenski S, Vellas B, Members TTF. International working group on Sarcopenia. J Nutr Health Aging. 2011;15(6):450–5.

103. Cesari M, Fielding RA, Pahor M, Goodpaster B, Hellerstein M, van Kan GA, Anker SD, Rutkove S, Vrijbloed JW, Isaac M, Rolland Y, M'Rini C, Aubertin-Leheudre M, Cedarbaum JM, Zamboni M, Sieber CC, Laurent D, Evans WJ, Roubenoff R, Morley JE, Vellas B. Biomarkers of sarcopenia in clinical trials-recommendations from the International Working Group on Sarcopenia. J Cachexia Sarcopenia Muscle. 2012;3(3):181–90.

104. Baumgartner RN, Koehler KM, Gallagher D, Romero L, Heymsfield SB, Ross RR, Garry PJ, Lindeman RD. Epidemiology of sarcopenia among the elderly in New Mexico. Am J Epidemiol. 1998;147(8):755–63.

105. Chen WT, Chou KH, Liu LK, Lee PL, Lee WJ, Chen LK, Wang PN, Lin CP. Reduced cerebellar gray matter is a neural signature of physical frailty. Hum Brain Mapp. 2015;36(9):3666–76.

106. McIsaac DI, Bryson GL, van Walraven C. Association of frailty and 1-year postoperative mortality following major elective non-cardiac surgery: a population-based cohort study. JAMA Surg. 2016;151(6):538–45.

107. Mosquera C, Spaniolas K, Fitzgerald TL. Impact of frailty on surgical outcomes: the right patient for the right procedure. Surgery. 2016;160(2):272–80.

108. Dahya V, Xiao J, Prado CM, Burroughs P, McGee D, Silva AC, Hurt JE, Mohamed SG, Noel T, Batchelor W. Computed tomography-derived skeletal muscle index: a novel predictor of frailty and hospital length of stay after transcatheter aortic valve replacement. Am Heart J. 2016;182:21–7.

109. Falk RH, Dubrey SW. Amyloid heart disease. Prog Cardiovasc Dis. 2010;52(4):347–61.

110. Shah KB, Inoue Y, Mehra MR. Amyloidosis and the heart: a comprehensive review. Arch Intern Med. 2006;166(17):1805–13.

111. Sun JP, Stewart WJ, Yang XS, Donnell RO, Leon AR, Felner JM, Thomas JD, Merlino JD. Differentiation of hypertrophic cardiomyopathy and cardiac amyloidosis from other causes of ventricular wall thickening by two-dimensional strain imaging echocardiography. Am J Cardiol. 2009;103(3):411–5.

112. Glaudemans AW, Slart RH, Zeebregts CJ, Veltman NC, Tio RA, Hazenberg BP, Dierckx RA. Nuclear imaging in cardiac amyloidosis. Eur J Nucl Med Mol Imaging. 2009;36(4):702–14.

113. Gillmore JD, Maurer MS, Falk RH, Merlini G, Damy T, Dispenzieri A, Wechalekar AD, Berk JL, Quarta CC, Grogan M, Lachmann HJ, Bokhari S, Castano A, Dorbala S, Johnson GB, Glaudemans AW, Rezk T, Fontana M, Palladini G, Milani P, Guidalotti PL, Flatman K, Lane T, Vonberg FW, Whelan CJ, Moon JC, Ruberg FL, Miller EJ, Hutt DF, Hazenberg BP, Rapezzi C, Hawkins PN. Nonbiopsy diagnosis of cardiac transthyretin amyloidosis. Circulation. 2016;133(24):2404–12.

114. American College of O, Gynecologists' Committee on Obstetric P. Committee opinion no. 656: guidelines for diagnostic imaging during pregnancy and lactation. Obstet Gynecol. 2016;127(2):e75–80.

115. Committee on Obstetric P. Committee opinion no. 723: guidelines for diagnostic imaging during pregnancy and lactation. Obstet Gynecol. 2017;130(4):e210–6.

116. Leyendecker JR, Gorengaut V, Brown JJ. MR imaging of maternal diseases of the abdomen and pelvis during pregnancy and the immediate postpartum period. Radiographics. 2004;24(5):1301–16.

117. Chen MM, Coakley FV, Kaimal A, Laros RK Jr. Guidelines for computed tomography and magnetic resonance imaging use during pregnancy and lactation. Obstet Gynecol. 2008;112(2 Pt 1):333–40.

118. Expert Panel on MRS, Kanal E, Barkovich AJ, Bell C, Borgstede JP, Bradley WG Jr, Froelich JW, Gimbel JR, Gosbee JW, Kuhni-Kaminski E, Larson PA, Lester JW Jr, Nyenhuis J, Schaefer DJ, Sebek EA, Weinreb J, Wilkoff BL, Woods TO, Lucey L, Hernandez D. ACR guidance document on MR safe practices: 2013. J Magn Reson Imaging. 2013;37(3):501–30.

119. Patel SJ, Reede DL, Katz DS, Subramaniam R, Amorosa JK. Imaging the pregnant patient for nonobstetric conditions: algorithms and radiation dose considerations. Radiographics. 2007;27(6):1705–22.

120. Gjelsteen AC, Ching BH, Meyermann MW, Prager DA, Murphy TF, Berkey BD, Mitchell LA. CT, MRI, PET, PET/CT, and ultrasound in the evaluation of obstetric and gynecologic patients. Surg Clin North Am. 2008;88(2):361–90, vii.

121. Webb JA, Thomsen HS, Morcos SK, Members of Contrast Media Safety Committee of European Society of Urogenital R. The use of iodinated and gadolinium contrast media during pregnancy and lactation. Eur Radiol. 2005;15(6):1234–40.

122. Morel DR, Schwieger I, Hohn L, Terrettaz J, Llull JB, Cornioley YA, Schneider M. Human pharmacokinetics and safety evaluation of SonoVue, a new contrast agent for ultrasound imaging. Invest Radiol. 2000;35(1):80–5.

123. Broome DR, Girguis MS, Baron PW, Cottrell AC, Kjellin I, Kirk GA. Gadodiamide-associated nephrogenic systemic fibrosis: why radiologists should be concerned. Am J Roentgenol. 2007;188(2):586–92.

124. Marckmann P, Skov L, Rossen K, Dupont A, Damholt MB, Heaf JG, Thomsen HS. Nephrogenic systemic fibrosis: suspected causative role of gadodiamide used for contrast-enhanced magnetic resonance imaging. J Am Soc Nephrol. 2006;17(9):2359–62.

125. Rahatli FK, Donmez FY, Kibaroglu S, Kesim C, Haberal KM, Turnaoglu H, Agildere AM. Does renal function affect gadolinium deposition in the brain? Eur J Radiol. 2018;104:33–7.

126. Gulani V, Calamante F, Shellock FG, Kanal E, Reeder SB. Gadolinium deposition in the brain: summary of evidence and recommendations. Lancet Neurol. 2017;16(7):564–70.

127. van der Molen AJ, Reimer P, Dekkers IA, Bongartz G, Bellin MF, Bertolotto M, Clement O, Heinz-Peer G, Stacul F, Webb JAW, Thomsen HS. Post-contrast acute kidney injury—Part 1: definition, clinical features, incidence, role of contrast medium and risk factors: recommendations for updated ESUR Contrast Medium Safety Committee guidelines. Eur Radiol. 2018;28(7):2845–55.

128. van der Molen AJ, Reimer P, Dekkers IA, Bongartz G, Bellin MF, Bertolotto M, Clement O, Heinz-Peer G, Stacul F, Webb JAW, Thomsen HS. Post-contrast acute kidney injury.

Part 2: risk stratification, role of hydration and other prophylactic measures, patients taking metformin and chronic dialysis patients: Recommendations for updated ESUR Contrast Medium Safety Committee guidelines. Eur Radiol. 2018;28(7):2856–69.

129. EANM procedural guidelines for radionuclide myocardial perfusion imaging with SPECT and SPECT/CT: 2015 revision. Eur J Nucl Med Mol Imaging. 2015;42(12):1929–40.

130. Luechinger R, Duru F, Scheidegger MB, Boesiger P, Candinas R. Force and torque effects of a 1.5-Tesla MRI scanner on cardiac pacemakers and ICDs. Pacing Clin Electrophysiol. 2001;24(2):199–205.

131. Nordbeck P, Weiss I, Ehses P, Ritter O, Warmuth M, Fidler F, Herold V, Jakob PM, Ladd ME, Quick HH, Bauer WR. Measuring RF-induced currents inside implants: impact of device configuration on MRI safety of cardiac pacemaker leads. Magn Reson Med. 2009;61(3):570–8.

132. Luechinger R, Zeijlemaker VA, Pedersen EM, Mortensen P, Falk E, Duru F, Candinas R, Boesiger P. In vivo heating of pacemaker leads during magnetic resonance imaging. Eur Heart J. 2005;26(4):376–83; discussion 325–7.

133. Luechinger R, Duru F, Zeijlemaker VA, Scheidegger MB, Boesiger P, Candinas R. Pacemaker reed switch behavior in 0.5, 1.5, and 3.0 Tesla magnetic resonance imaging units: are reed switches always closed in strong magnetic fields? Pacing Clin Electrophysiol. 2002;25(10):1419–23.

134. Gimbel JR. Unexpected asystole during 3T magnetic resonance imaging of a pacemaker-dependent patient with a 'modern' pacemaker. Europace. 2009;11(9):1241–2.

135. Ainslie M, Miller C, Brown B, Schmitt M. Cardiac MRI of patients with implanted electrical cardiac devices. Heart. 2014;100(5):363–9.

136. Indik JH, Gimbel JR, Abe H, Alkmim-Teixeira R, Birgersdotter-Green U, Clarke GD, Dickfeld TL, Froelich JW, Grant J, Hayes DL, Heidbuchel H, Idriss SF, Kanal E, Lampert R, Machado CE, Mandrola JM, Nazarian S, Patton KK, Rozner MA, Russo RJ, Shen WK, Shinbane JS, Teo WS, Uribe W, Verma A, Wilkoff BL, Woodard PK. 2017 HRS expert consensus statement on magnetic resonance imaging and radiation exposure in patients with cardiovascular implantable electronic devices. Heart Rhythm. 2017;14(7):e97–e153.

137. Cao G, Chen W, Pan K, Sun H, Wang Z. Reduced artifacts and improved diagnostic value of 640-slice computed tomography in patients with cardiac pacemakers. J Int Med Res. 2019;47:1916–26.

138. Takayanagi T, Arai T, Amanuma M, Sano T, Ichiba M, Ishizaka K, Sekine T, Matsutani H, Morita H, Takase S. Pacemaker-induced metallic artifacts in coronary computed tomography angiography: clinical feasibility of single energy metal artifact reduction technique. Nihon Hoshasen Gijutsu Gakkai Zasshi. 2017;73(6):460–6.

139. Marbach JR, Sontag MR, Van Dyk J, Wolbarst AB. Management of radiation oncology patients with implanted cardiac pacemakers: report of AAPM Task Group No. 34. American Association of Physicists in Medicine. Med Phys. 1994;21(1):85–90.

Planning the Procedure

3

Gudrun Feuchtner, Edwin Ho, Alberto Pozzoli,
Mizuki Miura, Thomas Senoner, Ricarda Hinzpeter,
Fabian Morsbach, Philipp Haager, Hans Rickli,
Mara Gavazzoni, Michel Zuber, Gräni Christoph,
Buechel Ronny, Philipp Kaufmann, Francesco Maisano,
and Hatem Alkadhi

3.1 Introduction

The percutaneous approach for transcatheter aortic valve implantation (TAVI) is becoming increasingly more common for high-, intermediate- and even low-risk aortic stenosis (AS) patients, always following heart team discussion. However, conventional surgical approach is still used nowadays for aortic valve replacement (AVR) at many institutions. Because of the continuous trend towards less invasive procedures, cardiac operations have become increasingly more sophisticated and complex [1].

Minimally invasive techniques in cardiac operations require higher surgical abilities to accomplish the same quality compared with the traditional procedures with cardio-pulmonary bypass (CPB) or sternotomy. Since early beginning of the 2000, minimally invasive aortic valve replacement (through a lateral right minithoracotomy or ministernotomy), became a favourable approach [2].

These surgical approaches limit the view of the surgeons and the space of the operating field, which result in a more challenging procedure.

Transthoracic ultrasound in this case provides important details about the anatomy of the valve, the configuration of the cusps and the state of the walls of both the root and the ascending aorta. For surgical planning *per se*, the echo information could become particularly operator dependent and should be integrated with CTA analysis.

Indeed, an optimal mental and anatomical preparation can support the surgeon to better overcome the difficulties caused by the new modalities of minimally invasive surgery. Multislice computed tomography angiography (CTA) has already been used successfully as part of the clinical routine in cardiac operations for many different purposes, including detailed illustration of the anatomy of the heart, examination of coronary arteries, coronary bypass grafts, and the mitral and tricuspid heart valves [3, 4].

This imaging tool can be used for diagnostic and postoperative quality control as well as for preoperative planning. As discussed in the previous chapter, preoperative planning with CTA has shown to be a helpful tool in reoperations and minimally invasive cardiac operations demonstrating an improved orientation in the operating field and potentially preventing surgical errors [5].

G. Feuchtner · T. Senoner
Radiology Unit, Innsbruck University Hospital, Innsbruck, Austria
e-mail: gudrun.feuchtner@i-med.ac.at; thomas.senoner@i-med.ac.at

E. Ho · M. Miura · M. Gavazzoni
Heart Center, Zurich University Hospital, Zurich, Switzerland
e-mail: edwin.ho@usz.ch; mizuki.miura@usz.ch;
mara.gavazzoni@usz.ch

A. Pozzoli · F. Maisano
Heart Surgery Unit, Zurich University Hospital,
Zurich, Switzerland
e-mail: alberto.pozzoli@usz.ch; francesco.maisano@usz.ch

R. Hinzpeter · F. Morsbach · H. Alkadhi (✉)
Radiology Unit, University Hospital Zurich, Zurich, Switzerland
e-mail: ricarda.hinzpeter@usz.ch; fabian.morsbach@usz.ch;
hatem.alkadhi@usz.ch

P. Haager · H. Rickli
Cardiology Unit, Kantonsspital St. Gallen, St. Gallen, Switzerland
e-mail: philipp.haager@usz.ch; hans.rickli@kssg.ch

M. Zuber
Cardiology Unit, Zurich University Hospital, Zurich, Switzerland
e-mail: michel.zuber@usz.ch

G. Christoph · B. Ronny · P. Kaufmann
Nuclear Medicine Unit, Zurich University Hospital,
Zurich, Switzerland
e-mail: christoph.Graeni@usz.ch; buechel.ronny@usz.ch;
pak@usz.ch

3.2 Surgical Planning

3.2.1 Intro

Standard preoperative imaging for aortic valve surgery includes transthoracic echocardiography (TTE) and coronary catheterization for patients with any risk factors for coronary disease. This baseline imaging will reveal additional valve or coronary disease that requires intervention. Over the last two decades, advances in computed tomography technology have revolutionized the diagnosis of cardiovascular disease. In particular, CTA has reduced significantly and, for some clinical indications, eliminated the need for diagnostic arterial catheterization. In the process, CTA has become invaluable in making the right diagnosis and surgical planning. Of note, using the same CTA acquisition, native coronary imaging can be extended to coronary bypass grafts, the beating myocardium, valve motion, ventricular outflow tracks, and related lesions. In general, when patients require concomitant coronary artery bypass grafting, the combined operation will be performed through a full median sternotomy. Minimally invasive approaches to the aortic valve are becoming nowadays the preferred option for patients at reasonable risk for surgery. They provide safe and effective exposure for operations involving both the aortic valve and ascending aorta. Potential advantages over conventional median sternotomy include decreases in the length of hospital stay, hospital costs, pain, recovery time and requirement for transfusions. The mini-sternotomy extends from the sternal notch to the right fourth intercostal space. The feasibility of this approach relies mostly on the proximity of the aortic valve to the fourth intercostal space. Variations in the location of the valve along the cranial-caudal or lateral planes can increase the complexity of the procedure. The preoperative imaging also allows the surgeon to plan cannulation and cardioprotection strategy. Induction cardioplegia is administered through an antegrade cannula in the proximal ascending aorta, either as a single dose solution or followed by intermittent maintenance doses directly into the coronary ostia depending on the surgeon's choice. If there is insufficient room for the ascending aortic cannula, femoral arterial and venous access should be considered.

3.2.2 Annular Sizing for SAVR

3.2.2.1 Intro

Surgical aortic valves come in an array of sizes and fitting the ideal valve for each patient is crucial for outcomes. A prosthetic valve that is too large may be difficult to implant and increase the risk of complications. One that is too small will have a higher residual gradient and potential patient prosthesis mismatch, both of which can correlate with symptoms or worse long term outcomes [6, 7]. In the era of transcatheter aortic valve replacement, prosthetic valve type and size are also important to consider in case a valve-in-valve implantation is needed in the future [8]. The largest possible valve and a mechanical structure that can expand may optimize the results of a transcatheter valve-in-valve and clinical outcomes [9].

The traditional method of sizing surgical valve replacement is direct inspection of the annulus at the time of surgery after the native valve has been excised. Specialized sterile sizer tools have been created to help select an appropriate prosthetic valve size. They are physically inserted into the annulus and the largest sizer that is able to complete fit is used to select the prosthesis size [10].

There may also be a role in pre-procedure evaluation and planning prior to aortic valve replacement surgery. In this section, the use of different imaging modalities to assist with annular sizing before and at the time of surgery will be reviewed.

3.2.2.2 Echo

Transesophageal echocardiography is often done periprocedurally at the time of cardiac surgery and may provide annular sizing information either by 2-dimensional or 3-dimensional measurements. With that said, the gold standard for sizing the annulus is direct assessment using a physical surgical sizing tool.

The conventional way to measure the size of the aortic annulus is to perform a single linear measurement at the annulus in the zoomed long axis view of the aortic valve, preferably using transesophageal echocardiography due to increased spatial resolution. This may lack accuracy because of the variable position of the imaging plane within the annulus. Based on the knowledge gained from 3-dimensional assessment of the aortic annulus in transcatheter aortic valve replacement, the annulus is an irregular ovoid shape most of the time rather than the circular shape assumed in 2-dimensional echocardiography. Additionally, the annular plane is defined by the nadir of the three aortic cusps, which cannot be assessed easily with a single imaging plane.

3-dimensional echocardiography is likely a much better way to size the annulus. This can be done by obtaining a high resolution dataset on transesophageal echocardiography and then using a multi-planar reconstruction tool to generate a measurement plane at the aortic annulus. The true shape of the annulus can then be observed and respected.

Since direct assessment of the annulus is possible in surgery, the role in echocardiography to determine the prosthesis size is limited. However, important insights on accuracy of imaging measurement strategies are important because they may have direct implications on annular sizing for transcatheter aortic valve replacement, where direct annular measurement is not possible (Fig. 3.1).

3.2.3 Aortic Valve Repair and Replacement Planning

3.2.3.1 Introduction

Surgery of the aortic valve, combined with the one of the aortic root, the ascending aorta and the arch, is becoming increasingly commonplace as the population ages.

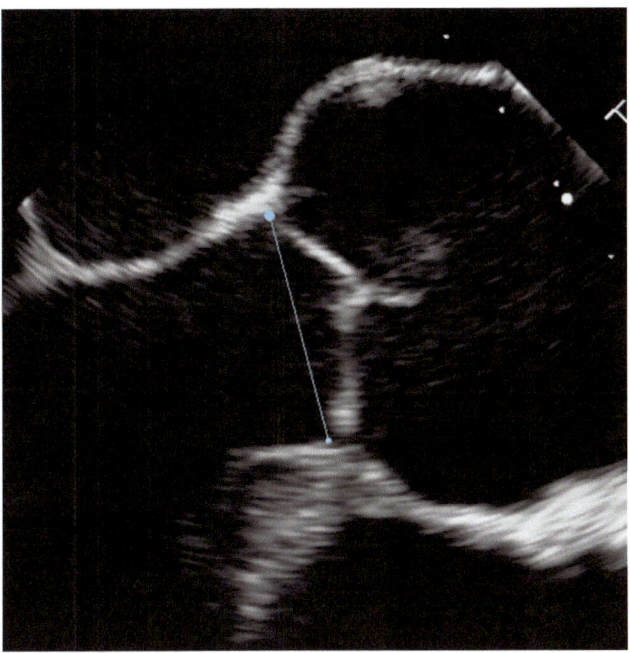

Fig. 3.1 2-dimensional measurement of the aortic annulus by transesophageal echocardiography on the long axis view

Transthoracic ultrasound in this context provides important details about the anatomy of the valve, the configuration of the cusps (tricuspid vs. bicuspid) and the state of the walls of both the root and the ascending aorta. For surgical planning *per se*, in challenging cases, the echo information could become particularly operator dependent and should be integrated with CTA analysis.

Leaflet morphology is assessed in short-axis projection of the aortic root. In contrast to the normal thin, uniform leaflets that open widely, the typically severely calcified and thickened leaflets in patients with severe aortic stenosis open in a restricted configuration with a stenotic aortic valve area.

Leaflet opening pattern is assessed using transthoracic echo. In aortic stenosis, the leaflets are thickened and calcified with decreased valvular excursion. Essential information are provided in aortic regurgitation, to assess possibility of repair, by the pliability of the aortic leaflets. If good pliability of the cusps is present, very well detected with ultrasounds in short axis, and the mechanism of regurgitation (including commissures orientation) is favourable, than an aortic repair procedure can be taken into consideration [11].

As discussed, CTA has high accuracy and reproducibility in detection and quantification of aortic calcification. These scans are not currently required as a standard of care for patients being evaluated for aortic valve surgery, however, patients with bicuspid valve disease often get them in order to exclude associated aortopathy. In particular, non–ECG-gated CTA is highly accurate in assessment of the aortic arch and descending thoracic aorta because they are not subject to significant cardiac motion. As said, nowadays any surgery

involving the aorta (whether the root, the arch, the ascending, or the descending portion) requires preoperative CTA for surgical decision-making.

The superior imaging of ECG-gated CTA better defines the pathology and hence facilitates preoperative planning. If portions of the aorta are calcified on CTA, then aortic cross-clamping and cannulation for cardiopulmonary bypass at those sites are contraindicated in order to avoid embolic phenomena and stroke. Thus preoperative cardiopulmonary bypass strategy and myocardial protection often are altered critically by preoperative CTA [12].

As with calcification, CTA is the most accurate modality to evaluate the aortic root, with both two-dimensional (2D) and three-dimensional (3D) visualization. Not only can the aortic root be sized from multiple imaging planes, but also the exact location of the aneurysmal pathology with respect to the valve and sinotubular junction often can be defined. This assessment is critical for preoperative decision making and surgical planning. In patients with ascending aortic aneurysms, if the aortic root is determined to be aneurysmal near the coronary ostia, surgical decision making changes from a simple tube-graft repair for the aneurysm to a much more complex composite root repair with coronary re-implantation. In patients with a sinus of Valsalva aneurysm, as opposed to a root aneurysm, CTA alters surgical strategy for repair.

For known ascending aortic aneurysms, CTA with 3D volume-rendered images give the surgeon preoperative visualization of aneurysm size and extent. The extension of an ascending aortic aneurysm into the arch can be showed, the expected location of aortic cross-clamping can be determined preoperatively. The location of normal aorta distally and the extent of arch involvement preoperatively will determine the arterial cardiopulmonary bypass cannulation site as well as the need for concomitant arch repair, circulatory arrest, or selective antegrade perfusion. Selective antegrade cerebral perfusion itself depends on intact right axillary and innominate arteries, and CTA is optimal for defining this anatomy. Since the success of a procedure can be compromised by unexpected intraoperative findings, CTA has contributed enormously to surgical planning by defining anatomy that would not be visualized preoperatively with any other imaging modality [12].

3.2.3.2 Functional Anatomy of the Aortic Valve for Repair

3.2.3.2.1 Intro
Surgical aortic valve repair may be preferable to surgical aortic valve replacement in some circumstances. This is because it avoids the potential morbidity associated with a prosthetic valve, such as thromboembolic complications, bleeding due to anticoagulation, patient prosthesis mismatch

or prosthetic valve dysfunction [13–16]. It may be particularly desirable in younger individuals who will have a higher cumulative risk of complications and definite need for reintervention due to prosthetic valve degeneration.

Situations in which repair may be feasible include bicuspid aortic valve with predominantly regurgitation or a trileaflet aortic valve with aortic root pathology but preserved leaflet integrity [17]. Valve repair may not be possible if the valve demonstrates advanced degenerative changes such as significant commissural fusion, thickening and calcification. Some surgical strategies may include prolapse plication and resuspension, shaving and decalcification, subcommissural annuloplasty, patch repair or remodeling of the sinotubular junction [18].

In the setting of a bicuspid valve, multiple surgical techniques can be used for valve repair. The strategy selected is based on the valve morphology and underlying mechanism of regurgitation. This is why understanding the functional anatomy is critical for planning surgical repair. The morphology of the aortic valve should be described using standardized terminology. The Schaefer classification is one way to describe a bicuspid aortic valve but is more limited in the variants that are included [19]. The Sievers classification is able to describe more forms of a bicuspid aortic valve and is therefore often preferred [20]. In addition to the cusp morphology, the primary mechanism of regurgitation should also be understood. This includes presence or absence of cusp prolapse, raphe fibrosis and calcification, aortic root pathology or insufficient leaflet tip coaptation. All of these features will help determine the surgical strategy [21, 22].

When the aortic valve is trileaflet, then careful evaluation of the aortic root and any leaflet abnormalities is important for surgical planning. The aortic annular and aortic dimensions should be clarified at the level of the Sinuses of Valsalva, sinotubular junction and proximal ascending aorta. The leaflets should be evaluated for any thickening or calcification that is impeding normal leaflet closure. Cusp prolapse, asymmetry or other abnormalities should also be well understood prior to an operation.

Multimodality imaging is helpful in understanding the valve morphology, function and associated aortic root or aortic pathology. The most commonly used methods for preoperative planning include echocardiography (both transthoracic and transesophageal) and computed tomography. The use of different modalities in understanding functional anatomy for planning a surgical repair of the aortic valve will be reviewed in this section (Fig. 3.2).

3.2.3.2.2 Echo

Echocardiography plays an important role in assessing the aortic valve for repair. First, the aortic valve morphology and pathology must be clarified. This can be done using a comprehensive transthoracic echocardiographic study but a

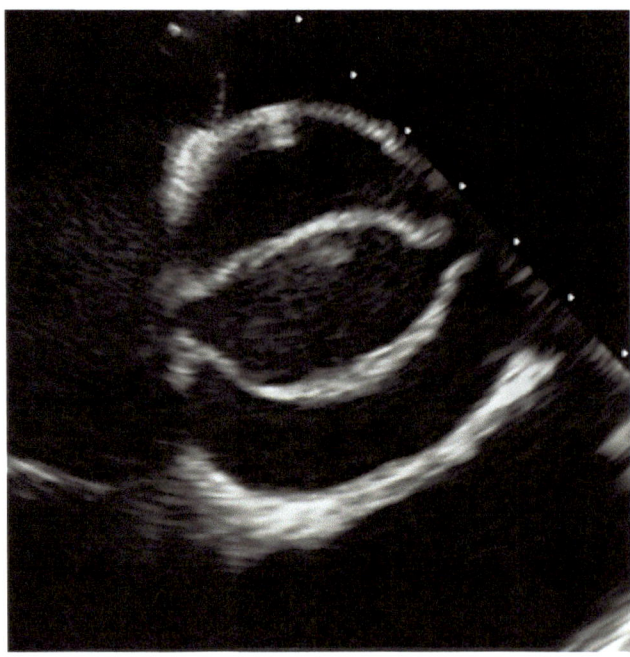

Fig. 3.2 An open bicuspid aortic valve seen in the short axis view on transesophageal echocardiography demonstrating a lack of significant calcification and commissure angle of 180°

transesophageal echocardiogram may be needed if the leaflet evaluation is difficult [23–25].

The aortic valve should be identified as trileaflet or bicuspid. If it is a bicuspid valve, then the leaflet morphology should be described based on standardized classification schemes, such as the one Sievers or Schaefer classifications [19, 20]. The degree of stenosis and regurgitation should also be assessed and described in accordance with guideline publications [26–28]. The context of the valve disease should also be understood, including chamber enlargement, ventricular disease, other valve pathology and any dilation of the aortic annulus, aortic root or proximal ascending aorta [29].

Specific echocardiographic features related to valve repair should also be considered. In one surgical series, echocardiographic predictors of successful repair for a regurgitant bicuspid aortic valve included an eccentric jet direction, no cusp thickening, no cusp calcification and lack of commissural thickening [22]. Another case series reported that cusp restriction and tissue deficiency were the main limitations of repairability [21].

Other centers have found that predictors of reoperation due to failed repair or one that was not durable included younger age, larger aortic annular dimension, lower cusp effective height and the need for a pericardial patch in the repair strategy [30, 31]. Cusp effective height is defined as the distance between the ventricular-arterial junction and the leaflet tip. Leaflet billowing, which has been defined one group as when the nadir of the aortic leaflet body lies on the ventricular side of the ventricular-arterial junction, has also been found to be a predictor of aortic valve repair failure [32].

Commissural orientation may also be associated with likelihood of successful repair. Although not studied extensively, one group found that when the commissures were not symmetric and were at an angle of <160° from one another, this finding was associated with need for reoperation [33].

In the setting of a trileaflet aortic valve, the aortic root size is likely the most important measure. Of course, significant leaflet abnormalities may preclude a valve sparing operation altogether. One large surgical series reported that in patients with an aortic annular diameter of 28 mm or greater, measured on the zoomed long axis view of the aortic valve by transesophageal echocardiography, valve sparing reimplantation was superior to subcommissural annuloplasty in terms of residual aortic regurgitation after repair [15].

It should be noted that although individual case series have reported echocardiographic parameters that are important to assess when aortic valve repair is considered, all data is observational and based on individual surgical programs. Given the heterogeneity of surgical strategy and technique, these findings have not been validated across multiple centres and may therefore have limited generalizability (Figs. 3.3 and 3.4).

3.2.3.3 Choosing the Ideal Prosthesis

3.2.3.3.1 Intro

The surgical planning in the choice of the prosthesis is certainly carried out with the utmost precision by the use of the CTA. The echocardiogram is an essential but comple-

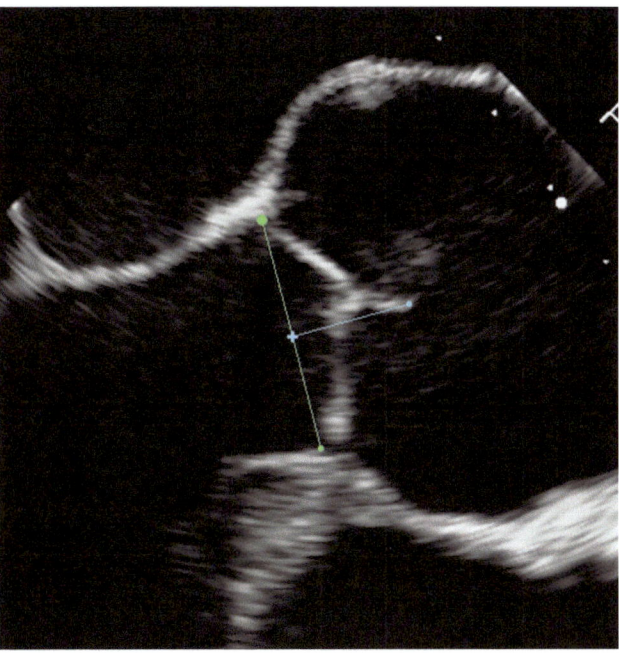

Fig. 3.4 Measurement of aortic valve leaflet effective height on the long axis view of a transesophageal echocardiogram

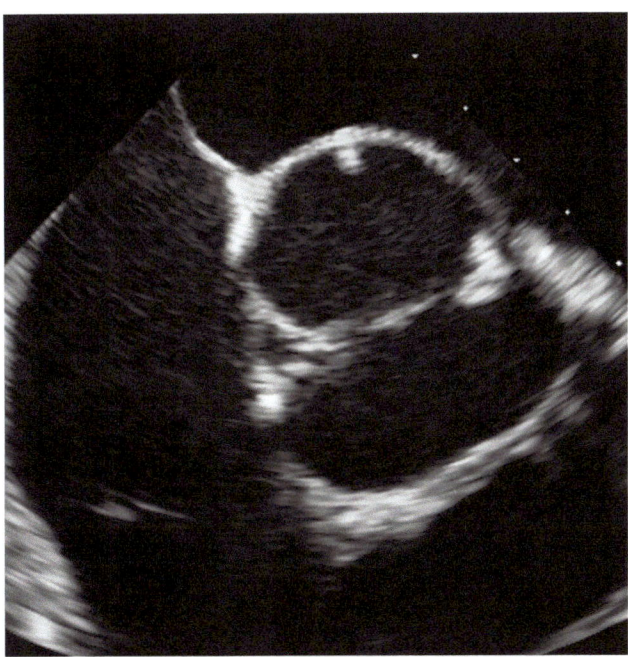

Fig. 3.3 A closed bicuspid aortic valve seen in the short axis view on transesophageal echocardiography demonstrating a lack of significant calcification and commissure angle of 180°

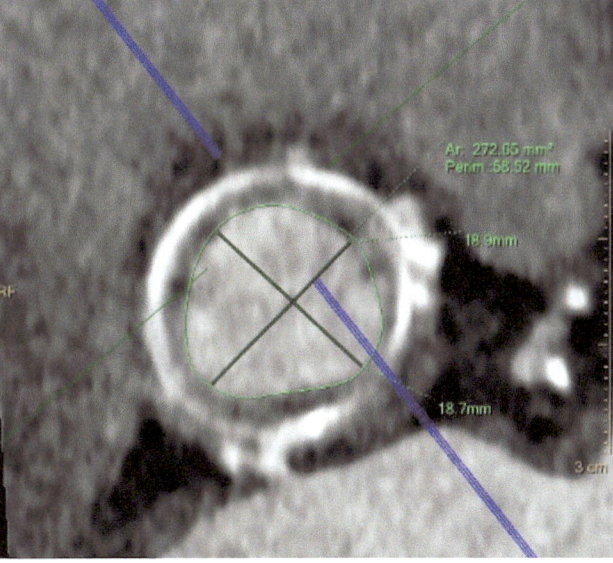

Fig. 3.5 Computed tomography during planning re-interventions: every detail regarding the previous implanted prosthesis can be quantified, in order to reach the best the height of the coronaries in respect to the aortic annulus and valvular plane

mentary method, being burdened by a greater number of artifacts and the difficulty of finding a cutting plane of the image reproducible with the same precision as the CTA (Fig. 3.5). With dedicated imaging programs and softwares, radiologists, but especially cardiac surgeons with advanced imaging knowledge, can perform accurate planning for the optimal choice of prosthesis. The degree of calcification of the aortic cusps, the size and arrangement of the calcifications of the aortic ring, the size of the Valsalva Sinuses and the height of the two coronary ostia relative to the valvular plane, are the main factors that guide the choice of the ideal prosthesis. Especially in all cases of patients with very small aortic rings, it will be possible to plan additional surgical maneuvers, such as root enlargement, in order to avoid problems of patient-prosthesis mismatch due to small prostheses.

3.2.3.3.2 Echo

When choosing a surgical aortic valve prosthesis, the role of echocardiography is limited. The replacement is done under cardioplegia with the aorta open, making live echocardiography at the time of replacement impossible. Sizing of the valve is done using direct physical evaluation of the annulus using specialized sizing tools. Echocardiography also suffers from limitations in accuracy when sizing the annulus, especially if done with 2-dimensional measurements only and before a disease valve is excised due to the degree of fibrosis and calcium [34].

Some characteristics that can be seen by echocardiography can be factored into the surgical management plan. For example, if the aortic annulus is noted to be small before the operation and there is a concern that only a small valve can be used with a significant risk of patient-prosthesis mismatch, then aortic root enlargement can be pre-planned and discussed with the patient. This can be assessed by an annular diameter by transthoracic or transeophageal 2-dimensional echocardiography in a zoomed long axis view of the aortic valve [23–25]. This dimension can then be compared to the dimensions of a desired prosthetic valve size to achieve an effective orifice area of greater than 0.85 cm^2 per square meter of body surface area. If needed, aortic root enlargement can be performed safely to allow for a larger prosthesis [35, 36].

3.2.3.4 Reintervention

3.2.3.4.1 Introduction

The number of patients undergoing reoperation for valvular heart disease is increasing and will continue to increase as the general population ages.

Reoperations are technically more difficult than primary operations because of adhesions around the heart with an associated risk of reentry, the presence of more advanced cardiac pathology, and the existence of more frequent comorbidities such as pulmonary hypertension. Important to know, re-operative replacement operations often are performed in functionally compromised patients who tolerate complications poorly.

More, redo cardiac surgery with patent coronary artery grafts after previous coronary artery bypass graft represents one of the most difficult problems in cardiac surgery.

Preoperative identification of all structures at risk is mandatory, and different, specific operative approaches always remain in consideration.

Recent reported experience suggests that preoperative cardiac CTA will lead to a modification in surgical strategy for 1 in 5 patients undergoing redo cardiac surgery (Fig. 3.6) [37].

For example, if CTA demonstrates a patent left internal mammary artery is close to the midline or a right ventricle directly adherent to the posterior table of the sternum, cardiopulmonary bypass is instituted prior to reentry. Definition of live grafts with respect to their proximal placement on the aorta is instrumental in determining, before the operation, the precise manner in which those grafts will be handled. For example, in reoperative surgery for AVR in the setting of live grafts, CTA allows the surgeon to plan preoperatively whether or not those grafts will have to be divided in carrying out the aortotomy for the AVR. As described earlier, CTA also allows the cardiac surgeon to plan the precise location of the aortotomy itself preoperatively.

3.2.3.4.2 Assessment of Adhesions

Intro

CT has been revolutionary in precisely defining the relationship of important structures (e.g, the aorta, right ventricle, or live grafts) to the midline and sternum for re-entry planning. In the context of reinterventions after isolated aortic valve surgery, fibrotic adhesions at the level of the sternal manu-

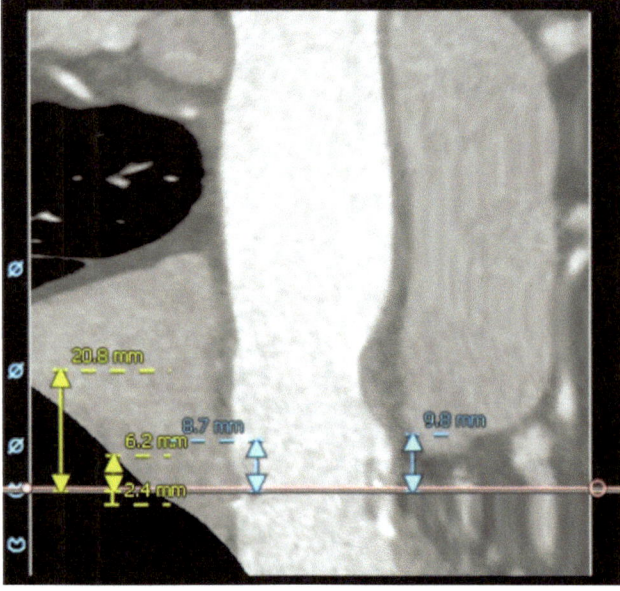

Fig. 3.6 Computed tomography is an essential tool during the preoperative planning of re-interventions, to quantify the height of the coronaries in respect to the aortic annulus and valvular plane. The dimension of the aortic root can be so narrow that a transcatheter intervention rather than a surgical one can be evaluated for the best treatment

brium (anonymous vein—left brachiocephalic venous trunk), at the level of the free wall of the right ventricle and their relationship with the sternal wires and the posterior wall of the sternum are particularly important (Figs. 3.7 and 3.8). This information, as already specified, is derived from the information derived from the CTA, which is much more complete and specific than the ultrasound.

Another interesting finding concerns the type of prosthesis in the aortic site, as well as the presence of any aortic vascular graft. In the specific case of some homograft pros-

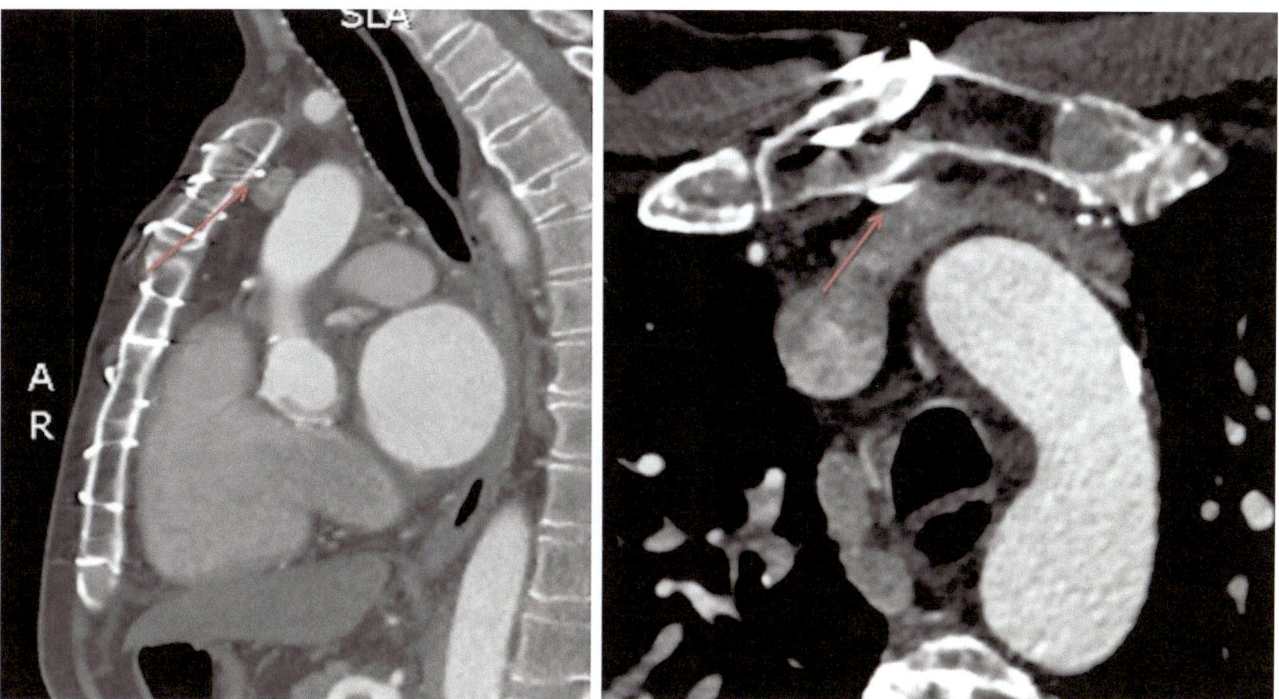

Fig. 3.7 In redo surgery, during re-sternotomy, one of the structures at highest risk of rupture is the left venous brachiocephalic trunk, or left anonymous vein (red arrow). Its course lies right behind the sternal manubrium, in contact most of the times with one of the upper sternal wires

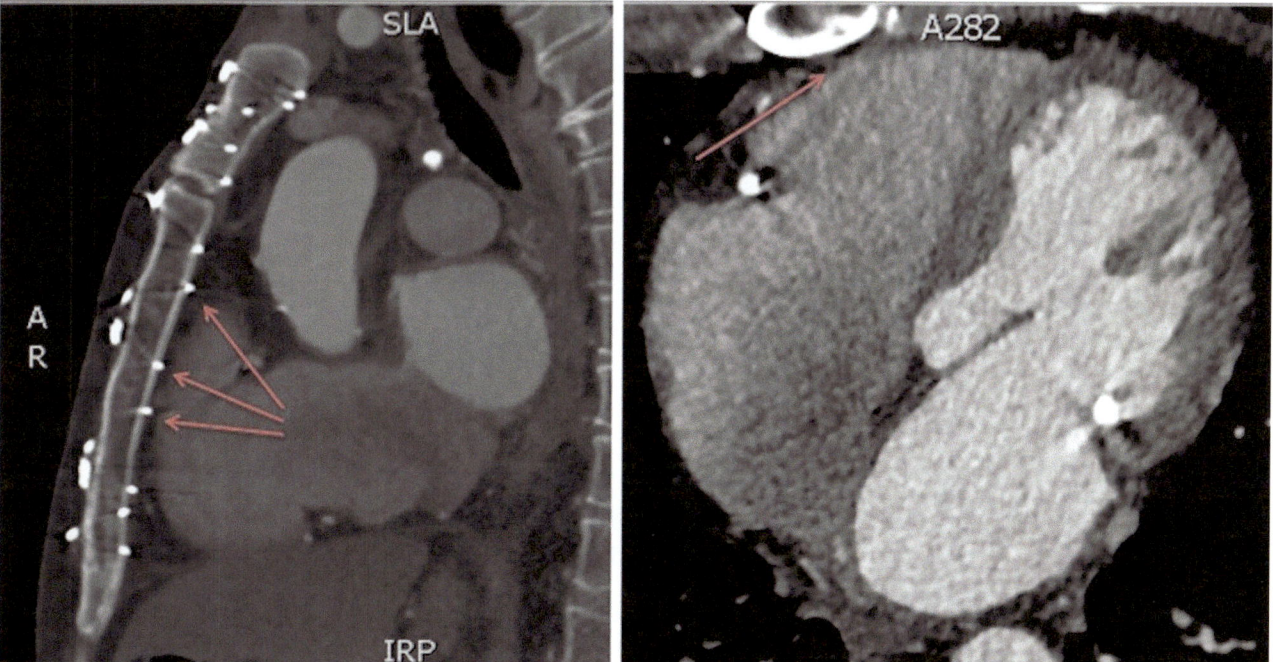

Fig. 3.8 In redo surgery, during re-sternotomy, another of the structures at highest risk of rupture, going down cranio-caudally, is the anterior free wall of the right ventricle (red arrows). Most of the times it is in contact with one of the metal sternal wires and the wall against the posterior wall of the sternum. Computed tomography is very helpful to rule out dangerous adhesions

theses, the calcific process visible to the CTA is so extensive that it involves the root itself and makes the reintervention extremely complex and high-risk.

Coronary Artery By-Pass Assessment with Angiography

The most high-risk reinterventions are those in which there is the presence of patent coronary artery bypass grafts. Intra-hospital mortality in case of bypass lesions during re-opening could be more than 50%. To this purpose, it is essential to understand the course of the arterial and venous grafts, the disposition, so as to be able to avoid and carefully isolate them during re-opening. Fundamental information is obtained with pre-intervention coronary angiography, in which the residual native coronary circulation, the course of the internal thoracic artery (left and right mammary, depending on the construction of the bypass), as well as the venous grafts are properly visualized (Fig. 3.9). The same information can be obtained with even greater accuracy through the use of contrast enhanced CTA scan (Fig. 3.10).

3.2.3.4.3 Access Choice

Intro

Reoperative sternotomy is challenging secondary to adhesions, loss of tissue planes, and the potential for injury to patent grafts, the aorta, and the right ventricle. Concerning other approaches, lateral thoracotomy, for example, was used extensively in the past, to obtain access to mediastinal

structures. For redo surgical cases, however, repeating the sternotomy could be a valuable and effective option [38].

Angiography

Biplane aortography with the first 1–2 heart cycles documented without contrast allows the assessment of the aortic annulus, aortic root, ascending aorta and aortic arch. During the first seconds the presence and location of calcium can be evaluated. If necessary, a rotational angiography without contrast and enhanced X-ray dosage can be added for better sensitivity and exact localization of the calcification. To evaluate the luminal sizes, contrast application is still necessary using Angiography as a luminography method. Strong lateral projection allows to evaluate the distance between sternum and aorta. If the swan-ganz catheter from right heart catheterization is still in place, the relationship to the right pulmonary artery and pulmonary trunk can be evaluated. Depending on the surgical strategy it can be necessary to add a peripheral angiography for peripheral cannulation. Calcifications, minimal luminal diameter and tortuosity of the vessel are in focus during exploration.

3.2.3.5 Access for Minimally Invasive SAVR

3.2.3.5.1 Planning a Ministernotomy and Right Minithoracotomy

In these minimally invasive procedures, both ministernotomy and right thoracotomy, it is critical to understand the

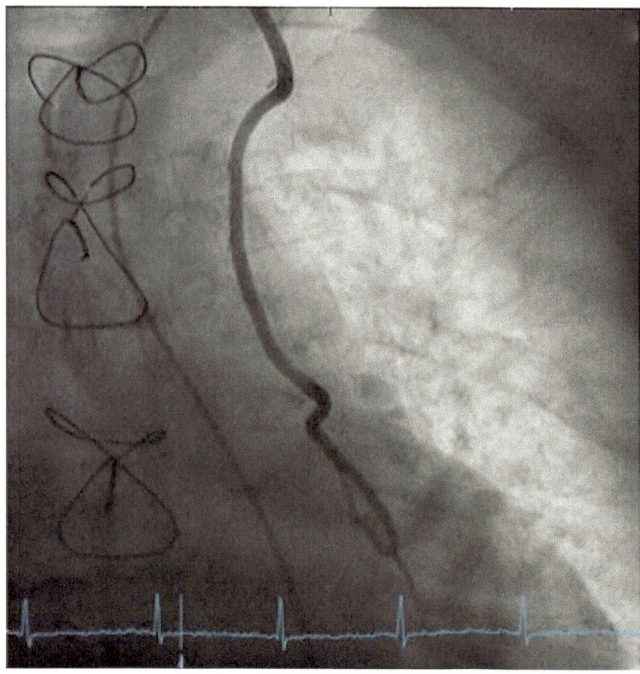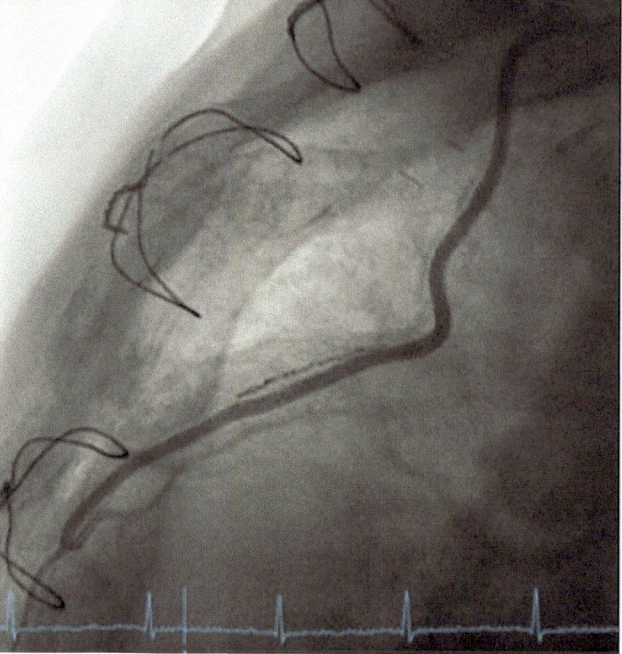

Fig. 3.9 Complementary to computed tomography, angiography is the other favoured imaging modality for those redo patients who received coronary artery bypass. They have patent grafts at the time of re-intervention, angio lets properly visualize the retrosternal course of the left internal mammary artery

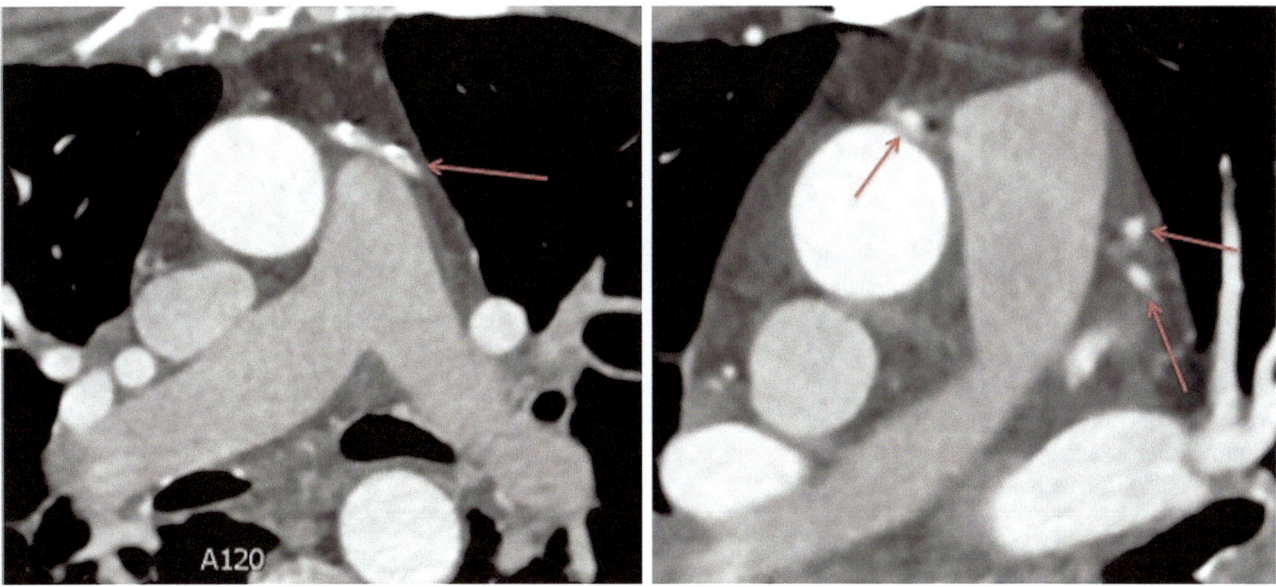

Fig. 3.10 In redo surgery, during re-sternotomy in presence of patent grafts, contrasted computed tomography is the ideal imaging modality to understand the localisation and their course in respect to other mediastinal structures and the sternum

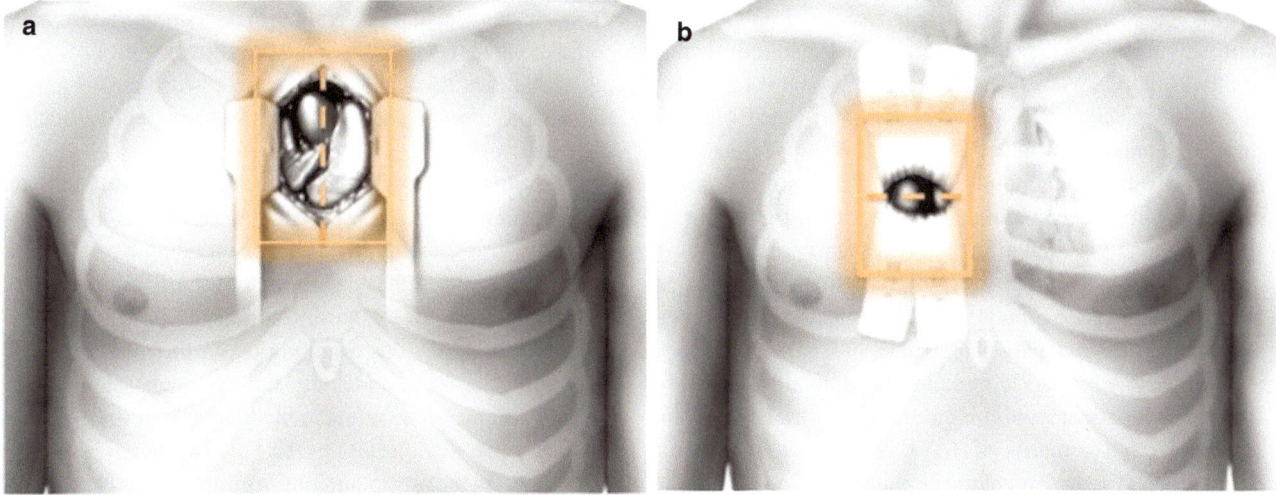

Fig. 3.11 Comparison of minimally invasive approaches for the surgical management of the aortic valve, panel A the right minitoracothomy and in panel B the upper ministernotomy

relationship of the valve to some targets on the bony thorax, the presence of calcification on the ascending aorta and, crucial, the conditions of groin vessels, if required for peripheral cannulation (Fig. 3.11). An horizontal aorta in normally not enhancing the exposure. If the patient's glomerular filtration and renal function is good, a contrast enhanced CTA scan with 3D reconstruction provides the best picture of the intrathoracic structures. If peripheral cannulation is scheduled, the CTA will involve the entire aorta until the femoral axis or otherwise a femoral arterial duplex may be obtained to show their quality. Reoperative procedures are challenging owing to diffuse mediastinal and pericardial adhesions.

A large incision that increases the operative exposure also has been associated with a higher risk of injury to cardiac structures and coronary artery bypass grafts and results in greater bleeding with its associated transfusion requirements [39].

A smaller incision with a limited sternotomy, on the other hand, reduces the area of pericardiolysis, thus mitigating these effects. The intact lower sternum that remains also preserves the integrity of the caudal chest wall, thereby enhancing sternal stability and promoting earlier extubation. Minimally invasive valve procedures gradually have become more accepted as new technologies and instrumentation have been developed. Reoperative procedures in which there is risk for graft injury are an area where minimally invasive strategies may be of direct benefit.

3.2.3.5.2 Planning a Left Thoracotomy

Intro

The left thoracotomy in the case of aortic surgery reintervention is not considered a choice approach, not offering particular advantages but on the contrary a suboptimal surgical exposure. It can be considered an alternative surgical access in some cases of reintervention of mitral surgery and in the case of reoperative descending thoracic aorta or thoracoabdominal aortic aneurysm surgery, which represent a challenge because of increased risk of lung injury and diffuse bleeding.

3.3 Interventional Planning

3.3.1 Introduction

Symptomatic severe aortic stenosis (AS) is the most common valvular heart disease requiring interventional therapy in the developed world. Although conventional surgical aortic valve replacement (AVR) has been performed for more than 50 years, the introduction and validation of transcatheter aortic valve implantation (TAVI) has led to a dramatic change in the management of AS over the past few years. A robust clinical research effort, including multiple, large randomized trials, has established TAVI as the preferred treatment for high-risk AS patients and an alternative to surgery for intermediate-risk patients [40, 41].

Currently, while AVR remains the standard of care for low-risk AS patients, on-going randomized trials are examining the relative merits of TAVI versus AVR in low-risk populations. Therapy recommendations have been incorporated in the most recent guidelines for the management of patients with AS in both european and the american guidelines [42, 43].

High-quality national and international registries will be needed to check these trends and to ensure adequate clinical outcomes in real-world practice. Concerning the best TAVI access, data from the randomized PARTNER 2 trial showed that the transfemoral (TF) route should be the preferred route during TAVI, since it is associated with reduced mortality compared with alternative "intra-thoracic" accesses, such as transapical and trans-aortic routes [44].

Current second-generation TAVI systems were modified to reduce the incidence of the common complications associated with first-generation devices, by improving sealing mechanisms, reducing the delivery system profile and making it easier to more precisely implant the device. In addition, the repositionability and retrievability of some of the newer devices have drastically reduced the risk of valve malpositioning.

3.3.2 Annular Sizing for TAVI

3.3.2.1 Intro

The assessment of the aortic annulus and root dimensions represents the key aspect in pre-procedural imaging, as these measurements determine the appropriate device size.

Self-expandable and balloon expandable valves are available in many sizes which should be perfectly adapted to patients. Undersizing of the prosthetic valve increases the risk of paravalvular regurgitation, while oversizing increases the risk of coronary occlusion or rupture of the annulus area.

The anatomy of the aortic root which includes the sinotubular junction, the aortic sinus containing the sinuses of Valsalva, and the aortic annulus, which represent the most relevant dimensions in pre-procedural planning of TAVI. The aortic annulus is a virtual basal ring formed by the nadirs of the aortic leaflets and is of rather ovoid configuration.

Several studies demonstrated the superiority of 3D imaging modalities such as CTA for the assessment of annular dimensions compared to 2D imaging modalities such as 2D-transesophageal echocardiography [45].

Traditionally, echocardiography has been used to determine feasibility of the aortic annulus und the aortic root for TAVI; however, variability of measurements have favoured during time the routinary adoption of CTA [46].

For evaluation of the aortic annulus, double oblique multiplanar reconstructions orienting two orthogonal planes for measuring the short and long diameters are required. The vertical oblique plane refers to the long axis of the aorta, and the transverse plane refers to the base of the cusps, thus an axial view of the aortic annulus with the lowest cusp insertion points of all three leaflets can be obtained. Based on the double oblique multiplanar reconstructions, several measurements can be taken of the aortic root dimension for TAVI planning: the area-based effective diameter and perimeter-derived measurements determined in CTA are the preferred parameters for the calculation of device size with high correlation. Besides prosthesis sizing, the distances from the aortic annulus to the coronary ostium of the right coronary artery (RCA) and to the ostium of the left coronary artery (LCA) are relevant in order to select a suitable device system. Lower distance of coronary ostia (<10 mm) and the implantation have been described as possible risk factors for coronary obstruction with some prosthesis and are associated with higher acute and late mortality rates [47].

Bicuspid aortic valve (BAV) associated stenosis is relatively common, interestingly enough, more so in the Asian population where up to half of those undergoing TAVR have concurrent BAV [48].

The early identification and characterization of BAV morphology has been shown to be highly important to help stratify risk and define treatment decision making.

Importantly, MDCT offers incremental information beyond echocardiography for the characterization and classification of bicuspid valvular disease. Pre-procedural identification of such morphology is enabled by MDCT, because of better resolution. The presence and arrangement of cusp fusion is often readily identifiable in a reconstructed transverse axial plane, as is the determination of the number of cusps, and intercommissural distance—factors described either in current or recently proposed BAV classification schemes.

3.3.2.2 CT

Computed tomography is ideally suited for the anatomic assessment of the aortic valve, as it provides isotropic voxels within the submillimetre range which allows for multiplanar reformation of images. ECG-synchronisation of the CT scan provides images without motion blurring or double contours. Individually tailored CT protocols allow for reliable and reproducible measurements which depend on sufficient contrast attenuation of the aortic root, adequate reduction of image noise and the absence of motion artefacts (Fig. 3.12).

The aortic annulus plane is defined as a virtual plane through the most basal attachment ("hinge points") of the aortic leaflets (Fig. 3.13). Identification of the annulus plane can be performed manually or software-based with semi-automatic or automatic anatomical segmentation. Annular contouring is performed along the blood pool-tissue interface. In case of annular calcification, the annulus contour is drawn as if no calcium is present. When a valve is deployed which is larger than the aortic annulus it is called oversizing. Oversizing is calculated as a percentage [%], as follows:

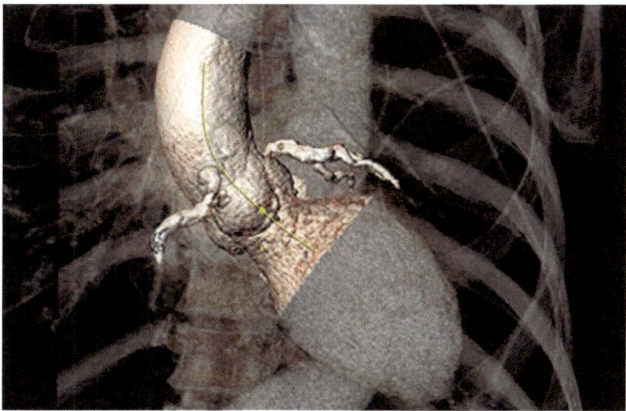

Fig. 3.12 CT assessment of the aortic root. Computed tomography is ideally suited for the anatomic assessment of the aortic valve as it allows for 2D and 3D image reconstructions and reformations

Oversizing [%] = (Valve nominal measurement/annular measurement−1) × 100.

Quantification of the annular dimension provides area and perimeter measurements which are most suitable for valve sizing. The ratio of short to long axis provides information about the sphericity of the aortic annulus. Usually, the decrease of the aortic annulus sphericity during systole due to the bulging of the aortomitral continuity towards the left atrium results in larger annulus area and perimeter compared to diastolic diastole. Therefore, systolic measurements are preferred for valve sizing. However, images acquired during systole are more prone to motion artefacts.

3.3.2.3 Echo

Annular sizing for transcatheter aortic valve replacement by echocardiography was of great interest to the valvular heart disease community because this procedure was initially done under transesophageal echocardiographic guidance and under general anesthesia. Additionally, the aortic annulus cannot be inspected and measured directly like it can be in the case of surgical aortic valve replacement. However, the procedure has been simplified over the years and most centers now perform this procedure using minimal sedation and without transesophageal echocardiography [49, 50].

Computed tomography scanning provides more information relevant to the entire procedure and allows for multiplanar reconstruction of the 3-dimensional dataset to incorporate the irregular shape of the aortic annulus into measurements [34]. Additionally, there is data to suggest that computed tomography is more accurate than echocardiography and reduces the incidence of paravalvular regurgitation [51]. This is why it is the preferred imaging modality for planning. However, when computed tomography is not available, such as in urgent or unstable cases, then transesophageal echocardiography is important in annular sizing and valve selection.

On transesophageal echocardiography, the annulus can be measured as a single 2-dimensional diameter in the zoomed long axis view of the aortic valve [49, 52]. A much more accurate measurement would be to use 3-dimensional echocardiography and measure the annulus using multi-planar reconstruction of a zoomed 3-dimensional volume of the aortic valve including at least some of the left ventricular outflow tract and aortic root. The greatest accuracy to direct annular measurements are obtained in mid-systole [51]. This is when the annulus is largest and most circular. Still, the anterior-posterior diameter tends to be the smaller diameter of the oval shaped aortic annulus. The reconstruction planes can be aligned so that a cross-sectional short axis plane is located at the basal ring defined by the nadir of the aortic leaflet hinge points. Ideally, this should be done using a single beat acquisition since stitch artifact in multi-beat acquisitions can introduce significant measurement error in this

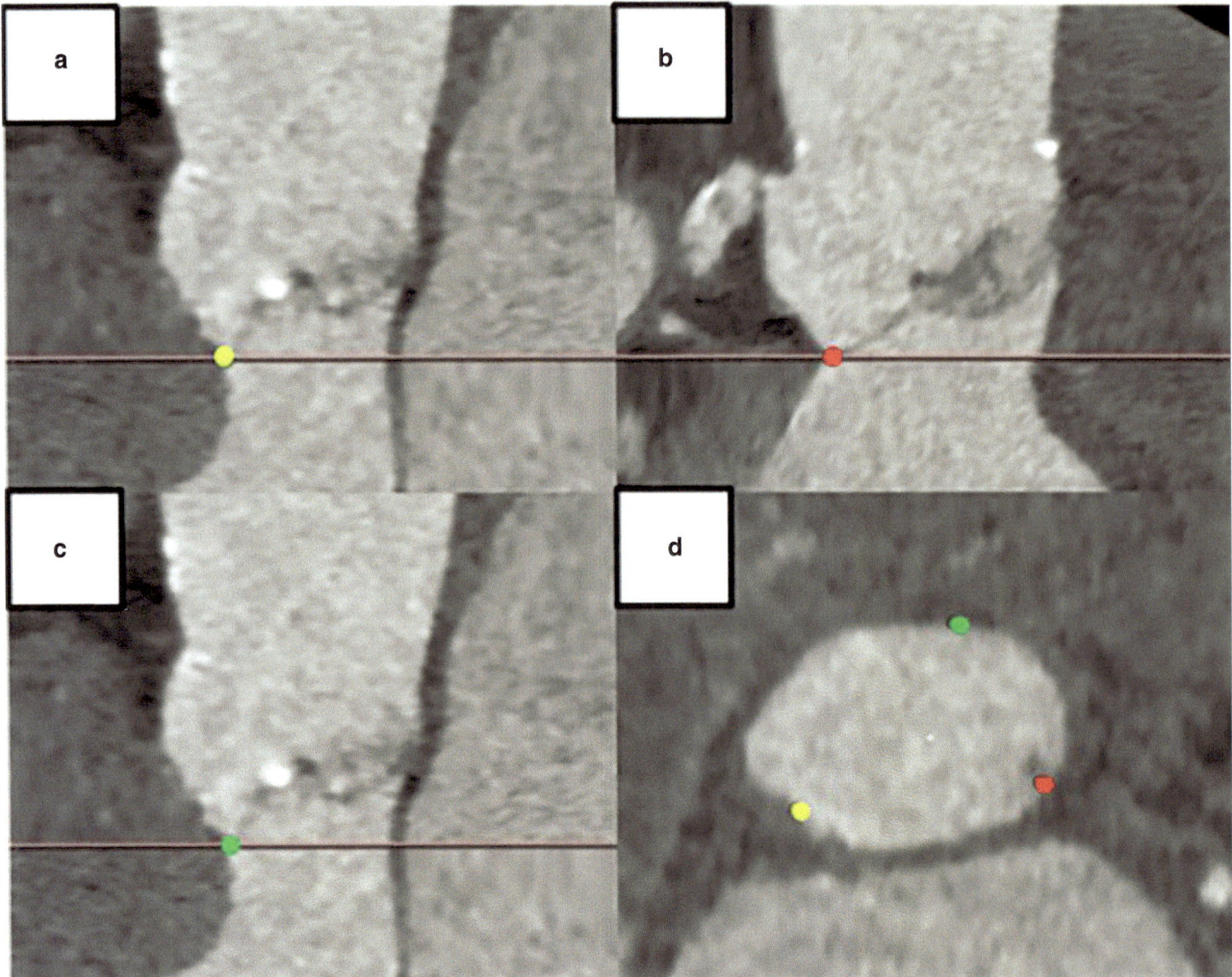

Fig. 3.13 Definition of the aortic annulus plane. The aortic annuls plane (**d**) is defined as a virtual plane through the hinge points of each aortic leaflet (**a–c**)

critical value. The technique to identify this plane using multi-planar reconstruction is to align as best as possible to just under the leaflet hinge based on the long axis views, and then to rotationally sweep across the three cusps using the short axis plane to ensure that this short axis plane is actually located just below the leaflet hinge points [52–55].

Once the proper measurement plane is defined, the maximal and minimal diameters as well as the circumference can be measured using standard tools built into most 3-dimensional echocardiographic analysis packages. The circumference-derived diameter can also be calculated and may be a more accurate dimension to use for valve sizing in transcatheter aortic valve replacement [53]. Unfortunately, the data still suggests that direct planimetry tends to underestimate the annulus size compared to computed tomography (a recognized gold standard) and is less reproducible. Dense calcification also makes visualization of the annulus and direct planimetry more challenging. The use of fully auto-

mated and semi-automated 3-dimensional echocardiography planimetry may be more accurate and preferred for procedural guidance (Fig. 3.14) [56–58].

3.3.2.4 Angiography

Technique of choice to quantify aortic annulus in TAVI procedures is multiplanar reconstruction from multislice, ECG gated CT images. In certain circumstances this is not accessible for different reasons. During an emergency setting in the cathlab or operating room it is sometimes necessary to go straight forward for valve implantation and therefore every operator should be familiar using angiography for quantification of the annulus. Doing so, it is most likely to pick up the maximum diameter of the annulus in contrast to echocardiography. The limitation of this 2 dimensional measure it the fact, that depending on the X-ray angulation or perspective on the annulus, the diameter is smaller or bigger due to the fact, that not the full diameter is transected but

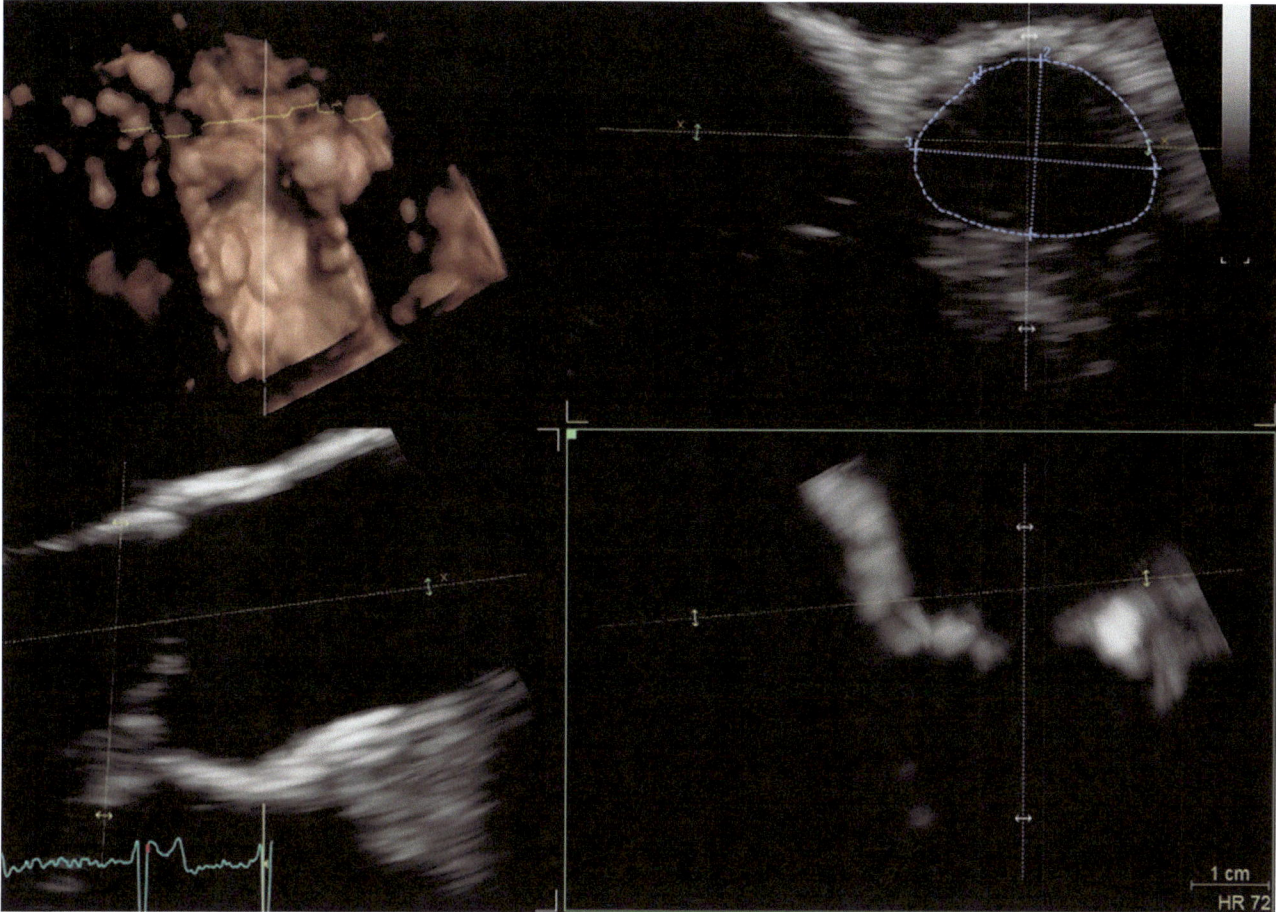

Fig. 3.14 Measurement of the aortic annulus using multi-planar reconstruction by 3-dimensional transesophageal echocardiography, a method that is more accurate than single 2-dimensional measurements

instead a tangent across the aortic root. In fact, the operator cannot realize which diameter he is measuring. This is nicely shown by Piazza et al. [59] Comparing 2D and 3D imaging techniques with standard angulations, sagittal diameters (LAO 90°) were smaller than coronal diameters (anterior-posterior) [60].

A new option for quantification during angiography is the rotational C-arm CT technique. In fact, contrast injection into the LV allows a better imaging of the anatomic annulus and measurements show a better to CT measurements as compared with injections into the ascending aorta [61].

In patients with severe kidney injury, today 3D TOE with multiplanar reconstruction of the annulus is the technique of choice (Fig. 3.15).

3.3.2.5 Balloon Sizing
Knowing the limitations of angiography based sizing of the annulus, balloon sizing is a valuable addition to determine the exact annulus size. Therefore an undersized balloon is used and contrast injection is performed during rapid pacing and balloon inflation with an almost perpendicular projec-

tion to the long axis of the balloon. Using the known sizes of the balloon as a reference, the annulus size can be measured in a single plain. Compared with TOE, Balloon Sizing results in about 1 mm bigger measurements of the annulus and in a different valve size in 26% [62]. Balloon sizing is of value in borderline big annuli and severe calcifications. It has been shown that the valve size differs in 30–50% of cases compared with CT, with significant higher aortic regurgitant index and no difference in other variables [63]. Today we use balloon sizing almost only in cases with borderline big annuli to decide whether or not we can treat the patient percutaneously in a hybrid OR setting with the capability for direct open heart surgery (Fig. 3.16).

3.3.3   Device Selection

3.3.3.1 Intro
Transcatheter aortic valve implantation (TAVI) has been successfully performed in inoperable, high-risk, intermediate-risk and even low-risk patients with low mortality and

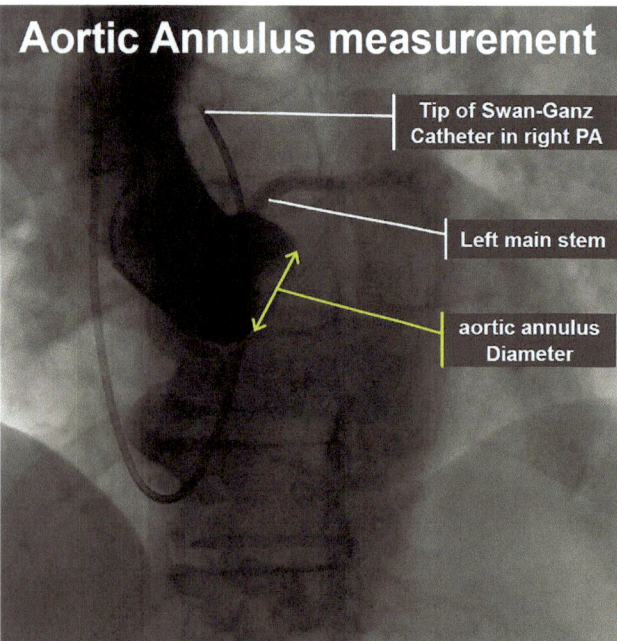

Fig. 3.15 Orthogonal angiography picks up the maximal diameter between non- and left coronary ostia. The relation to the left main can easily be identified and quantified. Normally, in contrast to echo, the maximal annulus diameter is picked up

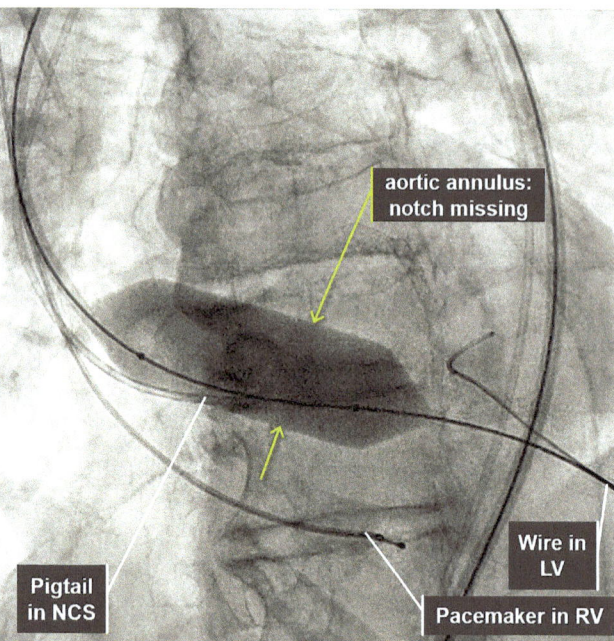

Fig. 3.16 Ballon sizing of the aortic annulus: Patient with severe renal insufficiency. The Ballon Size is lower than the annulus size (no notching of the annulus, ballon keeps moving during inflation). *NCS* non coronary sinus, *LV* left ventricle, *RV* right ventricle

complication rates [40, 64–67]. Most centers routinely implant different transcatheter heart valves (THVs) and a patient-tailored approach has become increasingly popular. Indeed, when chosing a particular THV, operators try to esti-

mate and balance the risk for annular rupture or other vascular complications, relevant paravalvular leak (PVL), need for a permanent pacemaker, the occurrence of patient prosthesis mismatch, coronary occlusion and other complications.

3.3.3.2 In Aortic Stenosis

Pre-procedural planning is probably the single most important element of a successful TAVI program. Multislice computed tomography (MSCT) of the chest, abdomen and pelvis with the ability to perform a 3-dimensional reconstruction has become the cornerstone of pre-procedural planning. Most of the available THVs are intended to be used in a broad range of anatomies, but certain features may influence device selection.

Device selection starts with measurement of the annular diameter, perimeter and area. In annuli with a mean diameter ranging from 29 to 30 mm, only the Medtronic CoreValve Evolut R 34 mm (Medtronic Inc., Minneapolis, USA) or the Edwards Sapien 3 29 mm (Edwards Lifesciences, Irvine, California, USA) are currently eligible. Based on the degree of calcification and the anatomy of the annulus and the left-ventricular outflow tranct (LVOT), the risk of the most devastating complication, annular rupture, should be estimated in every patient. The risk may be highest in patients with heavily calcified leaflets extending into the LVOT, and a shallow aortic root undergoing TAVI with a balloon-expandable valve (Fig. 3.17). Excessive oversizing, particularly of balloon-expandable THVs, has been closely linked to annular rupture [68]. Similarly, post-dilatation of self-expanding valves using large balloons carries the same risk. On the other hand, evidence indicates that the risk for relevant paravalvular regurgitation in patients with heavily calcified valves is higher with self-expanding than with balloon-expandable or mechanically expanded valves [69]. In patients with mild to moderate calcification, the difference in the degree of paravalvular regurgitation evens out. External sealing-skirts are currently added to many of the self-expanding THVs. If they are able to reduce the degree of paravalvular regurgitation even in the presence of heavy calcification remains to be proven.

In patients with low coronary artery ostia, a repositionable and retrievable THV such as the CoreValve Evolut R/Pro, the Portico (Abbott, Abbott Park, Illinois, USA), or the Lotus (Boston Scientific, Marlborough, Massachusetts, USA) may be preferred. In the presence of narrow iliofemoral arteries, there may be some delivery systems with a slight advantage. An outer diameter of 18F is now standard, but some devices such as the CoreValve Evolut R with it's inline sheath may offer a slight advantage, although the diameter has increased with the latest iteration, the Evolut PRO. Another factor to consider may be the presence of pre-existing conduction disorders (i.e. a right bundle branch block or a first degree atrioventricular block). In this patient population, a THV with a very low pacemaker rate such as

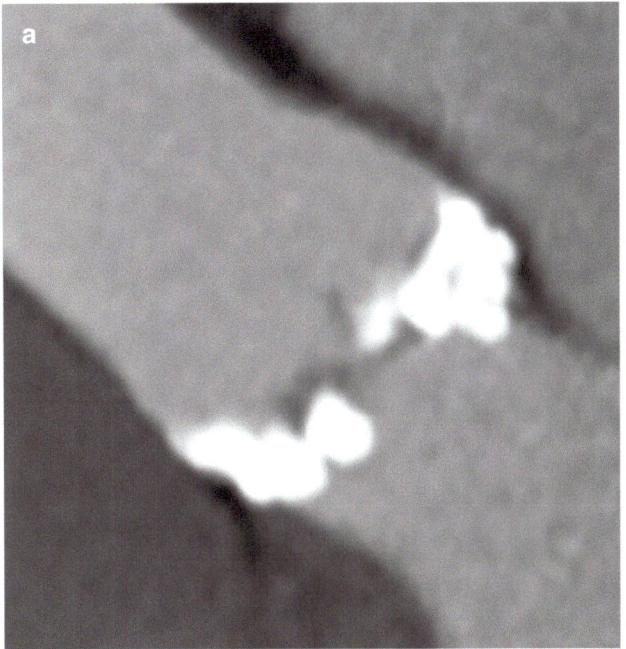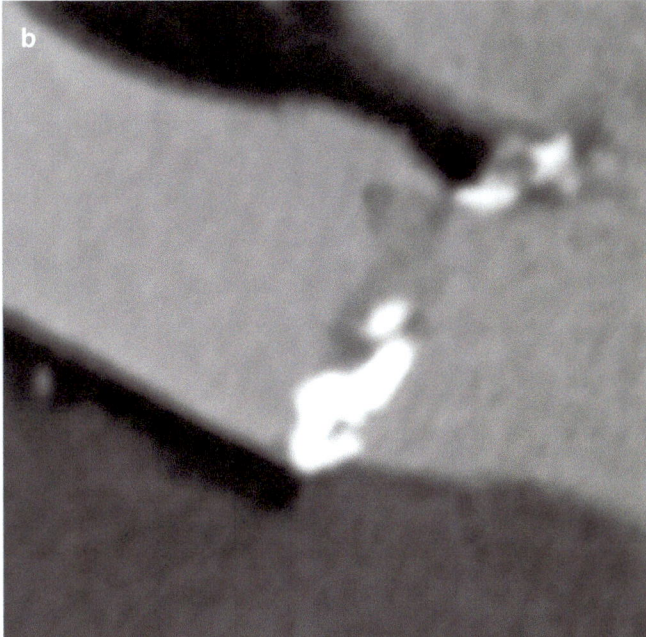

Fig. 3.17 A patient at very high risk for annular rupture. Note the heavy calcification of the leaflets extending into the left-ventricular outflow tract and the shallow sinus. In this patient, careful predilatation with a small balloon and implantation of a self-expanding THV may be preferred over implantation of a balloon-expandable THV, although the risk for paravalvular regurgitation remains considerable

the ACURATE neo may lead to a reduction in new permanent pacemaker rates [70].

3.3.3.3 In Aortic Regurgitation

Most of the current THVs have been developed for patients with aortic stenosis and rely on calcification of the native valve annulus to anchor the THV. While open heart surgery remains the gold-standard for most of these patients, TAVI has been performed off-label to treat patients at high surgical risk [71–74]. In aortic regurgitation, the annuli are often large and the leaflets are uncalcified or with minimal calcification (Fig. 3.18).

Accordingly, there is a high risk for ventricular embolization after release of the THV [75]. Some valves such as the JenaValve (JenaValve Technology, Irvine, California, USA) or the J-Valve (JieCheng Medical Technology Co., Suzhou, China) have been designed with a different anchoring (clasping) mechanism that does not rely on calcification of the native valve. However, they are currently not available for transfemoral access [76]. However, a first successful transfemoral implantation of the JenaValve has been described in a patient with pure aortic regurgitation [77]. At the current stage, no definitive recommendation regarding valve choice for transfemoral TAVI for the treatment of aortic regurgitation can be made. Nevertheless, the self-expanding ACURATE neo has an x-shaped design of the frame with an upper crown 5 mm larger than the nominal THV diameter which may help to anchor the prosthesis even in the absence of calcification [78]. The current evidence is scarce, but according to a recent publication, oversizing by the perime-

ter derived diameter of at least 2 mm is required and initial position should be 5 mm instead of 7 mm below the annulus. Furthermore, rapid pacing may be used to allow better stability and visualization during deployment [75].

3.3.4 Access Choice and Planning

3.3.4.1 Intro

Vascular access is the first step of the procedure itself and almost as important as valve implantation itself. Failure at this point can compromise the whole procedure and lead to live threatening situations.

First TAVI was done using the most complex access route from the femoral vein transseptal through the mitral valve in an antegrade fashion. This approach was overcome by developing stiffer and steerable delivery systems providing the possibility for retrograde access. In parallel, transapical access was promoted as an alternative antegrade access mainly by surgical colleagues [79]. Straight antegrade access was easy to perform and device size was not an issue. Different techniques have been developed to close the left ventricular apex. However, impact on left ventricular function is significant compared with transfemoral access [80]. Looking for alternatives, subclavian access with surgical cut down was used in patients with severe peripheral artery disease. First experiences started early and have been described in 2010 [81]. It can be used with local anesthesia only. In parallel, as an alternative to subclavian access, transcarotid approach was first performed in 2010 [82]. Surgical direct

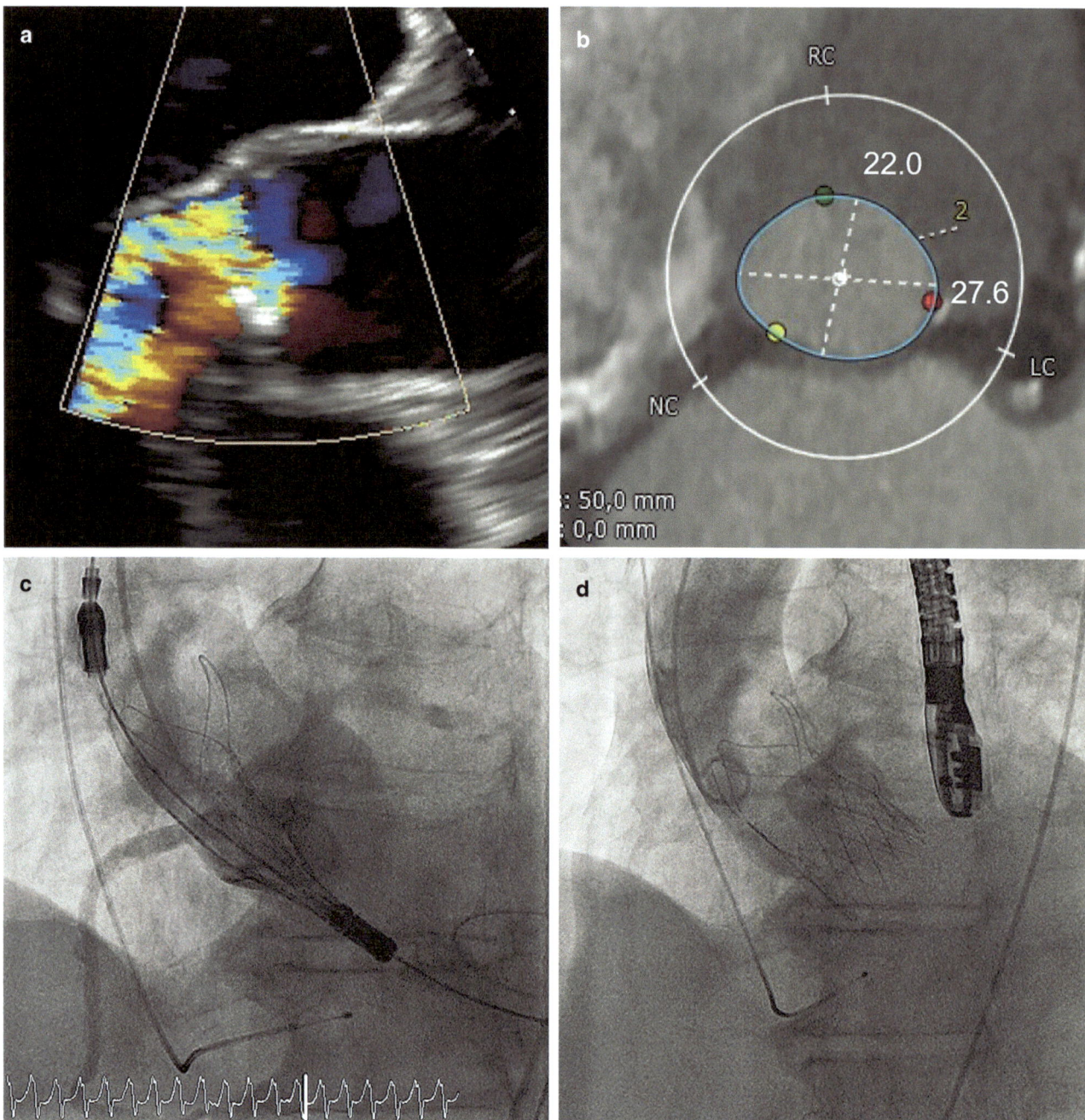

Fig. 3.18 TAVI in a patient with pure aortic regurgitation. The patient had an eccentric jet due to prolapse of the right coronary cusp (**a**). Annular measurement was performed in standard fashion (**b**). An ACURATE neo was positioned under semi-rapid pacing (**c**). Final result after release of the THV (**d**)

transthoracic access was also used. It is limited due to the short distance between the puncture side and the aortic valve. Puncture side has to be free of disease [83]. Latest, a venous transcaval transaortic approach was used in a multicenter, single-arm trial with 100 patients showing device success in 98 of 99 patients, 30d survival was 92% [84].

Planning of vascular access therefore needs to be done carefully. Transfemoral access is today the method of choice today and is the way in which TAVI has shown its superiority compared with surgery in intermediate and low risk patients [1, 41, 85]. Imaging is the key for understanding the optimal way of access and to choose the best prosthesis matching the individual patient with lowest risk.

First of all, CT protocols for TAVI include CT angiography of the great vessels including left and right subclavian artery, the carotids, the complete aorta down to the iliac and femoral vessels. With this examination every possible access can be evaluated. If not available, also angiography can be used. In patients with severe renal failure, ultrasound imaging is in favor to avoid contrast application. Native CT can give information about calcification but lumen assessment is not feasible enough. MRI angiography is a possible alternative, but Gadolinium i.v. is also a constrain in renal failure and overall accessibility is limited.

Surgical cut-down was used in the beginning of TAVR does not play an important role today anymore. Still, it can be used in problematic patient subsets and should be discussed in advance.

3.3.4.1.1 Femoral Access Assessment

Intro

Femoral access is for several reasons the main access for TAVR nowadays. First, all interventionalists are familiar with femoral access, even if radial approach gains to be more and more popular in coronary artery disease. Second, the overall setup is comfortable for a safe procedure with good X-ray protection for the interventionalist and less for assisting staff. Third, almost all devices can be used from femoral access and

the operator can choose the optimal solution for the individual patient. Fourth, several different closing devices to use solely or in combination are available and finally, manual compression is still possible. Fifth, different imaging modalities can be used to plan and even to guide secure puncture.

Older Patients with aortic stenosis have a higher prevalence of symptomatic peripheral artery disease (PAD) compared with the same age group without aortic stenosis [86]. Screening exams are essential to gather all available information to choose the correct technique. The different methodologies are discussed below with a big advantage for CT assessment as it allows a 3D assessment of the vessel with a clear idea of calcium distribution as the main factor driving vascular difficulties and complications. Vessel tortuosity can nicely picked up from the reconstructed images. The price to pay is a relatively high amount of contrast to be used.

CT

CT angiography provides non-invasive assessment of the anatomy of the iliofemoral vessels as well as the aorta (Fig. 3.19). Pre-procedural screening of the femoral access

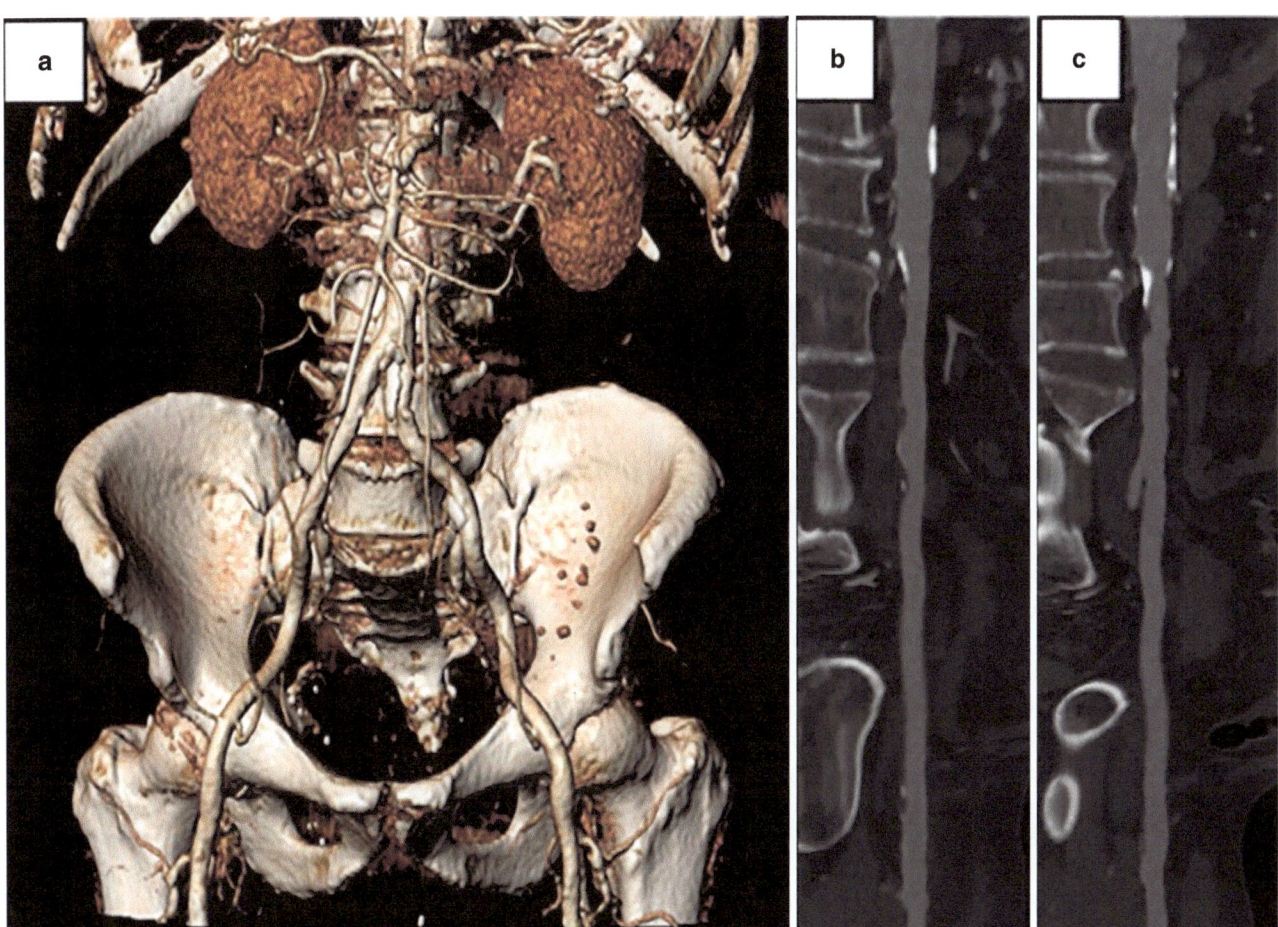

Fig. 3.19 Femoral access assessment via CT. CT angiography provides non-invasive assessment of the anatomy of the iliofemoral vessels via 3D reconstructions (**a**) as well as 2D multiplanar image reformations (**b** and **c**)

route depends on the assessment of vessel size, tortuosity and atheromatous plaques. Furthermore, CT could depict aneurysms and dissections in the access pathway and a high femoral artery bifurcation. Vascular pathologies can be related to fluoroscopically identifiable anatomical landmarks. Risk factors for major vascular complications are an external sheath diameter that exceeds the minimal artery diameter, moderate or severe calcification and vessel tortuosity. Recently, it was reported that an external sheath-to-iliofemoral-artery-ratio (SIFAR) <1.12 provides safe access for TAVR.

Angiography

Direct visualization of the common femoral artery (CFA) using angiography can be done during diagnostic work up or just before intervention. The advantage of angiography is its high spatial resolution and it is available during the procedure and guides also peripheral interventions.

A calibrated pigtail is placed above the bifurcation in the abdominal aorta. 20–30 cc of contrast are injected during 2 s to visualize both iliac and femoral arteries. With the markers of the pigtail, calibration of the system allows easy and exact measurements of the vessel size. Interestingly enough, if compared with CT images, angiographic measurements show up to 10% bigger vessel diameters. If image intensifier size is small it can be necessary to do left and right side sequentially with less amount of contrast for each side. The common femoral artery and the bifurcation into superficial and profunda femoris and its relationship to the femoral head and the inferior border (not the vessel origin) of the inferior epigastric artery needs to be identified. Ideal puncture side is above the bifurcation to permit stent implantation without compromising the profunda femoris in case of severe bleeding after TAVI. The proximal limit of the puncture side is the inferior border of the inferior epigastric artery. Higher punctures increase significant the risk of retroperitoneal bleeding. At the side of puncture, no calcifications should be present to allow vessel closure after the procedure. In case of calcium, a rotational angiography of the zoomed image from RAO to LAO or vice versa is recommended to identify the location of the calcium relative to the vessel lumen (anterior, posterior, medial or lateral). This can also be used as a landmark for the puncture itself. Digital subtraction angiography is the preferred technique to save the amount of contrast. Care must be taken to visualize the amount of Calcium because it is also subtracted from the images. Also landmarks are often more difficult to identify (Fig. 3.20) [87, 88].

Other

2D ultrasound imaging with additional color doppler imaging is the method of choice to examine vascular access in patients with severe renal impairment. Limitations are due to total reflections of the ultrasound signal in air filled bowel segments

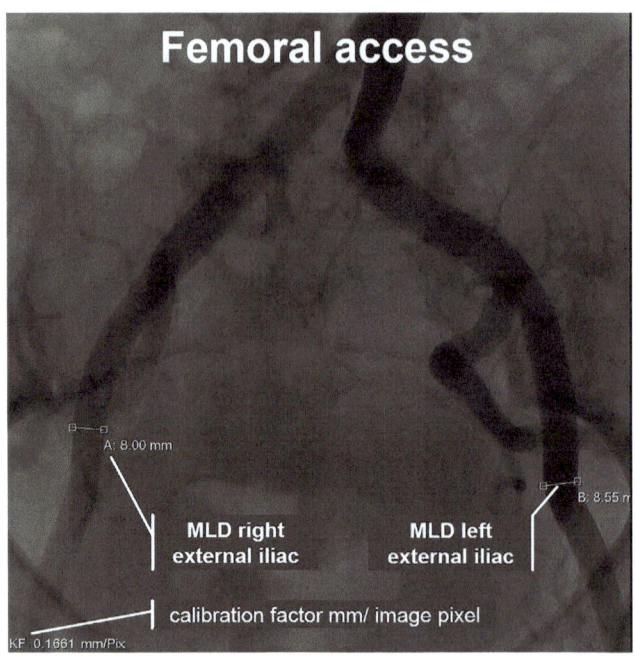

Fig. 3.20 Angiography of the iliac vessels using contrast injection into the distal above the bifurcation: overview is limited by the size of the image intensifier (here a 25 cm coronary system is used) with the necessity to pan the table to catch all areas of interest. Using geometric or catheter based calibration, measurements of the lumen can be easily done. Access is feasible from both sides in this case with an advantage to to the right with a less curved access

avoiding visualization of the iliac vessels. Fastening conditions are recommended for Ultrasound examination. Calcifications of the anterior wall can induce severe shadowing of the signal and prohibiting the visualization of the vessel itself. A systematic approach to the vessel anatomy and a clear language describing the vessel segments from the infrarenal aortic artery down to the femoral vessels of both sides is necessary within the screening process. In addition, minimal luminal diameter has to be reported, if necessary at every level of the vessel. Using additional functional Doppler modalities like pulse-wave Doppler and color coded Doppler, also the functional implications of existing plaques and possible stenosis can be evaluated. This is an important baseline status to evaluate possible post-procedure complications like activated plaques, prosthetic material from closure devices and impaired vessel morphology due to tightened sutures. As shown in Fig. 3.21, a comprehensive evaluation of the vessel can be done. Also the puncture side is easy to identify using the femoral head and the femoral bifurcation as landmark. Important is also to notice and describe the presence and course of the accompanying vein. This helps to avoid later complications due to wrong punctures. Veins can be easily identified as compressible. Also the artery can be compressed, but with much more force. In addition, the pulsation of the artery can be picked up already with 2D imaging. With color Doppler, it is easy to differentiate both entities (Fig. 3.22) [89].

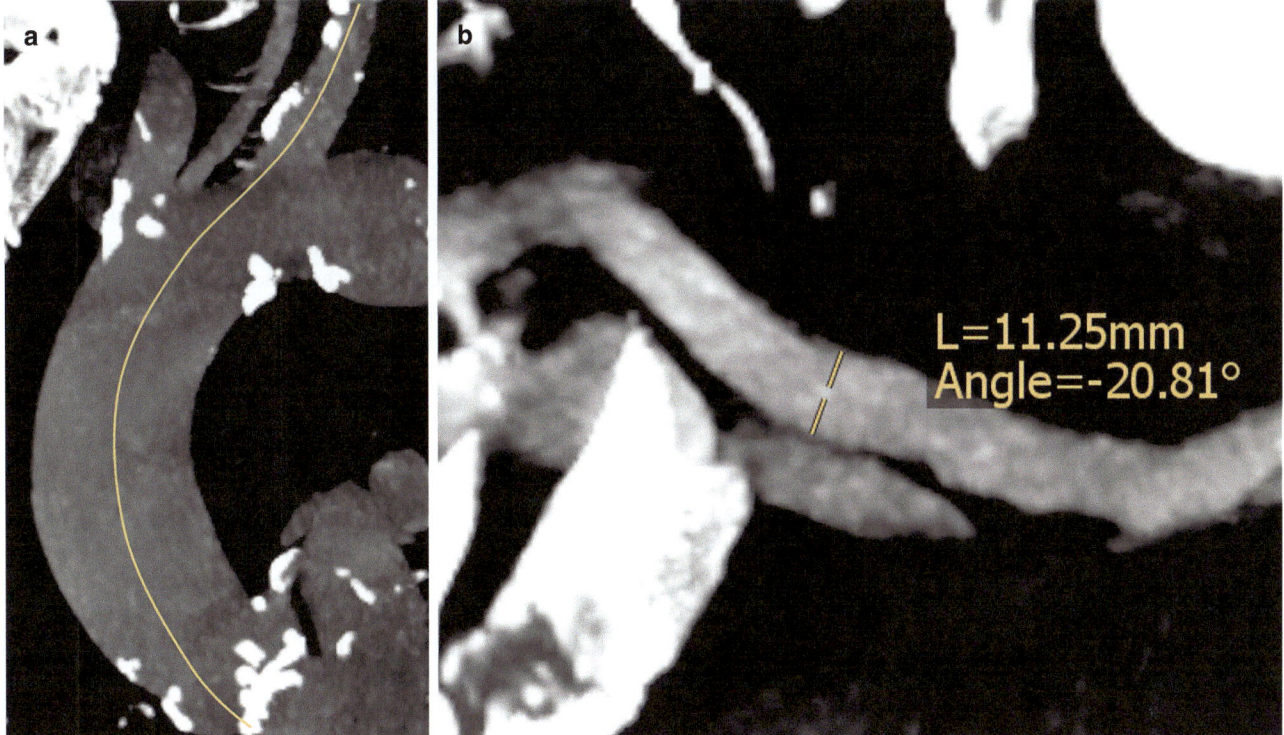

Fig. 3.21 Trajectory from the left subclavian artery to the aortic valve (**a**). Measurement of the axillary artery diameter at the intended puncture site (**b**)

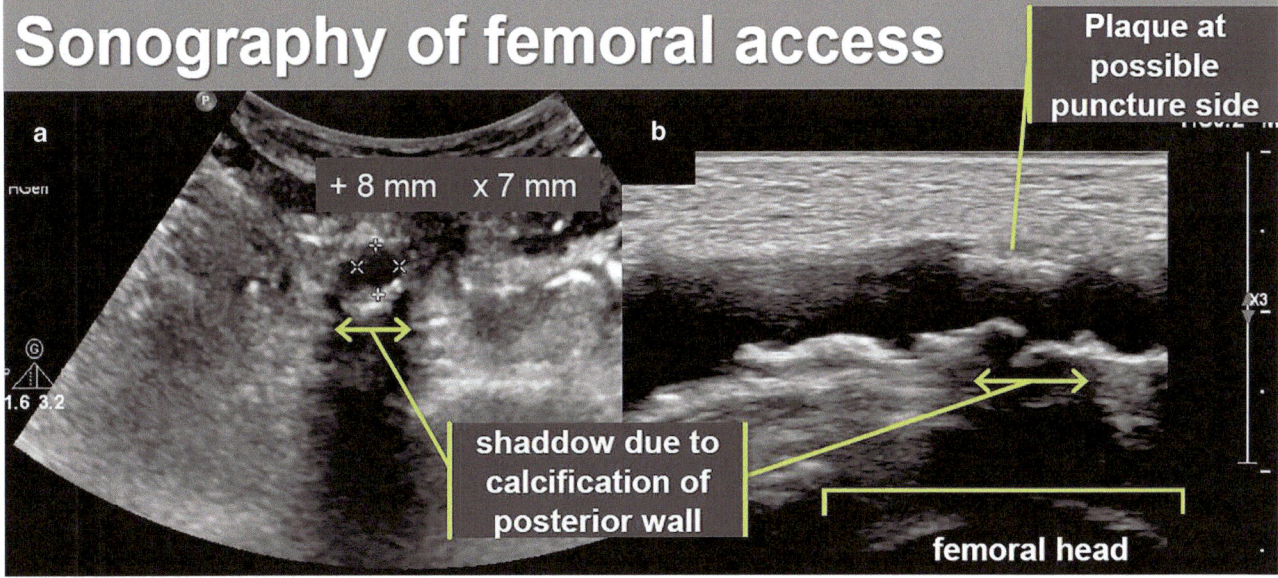

Fig. 3.22 Sonographic exploration of iliac and femoral vessels. Using short (**a**) and longaxis (**b**) imaging, accurate vessel assessment including measurements and functional variables (Doppler not shown) can be done. A right common iliac artery, B right common femoral artery. Shadowing of Echo Signal due to calcifications is shown. Notice the femoral head which can be picked up by ultrasound as anatomical landmark

3.3.4.1.2 Subclavian/Axillary Access Assessment

Intro
As delivery systems have become smaller, corresponding sheath sizes have also evolved facilitating higher rates of trans-femoral procedures. In parralel, however, smaller access sheaths facilitate greater use of non-femoral access when femoral access is prohibitive [90]. The main challenge with most traditional alternative access routes such as the transapical or direct aortic approach is that the access site is non-compressible.

This is not entirely true for the axillary artery, which is at least partially compressible. In most cases, an open surgical access and closure is performed for the subclavian/axillary access, but completely percutaneous cases have been performed [90, 91].

CT

The subclavian artery is an intra-thoracic structure that becomes the extra-thoracic axillary artery at the lateral border of the first rib. Usually, the proximal portion of the axillary artery is the optimal access site due to its invariant anatomy and absence of side-branches (Fig. 3.21).

In that sense, transsubclavian TAVI is a misnomer, as the vast majority of patients are treated via an axillary approach. A left-sided approach is used in the majority of cases due to the favorable orientation with regard to the aortic valve with a less tortuous trajectory [90, 91]. It should be mentioned that the axillo-subclavian artery is not as muscular as the femoral artery and may therefore be more prone to dissection or rupture. On the other hand, the vessel is usually less diseased compared to the iliofemoral arteries [92].

If a transsubclavian/transaxillary approach is planned, a computed tomography should be performed with image acquisition cranial enough to screen for anatomic factors such as vessel tortuosity, inadequate vessel size, especially in patients with a left internal mammary artery (LIMA) graft, and steep subclavian to aortic arch angulation [93]. The same techniques and reporting parameters of the iliofemoral vessels should be used [94].

Angiography

Both arteries can be visualized during diagnostic angiography with selective contrast injections. With radial approach, the intubation of the contralateral subclavian artery can be a challenge. The left subclavian artery is used for access in most of the cases, Petronio et al. reported 96% in the Italian registry [95]. Approach from the right subclavian artery is challenged by the tortuosity and higher bending of the sheath with difficulties to advance at the jugular angle. In addition, the origin of the right carotid artery is more exposed to the procedure.

Interestingly, in most of the cases not the subclavian, but the axillary artery is punctured. The subclavian artery is very much medial and defined by the segment of the vessel medial from the crossing with the first rib. Therefore the axillary artery has also to be taken in account.

Minimal luminal diameter is measured and care is taken to visualize calcifications, especially at the level of the aortic arch. Presence of a patent left or right mammary bypass is a relative contraindication and has to be included into the discussion about the best individual strategy. Within the Italian registry, only a few cases have been treated with ipsilateral mammary bypass. They recommended a minimal luminal diameter 1 mm above the maximal sheath size to avoid periprocedural ischemia. Nevertheless, there is also the risk of

dissection or vessel tear within the treated segment which was less as compared to femoral but still recognizable with 5% major and 7.1% minor vascular complications [95] (Fig. 3.23).

Other

Intensive care medicine has developed a huge experience with ultrasound guided punctures during the last years to improve safety and success for all kind of venous and arterial lines used for monitoring and therapy. Petzoldt described first in 1980 [96] the possibility of ultrasound guided puncture and opened up the perspective of its use today. Fragou published an randomized trial of ultrasound-guided subclavian vein-cannulation versus the traditional landmark method in critical care patients. With this technique they have been able to gain a 100% success rate in the ultrasound group as compared with 87.6% in the traditional landmark one (p < 0.05). Access time and number of attempts were significantly reduced, only 0.5% arterial puncture (5.4%), 1.5% hematoma (5.4%), 0% Pneumothorax (4.9%) and 0% hemothorax (4.4%) were described in the ultrasound group (landmark group). Rare data are available regarding the direct arterial access. Hayashi from Japan described their experience with ultrasound guided puncture of the artery to deliver 5F arterial lines within the tumor-supplying arteries for transarterial chemotherapy. They have been successful in 26 out of 29 cases. Catheter dislodgement was seen in 3 cases, 3 local hematomas and one wound infection was described. This are encouraging results and Schaefer et al.

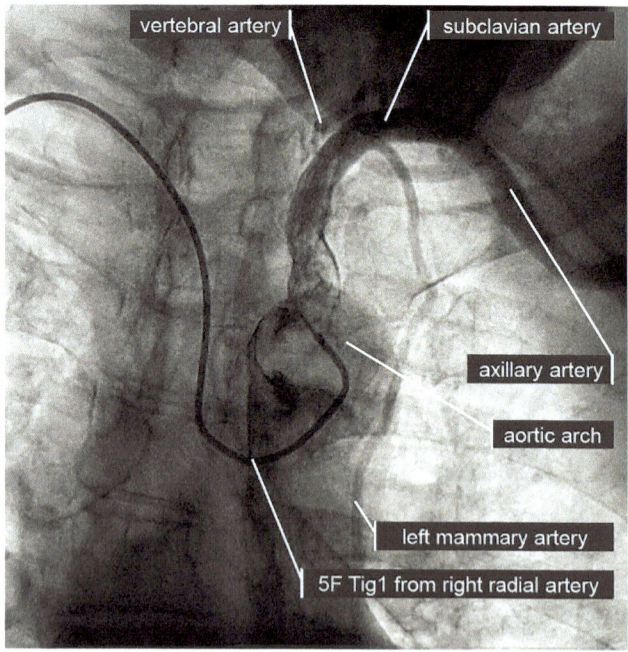

Fig. 3.23 Angiography of left subclavian artery. Some atherosclerosis close to the origin of the aortic arch. Distal from the lateral border of the first rib she continues as axillary artery. Recognize the offtake of the vertebral and mammary artery

reported their early experience with soley percutaneous transaxillary access and closure using different TAVI devices and the Manta closure system [97]. We can assume that different groups will follow this track in future.

3.3.4.1.3 Transapical Access Assessment

Intro

For a quite long time, transapical TAVI used to be and still is the standard alternative access in many centers. In the landmark PARTNER 1A trial published in 2011, as many as 30% of patients underwent TAVI via the transapical route [64]. Owing to the high proportion of patients amendable to the transfemoral approach, access site complications, and the advent of a variety of alternative access strategies, this rate has declined during the past years [98]. In Switzerland, as an example, the rate of patients undergoing transapical TAVI has continously declined from 18% in 2012 to 4% in 2017 (Fig. 3.24).

CT

In addition to annular assessment, MSCT allows assessment of the relationship and distance of the apex to the chest wall and the angle of the trajectory from the apex to the aortic annulus. It visualizes the left anterior descending coronary artery and the diagonal branches, which should be avoided when performing the purse-string sutures. Furthermore, computed tomography visualizes the presence or absence of septal hypertrophy which can sometimes hinder antegrade crossing of the aortic valve.

Echo

Although the use of transapical access for transcatheter aortic valve replacement is decreasing in favour of the transfemoral approach, there are some situations where it is still necessary. These procedures are performed under general anesthesia with live transesophageal echocardiographic guidance.

Access is obtained through an anterolateral minithoracotomy. The site is determined by palpation of the cardiac apex. This can also be confirmed using transthoracic echocardiography prior to the procedure. Guidelines recommend obtaining two orthogonal apical views of the left ventricle to determine the true location of the apex by echocardiography [99]. Using this information, the optimal rib space for the mini-thoractomy can be determined.

After the site is opened, a sheath is inserted into the ventricular apex. The sheath insertion site is not typically guided by a finger push on the apex that is visualized and assessed on transesophageal echocardiography like in some transapi-

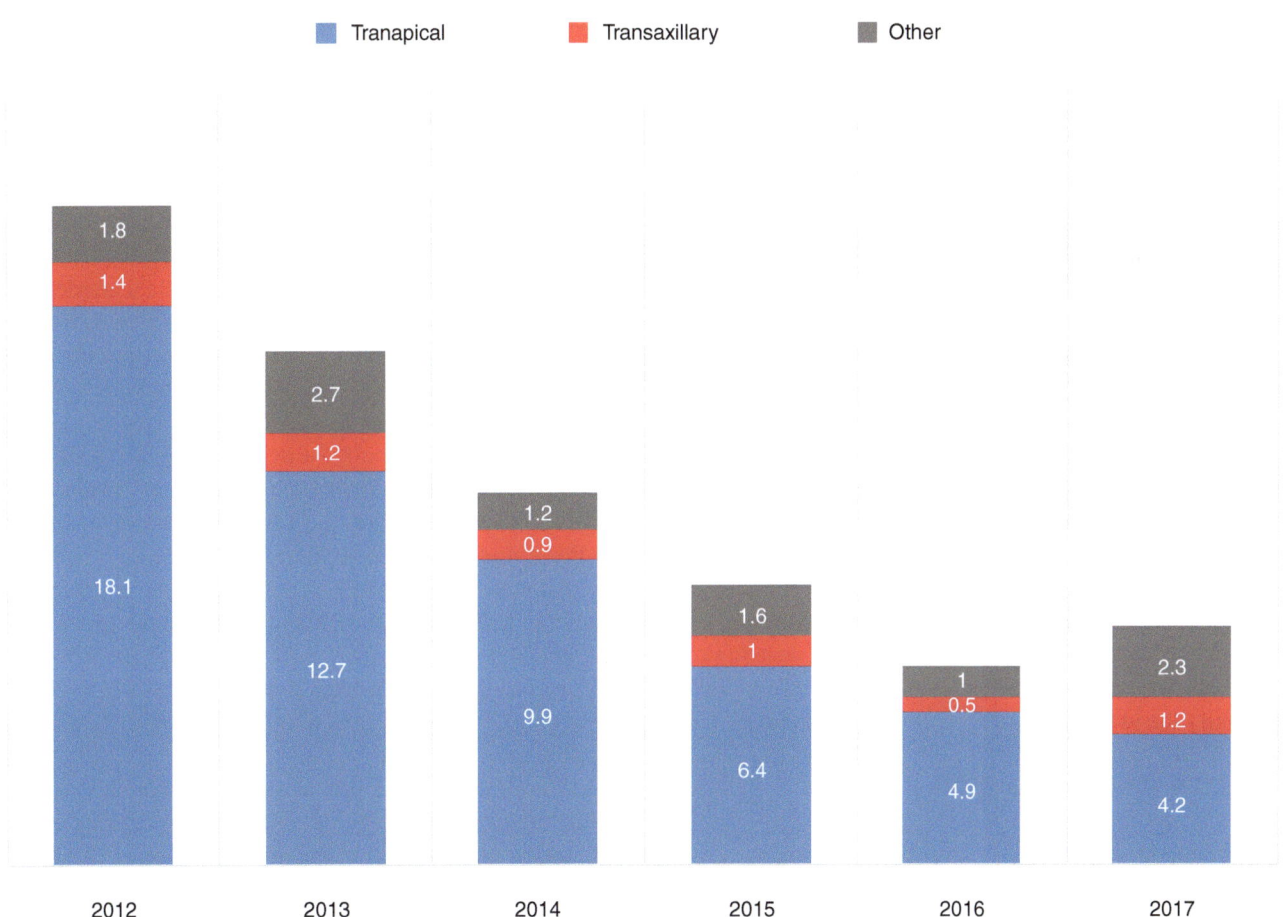

Fig. 3.24 Rate of non-transfemoral access in Switzerland. Between 2012 and 2017, the rate of transapical access has dropped from 18 to 4% (SwissTAVI registry)

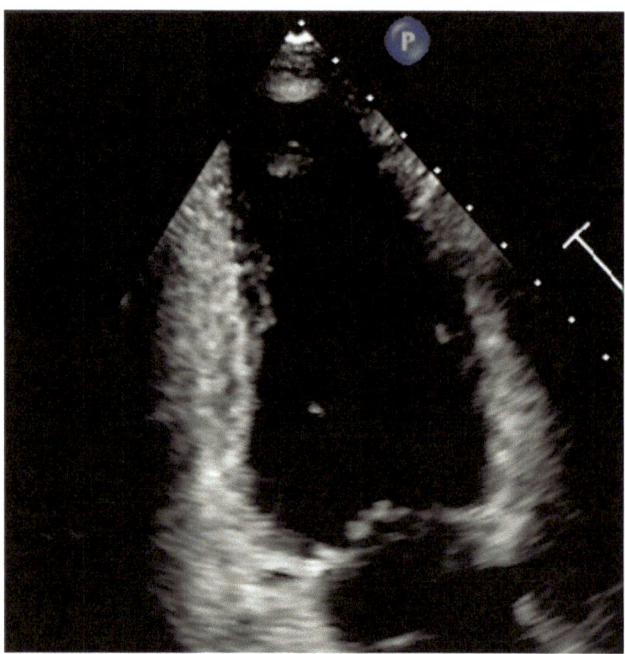

Fig. 3.25 Apical transthoracic echocardiography to verify the position of the left ventricular apex in preparation for transapical access for a valve replacement

cal transcatheter mitral valve devices. However, there is evidence that the trajectory of the device relative to the native aortic annulus, as determined by the angle between the left ventricular and left ventricular outflow tract axes by computed tomography, has been associated with the degree of paravalvular regurgitation [100]. Based on this, the strategy of using a finger-push test to optimize the apical puncture for trajectory could translate to transcatheter aortic valve replacement as well (Fig. 3.25).

Other

Aside from conventional imaging modalities, the transapical access site can be assessed using palpation for the apical impulse. There is no evidence comparing this strategy to an imaging based access assessment.

In the future, fusion imaging platforms and augmented reality technologies may be able to help facilitate transapical access site assessment. A live imaging overlay of a heart model from computed tomography data superimposed onto live transesophageal echocardiography and projected on the patient's chest to represent the true anatomic location of the left ventricle and apex would be an intuitive way to quickly identify the ideal rib space for a mini-thoractomy.

3.3.4.1.4 Direct Aortic and Other Accesses

Introduction

Other alternative access routes include the direct aortic, the transcarotid and the transcaval access. The direct aortic access requires a partial J-ministernotomy or a right anterior mini-

thoracotomy in the second intercostsal space. Then, puncture is performed through double string sutures and the ascending aorta is cannulated using the Seldinger technique [101]. One of the challenges with this access is that the risk for access-site complications in elderly, frail patients is not negligible as the aortic artery wall is often thin and frail in such patients.

The transcarotid access has gained popularity mainly in France [102]. Given suitable anatomy, this procedure can be performed in both general and local anesthesia. If pre-screening (see section "CT" below) is done carefully, the stroke rate does not appear to be higher than with other access routes.

Recently, the transcaval access has emerged as another alternative. This access really is a transfemoral access where the sheath is inserted through the femoral vein. Then, a passage and fistula from the inferior vena cava through the retroperitoneal space to the abdominal aorta is created in order to advance the large bore sheath. Following TAVI, the shunt is closed with a nitinol occluder [84].

CT

For planning of the direct aortic access, MSCT is of importance. The intended puncture site should be identified before starting the procedure. Ideally, the puncture should occur as far away from the aortic annulus (at least 6 cm in case a CoreValve is implanted) as possible and should be free of calcification [103]. In case the ascending aorta is located more on the right side of the sternum, a right anterior mini-thoracotomy may be performed by the surgeon. If the aorta is located more in the middle or on the left side, a partial left-sided J-sternotomy may be preferred.

For planning of the transcarotid access, MSCT image acquisition should be extended to visualize the supra-aortic anatomy. The dimensions of the carotid arteries should be assessed, as well as the subclavian and vertebral arteries. The carotid arteries are screened for the presence of stenosis or plaque at high risk of embolisation. In addition, patency of the circle of Willis is assessed to grant collateral blood flow during ipsilateral carotid clamping and obstruction by the delivery catheter [102]. If both carotid arteries are eligible, the left side is usually favored because it provides better coaxial alignment between the aortic root and the THV during deployment.

Planning of a transcaval procedure involves assessment of the abdominal aorta, which should ideally be calcium- and side-branch free at the zone where the puncture is performed. Furthermore, no obstacles such as interposed bowel or pedunculated aortic atheroma should be present [104].

Angiography

In most of the cases, CT provides enough information. If not available or not done due to other reasons, conventional angiographic evaluation of the ascending aorta is optimally done in a biplane fashion with ap and strong lateral projection. Digital Subtraction Angiography is not helpful due to missing landmarks, even though it is very helpful in contrast saving. Important is imaging in expiration to avoid a falsely deep access. Careful review for calcifications is necessary to identify the sweet spot for access. Rotational angiography without contrast has its role here too. Measurements have to be done depending on the device used as mentioned above. Access point is marked by the dedicated intercostal space.

For carotid access selective angiography is possible, even if it is third if not fourth line diagnostic approach in these patients. Drawback is a higher embolic and in rare cases also the risk of vessel dissections.

For transcaval access, angiography is necessary for the procedure, but not for the planning of the procedure itself. In principle it would be feasible even when it will be challenging to synchronize venous and arterial contrast delivery to obtain good images within the optimal contrast phase. Careful investigation of calcifications, side-branch vessels in case of emergency stenting and interposition of bowl or other structures within cava and aorta.

Other

Ultrasound is the method of choice to access the carotid arteries, both anatomically but also functionally with intracranial Doppler measurements to explore the collateral function of the circle of Willis. Within aortic and caval access ultrasound has actually no role due to the limited access and image quality.

3.3.5 Prevention of TAVR Complications

3.3.5.1 CT

Coronary ostium occlusion is a severe complication during TAVR, which occurs at a low prevalence of less than 1% [105],

however outcomes are adversewith 30 day mortality rates of up to 40.9% [94]. In case of a total LCA occlusion, acute ischemia in the anterior territiorium ensues, which poses the patient at increased risk of requiring emergency double CABG grafting including a sternotomy. Imaging plays the key role to prevent this potentially fatal complication.

There are 3 main reasons for an acute coronary ostium occlusion during the procedure. First, if the prosthesis stent length exceeds the coronary ostium height, and subsequently occludes the coronary ostium. This complication can be avoided by careful planning and sizing of the coronary ostium height, defined as the distance from annulus plane, as outlined below, using computed tomography (CT), or alternatively, transesophageal echocardiography.

Second, dislocation of valve leaflet calcifications into the left coronary artery (LCA) ostium may occur, leading to acute obstruction during stent implantation. Very long leaflets and mobile calcifications are risk factors that can be well visualized by CTA and can aid the surgeon to prevent this complication. Third, a large sinus valsalva diameter of >30 mm has been associated with an increased risk of coronary ostium obstruction [94].

How to size the coronary ostia using CT: Both left and right coronary ostia can be measured accurately with ECG-gated computed tomography (CT). The LCA ostium is sized on a left sagittal oblique view. The minimal distance from left coronary annulus to the lower margin of the LCA ostium circumference should be drawn using a digital caliper perpendicular to the annulus plane (Fig. 3.26a). Analogous, the right coronary ostium (RCA) ostium should be measured on oblique sagittal views (3-Chamber views), by switching to the RCA ostium plane (Fig. 3.26b).

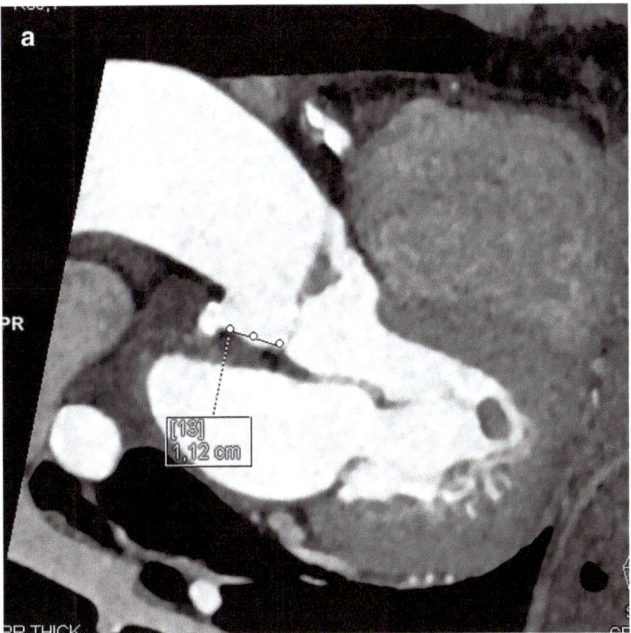 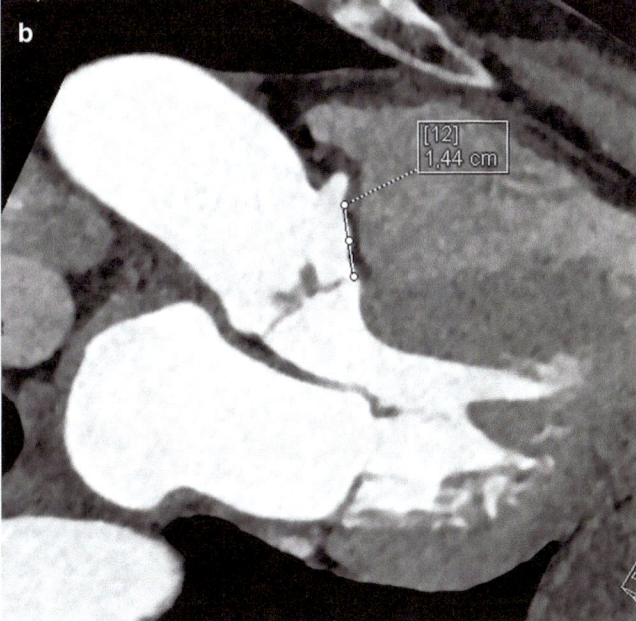

Fig. 3.26 Coronary height. (**a**) left coronary artery (LCA) ostium height, (**b**) right coronary artery (RCA) ostium height

Depending on the prosthesis type and size, the individual stent length is variable hence there is no absolute cut-off. In general, an ostium of less than 11 mm can be regarded as a "low ostium", applying for example to the 23 mm size prosthesis of one of the market leaders. For larger prosthesis models (e.g. 26 mm), a coronary ostium length of less than 13 mm may already be regarded as "low". The definition of a "low-ostium" will be made by the interdisciplinary heart-team with regards to the selected prosthesis model.

Inconclusion, accurate sizing of LCA and RCA coronary ostium height using computed tomography is mandatory prior to TAVR, in order to prevent overstenting of the coronary ostia and subsequent occlusion with potentially fatal myocardial ischemia.

3.3.5.2 Angiography

During diagnostic angiography, the distance between the annulus and the take-off of the coronaries can be easily assessed. Normally a left cranial angulation is the best projection to get an orthogonal view on the take-off of the ostia and to measure the correct distance. Normally the best projection is picked after the diagnostic angiogram. In this projection, if still necessary, an aortogram of the aortic sinus provides additional information of the size and shape of the left- and right sinus. Leaflet length, thickness and calcification to sinus high is the most important factor. If a good backwash is present, this information can already been taken from the diagnostic Angio.

3.3.5.3 Echo

The risk of coronary occlusion with transcatheter aortic valve replacement can be assessed by transesophageal echocardiography either pre- or peri-procedurally. The origin of the coronary arteries can usually be visualized in the zoomed long-axis view of the aortic valve and aortic root [49, 50, 55]. A height measurement of the ostia from the annulus can be measured, with lower heights increasing the risk of coronary occlusion.

Another strategy to find the coronary ostia is to use biplane imaging and sweep across the short axis view of the aortic valve. The subsequent long axis view can again be used to measure the coronary ostial height relative to the aortic annulus.

3-dimensional echocardiography with multi-planar reconstruction is another technique in which echocardiography can help assess the coronary ostia in relation to the annular plane [106, 107]. It is likely the most accurate, assuming spatial resolution is reasonable, since the annular plane is more easily defined and the coronary arteries can be brought into plane more easily. The need for adequate spatial resolution for this technique means that this evaluation is more feasible with transesophageal imaging compared to transthoracic echocardiography.

The calcium burden and distribution on the native aortic valve can also be noted. Large, relatively mobile nodules of thickening or calcification near the leaflet center of the leaflet tips of the left and right coronary cusp leaflets may increase the risk of obstruction if they are pushed towards the coronary artery ostia in the setting of a shallow sinus.

3.3.5.4 Assessment of Risk of Annulus Rupture

3.3.5.4.1 CT

Annulus rupture is a rare but potentially letal complication during TAVR [94], and the most common cause for emergent cardiac surgery (ECS) with 21.1%, besides left ventricular perforation [108].

There are 2 major risk factor [94]: First, severe annular and landing zone and/or left ventricular outflow tract (LVOT) calcification [108] and second, prosthetic heart valve (PHV) oversizing in relation to the effective annulus size, as well as overexpansion due to forced balloon post-dilatations after implantation.

Barbanti et al. [109] identified large annulus and subannular/LVOT calcification as significant predictors for annulus rupture. Accordingly, the classification of "severe", "moderate" and "mild" calcifications, in a subjective fashion, is recommended, based on circumferential extent, depth and their extension into the LVOT [94]. In clinical practice, it is further advised to distinguish between annular and subannular (upper 4–5 mm of LVOT) calcifications [94] and label them as crescent/flat/adherent or protruding. Further, their relation to the aortic valve cusps is suggested to be reported. The location of calcification is highly variable. Especially calcification of the upper part of the LVOT, particularly when immediately below the non-coronary cusp, are more likely causing annulus rupture [94] than others.

Commonly, the non-coronary and the left coronary annulus, including the intervalvular fibrosa, are most frequently affected from more severe calcification. Large protruding calcifications (>8 mm size) increase the risk of annular rupture [109], particularly with balloon expandable valves and should thus be specifically mentioned in a structured TAVR report.

Finally, the device landing zone is in close proximity with the conduction system, hence the risk of atrioventricular block and pacemaker implantation is supposed to be amplified, especially in the presence of pre-existent right bundle branch block [94].

Second, prosthesis heart valve (PHV) oversizing increases the risk of annulus rupture. Hence, accurate sizing by CT is crucial and of utmost importance. The aortic annulus size may change over the cardiac cycle, with no or up to 1–2 mm differences in annulus dimensions, and with a trend to larger values during systolic phase. The dynamics of annular extension during systole is pending on its rigidity, defined by the severity of calcification, but also by left atrial size and pressure. Due to compression from the left atrium, especially the anterior-posterior annulus diameter is prone to be smaller during diastolic phase as compared to the medio-lateral diameter. Accordingly, eccentricity ("ellipticity") of the annulus is enhanced during diastole, and rather vanishes during systole. This annular dynamics has significant implications for PHV sizing with tendency towards PHV undersizing if based on diastolic phase selection alone [94].

Area-based sizing is recommended for balloon-expandable devices, with relative PHV oversizing to the annulus by 0–10%, and for self-expandable valves, perimeter based oversizing of 10–25%, depending on the specific valve system. Excessive oversizing, particularly of balloon-expandable PHV, is closely associated with annular rupture [68] (>20% oversizing) [94].

In conclusion, CTA plays a pivotal role to prevent aortic annulus rupture and subsequent ECS during TAVR (Fig. 3.27a–c).

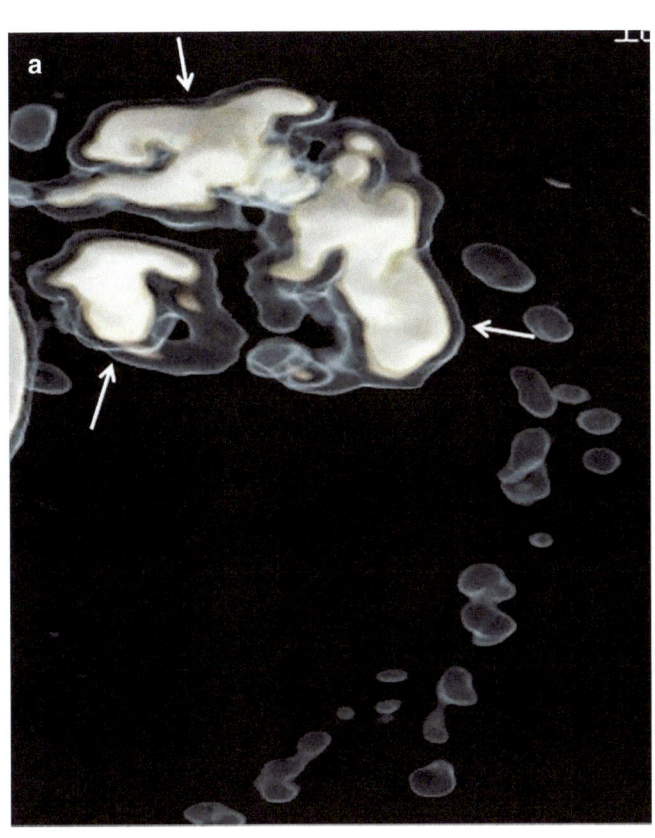

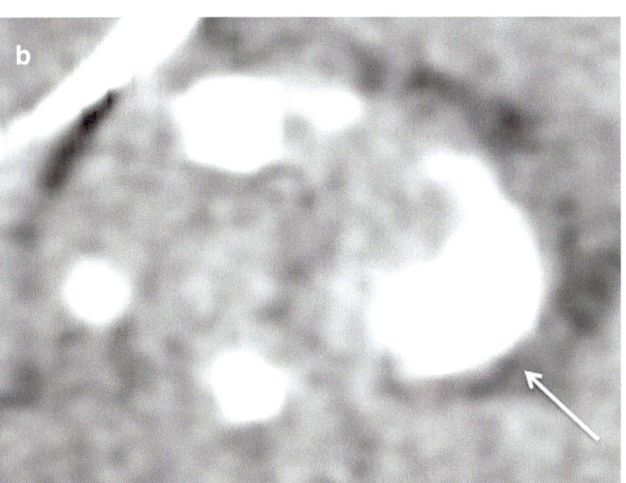

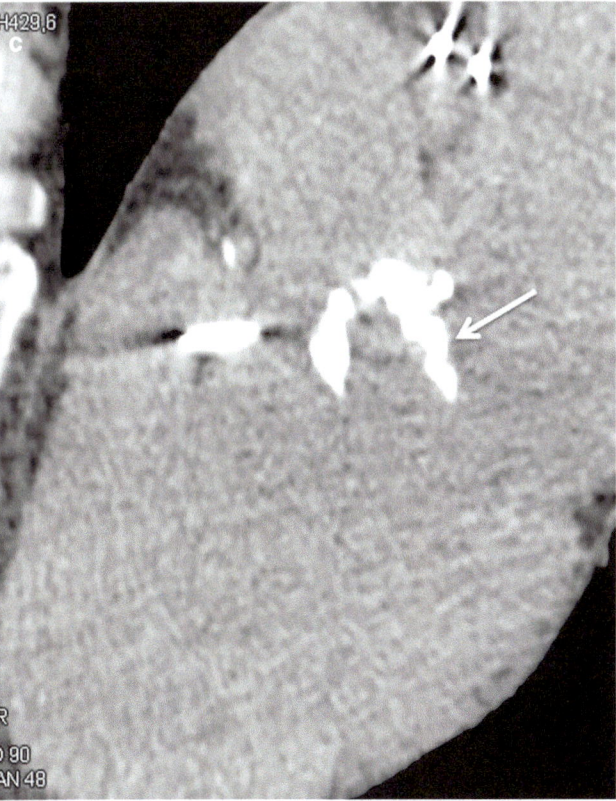

Fig. 3.27 Severe Calcification of all 3 cusps, left-coronary annulus and LVOT calcification. (**a**) 3D VRT shows severe calcification of all 3 cusps (arrows). (**b**) Axial unenhanced CT shows severe left coronary annulus calcium (white arrow). (**c**) left sagittal oblique view illustrates LVOT calcification extending below the annulus plane (white arrow)

3.3.5.4.2 Echo

Features associated with the risk for aortic annular rupture have been traditionally derived from computed tomography data, but are also visible by echocardiography. For example, in a computed tomography based analysis, calcification extending in the left ventricular outflow tract has been found to be a risk factor for annular rupture [109]. This characteristic should be easily seen by transesophageal echocardiography as well. On a zoomed long-axis view of the aortic valve or by sliding in and out of the esophagus to sweep through the short axis view, the pattern and extent of calcification can be seen by noting areas of higher echodensity. Excessive device oversizing compared to the annular measurement is also a risk factor for annular rupture during transcatheter aortic valve replacement [68, 109]. Echocardiographic annular measurements, even when done by multi-planar reconstruction to try to maximize accuracy, is less reproducible than computed tomography based measurements. This is especially true when measurements were performed by a novice imager as opposed to an expert reader. Additionally, it has been found in one analysis that direct planimetry from 3-dimensional transesophageal echocardiography to size the aortic annulus results in percent oversizing ranges that may near those increasing the risk of annular rupture [56].

Overall, although computed tomography proven predictors of annular rupture may be seen on echocardiography, data from echocardiographic studies is limited and there may be risks if relying on echocardiographic annular measurements alone (Fig. 3.28).

3.3.5.4.3 Angiography

Presence and distribution of calcium within the LVOT, annulus, Sini and sinutubular junction is important for the risk assessment regarding annular rupture. Using angiography, care must be taken to identify these spots of calcification, ideally identified and discussed before on the planning CT. The step ahead from CT planning to angiography guided procedure is difficult for the beginners but most important for the success and safety of valve implantation. With angiography alone it is difficult to identify and localize the extent of calcium.

3.3.5.5 Assessment of Risk of Paravalvular Leak

3.3.5.5.1 Introduction

Occurrence of paravalvular leak (PVL) is much more common in transcatheter aortic valve implantation (TAVI) as in surgical aortic valve replacement (SAVR). With first- and second generation devices, several authors have found a correlation with increased mortality [64, 110]. Also mid- and longterm prognosis seems to be impaired [111, 112]. During this early aera at the beginning of TAVI, most of the mea-

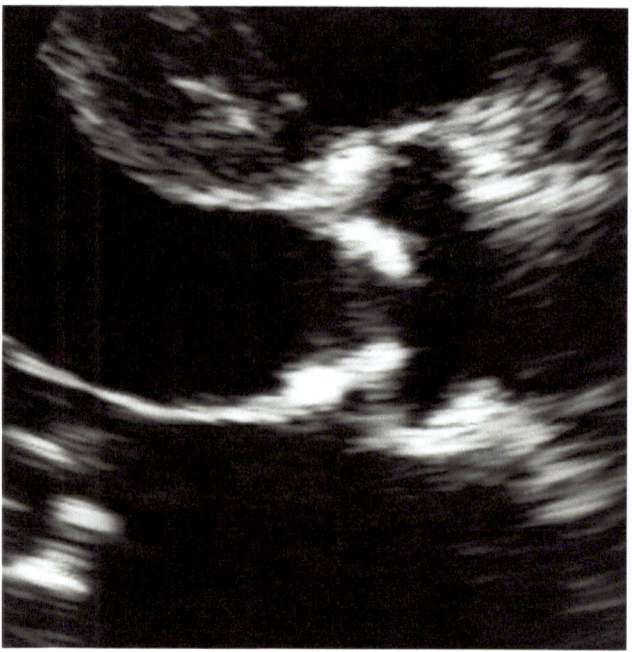

Fig. 3.28 Zoomed parasternal long axis view of the aortic valve on transthoracic echocardiography demonstrating significant aortic valve leaflet and annular calcification extending to the aortic root, left ventricular outflow tract and aortic-mitral continuity, potentially increasing the risk of annular rupture with transcatheter aortic valve replacement

surements have been done with Echo or transoesophageal echo. Incorrect or insufficient sizing was the major reason for PVL after the procedure at this time [113]. With better quantification of the native annulus after introducing the systematic use of CT and a systematic approach for annulus measurements, AR became less of a problem. This was in parallel with Device redesigns: almost all devices have a "sealing" skirt to improve sealing of the annulus.

Second issue is the calcification of the native annulus. Focal calcifications interfere with the skirt leading to circumscript PVL. Wide-spread calcifications of the annulus increases rigidity with possible incomplete valve expansion and relevant PVL due to in complete apposition. This can easily be detected by angiography during the procedure and careful post dilatation or a valve-in-Valve procedure is the method of choice.

Third issue is the geometric deformation away from a circle towards an elliptical or irregular shaped orifice. The most extreme form of this is a bicuspid valve, especially in the combination with severe calcifications.

Having these issues in mind it becomes evident, that a good morphologic exploration of the LVOT, annulus, aortic root, sinotubular junction, shape of the annulus and calcium distribution and the way of residual opening of the cusps is necessary to rank the risk of PVL after the procedure. As mentioned above, this is also a critical step to decide which prosthesis will fit best in the individual patient.

A good implantation technique itself to avoid malapposition is at the end of the day a precondition to achieve a good functional result. Too low implantation results in a PVL over the pericardial skirt, to high does not provide enough annulus sealing. Devices which allow a reposition after assessment are a big advantage (Lotus, Portico, from a historic perspective direct flow for example). If the valve cannot be repositioned, in most cases a second valve as valve-in-valve does solve the problem due to a broadened sealing skirt. A new developments is the 3D modelling of the annulus within the CT datasets to simulate the valve implantation with different valve types, sizes and implantation techniques. The challenge will be to reproduce the optimal implantation technique in real live.

Why is it important, to assess the risk of PVL in advance? Assessment of Regurgitation, especially paravalvular regurgitation is technically demanding and no gold standard exist. During valve implantation, aortic angiography is practically today the most widely and often only used technique due to the fact that most of the procedures are done with local anesthesia and therefore no transoesophageal echo is available. Decision making within the Hybrid suite is therefore limited.

Prior discharge and at follow up almost all patients are examined using transthoracic ultrasound. Both methods have a different sensitivity and their individual limitations. In fact, even in native Valves exact quantification the amount of regurgitation is difficult. With an aortic valve implanted this becomes even worth. Results are therefore not 1:1 comparable and have to be interpreted with caution [114]. In fact, most reliable data on assessment of PVL after TAVI are provided by the core lab analysis of the big randomized trials [115].

3.3.5.5.2 CT

Calcification of the aortic root at and below the level of the aortic annulus is not only associated with aortic rupture but is furthermore associated with the risk of post-procedural paravalvular regurgitation. Quantity and asymmetry of aortic valve calcification and calcification of the upper LVOT could predict greater than or equal to mild postprocedural paravalvular regurgitation or the need for postdilatation of the valve prosthesis (Fig. 3.29). Oversizing of the transcatheter aortic valve may reduce the risk of moderate or severe paravalvular leakage.

Aortic Valve Calcification

Echocardiographic diagnosis of low-flow, low-gradient aortic stenosis with preserved ejection fraction remains challenging. Quantification of Aortic valve calcification (AVC) by computed tomography (CT) has gained in importance, especially in patients with paradoxical low-flow, low-gradient aortic stenosis. Quantification of aortic valve calci-

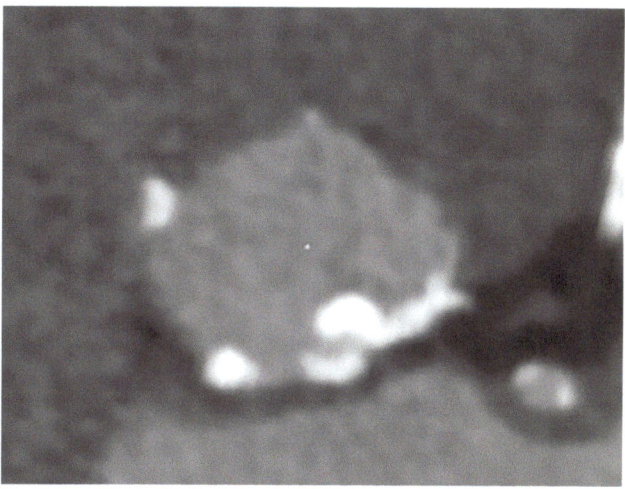

Fig. 3.29 Post-procedural paravalvular regurgitation. Quantity and asymmetry of aortic valve calcification and calcification of the upper LVOT (shown in the image) could predict greater than or equal to mild postprocedural paravalvular regurgitation or the need for postdilatation of the valve prosthesis

fication on CT is easy to perform and highly reproducible. Quantification of AVC with CT is performed using the method proposed by Agatston requiring the acquisition of a non-enhanced CT scan at 120 kVp. Previously, the European Society of Cardiology recommended cut-off values for the AVC Agatston Score to assess the likelihood of severe aortic stenosis according to AVC load. On contrast-enhanced CT, mathematical formulas may enable the quantification of aortic valve calcification even with variable degree of enhancement of the aortic root. The aortic valve quantification is performed using the same software and the same Hounsfield Unit threshold as for quantification of coronary calcifications (Fig. 3.30).

3.3.5.5.3 Echo

Paravalvular regurgitation following transcatheter aortic valve replacement is primarily assessed by echocardiography [7, 99, 116]. It is an important outcome to assess because moderate or greater paravalvular regurgitation is associated with worse clinical outcomes including death and heart failure hospitalizations [117, 118].

Guidelines have been published recognizing this unique form of regurgitation, which did not exist with the same incidence in surgical valve replacement because the prosthesis was sewn firmly into place on the annulus. Transcatheter valves are pressure fit into the annulus, creating the potential for small gaps between the prosthesis and native annulus. Newer generations of transcatheter devices have special features to minimize this risk of regurgitation and early reports are promising [119]. However, there is still a fine balance between placing too much pressure on the native annulus and potentially causing complete heart

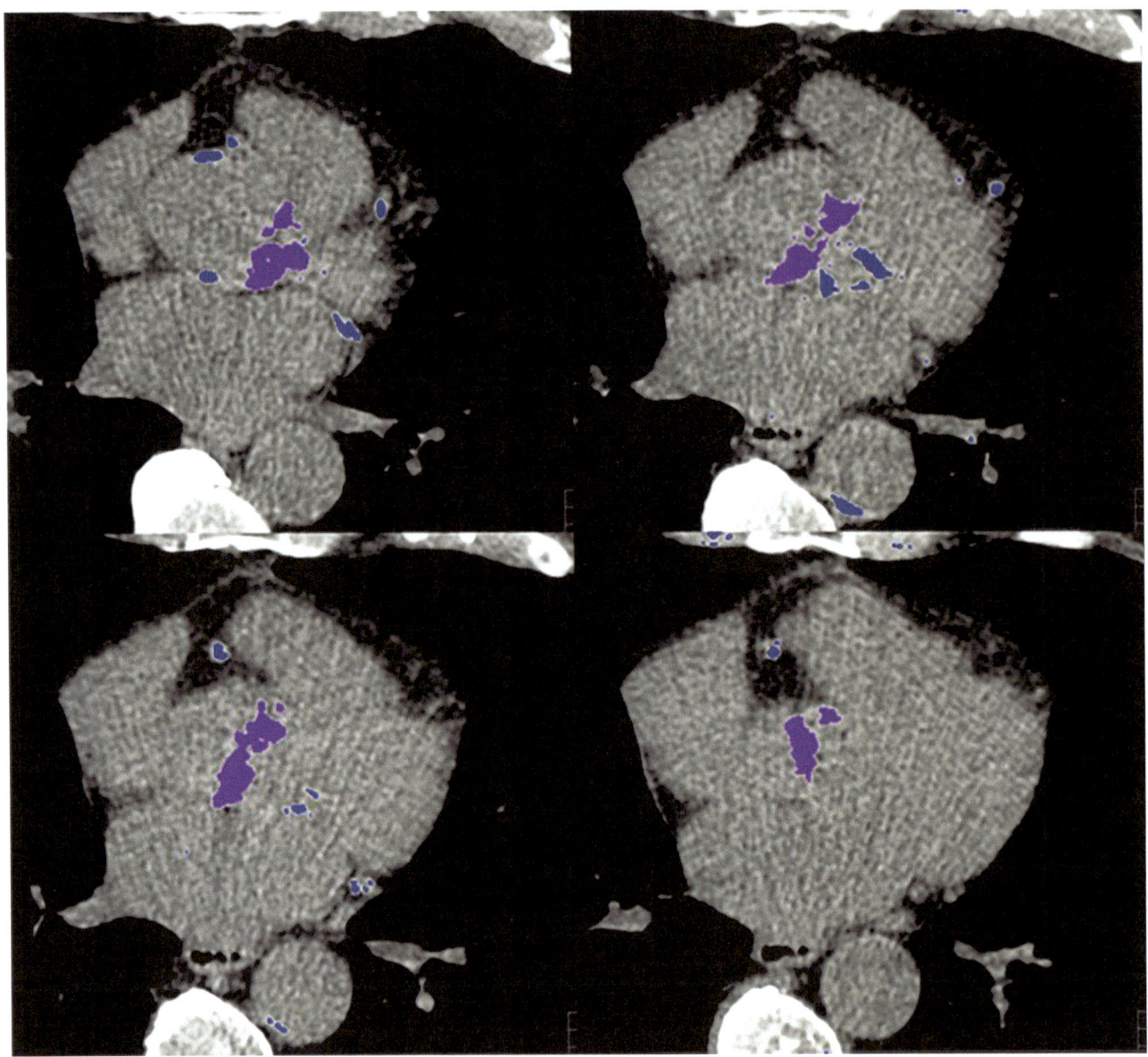

Fig. 3.30 Aortic valve calcification. The Agatston Score of aortic valve calcification is quantified using the same software and the same Hounsfield Unit threshold as for quantification of coronary calcifications

block or annular rupture, and too little pressure resulting in significant paravalvular regurgitation.

As a result of the above considerations, one of the most important aspects of paravalvular regurgitation risk in transcatheter aortic valve replacement is appropriate sizing of the prosthesis to the native annulus. While echocardiography is able to provide accurate sizing dimensions, especially when multiplanar reconstruction is used with semi-automated techniques, it has been found that accuracy is still limited and there is an increased risk of paravalvular regurgitation compared to sizing by computed tomography [51, 53, 56].

Other predictors of paravalvular regurgitation in transcatheter aortic valve replacement based on computed tomography characteristics include eccentricity of the left

ventricular outflow tract, device undersizing, high burden of leaflet calcification, and suboptimal implantation depth [118, 120]. Although studies specific to echocardiography using these parameters have not been reported, some of these characteristics can be assessed by echocardiography.

Quantification of calcium burden is not easily done by echocardiography without proprietary software algorithms [121]. However, one small study used a semi-quantitative echocardiographic score assessing the overall degree of calcium on and around the aortic valve and found that it was associated with moderate paravalvular regurgitation after transapical transcatheter aortic valve replacement [122]. Another group looked at pure echocardiographic features associated with significant post-procedural paravalvular regurgitation and found that commissural calcification, especially between the right and non-coronary cusps, was associated with paravalvular regurgitation [123].

Many heart valve centers of excellence perform transcatheter aortic valve replacement under conscious sedation rather than general anesthesia. From the echocardiographic perspective, this means that transesophageal echocardiography is rarely used and procedures are now performed using transthoracic echocardiography only. One study compared procedures guided by transesophageal echocardiography and those guided by transthoracic echocardiography and found no differences in paravalvular regurgitation at 30 day follow up [124]. This suggests that most procedures can continue to be performed without transesophageal echocardiography and more weight should be placed on the pre-procedural transthoracic echocardiogram and planning computed tomography scan for predicting the risk of paravalvular regurgitation (Fig. 3.31).

3.4 Planning the Associated Procedures

3.4.1 Introduction

We have to discuss arguments pro and contra a combined and additional or associated procedure in aortic valve therapies.

First, the indication of each procedure must be given independently. Second, also an indication must be given not to postpone one of both procedures. Third, the operator must be able to do each procedure in perfection.

From a patient's perspective, it sounds interesting, to get "everything fixed" at a single procedure. But in opposite to open heart surgery, percutaneous procedures have the unique feature that you do not have to fix everything "while the chest is open". The risk of a second procedure is not increased by the previous one in terms of difficult access like in open heart surgery.

Also from a procedure perspective, a PFO occlusion for example, needs a different set up in means of access as compared with transfemoral TAVI. On the other hand, if you are performing a Mitral Clip procedure and a clear indication is given for LAA closure, you spare the potential risk of a second transseptal puncture if you add the LAA occlusion at the end of the mitral clip procedure.

Therefore it is not necessary per se to get everything fixed during one single procedure. Interventional procedures offer the possibility to combine without the imperative to combine. A serious discussion with the patient about indication and possibilities is necessary with enough time to think about. Obviously, economic reasons normally prohibit procedure combinations due to restrictions in reimbursement.

3.4.2 LAA Occlusion

3.4.2.1 Introduction

Patients after TAVI who are in atrial fibrillation (AF) have a higher morbidity and mortality due to increased risk of stroke and of bleeding related to oral anticoagulation therapy [125, 126]. Additonally bleeding worsens 1 year mortality up to 4× compared with patients in sinus rhythm [127]. Optimal medical and device therapy is not yet well defined in this subsets of patients. In most cases we face Patients with a high thromboembolic risk expressed by a high CHADS2Vasc Score [128]. In Addition, the bleeding risk is also elevated due to the mostly very old and frail patients. The experience with dual antiplatelet therapy (DAPT) for 6 month was transferred from coronary stent implantation and adopted to TAVI and is actual the first line therapy after aortic valve implantation [115].

DAPT is not sufficient in Patients with AFib. Bleeding risk is same as with oral anticoagulation without effective antiischemic properties [129]. Patients already on oral anticoagulation with warfarin or Coumadin can be kept on this therapy without adding platelet inhibition. In fact, this can probably be the therapy of choice in all patients to reduce the risk of leaflet thickening or silent valve thrombosis and is recommended in patients with low bleeding risk for 3–6 months [130]. Coumadin is therapy of choice in patients with elevated valve gradients due to valve thrombosis [131]. Therapy of subclinical vavle thickening is yet still uncertain, but data are showing the positive effect of therapeutic oral anticoagulation here to [132]. Data with NOACS are more incongruent or still lacking. The combination of Xarelto and Aspirin was tested within the Galileo trial and increased both the bleeding- and the risk of thromboembolic events as compared with standard therapy of DAPT. The trial was stopped prematurely and is not yet published [133]. Dabigatran has had no effect in mechanical valve replacement and the trial was also stopped early [134].

Therefore the combination of Aortic valve implantation with closure of the left atrial appendage promise to be a elegant way to avoid excessive anticoagulation and therewith reducing bleeding risk while providing embolic risk protection by closing the most likely source of emboli. Care hast to be taken that a LAA thrombus pre interventional is not present by providing effective oral anticoagulation for >4 weeks or transoesophageal Echo before the intervention.

Until now systematic studies are missing. Small series are reported during valve. A randomized monocenter study in patients with atrial fibrillation undergoing TAVI with the Abbott Portico Device randomized to additional LAA occlusion with the Abbott Amulet Occluder or medical therapy only has finished inclusion (ClinicalTrials.gov Identifier NCT03088098).

Fig. 3.31 Zoomed short axis view of the aortic valve on transesophageal echocardiography demonstrating calcification predominantly affecting the commissure between the left and right coronary cusps, a potential risk factor for paravalvular regurgitation after transcatheter aortic valve replacement

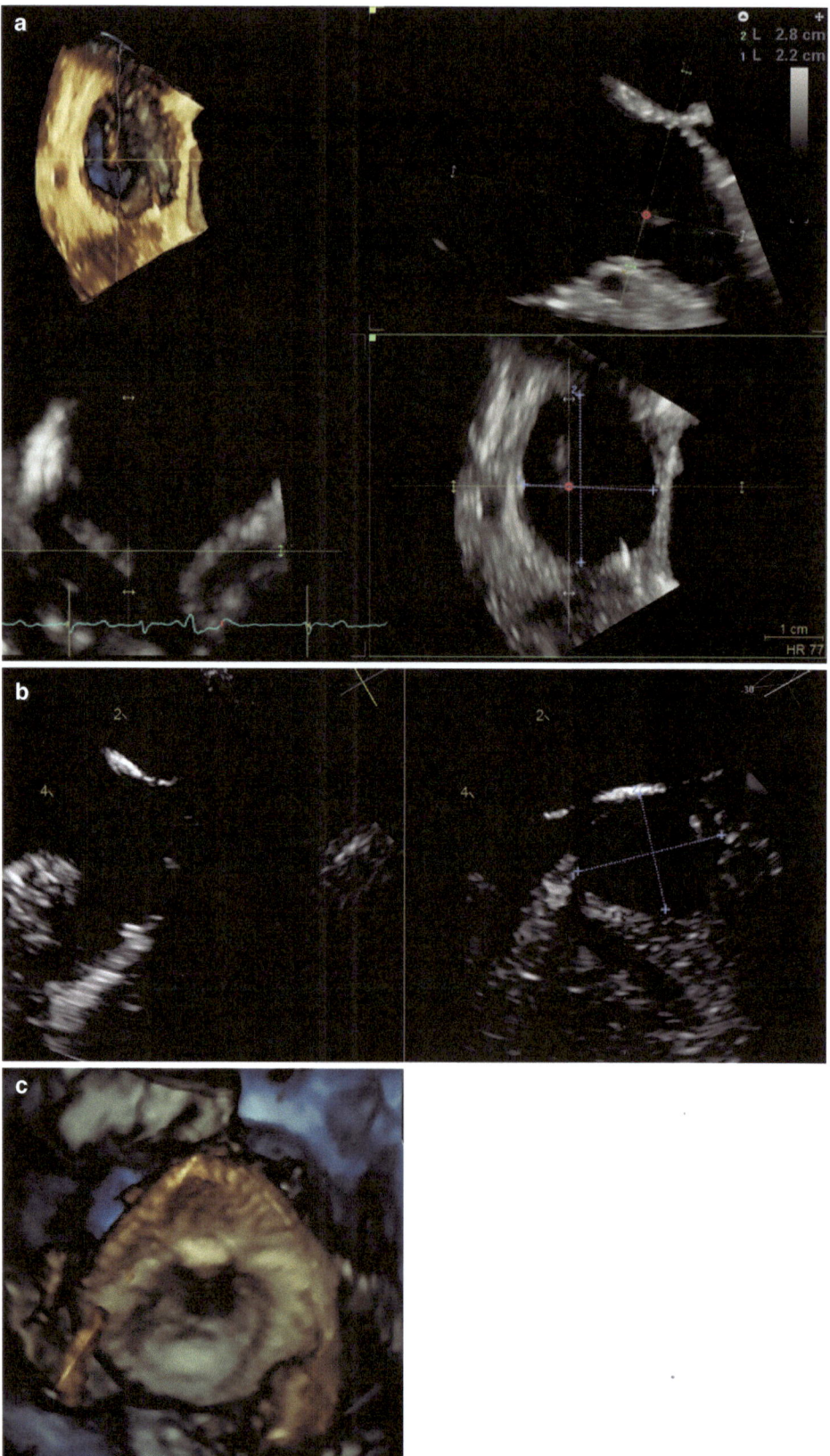

3.4.2.2 Echo

Left atrial appendage closure at the same time as transcatheter aortic valve replacement is feasible but requires either pre- or intra-procedural echocardiographic evaluation of the appendage [135, 136].

First, the appendage morphology and dimensions should be assessed to assist with device selection. The specific landing zone of the various devices dictate the location of key measurements. 3-dimensional transesophageal echocardiography or biplane imaging can often provide very accurate cross sectional dimensions that account for the non-circular shape of the appendage [137–139].

Next, thrombus in the left atrial appendage should be ruled out because of the manipulation inside the appendage that occurs during the procedure. Guide wires and the device will enter and could dislodge any thrombus that is present. Additionally, it is typical for angiography of the appendage to be performed as another assessment of appendage shape and size. Thrombus present in the appendage could also be dislodged due to the injection.

Since transcatheter left atrial appendage closure is often performed by femoral venous access and a transseptal approach, the interatrial septum and fossa ovalis should be assessed by echocardiography before the procedure. A patent foramen ovale or atrial septal defect may affect the location of crossing the septum. If the concomitant left atrial appendage closure is guided by live transesophageal echocardiography, then a targeted transseptal puncture location can be achieved. The ideal puncture site is usually in the inferior and posterior portion of the fossa. This optimizes the trajectory of the device and delivery catheter to the long axis of the left atrial appendage.

Positioning of the device in the left atrial appendage can be guided by live transesophageal echocardiography and optimized prior to deployment. Lastly, evaluation of the result after deployment in terms of stability, any evidence of a leak around the device, interference with surrounding cardiac structures (such as obstruction of the left upper pulmonary vein or with mitral valve function in devices with large discs that cover the opening of the appendage) and periprocedural complications can be performed (Fig. 3.32).

3.4.2.3 Angiography

Two steps have to be considered in this procedure, first transseptal puncture, second proper delivery of the device within the LAA. After placing the transseptal sheaths within the superior vena cava, a slow pullback is performed in PA X-ray position. The needle is oriented at 4–5 o'clock at the end of the catheter. As soon as the tip of the catheter is entering the fossa ovalis, a small jump is visible on the screen and a simi-

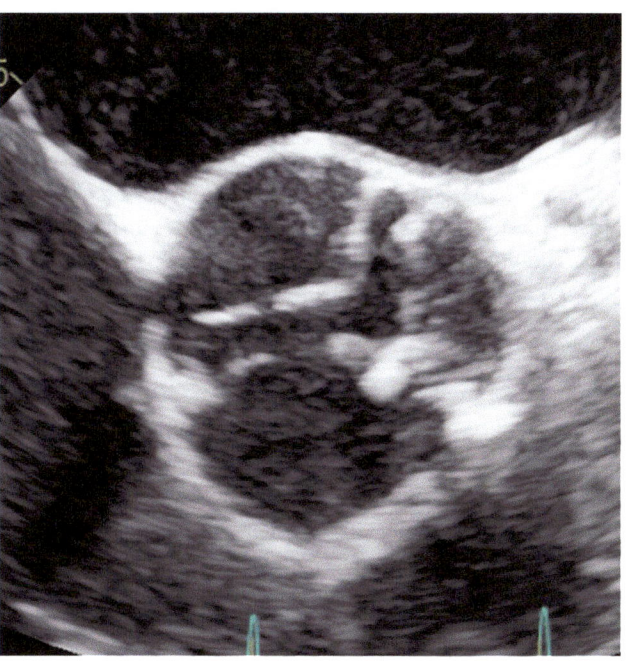

Fig. 3.32 Transcatheter left atrial appendage closure device landing zone sizing by transesophageal echocardiography using multi-planar reconstruction of a 3-dimensional data set (**a**) and simultaneous biplane imaging (**b**). Final 3-dimensional appearance of the closure device in place (**c**)

lar tactile feedback can be felt. Before puncture of the septum, correct posterior orientation of the needle has to be confirmed: On PA projection the tip is oriented to the right, on lateral projection it is oriented posterior. Very little contrast (about 0.5 cc) can be used to visualize the septum through the not yet puncturing needle. Within a TAVI native patient, a pigtail within the acoronary cusp could be helpful for orientation too. In our scenario, the just implanted TAVI prosthesis gives an perfect additional orientation and makes this step of the procedure more easy to take. After passing the septum only with the needle, LA positioning is confirmed with checking the blood pressure through the needle. If correct, the dilatator is advanced 2 cm within the LA, position fixed with on hand and the sheath advanced to the tip of the dilatator by pushing the first during pulling the last. A floppy guidewire is inserted and positioned within the left upper pulmonary vein. The sheath for intervention is positioned within the LA. To avoid perforation during intubation of the LAA, a pigtail can be used within the sheath and angiography can be done using the pigtail. LAA is visualized using a right caudal and a right cranial projection. RAO 30°, Caudal 20° often demonstrates best the body and tip of the LAA. Within RAO 30°, Cranial 10°, the LAA ostium and the neck is best visualized. Measurements are taken as recommended by the device companies and the recommended device is picked up. The tip of the guiding catheter is a perfect reference for exact calibration. Placement of the device differs. To implant a watchman device the sheath has to be advanced deeply into the LAA. This increases the potential of perforation. For the amulet device, the sheath is basically placed at the entrance of the LAA and the device is developed until it figures like a small ball at the tip of the catheter. Now it can be placed slowly at its final position. After a pull test, the position of the device is checked by additional contrast injections. Proper sealing of the LAA with avoiding pouches within the niche towards the Coumadin ridge has to be the goal of the procedure. Finally, closure of the femoral vein is done using a figure of 8 for 12–18 h. This is a cheap and effective solution (avoid deep stiches not to grasp the artery). Also a Perclose device can be used for venous closure. Too long compression of the femoral vein should be avoided not to risk venous thrombosis.

Anticoagulation regime depends on the clinical situation. Dual antiplatelet therapy (DAPT) is recommended for 3 month, Aspirin for 6 month. In patients who suffered from cerebral bleeding, even 1 month DAPT can be too long and Aspirin only has to be considered. Endocarditis prophylaxis is recommended for 6 month (same as with PFO or ASD closure).

3.4.3 Mitral Valve Regurgitation and Stenosis

3.4.3.1 Intro

For the planning of TAVI procedures with associated mitral insufficiency and/or stenosis the gold standard offers transesophageal echocardiography, which provides the highest degree of information on the quantification of insufficiency, etiology and mechanism (degenerative or functional), as well as biventricular function and associated pulmonary pressure.

From a purely technical point of view, if a concurrent intervention on the mitral valve or a transcatheter mitral replacement is to be planned, the key information comes from the radiological analysis by CTA (already done to quantify the aortic valve). With advanced imaging softwares, it is possible to reconstruct and calculate with extreme precision the degree and disposition of any calcifications, the valvular area, the course of the circumflex coronary artery towards the mitral annulus.

Of note, to overcome some inaccuracies of two-dimensional echocardiography in grading MR in TAVI patients, may be of help, similar to three-dimensional echocardiography, CTA provides volume-rendered images of the mitral valve that can be aligned parallel to the mitral regurgitant orifice enabling an *en face* view for direct assessment of the anatomic regurgitant orifice area.

3.4.3.2 Echo

Concomitant mitral regurgitation is not uncommon in the setting of severe aortic stenosis. There is a high burden of both conditions in population based studies and patient populations with each valve lesion tend to overlap [140]. While the high afterload state of severe aortic stenosis may exacerbate underlying mitral regurgitation, a significant proportion of patients continue to have severe mitral regurgitation after transcatheter aortic valve implantation [141, 142].

If both aortic valve disease and mitral regurgitation need to be treated, and the surgical risk is deemed too high for open aortic valve replacement, then the mitral valve will need to be evaluated for a percutaneous treatment option as well since the expected surgical risk should be similar. Several categories of transcatheter mitral repair devices exist but the most commonly used technique is edge-to-edge repair using the MitraClip device (Abbott, Santa Clara, California, United States of America) [143–145].

Echocardiographic assessment of the mitral valve to assess for suitability of edge-to-edge repair should be done using transthoracic and transesophageal echocardiography. The leaflets should be assessed for any thickening or calcification that may interfere with device grasping. Baseline mitral valve area and gradient should be evaluated to rule out mitral stenosis and assess for the risk of mitral stenosis with edge-to-edge repair, since the mitral valve area is expected to decrease by half following this type of procedure. The degree of mitral regurgitation should be quantified and the location of the predominant jet should be identified for procedural planning. In the case of a prolapse or flail mitral leaflet, the larger the prolapse width or flail gap, the more difficult it may be to successfully perform edge-to-edge repair. The EVEREST trials were the first trials to evaluate the MitraClip device and had a set of echocardiographic criteria for the procedure [146]. However, as worldwide experience increased, it was well recognized that a much wider range of mitral valve anatomy can be treated, although the difficulty may vary [147, 148]. Complete assessment of the mitral valve can also determine whether an alternative transcatheter mitral repair strategy is more appropriate in the event that edge-to-edge is not ideal. Other options include direct annuloplasty, indirect annuloplasty and transcatheter mitral valve replacement [149].

As the clinical indications expand for transcatheter aortic valve replacement and lower risk patients are given this option as an alternative to open surgical aortic valve replacement, the role of mitral valve disease will need to be evaluated in more detail. The durability and long-term outcomes of transcatheter mitral valve repair is not as well studied, so lower risk individuals needing multiple valve interventions may need conventional open surgery to best manage their valve disease.

Mitral stenosis is less common but may coexist with aortic valve disease in the setting of rheumatic valve disease with multiple valve involvement or severe valvular degneration and calcification. A mild degree of stenosis may not require intervention. Therefore, it is important to evaluate the etiology and severity of mitral stenosis [42, 150, 151].

Rheumatic mitral leaflets demonstrate thickening at the tips and commissural fusion. The posterior leaflet is often fixed and there may be associated thickening of the subvalvular apparatus. The severity should then be assessed by evaluating valve area by direct planimetry of a short axis view of the aortic valve at the level of the leaflet tips. In addition to this, transvalvular gradient in the context of the heart rate during the study should be traced using continuous wave spectral Doppler across the mitral valve. This tracing can also be used to calculate the mitral valve area by the pressure half time method as another estimate of the anatomic orifice area.

Based on the current guidelines, significant stenosis is defined as a valve area of less than 1.5 cm^2 and a pressure half time of 150 ms or greater [42, 151]. These parameters usually also correspond with a transvalvular gradient over 10 mmHg, but is highly dependent on the heart rate. If this is felt to be a contributor to active cardiac symptoms, percutaneous mitral balloon valvuloplasty can be considered for rheumatic mitral stenosis. This is generally a low risk procedure that is tolerated well. Echocardiographic signs associated with increased risk of a poor procedural outcome, usually failure to alleviate the stenosis and significant worsening of mitral regurgitation, include asymmetric valve thickening, asymmetric commissural fusion, significant valve thickening or calcification, marked mobility restriction of the leaflets and severe involvement of the subvalvular apparatus [152, 153]. The pre-procedural grade of mitral regurgitation should also be considered.

In the setting of calcific mitral stenosis, the valve commissures are not fused. Rather, significant calcification in the mitral annulus and body of the mitral valve leaflets restricts opening and can result in some degree of inflow obstruction. This is best appreciated on the parasternal long and short axis views of the mitral valve in addition to transesophageal evaluation of the valve. The same echocardiographic thresholds are used to define severity. Severe mitral stenosis due to this etiology is less common. If the degree of stenosis is severe and intervention is indicated, the treatment options are more limited when compared to rheumatic mitral stenosis. Surgical decalcification is high risk due to the possibility of cardiac rupture at the atrial ventricular junction [154, 155]. Transcatheter valve implantation using pre-existing aortic valve replacement devices can be done either through an open or transcatheter route, but the outcomes are suboptimal [156–158]. Dedicated transcatheter

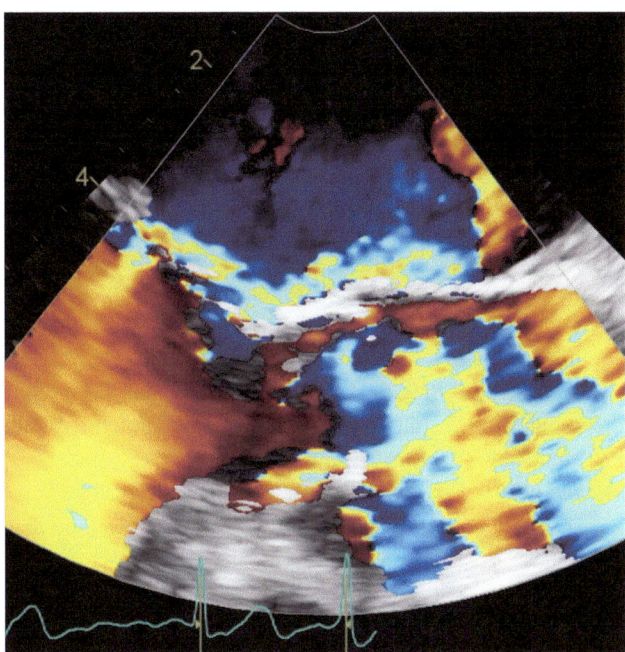

Fig. 3.33 Colour Doppler imaging on transesophageal echocardiography of the long axis view in mid systole demonstrating anteriorly directed eccentric mitral regurgitation in addition to flow acceleration across the aortic valve, both of which may be amenable to transcatheter intervention

mitral valve replacement devices that can be used for calcific mitral stenosis are early in development and considered investigational [159]. There are also procedural risks, including acute left ventricular outflow tract obstruction [160]. Echocardiographic features that may be associated with this risk include a small left ventricle, proximal septal thickening and pre-existing dynamic left ventricular outflow tract obstruction. Estimating risk of post-procedure obstruction using the predicted neo-left ventricular outflow tract size after prosthesis implantation has been studied in computed tomography but not yet by echocardiography (Fig. 3.33) [161, 162].

3.4.3.3 Angiography
Valvular regurgitation can be evaluated by angiography. Angiographic evaluation of regurgitant severity is based on ejection of contrast media into the left atrium, through the affected mitral valve, or into the left ventricle through the insufficient aortic valve [163].

The severity of regurgitation is graded on a semi quantitative scale of 0+ to 4+, in which a mild degree has contrast refluxes into the left atrium but clears on each beat, while severe has left atrium becomes **as dense as** the left ventricle on the first beat and contrast is seen refluxing into the pulmonary veins [164].

The distinction between the four several grades of regurgitation with this methodic is difficult and in most cases inaccurate. This methodic of estimation of degree of regurgitation has some important limitations, which limitate a lot its usefulness:

- the quantity of contrast material (volume and speed of injection): if this is reduced may underestimate the degree of regurgitation
- arrhythmias (ventricular extra-beats or atrial fibrillation, or even mechanical ones produced by the catheter itself) significantly affects the ventricular filling and subsequently the indicated grade of regurgitation
- although mild regurgitation is clearly distinct from severe regurgitation, intermediate grades may not be reliable calculated
- the position of catheter in the ventricle (for mitral valve) or in the aorta (for aortic valve), in relation to the site of valve
- the recorded plane of ventricle and/or atrium, to avoid overlapping. The proper projection for estimation of aortic regurgitation is that of 45° in left anterior oblique view with 10–15% of cranial angulation, while that for mitral regurgitation is a 30° in right anterior oblique view
- avoid the overlapping of descending thoracic aorta and left atrium which may overestimate the mitral regurgitation.

Angiography provides evaluation of grade of regurgitation in a small subset of patients, especially when the non-invasive evaluation is not clear-cut with the clinical findings.

References

1. Mack MJ, Leon MB, Thourani VH, Makkar R, Kodali SK, Russo M, Kapadia SR, Malaisrie SC, Cohen DJ, Pibarot P, Leipsic J, Hahn RT, Blanke P, Williams MR, McCabe JM, Brown DL, Babaliaros V, Goldman S, Szeto WY, Genereux P, Pershad A, Pocock SJ, Alu MC, Webb JG, Smith CR. Transcatheter aortic-valve replacement with a balloon-expandable valve in low-risk patients. N Engl J Med. 2019;380(18):1695–705.
2. Kypson AP. Recent trends in minimally invasive cardiac surgery. Cardiology. 2007;107(3):147–58.
3. Alkadhi H, Wildermuth S, Plass A, Bettex D, Baumert B, Leschka S, Desbiolles LM, Marincek B, Boehm T. Aortic stenosis: comparative evaluation of 16-detector row CT and echocardiography. Radiology. 2006;240(1):47–55.
4. Plass A, Scheffel H, Alkadhi H, Kaufmann P, Genoni M, Falk V, Grunenfelder J. Aortic valve replacement through a minimally invasive approach: preoperative planning, surgical technique, and outcome. Ann Thorac Surg. 2009;88(6):1851–6.
5. Wildermuth S, Leschka S, Duru F, Alkadhi H. 3-D CT for cardiovascular treatment planning. Eur Radiol. 2005;15(Suppl 4):D110–5.
6. Zoghbi WA, Chambers JB, Dumesnil JG, Foster E, Gottdiener JS, Grayburn PA, Khandheria BK, Levine RA, Marx GR, Miller FA Jr, Nakatani S, Quinones MA, Rakowski H, Rodriguez LL, Swaminathan M, Waggoner AD, Weissman NJ, Zabalgoitia

M. Recommendations for evaluation of prosthetic valves with echocardiography and doppler ultrasound: a report From the American Society of Echocardiography's Guidelines and Standards Committee and the Task Force on Prosthetic Valves, developed in conjunction with the American College of Cardiology Cardiovascular Imaging Committee, Cardiac Imaging Committee of the American Heart Association, the European Association of Echocardiography, a registered branch of the European Society of Cardiology, the Japanese Society of Echocardiography and the Canadian Society of Echocardiography, endorsed by the American College of Cardiology Foundation, American Heart Association, European Association of Echocardiography, a registered branch of the European Society of Cardiology, the Japanese Society of Echocardiography, and Canadian Society of Echocardiography. J Am Soc Echocardiogr. 2009;22(9):975–1014; quiz 1082–4.
7. Lancellotti P, Pibarot P, Chambers J, Edvardsen T, Delgado V, Dulgheru R, Pepi M, Cosyns B, Dweck MR, Garbi M, Magne J, Nieman K, Rosenhek R, Bernard A, Lowenstein J, Vieira ML, Rabischoffsky A, Vyhmeister RH, Zhou X, Zhang Y, Zamorano JL, Habib G. Recommendations for the imaging assessment of prosthetic heart valves: a report from the European Association of Cardiovascular Imaging endorsed by the Chinese Society of Echocardiography, the Inter-American Society of Echocardiography, and the Brazilian Department of Cardiovascular Imaging. Eur Heart J Cardiovasc Imaging. 2016;17(6):589–90.
8. Alnasser S, Cheema AN, Simonato M, Barbanti M, Edwards J, Kornowski R, Horlick E, Wijeysundera HC, Testa L, Bedogni F, Amrane H, Walther T, Pelletier M, Latib A, Laborde JC, Hildick-Smith D, Kim WK, Tchetche D, Agrifoglio M, Sinning JM, van Boven AJ, Kefer J, Frerker C, van Mieghem NM, Linke A, Worthley S, Asgar A, Sgroi C, Aziz M, Danenberg HD, Labinaz M, Manoharan G, Cheung A, Webb JG, Dvir D. Matched comparison of self-expanding transcatheter heart valves for the treatment of failed aortic surgical bioprosthesis: insights from the valve-in-valve International Data Registry (VIVID). Circ Cardiovasc Interv. 2017;10(4):e004392.
9. Pibarot P, Simonato M, Barbanti M, Linke A, Kornowski R, Rudolph T, Spence M, Moat N, Aldea G, Mennuni M, Iadanza A, Amrane H, Gaia D, Kim WK, Napodano M, Baumbach H, Finkelstein A, Kobayashi J, Brecker S, Don C, Cerillo A, Unbehaun A, Attias D, Nejjari M, Jones N, Fiorina C, Tchetche D, Philippart R, Spargias K, Hernandez JM, Latib A, Dvir D. Impact of pre-existing prosthesis-patient mismatch on survival following aortic valve-in-valve procedures. JACC Cardiovasc Interv. 2018;11(2):133–41.
10. George I, Guglielmetti LC, Bettinger N, Moss A, Wang C, Kheysin N, Hahn R, Kodali S, Leon M, Bapat V, Borger MA, Williams M, Smith C, Khalique OK. Aortic valve annular sizing: intraoperative assessment versus preoperative multidetector computed tomography. Circ Cardiovasc Imaging. 2017;10(5):e005968.
11. de Kerchove L, Mastrobuoni S, Froede L, Tamer S, Boodhwani M, van Dyck M, El Khoury G, Schafers HJ. Variability of repairable bicuspid aortic valve phenotypes: towards an anatomical and repair-oriented classification. Eur J Cardiothorac Surg. 2019.
12. Cohn LH. Cardiac surgery in the adult. 3rd ed. New York: McGraw and Hill; 2007.
13. Mankad S. Management of prosthetic heart valve complications. Curr Treat Options Cardiovasc Med. 2012;14(6):608–21.
14. Lim WY, Lloyd G, Bhattacharyya S. Mechanical and surgical bioprosthetic valve thrombosis. Heart. 2017;103(24):1934–41.
15. Rodriguez-Gabella T, Voisine P, Puri R, Pibarot P, Rodes-Cabau J. Aortic bioprosthetic valve durability: incidence, mechanisms, predictors, and management of surgical and transcatheter valve degeneration. J Am Coll Cardiol. 2017;70(8):1013–28.

16. Yanagawa B, Whitlock RP, Verma S, Gersh BJ. Anticoagulation for prosthetic heart valves: unresolved questions requiring answers. Curr Opin Cardiol. 2016;31(2):176–82.

17. Prodromo J, D'Ancona G, Amaducci A, Pilato M. Aortic valve repair for aortic insufficiency: a review. J Cardiothorac Vasc Anesth. 2012;26(5):923–32.

18. El Khoury G, Vanoverschelde JL, Glineur D, Pierard F, Verhelst RR, Rubay J, Funken JC, Watremez C, Astarci P, Lacroix V, Poncelet A, Noirhomme P. Repair of bicuspid aortic valves in patients with aortic regurgitation. Circulation. 2006;114(1 Suppl):I610–6.

19. Schaefer BM, Lewin MB, Stout KK, Gill E, Prueitt A, Byers PH, Otto CM. The bicuspid aortic valve: an integrated phenotypic classification of leaflet morphology and aortic root shape. Heart. 2008;94(12):1634–8.

20. Sievers HH, Schmidtke C. A classification system for the bicuspid aortic valve from 304 surgical specimens. J Thorac Cardiovasc Surg. 2007;133(5):1226–33.

21. Pettersson GB, Crucean AC, Savage R, Halley CM, Grimm RA, Svensson LG, Naficy S, Gillinov AM, Feng J, Blackstone EH. Toward predictable repair of regurgitant aortic valves: a systematic morphology-directed approach to bicommissural repair. J Am Coll Cardiol. 2008;52(1):40–9.

22. Nash PJ, Vitvitsky E, Li J, Cosgrove DM III, Pettersson G, Grimm RA. Feasibility of valve repair for regurgitant bicuspid aortic valves—an echocardiographic study. Ann Thorac Surg. 2005;79(5):1473–9.

23. Mitchell C, Rahko PS, Blauwet LA, Canaday B, Finstuen JA, Foster MC, Horton K, Ogunyankin KO, Palma RA, Velazquez EJ. Guidelines for performing a comprehensive transthoracic echocardiographic examination in adults: recommendations from the American Society of Echocardiography. J Am Soc Echocardiogr. 2019;32(1):1–64.

24. Hahn RT, Abraham T, Adams MS, Bruce CJ, Glas KE, Lang RM, Reeves ST, Shanewise JS, Siu SC, Stewart W, Picard MH. Guidelines for performing a comprehensive transesophageal echocardiographic examination: recommendations from the American Society of Echocardiography and the Society of Cardiovascular Anesthesiologists. Anesth Analg. 2014;118(1):21–68.

25. Flachskampf FA, Wouters PF, Edvardsen T, Evangelista A, Habib G, Hoffman P, Hoffmann R, Lancellotti P, Pepi M. Recommendations for transoesophageal echocardiography: EACVI update 2014. Eur Heart J Cardiovasc Imaging. 2014;15(4):353–65.

26. Zoghbi WA, Adams D, Bonow RO, Enriquez-Sarano M, Foster E, Grayburn PA, Hahn RT, Han Y, Hung J, Lang RM, Little SH, Shah DJ, Shernan S, Thavendiranathan P, Thomas JD, Weissman NJ. Recommendations for noninvasive evaluation of native valvular regurgitation: a report from the American Society of Echocardiography Developed in Collaboration with the Society for Cardiovascular Magnetic Resonance. J Am Soc Echocardiogr. 2017;30(4):303–71.

27. Baumgartner HC, Hung JC-C, Bermejo J, Chambers JB, Edvardsen T, Goldstein S, Lancellotti P, LeFevre M, Miller F Jr, Otto CM. Recommendations on the echocardiographic assessment of aortic valve stenosis: a focused update from the European Association of Cardiovascular Imaging and the American Society of Echocardiography. Eur Heart J Cardiovasc Imaging. 2017;18(3):254–75.

28. Lancellotti P, Tribouilloy C, Hagendorff A, Popescu BA, Edvardsen T, Pierard LA, Badano L, Zamorano JL. Recommendations for the echocardiographic assessment of native valvular regurgitation: an executive summary from the European Association of Cardiovascular Imaging. Eur Heart J Cardiovasc Imaging. 2013;14(7):611–44.

29. Lang RM, Badano LP, Mor-Avi V, Afilalo J, Armstrong A, Ernande L, Flachskampf FA, Foster E, Goldstein SA, Kuznetsova T, Lancellotti P, Muraru D, Picard MH, Rietzschel ER, Rudski L, Spencer KT, Tsang W, Voigt JU. Recommendations for cardiac chamber quantification by echocardiography in adults: an update from the American Society of Echocardiography and the European Association of Cardiovascular Imaging. Eur Heart J Cardiovasc Imaging. 2015;16(3):233–70.

30. Aicher D, Kunihara T, Abou Issa O, Brittner B, Graber S, Schafers HJ. Valve configuration determines long-term results after repair of the bicuspid aortic valve. Circulation. 2011;123(2):178–85.

31. Habertheuer A, Milewski RK, Bavaria JE, Siki M, Freas M, Desai N, Szeto W, Ram C, Hu R, Vallabhajosyula P. Predictors of recurrent aortic insufficiency in type I bicuspid aortic valve repair. Ann Thorac Surg. 2018;106(5):1316–24.

32. Ridley C, Sohmer B, Vallabhajosyula P, Augoustides JGT. Aortic leaflet billowing as a risk factor for repair failure after aortic valve repair. J Cardiothorac Vasc Anesth. 2017;31(3):1001–6.

33. de Kerchove L, Mastrobuoni S, Boodhwani M, Astarci P, Rubay J, Poncelet A, Vanoverschelde JL, Noirhomme P, El Khoury G. The role of annular dimension and annuloplasty in tricuspid aortic valve repair. Eur J Cardiothorac Surg. 2016;49(2):428–37; discussion 437-8.

34. Kempfert J, Van Linden A, Lehmkuhl L, Rastan AJ, Holzhey D, Blumenstein J, Mohr FW, Walther T. Aortic annulus sizing: echocardiographic versus computed tomography derived measurements in comparison with direct surgical sizing. Eur J Cardiothorac Surg. 2012;42(4):627–33.

35. Rocha RV, Manlhiot C, Feindel CM, Yau TM, Mueller B, David TE, Ouzounian M. Surgical enlargement of the aortic root does not increase the operative risk of aortic valve replacement. Circulation. 2018;137(15):1585–94.

36. Aggarwal N, Gadhinglajkar SV, Panicker VT, Sreedhar R, Babu S, Mathew DG, Prasannakumar CS. Posterior aortic root enlargement during aortic valve replacement: role of intraoperative transesophageal echocardiography. J Cardiothorac Vasc Anesth. 2017;31(4):1312–7.

37. Gasparovic H, Rybicki FJ, Millstine J, Unic D, Byrne JG, Yucel K, Mihaljevic T. Three dimensional computed tomographic imaging in planning the surgical approach for redo cardiac surgery after coronary revascularization. Eur J Cardiothorac Surg. 2005;28(2):244–9.

38. Pansini S, Ottino G, Forsennati PG, Serpieri G, Zattera G, Casabona R, di Summa M, Villani M, Poletti GA, Morea M. Reoperations on heart valve prostheses: an analysis of operative risks and late results. Ann Thorac Surg. 1990;50(4):590–6.

39. Tam RK, Garlick RB, Almeida AA. Minimally invasive redo aortic valve replacement. J Thorac Cardiovasc Surg. 1997;114(4):682–3.

40. Adams DH, Popma JJ, Reardon MJ, Yakubov SJ, Coselli JS, Deeb GM, Gleason TG, Buchbinder M, Hermiller J Jr, Kleiman NS, Chetcuti S, Heiser J, Merhi W, Zorn G, Tadros P, Robinson N, Petrossian G, Hughes GC, Harrison JK, Conte J, Maini B, Mumtaz M, Chenoweth S, Oh JK. Transcatheter aortic-valve replacement with a self-expanding prosthesis. N Engl J Med. 2014;370(19):1790–8.

41. Leon MB, Smith CR, Mack MJ, Makkar RR, Svensson LG, Kodali SK, Thourani VH, Tuzcu EM, Miller DC, Herrmann HC, Doshi D, Cohen DJ, Pichard AD, Kapadia S, Dewey T, Babaliaros V, Szeto WY, Williams MR, Kereiakes D, Zajarias A, Greason KL, Whisenant BK, Hodson RW, Moses JW, Trento A, Brown DL, Fearon WF, Pibarot P, Hahn RT, Jaber WA, Anderson WN, Alu MC, Webb JG. Transcatheter or surgical aortic-valve replacement in intermediate-risk patients. N Engl J Med. 2016;374(17):1609–20.

42. Baumgartner H, Falk V, Bax JJ, De Bonis M, Hamm C, Holm PJ, Iung B, Lancellotti P, Lansac E, Rodriguez Munoz D, Rosenhek R, Sjogren J, Tornos Mas P, Vahanian A, Walther T, Wendler O, Windecker S, Zamorano JL. 2017 ESC/EACTS guide-

lines for the management of valvular heart disease. Eur Heart J. 2017;38(36):2739–91.

43. Nishimura RA, Otto CM, Bonow RO, Carabello BA, Erwin JP III, Fleisher LA, Jneid H, Mack MJ, McLeod CJ, O'Gara PT, Rigolin VH, Sundt TM III, Thompson A. 2017 AHA/ACC focused update of the 2014 AHA/ACC guideline for the management of patients with valvular heart disease: a report of the American College of Cardiology/American Heart Association Task Force on Clinical Practice Guidelines. J Am Coll Cardiol. 2017;70(2):252–89.

44. Elmariah S, Fearon WF, Inglessis I, Vlahakes GJ, Lindman BR, Alu MC, Crowley A, Kodali S, Leon MB, Svensson L, Pibarot P, Hahn RT, Thourani VH, Palacios IF, Miller DC, Douglas PS, Passeri JJ. Transapical transcatheter aortic valve replacement is associated with increased cardiac mortality in patients with left ventricular dysfunction: insights from the PARTNER I trial. JACC Cardiovasc Interv. 2017;10(23):2414–22.

45. Tamborini G, Fusini L, Muratori M, Cefalu C, Gripari P, Ali SG, Pontone G, Andreini D, Bartorelli AL, Alamanni F, Fiorentini C, Pepi M. Feasibility and accuracy of three-dimensional transthoracic echocardiography vs. multidetector computed tomography in the evaluation of aortic valve annulus in patient candidates to transcatheter aortic valve implantation. Eur Heart J Cardiovasc Imaging. 2014;15(12):1316–23.

46. Storz C, Geisler T, Notohamiprodjo M, Nikolaou K, Bamberg F. Role of imaging in transcatheter aortic valve replacement. Curr Treat Options Cardiovasc Med. 2016;18(10):59.

47. Ribeiro HB, Webb JG, Makkar RR, Cohen MG, Kapadia SR, Kodali S, Tamburino C, Barbanti M, Chakravarty T, Jilaihawi H, Paradis JM, de Brito FS, Jr CSJ, Cheema AN, de Jaegere PP, del Valle R, Chiam PT, Moreno R, Pradas G, Ruel M, Salgado-Fernandez J, Sarmento-Leite R, Toeg HD, Velianou JL, Zajarias A, Babaliaros V, Cura F, Dager AE, Manoharan G, Lerakis S, Pichard AD, Radhakrishnan S, Perin MA, Dumont E, Larose E, Pasian SG, Nombela-Franco L, Urena M, Tuzcu EM, Leon MB, Amat-Santos IJ, Leipsic J, Rodes-Cabau J. Predictive factors, management, and clinical outcomes of coronary obstruction following transcatheter aortic valve implantation: insights from a large multicenter registry. J Am Coll Cardiol. 2013;62(17):1552–62.

48. Jilaihawi H, Chen M, Webb J, Himbert D, Ruiz CE, Rodes-Cabau J, Pache G, Colombo A, Nickenig G, Lee M, Tamburino C, Sievert H, Abramowitz Y, Tarantini G, Alqoofi F, Chakravarty T, Kashif M, Takahashi N, Kazuno Y, Maeno Y, Kawamori H, Chieffo A, Blanke P, Dvir D, Ribeiro HB, Feng Y, Zhao ZG, Sinning JM, Kliger C, Giustino G, Pajerski B, Imme S, Grube E, Leipsic J, Vahanian A, Michev I, Jelnin V, Latib A, Cheng W, Makkar R. A bicuspid aortic valve imaging classification for the TAVR era. JACC Cardiovasc Imaging. 2016;9(10):1145–58.

49. Hahn RT. Use of imaging for procedural guidance during transcatheter aortic valve replacement. Curr Opin Cardiol. 2013;28(5):512–7.

50. Vollema EM, Delgado V, Bax JJ. Echocardiography in transcatheter aortic valve replacement. Heart Lung Circ. 2019;28(9):1384–99.

51. Jilaihawi H, Kashif M, Fontana G, Furugen A, Shiota T, Friede G, Makhija R, Doctor N, Leon MB, Makkar RR. Cross-sectional computed tomographic assessment improves accuracy of aortic annular sizing for transcatheter aortic valve replacement and reduces the incidence of paravalvular aortic regurgitation. J Am Coll Cardiol. 2012;59(14):1275–86.

52. Bleakley C, Eskandari M, Monaghan M. 3D transoesophageal echocardiography in the TAVI sizing arena: should we do it and how do we do it? Echo Res Pract. 2017;4(1):R21–r32.

53. Hahn RT, Khalique O, Williams MR, Koss E, Paradis JM, Daneault B, Kirtane AJ, George I, Leon MB, Kodali S. Predicting paravalvular regurgitation following transcatheter valve replacement: utility of a novel method for three-dimensional echocardiographic measurements of the aortic annulus. J Am Soc Echocardiogr. 2013;26(9):1043–52.

54. Kasel AM, Cassese S, Bleiziffer S, Amaki M, Hahn RT, Kastrati A, Sengupta PP. Standardized imaging for aortic annular sizing: implications for transcatheter valve selection. JACC Cardiovasc Imaging. 2013;6(2):249–62.

55. Patel PA, Gutsche JT, Vernick WJ, Giri JS, Ghadimi K, Weiss SJ, Jagasia DH, Bavaria JE, Augoustides JG. The functional aortic annulus in the 3D era: focus on transcatheter aortic valve replacement for the perioperative echocardiographer. J Cardiothorac Vasc Anesth. 2015;29(1):240–5.

56. Khalique OK, Hamid NB, White JM, Bae DJ, Kodali SK, Nazif TM, Vahl TP, Paradis JM, George I, Leon MB, Hahn RT. Impact of methodologic differences in three-dimensional echocardiographic measurements of the aortic annulus compared with computed tomographic angiography before transcatheter aortic valve replacement. J Am Soc Echocardiogr. 2017;30(4):414–21.

57. Podlesnikar T, Prihadi EA, van Rosendael PJ, Vollema EM, van der Kley F, de Weger A, Ajmone Marsan N, Naji F, Fras Z, Bax JJ, Delgado V. Influence of the quantity of aortic valve calcium on the agreement between automated 3-dimensional transesophageal echocardiography and multidetector row computed tomography for aortic annulus sizing. Am J Cardiol. 2018;121(1):86–93.

58. Mediratta A, Addetia K, Medvedofsky D, Schneider RJ, Kruse E, Shah AP, Nathan S, Paul JD, Blair JE, Ota T, Balkhy HH, Patel AR, Mor-Avi V, Lang RM. 3D echocardiographic analysis of aortic annulus for transcatheter aortic valve replacement using novel aortic valve quantification software: comparison with computed tomography. Echocardiography. 2017;34(5):690–9.

59. Piazza N, de Jaegere P, Schultz C, Becker AE, Serruys PW, Anderson RH. Anatomy of the aortic valvar complex and its implications for transcatheter implantation of the aortic valve. Circ Cardiovasc Interv. 2008;1(1):74–81.

60. Altiok E, Koos R, Schroder J, Brehmer K, Hamada S, Becker M, Mahnken AH, Almalla M, Dohmen G, Autschbach R, Marx N, Hoffmann R. Comparison of two-dimensional and three-dimensional imaging techniques for measurement of aortic annulus diameters before transcatheter aortic valve implantation. Heart. 2011;97(19):1578–84.

61. Balzer JC, Boering YC, Mollus S, Schmidt M, Hellhammer K, Kroepil P, Westenfeld R, Zeus T, Antoch G, Linke A, Steinseifer U, Merx MW, Kelm M. Left ventricular contrast injection with rotational C-arm CT improves accuracy of aortic annulus measurement during cardiac catheterisation. EuroIntervention. 2014;10(3):347–54.

62. Babaliaros VC, Junagadhwalla Z, Lerakis S, Thourani V, Liff D, Chen E, Vassiliades T, Chappell C, Gross N, Patel A, Howell S, Green JT, Veledar E, Guyton R, Block PC. Use of balloon aortic valvuloplasty to size the aortic annulus before implantation of a balloon-expandable transcatheter heart valve. JACC Cardiovasc Interv. 2010;3(1):114–8.

63. Condado JF, Lerakis S, Stewart J, Jensen H, Henry TS, Ko SM, Stillman A, Rajaei MH, Mavromatis K, Devireddy C, Sarin E, Leshnower B, Guyton R, Kaebnick B, Thourani VH, Block PC, Babaliaros V. Balloon versus computed tomography sizing of the aortic annulus for transcatheter aortic valve replacement and the impact of left ventricular outflow tract calcification and morphology on sizing. J Invasive Cardiol. 2016;28(7):295–304.

64. Smith CR, Leon MB, Mack MJ, Miller DC, Moses JW, Svensson LG, Tuzcu EM, Webb JG, Fontana GP, Makkar RR, Williams M, Dewey T, Kapadia S, Babaliaros V, Thourani VH, Corso P, Pichard AD, Bavaria JE, Herrmann HC, Akin JJ, Anderson WN, Wang D, Pocock SJ. Transcatheter versus surgical aortic-valve replacement in high-risk patients. N Engl J Med. 2011;364(23):2187–98.

65. Kim WK, Hengstenberg C, Hilker M, Kerber S, Schafer U, Rudolph T, Linke A, Franz N, Kuntze T, Nef H, Kappert U, Zembala MO, Toggweiler S, Walther T, Mollmann H. The SAVI-TF registry: 1-year outcomes of the european post-market

registry using the ACURATE neo transcatheter heart valve under real-world conditions in 1,000 patients. JACC Cardiovasc Interv. 2018;11(14):1368–74.

66. Mack MJ, Leon MB, Thourani VH, Makkar R, Kodali SK, Russo M, Kapadia SR, Malaisrie SC, Cohen DJ, Pibarot P, Leipsic J, Hahn RT, Blanke P, Williams MR, McCabe JM, Brown DL, Babaliaros V, Goldman S, Szeto WY, Genereux P, Pershad A, Pocock SJ, Alu MC, Webb JG, Smith CR, Investigators P. Transcatheter aortic-valve replacement with a balloon-expandable valve in low-risk patients. N Engl J Med. 2019;380(18):1695–705.

67. Popma JJ, Deeb GM, Yakubov SJ, Mumtaz M, Gada H, O'Hair D, Bajwa T, Heiser JC, Merhi W, Kleiman NS, Askew J, Sorajja P, Rovin J, Chetcuti SJ, Adams DH, Teirstein PS, Zorn GL III, Forrest JK, Tchetche D, Resar J, Walton A, Piazza N, Ramlawi B, Robinson N, Petrossian G, Gleason TG, Oh JK, Boulware MJ, Qiao H, Mugglin AS, Reardon MJ, Evolut Low Risk Trial Investigators. Transcatheter aortic-valve replacement with a self-expanding valve in low-risk patients. N Engl J Med. 2019;380(18):1706–15.

68. Coughlan JJ, Kiernan T, Mylotte D, Arnous S. Annular rupture during transcatheter aortic valve implantation: predictors, management and outcomes. Interv Cardiol. 2018;13(3):140–4.

69. Rodriguez-Olivares R, El Faquir N, Rahhab Z, van Gils L, Ren B, Sakhi R, Geleijnse ML, van Domburg R, de Jaegere PPT, Zamorano Gomez JL, Van Mieghem NM. Impact of device-host interaction on paravalvular aortic regurgitation with different transcatheter heart valves. Cardiovasc Revasc Med. 2019;20(2):126–32.

70. Toggweiler S, Nissen H, Mogensen B, Cuculi F, Fallesen C, Veien KT, Brinkert M, Kobza R, Ruck A. Very low pacemaker rate following ACURATE neo transcatheter heart valve implantation. EuroIntervention. 2017;13(11):1273–80.

71. Webb JG, Htun N. Transcatheter options for the treatment of noncalcified aortic regurgitation. JACC Cardiovasc Interv. 2015;8(14):1850–3.

72. Yoon SH, Schmidt T, Bleiziffer S, Schofer N, Fiorina C, Munoz-Garcia AJ, Yzeiraj E, Amat-Santos IJ, Tchetche D, Jung C, Fujita B, Mangieri A, Deutsch MA, Ubben T, Deuschl F, Kuwata S, De Biase C, Williams T, Dhoble A, Kim WK, Ferrari E, Barbanti M, Vollema EM, Miceli A, Giannini C, Attizzani GF, Kong WKF, Gutierrez-Ibanes E, Jimenez Diaz VA, Wijeysundera HC, Kaneko H, Chakravarty T, Makar M, Sievert H, Hengstenberg C, Prendergast BD, Vincent F, Abdel-Wahab M, Nombela-Franco L, Silaschi M, Tarantini G, Butter C, Ensminger SM, Hildick-Smith D, Petronio AS, Yin WH, De Marco F, Testa L, Van Mieghem NM, Whisenant BK, Kuck KH, Colombo A, Kar S, Moris C, Delgado V, Maisano F, Nietlispach F, Mack MJ, Schofer J, Schaefer U, Bax JJ, Frerker C, Latib A, Makkar RR. Transcatheter aortic valve replacement in pure native aortic valve regurgitation. J Am Coll Cardiol. 2017;70(22):2752–63.

73. Sawaya FJ, Deutsch MA, Seiffert M, Yoon SH, Codner P, Wickramarachchi U, Latib A, Petronio AS, Rodes-Cabau J, Taramasso M, Spaziano M, Bosmans J, Biasco L, Mylotte D, Savontaus M, Gheeraert P, Chan J, Jorgensen TH, Sievert H, Mocetti M, Lefevre T, Maisano F, Mangieri A, Hildick-Smith D, Kornowski R, Makkar R, Bleiziffer S, Sondergaard L, De Backer O. Safety and efficacy of transcatheter aortic valve replacement in the treatment of pure aortic regurgitation in native valves and failing surgical bioprostheses: results from an International Registry Study. JACC Cardiovasc Interv. 2017;10(10):1048–56.

74. Urena M, Himbert D, Ohlmann P, Capretti G, Goublaire C, Kindo M, Morel O, Ghodbane W, Iung B, Vahanian A. Transcatheter aortic valve replacement to treat pure aortic regurgitation on noncalcified native valves. J Am Coll Cardiol. 2016;68(15):1705–6.

75. Toggweiler S, Cerillo AG, Kim WK, Biaggi P, Lloyd C, Hilker M, Almagor Y, Cuculi F, Brinkert M, Kobza R, Muller O, Ruck A, Corti R. Transfemoral implantation of the Acurate neo for the treatment of aortic regurgitation. J Invasive Cardiol. 2018;30(9):329–33.

76. Zhu D, Wei L, Cheung A, Guo Y, Chen Y, Zhu L, Liu H, Yang Y, Zhang J, Wang C. Treatment of pure aortic regurgitation using a second-generation transcatheter aortic valve implantation system. J Am Coll Cardiol. 2016;67(23):2803–5.

77. Schafer U, Schirmer J, Niklas S, Harmel E, Deuschl F, Conradi L. First-in-human implantation of a novel transfemoral selfexpanding transcatheter heart valve to treat pure aortic regurgitation. EuroIntervention. 2017;13(11):1296–9.

78. Schafer U, Conradi L, Diemert P, Deuschl F, Schofer N, Seiffert M, Lubos E, Schirmer J, Reichenspurner H, Blankenberg S, Treede H. Symetis ACURATE TAVI: review of the technology, developments and current data with this self-expanding transcatheter heart valve. Minerva Cardioangiol. 2015;63(5):359–69.

79. Walther T, Arsalan M, Kim W, Kempfert J. TAVI: transapical—what else? EuroIntervention. 2013;9(Suppl):S19–24.

80. Meyer CG, Frick M, Lotfi S, Altiok E, Koos R, Kirschfink A, Lehrke M, Autschbach R, Hoffmann R. Regional left ventricular function after transapical vs. transfemoral transcatheter aortic valve implantation analysed by cardiac magnetic resonance feature tracking. Eur Heart J Cardiovasc Imaging. 2014;15(10):1168–76.

81. Bruschi G, Fratto P, De Marco F, Oreglia J, Colombo P, Botta L, Cannata A, Moreo A, De Chiara B, Lullo F, Paino R, Martinelli L, Klugmann S. The trans-subclavian retrograde approach for transcatheter aortic valve replacement: single-center experience. J Thorac Cardiovasc Surg. 2010;140(4):911–5, 915.e1-2.

82. Modine T, Lemesle G, Azzaoui R, Sudre A. Aortic valve implantation with the CoreValve ReValving System via left carotid artery access: first case report. J Thorac Cardiovasc Surg. 2010;140(4):928–9.

83. Latsios G, Gerckens U, Grube E. Transaortic transcatheter aortic valve implantation: a novel approach for the truly "no-access option" patients. Catheter Cardiovasc Interv. 2010;75(7):1129–36.

84. Greenbaum AB, Babaliaros VC, Chen MY, Stine AM, Rogers T, O'Neill WW, Paone G, Thourani VH, Muhammad KI, Leonardi RA, Ramee S, Troendle JF, Lederman RJ. Transcaval access and closure for transcatheter aortic valve replacement: a prospective investigation. J Am Coll Cardiol. 2017;69(5):511–21.

85. Popma JJ, Deeb GM, Yakubov SJ, Mumtaz M, Gada H, O'Hair D, Bajwa T, Heiser JC, Merhi W, Kleiman NS, Askew J, Sorajja P, Rovin J, Chetcuti SJ, Adams DH, Teirstein PS, Zorn GL III, Forrest JK, Tchetche D, Resar J, Walton A, Piazza N, Ramlawi B, Robinson N, Petrossian G, Gleason TG, Oh JK, Boulware MJ, Qiao H, Mugglin AS, Reardon MJ. Transcatheter aortic-valve replacement with a self-expanding valve in low-risk patients. N Engl J Med. 2019;380(18):1706–15.

86. Aronow WS, Ahn C, Kronzon I. Association of valvular aortic stenosis with symptomatic peripheral arterial disease in older persons. Am J Cardiol. 2001;88(9):1046–7.

87. Toggweiler S, Leipsic J, Binder RK, Freeman M, Barbanti M, Heijmen RH, Wood DA, Webb JG. Management of vascular access in transcatheter aortic valve replacement: part 1: basic anatomy, imaging, sheaths, wires, and access routes. JACC Cardiovasc Interv. 2013;6(7):643–53.

88. Vavuranakis M, Kalogeras K, Vrachatis D, Kariori M, Voudris V, Aznaouridis K, Moldovan C, Vaina S, Lazaros G, Masoura K, Thomopoulou S, Stefanadis C. Inferior epigastric artery as a landmark for transfemoral TAVI. Optimizing vascular access? Catheter Cardiovasc Interv. 2013;81(6):1061–6.

89. Hwang JY. Doppler ultrasonography of the lower extremity arteries: anatomy and scanning guidelines. Ultrasonography. 2017;36(2):111–9.

90. Dahle TG, Kaneko T, McCabe JM. Outcomes following subclavian and axillary artery access for transcatheter aortic valve replacement: Society of the Thoracic Surgeons/American College of Cardiology TVT Registry Report. JACC Cardiovasc Interv. 2019;12(7):662–9.

91. De Palma R, Ruck A, Settergren M, Saleh N. Percutaneous axillary arteriotomy closure during transcatheter aortic valve replacement using the MANTA device. Catheter Cardiovasc Interv. 2018;92(5):998–1001.

92. Young MN, Singh V, Sakhuja R. A review of alternative access for transcatheter aortic valve replacement. Curr Treat Options Cardiovasc Med. 2018;20(7):62.

93. Bapat V, Tang GHL. Axillary/subclavian transcatheter aortic valve replacement: the default alternative access? JACC Cardiovasc Interv. 2019;12(7):670–2.

94. Blanke P, Weir-McCall JR, Achenbach S, Delgado V, Hausleiter J, Jilaihawi H, Marwan M, Norgaard BL, Piazza N, Schoenhagen P, Leipsic JA. Computed tomography imaging in the context of transcatheter aortic valve implantation (TAVI)/transcatheter aortic valve replacement (TAVR): an expert consensus document of the Society of Cardiovascular Computed Tomography. J Cardiovasc Comput Tomogr. 2019;13(1):1–20.

95. Petronio AS, De Carlo M, Bedogni F, Maisano F, Ettori F, Klugmann S, Poli A, Marzocchi A, Santoro G, Napodano M, Ussia GP, Giannini C, Brambilla N, Colombo A. 2-year results of CoreValve implantation through the subclavian access: a propensity-matched comparison with the femoral access. J Am Coll Cardiol. 2012;60(6):502–7.

96. Petzoldt R. Ultrasound-guided puncture of the subclavian vein. Intensive Care Med. 1980;7(1):39–40.

97. Schaefer A, Schirmer J, Schofer N, Schneeberger Y, Deuschl F, Blankenberg S, Reichenspurner H, Conradi L, Schafer U. Transaxillary transcatheter aortic valve implantation utilizing a novel vascular closure device with resorbable collagen material: a feasibility study. Clin Res Cardiol. 2019;108(7):779–86.

98. Lanz J, Greenbaum A, Pilgrim T, Tarantini G, Windecker S. Current state of alternative access for transcatheter aortic valve implantation. EuroIntervention. 2018;14(AB):AB40–52.

99. Zamorano JL, Badano LP, Bruce C, Chan KL, Goncalves A, Hahn RT, Keane MG, La Canna G, Monaghan MJ, Nihoyannopoulos P, Silvestry FE, Vanoverschelde JL, Gillam LD. EAE/ASE recommendations for the use of echocardiography in new transcatheter interventions for valvular heart disease. Eur Heart J. 2011;32(17):2189–214.

100. Foldyna B, Hansig M, Lucke C, Holzhey D, Andres C, Grothoff M, Linke A, Mohr FW, Gutberlet M, Lehmkuhl L. Access path angle in transapical aortic valve replacement: risk factor for paravalvular leakage. Ann Thorac Surg. 2014;98(5):1572–8.

101. Bruschi G, de Marco F, Botta L, Cannata A, Oreglia J, Colombo P, Barosi A, Colombo T, Nonini S, Paino R, Klugmann S, Martinelli L. Direct aortic access for transcatheter self-expanding aortic bioprosthetic valves implantation. Ann Thorac Surg. 2012;94(2):497–503.

102. Overtchouk P, Folliguet T, Pinaud F, Fouquet O, Pernot M, Bonnet G, Hubert M, Lapeze J, Claudel JP, Ghostine S, Azmoun A, Caussin C, Zannis K, Harmouche M, Verhoye JP, Lafont A, Chamandi C, Ruggieri VG, Di Cesare A, Leclercq F, Gandet T, Modine T. Transcarotid approach for transcatheter aortic valve replacement with the Sapien 3 prosthesis: a Multicenter French Registry. JACC Cardiovasc Interv. 2019;12(5):413–9.

103. Bapat VN, Attia RQ, Thomas M. Distribution of calcium in the ascending aorta in patients undergoing transcatheter aortic valve implantation and its relevance to the transaortic approach. JACC Cardiovasc Interv. 2012;5(5):470–6.

104. Lederman RJ, Greenbaum AB, Rogers T, Khan JM, Fusari M, Chen MY. Anatomic suitability for transcaval access based on computed tomography. JACC Cardiovasc Interv. 2017;10(1):1–10.

105. Jabbour RJ, Tanaka A, Finkelstein A, Mack M, Tamburino C, Van Mieghem N, de Backer O, Testa L, Gatto P, Purita P, Rahhab Z, Veulemans V, Stundl A, Barbanti M, Nerla R, Sinning JM, Dvir D, Tarantini G, Szerlip M, Scholtz W, Scholtz S, Tchetche D,

Castriota F, Butter C, Sondergaard L, Abdel-Wahab M, Sievert H, Alfieri O, Webb J, Rodes-Cabau J, Colombo A, Latib A. Delayed coronary obstruction after transcatheter aortic valve replacement. J Am Coll Cardiol. 2018;71(14):1513–24.

106. Mukherjee C, Hein F, Holzhey D, Lukas L, Mende M, Kaisers UX, Ender J. Is real time 3D transesophageal echocardiography a feasible approach to detect coronary ostium during transapical aortic valve implantation? J Cardiothorac Vasc Anesth. 2013;27(4):654–9.

107. Tamborini G, Fusini L, Gripari P, Muratori M, Cefalu C, Maffessanti F, Alamanni F, Bartorelli A, Pontone G, Andreini D, Bertella E, Fiorentini C, Pepi M. Feasibility and accuracy of 3DTEE versus CT for the evaluation of aortic valve annulus to left main ostium distance before transcatheter aortic valve implantation. JACC Cardiovasc Imaging. 2012;5(6):579–88.

108. Eggebrecht H, Vaquerizo B, Moris C, Bossone E, Lammer J, Czerny M, Zierer A, Schrofel H, Kim WK, Walther T, Scholtz S, Rudolph T, Hengstenberg C, Kempfert J, Spaziano M, Lefevre T, Bleiziffer S, Schofer J, Mehilli J, Seiffert M, Naber C, Biancari F, Eckner D, Cornet C, Lhermusier T, Philippart R, Siljander A, Giuseppe Cerillo A, Blackman D, Chieffo A, Kahlert P, Czerwinska-Jelonkiewicz K, Szymanski P, Landes U, Kornowski R, D'Onofrio A, Kaulfersch C, Sondergaard L, Mylotte D, Mehta RH, De Backer O. Incidence and outcomes of emergent cardiac surgery during transfemoral transcatheter aortic valve implantation (TAVI): insights from the European Registry on Emergent Cardiac Surgery during TAVI (EuRECS-TAVI). Eur Heart J. 2018;39(8):676–84.

109. Barbanti M, Yang TH, Rodes Cabau J, Tamburino C, Wood DA, Jilaihawi H, Blanke P, Makkar RR, Latib A, Colombo A, Tarantini G, Raju R, Binder RK, Nguyen G, Freeman M, Ribeiro HB, Kapadia S, Min J, Feuchtner G, Gurtvich R, Alqoofi F, Pelletier M, Ussia GP, Napodano M, de Brito FS Jr, Kodali S, Norgaard BL, Hansson NC, Pache G, Canovas SJ, Zhang H, Leon MB, Webb JG, Leipsic J. Anatomical and procedural features associated with aortic root rupture during balloon-expandable transcatheter aortic valve replacement. Circulation. 2013;128(3):244–53.

110. Abdel-Wahab M, Zahn R, Horack M, Gerckens U, Schuler G, Sievert H, Eggebrecht H, Senges J, Richardt G. Aortic regurgitation after transcatheter aortic valve implantation: incidence and early outcome. Results from the german transcatheter aortic valve interventions registry. Heart. 2011;97(11):899–906.

111. Gilard M, Eltchaninoff H, Iung B, Donzeau-Gouge P, Chevreul K, Fajadet J, Leprince P, Leguerrier A, Lievre M, Prat A, Teiger E, Lefevre T, Himbert D, Tchetche D, Carrie D, Albat B, Cribier A, Rioufol G, Sudre A, Blanchard D, Collet F, Dos Santos P, Meneveau N, Tirouvanziam A, Caussin C, Guyon P, Boschat J, Le Breton H, Collart F, Houel R, Delpine S, Souteyrand G, Favereau X, Ohlmann P, Doisy V, Grollier G, Gommeaux A, Claudel JP, Bourlon F, Bertrand B, Van Belle E, Laskar M. Registry of transcatheter aortic-valve implantation in high-risk patients. N Engl J Med. 2012;366(18):1705–15.

112. Kodali SK, Williams MR, Smith CR, Svensson LG, Webb JG, Makkar RR, Fontana GP, Dewey TM, Thourani VH, Pichard AD, Fischbein M, Szeto WY, Lim S, Greason KL, Teirstein PS, Malaisrie SC, Douglas PS, Hahn RT, Whisenant B, Zajarias A, Wang D, Akin JJ, Anderson WN, Leon MB. Two-year outcomes after transcatheter or surgical aortic-valve replacement. N Engl J Med. 2012;366(18):1686–95.

113. Detaint D, Lepage L, Himbert D, Brochet E, Messika-Zeitoun D, Iung B, Vahanian A. Determinants of significant paravalvular regurgitation after transcatheter aortic valve: implantation impact of device and annulus discongruence. JACC Cardiovasc Interv. 2009;2(9):821–7.

114. van Gils L, Wohrle J, Hildick-Smith D, Bleiziffer S, Blackman DJ, Abdel-Wahab M, Gerckens U, Brecker S, Bapat V, Modine

T, Soliman OI, Nersesov A, Allocco D, Falk V, Van Mieghem NM. Importance of contrast aortography with lotus transcatheter aortic valve replacement: a post hoc analysis from the RESPOND Post-Market Study. JACC Cardiovasc Interv. 2018;11(2):119–28.

115. Leon MB, Smith CR, Mack M, Miller DC, Moses JW, Svensson LG, Tuzcu EM, Webb JG, Fontana GP, Makkar RR, Brown DL, Block PC, Guyton RA, Pichard AD, Bavaria JE, Herrmann HC, Douglas PS, Petersen JL, Akin JJ, Anderson WN, Wang D, Pocock S. Transcatheter aortic-valve implantation for aortic stenosis in patients who cannot undergo surgery. N Engl J Med. 2010;363(17):1597–607.

116. Pibarot P, Hahn RT, Weissman NJ, Monaghan MJ. Assessment of paravalvular regurgitation following TAVR: a proposal of unifying grading scheme. JACC Cardiovasc Imaging. 2015;8(3):340–60.

117. Pibarot P, Hahn RT, Weissman NJ, Arsenault M, Beaudoin J, Bernier M, Dahou A, Khalique OK, Asch FM, Toubal O, Leipsic J, Blanke P, Zhang F, Parvataneni R, Alu M, Herrmann H, Makkar R, Mack M, Smalling R, Leon M, Thourani VH, Kodali S. Association of paravalvular regurgitation with 1-year outcomes after transcatheter aortic valve replacement with the SAPIEN 3 valve. JAMA Cardiol. 2017;2(11):1208–16.

118. Athappan G, Patvardhan E, Tuzcu EM, Svensson LG, Lemos PA, Fraccaro C, Tarantini G, Sinning JM, Nickenig G, Capodanno D, Tamburino C, Latib A, Colombo A, Kapadia SR. Incidence, predictors, and outcomes of aortic regurgitation after transcatheter aortic valve replacement: meta-analysis and systematic review of literature. J Am Coll Cardiol. 2013;61(15):1585–95.

119. Tchetche D, Windecker S, Kasel AM, Schaefer U, Worthley S, Linke A, Abdel-Wahab M, Le Breton H, Sondergaard L, Spence MS, Petronio S, Baumgartner H, Hovorka T, Blanke P, Reichenspurner H. 1-year outcomes of the CENTERA-EU trial assessing a novel self-expanding transcatheter heart valve. JACC Cardiovasc Interv. 2019;12(7):673–80.

120. Tang GHL, Zaid S, Schnittman SR, Ahmad H, Kaple R, Undemir C, Dutta T, Poniros A, Bennett J, Feng C, Cohen M, Lansman SL. Novel predictors of mild paravalvular aortic regurgitation in SAPIEN 3 transcatheter aortic valve implantation. EuroIntervention. 2018;14(1):58–68.

121. d'Humieres T, Faivre L, Chammous E, Deux JF, Bergoend E, Fiore A, Radu C, Couetil JP, Benhaiem N, Derumeaux G, Dubois-Rande JL, Ternacle J, Fard D, Lim P. A new three-dimensional echocardiography method to quantify aortic valve calcification. J Am Soc Echocardiogr. 2018;31(10):1073–9.

122. Colli A, D'Amico R, Kempfert J, Borger MA, Mohr FW, Walther T. Transesophageal echocardiographic scoring for transcatheter aortic valve implantation: impact of aortic cusp calcification on postoperative aortic regurgitation. J Thorac Cardiovasc Surg. 2011;142(5):1229–35.

123. Gripari P, Ewe SH, Fusini L, Muratori M, Ng AC, Cefalu C, Delgado V, Schalij MJ, Bax JJ, Marsan NA, Tamborini G, Pepi M. Intraoperative 2D and 3D transoesophageal echocardiographic predictors of aortic regurgitation after transcatheter aortic valve implantation. Heart. 2012;98(16):1229–36.

124. Hayek SS, Corrigan FE III, Condado JF, Lin S, Howell S, MacNamara JP, Zheng S, Keegan P, Thourani V, Babaliaros VC, Lerakis S. Paravalvular regurgitation after transcatheter aortic valve replacement: comparing transthoracic versus transesophageal echocardiographic guidance. J Am Soc Echocardiogr. 2017;30(6):533–40.

125. Urena M, Webb JG, Eltchaninoff H, Munoz-Garcia AJ, Bouleti C, Tamburino C, Nombela-Franco L, Nietlispach F, Moris C, Ruel M, Dager AE, Serra V, Cheema AN, Amat-Santos IJ, de Brito FS, Lemos PA, Abizaid A, Sarmento-Leite R, Ribeiro HB, Dumont E, Barbanti M, Durand E, Alonso Briales JH, Himbert D, Vahanian A, Imme S, Garcia E, Maisano F, del Valle R, Benitez LM, Garcia del Blanco B, Gutierrez H, Perin MA, Siqueira D, Bernardi G,

Philippon F, Rodes-Cabau J. Late cardiac death in patients undergoing transcatheter aortic valve replacement: incidence and predictors of advanced heart failure and sudden cardiac death. J Am Coll Cardiol. 2015;65(5):437–48.

126. Stortecky S, Buellesfeld L, Wenaweser P, Heg D, Pilgrim T, Khattab AA, Gloekler S, Huber C, Nietlispach F, Meier B, Juni P, Windecker S. Atrial fibrillation and aortic stenosis: impact on clinical outcomes among patients undergoing transcatheter aortic valve implantation. Circ Cardiovasc Interv. 2013;6(1):77–84.

127. Genereux P, Cohen DJ, Mack M, Rodes-Cabau J, Yadav M, Xu K, Parvataneni R, Hahn R, Kodali SK, Webb JG, Leon MB. Incidence, predictors, and prognostic impact of late bleeding complications after transcatheter aortic valve replacement. J Am Coll Cardiol. 2014;64(24):2605–15.

128. Lip GY, Nieuwlaat R, Pisters R, Lane DA, Crijns HJ. Refining clinical risk stratification for predicting stroke and thromboembolism in atrial fibrillation using a novel risk factor-based approach: the euro heart survey on atrial fibrillation. Chest. 2010;137(2):263–72.

129. Kirchhof P, Benussi S, Kotecha D, Ahlsson A, Atar D, Casadei B, Castella M, Diener HC, Heidbuchel H, Hendriks J, Hindricks G, Manolis AS, Oldgren J, Popescu BA, Schotten U, Van Putte B, Vardas P. 2016 ESC guidelines for the management of atrial fibrillation developed in collaboration with EACTS. Eur Heart J. 2016;37(38):2893–962.

130. Nijenhuis VJ, Brouwer J, Sondergaard L, Collet JP, Grove EL, Ten Berg JM. Antithrombotic therapy in patients undergoing transcatheter aortic valve implantation. Heart. 2019;105(10):742–8.

131. Latib A, Naganuma T, Abdel-Wahab M, Danenberg H, Cota L, Barbanti M, Baumgartner H, Finkelstein A, Legrand V, de Lezo JS, Kefer J, Messika-Zeitoun D, Richardt G, Stabile E, Kaleschke G, Vahanian A, Laborde JC, Leon MB, Webb JG, Panoulas VF, Maisano F, Alfieri O, Colombo A. Treatment and clinical outcomes of transcatheter heart valve thrombosis. Circ Cardiovasc Interv. 2015;8(4):e001779.

132. Makkar RR, Fontana G, Jilaihawi H, Chakravarty T, Kofoed KF, De Backer O, Asch FM, Ruiz CE, Olsen NT, Trento A, Friedman J, Berman D, Cheng W, Kashif M, Jelnin V, Kliger CA, Guo H, Pichard AD, Weissman NJ, Kapadia S, Manasse E, Bhatt DL, Leon MB, Sondergaard L. Possible subclinical leaflet thrombosis in bioprosthetic aortic valves. N Engl J Med. 2015;373(21):2015–24.

133. Windecker S, Tijssen J, Giustino G, Guimaraes AH, Mehran R, Valgimigli M, Vranckx P, Welsh RC, Baber U, van Es GA, Wildgoose P, Volkl AA, Zazula A, Thomitzek K, Hemmrich M, Dangas GD. Trial design: rivaroxaban for the prevention of major cardiovascular events after transcatheter aortic valve replacement: rationale and design of the GALILEO study. Am Heart J. 2017;184:81–7.

134. Jaffer IH, Stafford AR, Fredenburgh JC, Whitlock RP, Chan NC, Weitz JI. Dabigatran is less effective than warfarin at attenuating mechanical heart valve-induced thrombin generation. J Am Heart Assoc. 2015;4(8):e002322.

135. Bogunovic N, Scholtz W, Prinz C, Faber L, Horstkotte D, van Buuren F. Percutaneous closure of left atrial appendage after transcatheter aortic valve implantation—an interventional approach to avoid anticoagulation therapy in elderly patients: TAVI and closure of LAA to avoid warfarin therapy. EuroIntervention. 2012;7(11):1361–3.

136. Khattab AA, Gloekler S, Sprecher B, Shakir S, Guerios E, Stortecky S, O'Sullivan CJ, Nietlispach F, Moschovitis A, Pilgrim T, Buellesfeld L, Wenaweser P, Windecker S, Meier B. Feasibility and outcomes of combined transcatheter aortic valve replacement with other structural heart interventions in a single session: a matched cohort study. Open Heart. 2014;1(1):e000014.

137. Asmarats L, Rodes-Cabau J. Percutaneous left atrial appendage closure: current devices and clinical outcomes. Circ Cardiovasc Interv. 2017;10(11):e005359.

138. Jazayeri MA, Vuddanda V, Parikh V, Lakkireddy DR. Percutaneous left atrial appendage closure: current state of the art. Curr Opin Cardiol. 2017;32(1):27–38.

139. Beigel R, Wunderlich NC, Ho SY, Arsanjani R, Siegel RJ. The left atrial appendage: anatomy, function, and noninvasive evaluation. JACC Cardiovasc Imaging. 2014;7(12):1251–65.

140. Nkomo VT, Gardin JM, Skelton TN, Gottdiener JS, Scott CG, Enriquez-Sarano M. Burden of valvular heart diseases: a population-based study. Lancet. 2006;368(9540):1005–11.

141. Giordana F, Capriolo M, Frea S, Marra WG, Giorgi M, Bergamasco L, Omede PL, Sheiban I, D'Amico M, Bovolo V, Salizzoni S, La Torre M, Rinaldi M, Marra S, Gaita F, Morello M. Impact of TAVI on mitral regurgitation: a prospective echocardiographic study. Echocardiography. 2013;30(3):250–7.

142. Cortes C, Amat-Santos IJ, Nombela-Franco L, Munoz-Garcia AJ, Gutierrez-Ibanes E, De La Torre Hernandez JM, Cordoba-Soriano JG, Jimenez-Quevedo P, Hernandez-Garcia JM, Gonzalez-Mansilla A, Ruano J, Jimenez-Mazuecos J, Castrodeza J, Tobar J, Islas F, Revilla A, Puri R, Puerto A, Gomez I, Rodes-Cabau J, San Roman JA. Mitral regurgitation after transcatheter aortic valve replacement: prognosis, imaging predictors, and potential management. JACC Cardiovasc Interv. 2016;9(15):1603–14.

143. Feldman T, Kar S, Rinaldi M, Fail P, Hermiller J, Smalling R, Whitlow PL, Gray W, Low R, Herrmann HC, Lim S, Foster E, Glower D. Percutaneous mitral repair with the MitraClip system: safety and midterm durability in the initial EVEREST (Endovascular Valve Edge-to-Edge REpair Study) cohort. J Am Coll Cardiol. 2009;54(8):686–94.

144. Nickenig G, Estevez-Loureiro R, Franzen O, Tamburino C, Vanderheyden M, Luscher TF, Moat N, Price S, Dall'Ara G, Winter R, Corti R, Grasso C, Snow TM, Jeger R, Blankenberg S, Settergren M, Tiroch K, Balzer J, Petronio AS, Buttner HJ, Ettori F, Sievert H, Fiorino MG, Claeys M, Ussia GP, Baumgartner H, Scandura S, Alamgir F, Keshavarzi F, Colombo A, Maisano F, Ebelt H, Aruta P, Lubos E, Plicht B, Schueler R, Pighi M, Di Mario C. Percutaneous mitral valve edge-to-edge repair: in-hospital results and 1-year follow-up of 628 patients of the 2011-2012 Pilot European Sentinel Registry. J Am Coll Cardiol. 2014;64(9):875–84.

145. Stone GW, Lindenfeld J, Abraham WT, Kar S, Lim DS, Mishell JM, Whisenant B, Grayburn PA, Rinaldi M, Kapadia SR, Rajagopal V, Sarembock IJ, Brieke A, Marx SO, Cohen DJ, Weissman NJ, Mack MJ. Transcatheter mitral-valve repair in patients with heart failure. N Engl J Med. 2018;379(24):2307–18.

146. Mauri L, Garg P, Massaro JM, Foster E, Glower D, Mehoudar P, Powell F, Komtebedde J, McDermott E, Feldman T. The EVEREST II trial: design and rationale for a randomized study of the evalve mitraclip system compared with mitral valve surgery for mitral regurgitation. Am Heart J. 2010;160(1):23–9.

147. Lesevic H, Karl M, Braun D, Barthel P, Orban M, Pache J, Hadamitzky M, Mehilli J, Stecher L, Massberg S, Ott I, Schunkert H, Kastrati A, Sonne C, Hausleiter J. Long-term outcomes after MitraClip implantation according to the presence or absence of EVEREST inclusion criteria. Am J Cardiol. 2017;119(8):1255–61.

148. Nyman CB, Mackensen GB, Jelacic S, Little SH, Smith TW, Mahmood F. Transcatheter mitral valve repair using the edge-to-edge clip. J Am Soc Echocardiogr. 2018;31(4):434–53.

149. Maisano F, Alfieri O, Banai S, Buchbinder M, Colombo A, Falk V, Feldman T, Franzen O, Herrmann H, Kar S, Kuck KH, Lutter G, Mack M, Nickenig G, Piazza N, Reisman M, Ruiz CE, Schofer J, Sondergaard L, Stone GW, Taramasso M, Thomas M, Vahanian A, Webb J, Windecker S, Leon MB. The future of transcatheter mitral

150. valve interventions: competitive or complementary role of repair vs. replacement? Eur Heart J. 2015;36(26):1651–9.

150. Nishimura RA, Otto CM, Bonow RO, Carabello BA, Erwin JP III, Fleisher LA, Jneid H, Mack MJ, McLeod CJ, O'Gara PT, Rigolin VH, Sundt TM III, Thompson A. 2017 AHA/ACC focused update of the 2014 AHA/ACC guideline for the Management of Patients with Valvular Heart Disease: a report of the american College of Cardiology/American Heart Association task force on clinical practice guidelines. Circulation. 2017;135(25):e1159–95.

151. Nishimura RA, Otto CM, Bonow RO, Carabello BA, Erwin JP III, Guyton RA, O'Gara PT, Ruiz CE, Skubas NJ, Sorajja P, Sundt TM III, Thomas JD. 2014 AHA/ACC guideline for the management of patients with valvular heart disease: a report of the American College of Cardiology/American Heart Association Task Force on Practice Guidelines. J Am Coll Cardiol. 2014;63(22):e57–185.

152. Nunes MC, Tan TC, Elmariah S, do Lago R, Margey R, Cruz-Gonzalez I, Zheng H, Handschumacher MD, Inglessis I, Palacios IF, Weyman AE, Hung J. The echo score revisited: impact of incorporating commissural morphology and leaflet displacement to the prediction of outcome for patients undergoing percutaneous mitral valvuloplasty. Circulation. 2014;129(8):886–95.

153. Wilkins GT, Weyman AE, Abascal VM, Block PC, Palacios IF. Percutaneous balloon dilatation of the mitral valve: an analysis of echocardiographic variables related to outcome and the mechanism of dilatation. Br Heart J. 1988;60(4):299–308.

154. Bertrand PB, Mihos CG, Yucel E. Mitral annular calcification and calcific mitral stenosis: therapeutic challenges and considerations. Curr Treat Options Cardiovasc Med. 2019;21(4):19.

155. Okada Y. Surgical management of mitral annular calcification. Gen Thorac Cardiovasc Surg. 2013;61(11):619–25.

156. Polomsky M, Koulogiannis KP, Kipperman RM, Cohen BM, Magovern CJ, Slater JP, Xydas S, Marcoff L, Brown JM. Mitral valve replacement with Sapien 3 transcatheter valve in severe mitral annular calcification. Ann Thorac Surg. 2017;103(1):e57–9.

157. Murashita T, Suri RM, Daly RC. Sapien XT transcatheter mitral valve replacement under direct vision in the setting of significant mitral annular calcification. Ann Thorac Surg. 2016;101(3):1171–4.

158. Guerrero M, Dvir D, Himbert D, Urena M, Eleid M, Wang DD, Greenbaum A, Mahadevan VS, Holzhey D, O'Hair D, Dumonteil N, Rodes-Cabau J, Piazza N, Palma JH, DeLago A, Ferrari E, Witkowski A, Wendler O, Kornowski R, Martinez-Clark P, Ciaburri D, Shemin R, Alnasser S, McAllister D, Bena M, Kerendi F, Pavlides G, Sobrinho JJ, Attizzani GF, George I, Nickenig G, Fassa AA, Cribier A, Bapat V, Feldman T, Rihal C, Vahanian A, Webb J, O'Neill W. Transcatheter mitral valve replacement in native mitral valve disease with severe mitral annular calcification: results From the First Multicenter Global Registry. JACC Cardiovasc Interv. 2016;9(13):1361–71.

159. Sorajja P, Gossl M, Bae R, Tindell L, Lesser JR, Askew J, Farivar RS. Severe mitral annular calcification: first experience with transcatheter therapy using a dedicated mitral prosthesis. JACC Cardiovasc Interv. 2017;10(11):1178–9.

160. Guerrero M, Wang DD, Himbert D, Urena M, Pursnani A, Kaddissi G, Iyer V, Salinger M, Chakravarty T, Greenbaum A, Makkar R, Vahanian A, Feldman T, O'Neill W. Short-term results of alcohol septal ablation as a bail-out strategy to treat severe left ventricular outflow tract obstruction after transcatheter mitral valve replacement in patients with severe mitral annular calcification. Catheter Cardiovasc Interv. 2017;90(7):1220–6.

161. Wang DD, Eng MH, Greenbaum AB, Myers E, Forbes M, Karabon P, Pantelic M, Song T, Nadig J, Guerrero M, O'Neill WW. Validating a prediction modeling tool for left ventricular outflow tract (LVOT) obstruction after transcatheter mitral valve replacement (TMVR). Catheter Cardiovasc Interv. 2018;92(2):379–87.

162. Yoon SH, Bleiziffer S, Latib A, Eschenbach L, Ancona M, Vincent F, Kim WK, Unbehaum A, Asami M, Dhoble A, Silaschi M, Frangieh AH, Veulemans V, Tang GHL, Kuwata S, Rampat R, Schmidt T, Patel AJ, Nicz PFG, Nombela-Franco L, Kini A, Kitamura M, Sharma R, Chakravarty T, Hildick-Smith D, Arnold M, de Brito FS Jr, Jensen C, Jung C, Jilaihawi H, Smalling RW, Maisano F, Kasel AM, Treede H, Kempfert J, Pilgrim T, Kar S, Bapat V, Whisenant BK, Van Belle E, Delgado V, Modine T, Bax JJ, Makkar RR. Predictors of left ventricular outflow tract obstruction after transcatheter mitral valve replacement. JACC Cardiovasc Interv. 2019;12(2):182–93.

163. Otto C. Valvular heart disease. Philadelphia: Saunders an Imprint of Elsevier; 2004. p. 404–5.

164. Grossman W. Profiles in valvular heart disease. Grossman's cardiac catheterization, angiography and intervention. Philadelphia: Williams and Wilkins; 2000. p. 759–84.

Intraprocedural Guidance and Monitoring

4

Mara Gavazzoni, Alberto Pozzoli, Mizuki Miura, Edwin Ho,
Maurizio Taramasso, André R. Plass, Philipp Haager,
Hans Rickli, Michel Zuber, and Francesco Maisano

4.1 Intro

Currently, aortic stenosis (AS) is the most common cause of valve replacement in Europe and North America [1] where the most frequent cause is degenerative.

Aortic regurgitation (AR) can be due to primary disease of the aortic valve cusps and/or of the aortic root and ascending aorta. Two-thirds of the underlying aetiology of aortic regurgitation in the Euro Heart Survey are degenerative. Other causes include infective and rheumatic and degeneration of previous AV prosthesis [2, 3].

Treatment of aortic valve disease is mostly carried out by surgical aortic valve replacement (SAVR). The option of repairing a stenotic aortic valve is limited to specific situations, mostly in case of pure AR [4].

The presence of symptoms is the most important factor for referring patients to interventions when the severity of pathological process is known. Other factors are: indices of left ventricle remodelling (reduced ejection fraction LVEF, increased end diastolic or systolic volumes and diameters, EDVi, ESVi mL/m^2), exercise response for AS, concomitant need for other cardiac surgery, progression of severity during follow up, subclinical congestion (N-terminal pro b-type natriuretic peptide, NT-proBNP, and pulmonary arterial systolic pressure). When one of these occurs in setting of severe

aortic valve disease, patient should be referred to specialized centres and Heart Team would define the following diagnostic and therapeutic process.

Current indication for interventions in aortic valve diseases (AS and AR) are summarized in Table 4.1.

First described invervention in the history of heart valve surgery was on aortic stenosis and was attributed to Theodore Tuffier (1857–1929). At that time, without cardioplegia

M. Gavazzoni · A. Pozzoli · M. Miura · E. Ho · M. Taramasso
A. R. Plass · F. Maisano (✉)
Heart Surgery Unit, Zurich University Hospital,
Zurich, Switzerland
e-mail: mara.gavazzoni@usz.ch; alberto.pozzoli@usz.ch;
mizuki.miura@usz.ch; edwin.ho@usz.ch;
maurizio.taramasso@usz.ch; andre.plass@usz.ch;
francesco.maisano@usz.ch

P. Haager · H. Rickli
Cardiology Unit, Kantonsspital St. Gallen, St. Gallen, Switzerland
e-mail: philipp.haager@usz.ch; hans.rickli@kssg.ch

M. Zuber
Cardiology Unit, Zurich University Hospital, Zurich, Switzerland
e-mail: michel.zuber@usz.ch

Table 4.1 Current European guidelines for treatment of aortic stenosis and aortic regurgitation

Indications for surgery in severe aortic stenosis	
Intervention is indicated	
Intervention is indicated in symptomatic patients with severe, high-gradient aortic stenosis (mean gradient ≥ 40 mmHg or peak velocity ≥ 4.0 m/s)	IB
Intervention is indicated in symptomatic patients with severe low-flow, low-gradient (<40 mmHg) aortic stenosis with reduced ejection fraction and evidence of flow (contractile) reserve excluding pseudosevere aortic stenosis	IC
SAVR is indicated in asymptomatic patients with severe aortic stenosis and systolic LV dysfunction (LVEF <50%) not due to another cause	IC
SAVR is indicated in asymptomatic patients with severe aortic stenosis and abnormal exercise test showing symptoms on exercise clearly related to aortic stenosis	IC
SAVR is indicated in asymptomatic patients with severe aortic stenosis undergoing CABG or surgery of the ascending aorta or of another valve	IC
Intervention should be considered	
SAVR should be considered in asymptomatic patients with severe aortic stenosis and an abnormal exercise test showing a decrease in blood pressure below baseline	IIaC
SAVR should be considered in asymptomatic patients with normal ejection fraction if the surgical risk is low and one of the following findings is present: • Very severe aortic stenosis defined by a Vmax > 5.5 m/s • Severe valve calcification and a rate of Vmax progression ≥ 0.3 m/s/year • Markedly elevated BNP levels (>threefold age- and sex-corrected normal range) confirmed by repeated measurements without other explanations	IIaC

(continued)

F. Maisano et al. (eds.), *Multimodality Imaging for Cardiac Valvular Interventions, Volume 1 Aortic Valve*,
https://doi.org/10.1007/978-3-030-27584-6_4

Table 4.1 (continued)

Indications for surgery in severe aortic stenosis

- Severe pulmonary hypertension (systolic pulmonary artery pressure at rest >60 mmHg confirmed by invasive measurement) without other explanation

SAVR should be considered in patients with moderate aortic stenosise undergoing CABG or surgery of the ascending aorta or of another valve after Heart Team decision	IIaC

Intervention is not recommended

Intervention should not be performed in patients with severe comorbidities when the intervention is unlikely to improve quality of life or survival	III

Indications for surgery in (A) severe aortic regurgitation and (B) aortic root disease (irrespective of the severity of aortic regurgitation)

(A) Severe aortic regurgitation

Surgery is indicated in symptomatic patients	IB
Surgery is indicated in asymptomatic patients with resting LVEF ≤ 50%	IB
Surgery is indicated in patients undergoing CABG or surgery of the ascending aorta or of another valve	IC
Heart Team discussion is recommended in selected patients in whom aortic valve repair may be a feasible alternative to valve replacement	IC
Surgery should be considered in asymptomatic patients with resting ejection fraction >50% with severe LV dilatation: LVEDD >70 mm or LVESD >50 mm (or LVESD >25 mm/m^2 BSA in patients with small body size)	IIaB

(B) Aortic root or tubular ascending aortic aneurysm (irrespective of the severity of aortic regurgitation)

Aortic valve repair, using the reimplantation or remodelling with aortic annuloplasty technique, is recommended in young patients with aortic root dilation and tricuspid aortic valves, when performed by experienced surgeons.	IC
Surgery is indicated in patients with Marfan syndrome who have aortic root disease with a maximal ascending aortic diameter ≥ 50 mm	IC
Surgery should be considered in patients who have aortic root disease with maximal ascending aortic diameter:	IIaC

- ≥45 mm in the presence of Marfan syndrome and additional risk factors or patients with a TGFBR1 or TGFBR2 mutation (including Loeys–Dietz syndrome)
- ≥50 mm in the presence of a bicuspid valve with additional risk factors or coarctation
- ≥55 mm for all other patients

When surgery is primarily indicated for the aortic valve, replacement of the aortic root or tubular ascending aorta should be considered when ≥45 mm, particularly in the presence of a bicuspid valve	IIaC

(close heart surgery) and without echocardiographic evaluation of aortic valve (AV), the invagination of the aortic wall with the index finger and tearing of the was the only one way to solve the stenosis.

After advent of cardioplegia, heart and lung machine, heparin and the modern cardiac surgery was developed. At that time patients were referred to generalist practitioners or specialists for symptoms and then, when cardiac murmur was found and clinical details supported the suspected valvulopathy, patients were candidate to intervention. The only available view of the valve pathology was the intraoperative surgical one. Development and spreading of imaging techniques (cardioscopies first and then echocardiography) created the real revolution in the continuity of care for the patients: with technical improvement of imaging techniques, the possibility to integrate different modalities, and the increase amount of less-operator dependent parameters cardiac and vascular imaging have become pivotal for patient-centred Heart Team (Fig. 4.1).

In pre-procedural phase a carefully analysis of results of different tools is needed and includes evaluation of transthoracic and transoesophageal echocardiography (TTE, TEE), coronary angiography (CA), multi slice computerized tomography (MSCT). Cardiac magnetic resonance (CMR) has a role in valvular disease in specific cases of contraindication to ultrasound technique or technical un-feasibility [5]. MSCT clearly evaluates the morphology of AV when some doubts persist after TTE/TEE evaluation, amount and distribution of aortic calcification, coronary arteries abnormalities, the diameters of aortic root and ascending aorta and all those characteristics that have an impact on the risk of complications after extra-corporeal circulation (ECC) and aortic clamping (AC). MSCT is even more important in transcatheter interventions for planning interventions and predicting the outcome [6, 7]. Coronary angiography (CA) is indicated before AV interventions for diagnosis of coronary artery disease (CAD) in patients with history of cardiovascular disease; suspected myocardial ischaemia, LV systolic dysfunction, and In patients who are at least intermediate cardiovascular risk score (class of recommendation: IA). A coronary computed tomography angiography should be considered as alternative to CA before valve surgery in patients with severe aortic stenosis and low probability of CAD or in whom CA is technically not feasible (class IIa) [8].

After procedural planning and heart team discussion, when the procedure is ongoing, the most important tools for immediate pre-procedural and for intra-procedural monitoring purpose should be functional and dynamic. Currently, TEE, intracardiac and epicardial echocardiography (ICE, ECE) are used for this aims and in the specific setting of AV interventions indications for intraoperative use of cardiac ultrasound techniques include both elective and urgent situations. TEE was introduced in open heart surgery in the early 1980s and since that time many guidelines and consensus documents have been written increasing its utility to facilitate surgical decision making. A specific training is now supposed for specialists that are going to perform perioperative transesophageal echocardiography [9–13].

When a TEE probe cannot be inserted, epicardial echocardiography (ECE) can be used for intraoperative use in open heart surgery (after heart surface is exposed); in the field of transcatheter interventions when TEE is contraindicated or anaesthesia cannot be performed, intracardiac

Fig. 4.1 Imaging is the basis or the multidisciplinary heart team

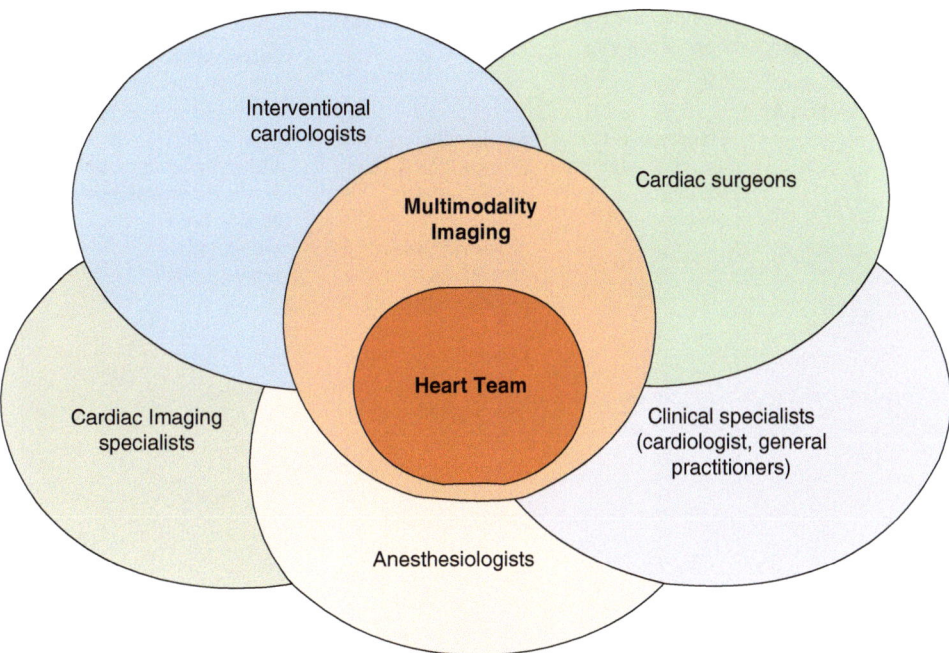

echocardiography (ICE) can be used by operators in hybrid room for intraoperative guidance [14–17].

X-ray fluoroscopy and CA are mainly important in the setting of transcatheter therapies and ultrasound techniques have a central role either in open heart surgery and transcatheter interventions. X-ray fluoroscopy is considered the current modality for real time imaging during transcatheter interventions. It provides optimal spatial and temporal resolution but the main limits remain: poor soft tissue characterization, lack of quantitative physiologic information, exposure of patients and staff to ionizing radiation. CA during transcatheter AV procedures, CA and aortography are currently used for assessing results of AV transcatheter procedures and complications, even if the risk of coronary arteries occlusion is low when native host AV is treated (0.3%, increasing at 3–4% in case of degeneration of bioprosthesis requiring valve in valve procedures) [18].

The most important advantage of using these techniques is that they allow a real-time and dynamic visualization of cardiac structures and function at the time of procedure with the specific hemodynamic conditions in which operators will deal, that are changing continuously during interventions.

Moreover, using TEE guidance, an effective communication between imaging specialist and surgeons can be achieved immediately before the interventions, giving to both of them the possibility to have real-time feedback of what is going to happen. TEE findings and surgical findings can be complementary for getting the best treatment for the patient and the best assessment of results at the end of intervention. This cooperation becomes necessary and should be even more effective during transcatheter interventions.

Intraoperative TEE should be complementary to more comprehensive preoperative TEE because it is supposed to have other aims than diagnosis: assessing of right and left ventricular function at different procedural steps, monitoring valves function, checking volume state and load conditions, evaluating pericardial integrity. These main targets are needed for evaluation of procedural success and complications.

Finally, for transcatheter interventions a novel imaging technique has been developed: Fusion Imaging with Echo-Navigator (Philips Medical System, Best, the Netherlands). This is able to acquire patient-specific imaging data from both fluoroscopic projections and bi-dimensional and 3D TEE volumetric data set. The result is sort of 'hybrid image' so-called 'fusion image'. Fusion images are currently used for facilitate catheters' and devices' manipulation during catheter-based structural heart disease, especially for aortic and mitral para-valvular leak closure and mitral valve intervention [19].

Table 4.2 summarized the role of imaging tools currently used for aortic intervention.

4.2 Intraoperatory Echocardiography for Surgical Procedures

4.2.1 Intro

Surgery of the aortic valve is now a routine cardiac procedure performed in most of cardiac surgery centers [19, 20]. Before 1950, rheumatic aortic valve disease after rheumatic fever due to streptococcal infection was the most frequent etiology for aortic valve disease before 1950. After the intro-

Table 4.2 Imaging modalities used in AV interventions planning, intraprocedural guidance and monitoring

Table 4.2 (continued)

Transesophageal echocardiography	Time-points of TEE	
	Preoperative TEE assessment (before starting interventions)	All situations in which pre-operative TTE is non-diagnostic
		Anatomic issues of AV (morphology, calcifications, coronary ostia)
		Evaluation of prosthetic valve, cusps mobility and paravalvular leak
		Assessing contomitant other valve pathologies (mitral, tricuspid) and LV and RV function
		Patients on ventilators or poor thoracic impedance for adequate TTE or unable to move into lateral position
		Routine basic TEE in all open heart and thoracic aortic surgical procedures (and for some aorto-coronary by pass)
		Comprehensive pre-procedural TEE is performed when complex pathology is suspected
		Non cardiac surgery when patients have known cardiovascular pathology that could impact outcomes (es. patients with known aortic stenosis)
	Transcatheter procedures guidance	TEE during balloon dilatation
		TEE during valve deployment
	Post-procedural outcomes	Assessment of valve prosthesis function in aortic position (position, cusps mobility, leak)
		Assessment of other valvulopathies (changements in degree)
		Assessment of complications
Epicardial echocardiography	Is used for the same purpose of pre-intra and post operative TEE in open heart surgery when TEE is contraindicated and heart surface is accessible	

Intracardiac echocardiography	Is used for the same purpose of pre-intra and post operative TEE in transcatheter AV interventions when TEE or general anesthesia is contraindicated	
Other imaging modalities used in AV interventions planning, intraprocedural guidance and monitoring		
Multi-sliced computed tomography	Pre-operative assessment	Amount and distribution of AV calcifications
		Aortic Root anatomy and dimensions
		Coronary ostia-annulus distance (for TAVI)
		Access route for transcatheter interventions
		Planning optimal fluoroscopy view for guiding interventions
		Contraindication to aortic clamping (open heart surgery)
Fluoroscopy		Real-time monitoring and guidance of transcatheter navigation for AV interventions
Coronary angiography	Pre-procedural assessment	Evaluation of concomitant coronary disease
	Intraprocedural guidance	Real time monitoring of position and patency of coronaries during interventions
Fusion imaging	Intra-procedural guidance	

duction of penicillin prophylaxis and treatment, rheumatic heart valve disease was reduced in developed countries and calcified aortic valve stenosis currently represents the most frequent form of aortic valve disease [21, 22].

The nature of aortic valve disease carrying patients to intervention is either aortic valve stenosis, aortic regurgitation (AR), or a combination of these. Current typologies of aortic interventions for AR are summarized in (Fig. 4.2).

In these case SAVR options include mechanical or biological prostheses. When AV replacement is the choice, the risk/benefit ratio of mechanical and bioprosthetic valves should be evaluated and the following considerations have been suggested by European and American Society of Cardiology and Cardio-Thoracic Surgery (ESC/EACTS/ASE) for the choice of appropriate prosthesis: (1) life expectancy and age of patients: use of mechanical aortic valve prostheses in patients younger than 60 years of age and bioprosthetic valve are above the age of 65 in European guidelines and above the age of 70 in American guidelines;

Fig. 4.2 Echocardiographic evaluation for pre-procedural planning in AV surgery and surgery on aorta (∗ valve is repairable when one of the following occurs: prolapse of one cusp, dilatation of sinus-tubular junction, commissural non restrictive lesions, perforation or annular dilatation; STJ Sinus-Tubular-junction)

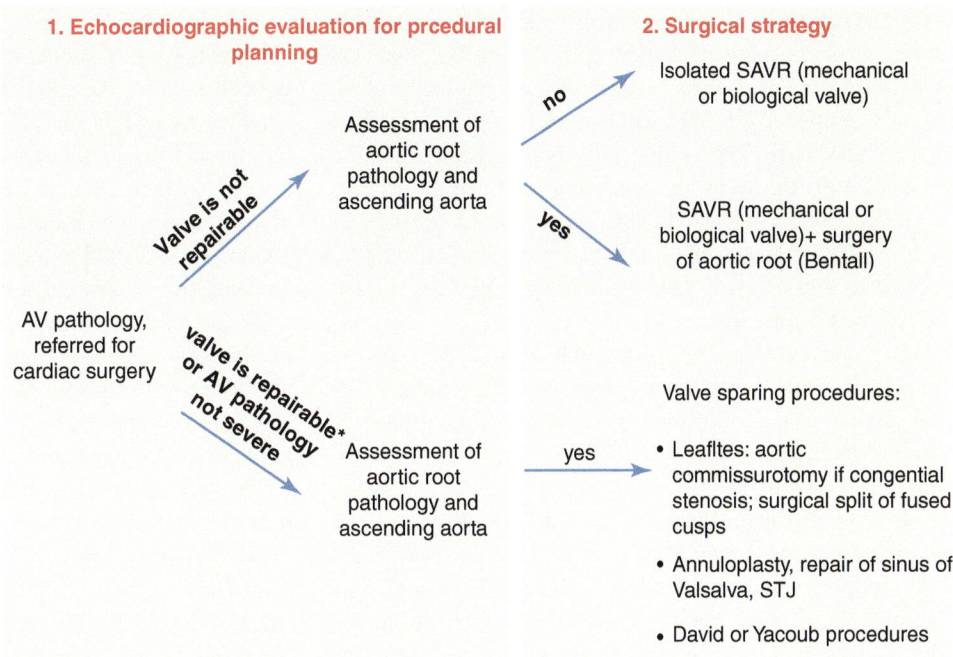

(2) the estimated risk of a potential reoperation in the future, related to age, risk factors and presence of other valve disease; (3) bleeding risk, which may be higher because of specific comorbidities, compliance concerns, lifestyle and occupational conditions; (4) concomitant atrial fibrillation (AF) or a hypercoagulable state and other conditions that require use of oral anticoagulation; (5) the risk of degeneration of bioprosthetic valves that may be accelerated in young patients with hyperparathyroidism or renal failure; (6) the wish of a patient to become pregnant; and (7) patient preferences. American guidelines add the expected haemodynamics for a specific valve type and size as an important factor when considering the type of prosthesis [8, 23, 24].

Biological prostheses are available as stented valves, stentless or sutureless. In stented prostheses the biological tissue of the valve is mounted on a frame stent while stentless valves by definition do not possess a rigid stent frame and they can be surgically implanted with a subcoronary placement full root replacement. The advantage of respecting native root is guarantee that physiological movements of this wall, so reducing risk of future chronic enlargement.

A repair of stenotic AV might be attempted when fusion of free margin of cusps is the main pathogenic mechanism of valve stenosis and when AV leaflets tissue is not retracted, thickened or calcified. A sharp separation of the fused or non-separated free margins of the cusps is the best surgical option for increasing valve opening area and ameliorating functioning. AV repair is nowadays very rarely performed for AS. Therefore it has still a role in AR when the cause is one of: prolapse of one cusp, dilatation of sinus-tubular junc-

tion, commissural non restrictive lesions, perforation or annular dilatation. Indeed, these are predictors for good result of AV repair in AR. When combined lesions coexist, calcifications, thickening or prolapse of more than one cusps in tricuspid valve the probability of good result for AV repair is low and surgeon should plan SAVR [25].

Reparability of AV is a central issue in case of pathology of AV and root. In such cases, when AV can be saved, the type of intervention depends on whether only the tubular part of the ascending aorta or the complete aortic root should be replaced.

The Bentall procedures with reimplantation of the coronary arteries for the complete replacement of the aortic root and the ascending aorta can be performed with a composite mechanical valve-graft conduit or in combination with a stented biological valve ("bio Bentall"); it has been demonstrated to have good long term results; [26, 27] stentless biological valve and dacron prostheses for aortic root surgery can be used [28]. If aortic root is not pathological, a conventional aortic valve and ascending aorta replacement should be done for simplifying the procedure [29]. Finally, when aortic root is mild dilated or only ectasic, an aortoplasty can be performed. When aortic valve can be saved and aortic root needs to be replaced, valve sparing interventions include David and Yacoub procedures [30–32].

Other following concomitant pathogenic issue must be pointed out before intervention to have a complete pre-procedural planning.

In case of concomitant significant left ventricular hypertrophy coexisting, the evaluation of morphology

and distribution of this hypertrophy should be carefully done. In some patients hypertrophy of the bulbo-spiralis muscle in the left ventricular outflow tract can lead to additional significant left ventricular outflow tract obstruction. When ARV is performed, the subvalvular gradient is automatically increased by the reduction of downstream pressure. This condition could be very deleterious for the patients, it is typical of advanced ages because of more stiffned left ventricles and can lead to immediate post operative pulmonary oedema and crush.

To avoid a residual left ventricular outflow tract obstruction after aortic valve replacement, an enlargement of the subvalvular part is indicated, via a myectromy similar but limited compared to that described by Morrow for hypertrophic cardiomyopathy [33].

In case of concomitant coronary arteries disease, coronary artery by pass graft (CABG) should be performed; first the aortic valve is excised to allow for manipulation of the heart during CABG without the calcium embolization; then distal anastomosis is performed, then AV is replaced and finally proximal anastomosis is done [30].

In case of multiple valve diseases requiring surgical attention calcified aortic valve is excised at first, in order to avoid embolization, then mitral valve is repaired or replaced if needed because mitral valve annulus replacement can lead to reduction of the aortic valve diameter that should be measured after mitral intervention. Last, aortic valve is treated and at the end tricuspid valve if needed [5].

4.2.2 Preoperative Echo Assessment

4.2.2.1 Intro

The last version of consensus statement of the American Society of Echocardiography and the Society of Cardiovascular Anaesthesiologists recommends that a basic perioperative echocardiography should be performed and reported every time the nature of planned surgery might result in severe hemodynamic, pulmonary, neurologic compromise [34].

Intra procedural TEE during cardiac surgery is relatively safe and has been associated with overall mortality of <1 per 10,000 patients and morbidity of 2–5 per 1000 patients [35, 36]. The incidence of complications is related to duration of intervention and probe manipulation. Perioperative echocardiography has been shown to influence cardiac anesthetic choice and surgical management in 50% of cases [37, 38].

A complete pre-operative echocardiographic evaluation is performed on beating heart after general anaesthesia and before cardioplegia. At this temporal frame cardiac performance and valve function could be influenced by general anesthesia and positive end-expiratory pressure due to mechanical ventilatory support.

For AV interventions, it is expected that preoperative echocardiography should allow to clarify **all the following concerns**: (1) valve anatomy, number of cusps, tissue characterization and integrity, amount of calcification and distribution; (2) aortic root and ascendant aorta anatomy and sizing; (3) biventricular function and concomitant secondary/primary valve disease (mitral valve regurgitation); (4) abnormalities in left ventricle outflow tract: assessing gradient and site of systolic obstruction; establishing the wall thickness of LV (5) in case of combined valvular vitium, quantitation of concomitant AR for cardioplegia; (6) amount and extension of aortic plaque and calcification for clamping; (7) assessing the right placement of left venting (retrograde or anterograde cardioplegia).

The **recommended views for perioperative TEE** are: mid-esophageal (ME) four-chamber view, ME two chamber view, ME aortic valve (AV) long axis (LAX) view, ME Ascending Aorta LAX View, ME Ascending Aorta short axis (SAX) View, ME AV SAX view, ME RV Inflow-Outflow View, ME Bicaval View, transgastric (TG) Midpapillary SAX View, descending aorta SAX and LAX Views.

The role of TEE for specific purpose of AV is more important in the morphologic assessment rather than the functional assessment of the native AV. Indeed, it is sometimes more difficult to have good alignment across AV with TEE rather than TTE. 2D TEE and TTE remain the gold standard for morphologic assessment of the AV and root, while 3D TEE improves assessment of LVOT and AV annulus shape and dimensions, since it overcomes the geometrical assumption of circularity [12, 39, 40]. **From the ME AV SAX view** AV cusp number and AV planimetric area (AVA) can be measured. The cusp adjacent to the atrial septum is the noncoronary cusp, the most anterior cusp is the right coronary cusp, and the other is the left coronary (Fig. 4.3).

The ME AV LAX view is particularly important to appreciate the presence of basal septal hypertrophy and allows imaging of LVOT, AV, annulus, and aortic root diameters. It has to be noted that in **ME AV LAX** the cusp of the AV that appears anteriorly or toward the bottom of the display is always the right coronary cusp, but the cusp that appears posteriorly in this cross-section may be the left or the non-coronary cusp, depending on the exact location of the imaging plane as it passes through the valve. The annulus is identified as the points of attachment of the AV cusps (or hinge point) and is normally between 1.8 and 2.5 cm and it is measured in mid-systole. Measurements of the aortic root usually are made at (1) the AV annulus level (2) the maximal diameter in the sinuses of Valsalva, and (3) the sinotubular junction (at distal ending of sinuses of Valsalva when tubular portion of the ascending aorta appears) [41]. 2D measurement of the LVOT should be performed in early to mid-systole, typically within 5 mm of the annulus.

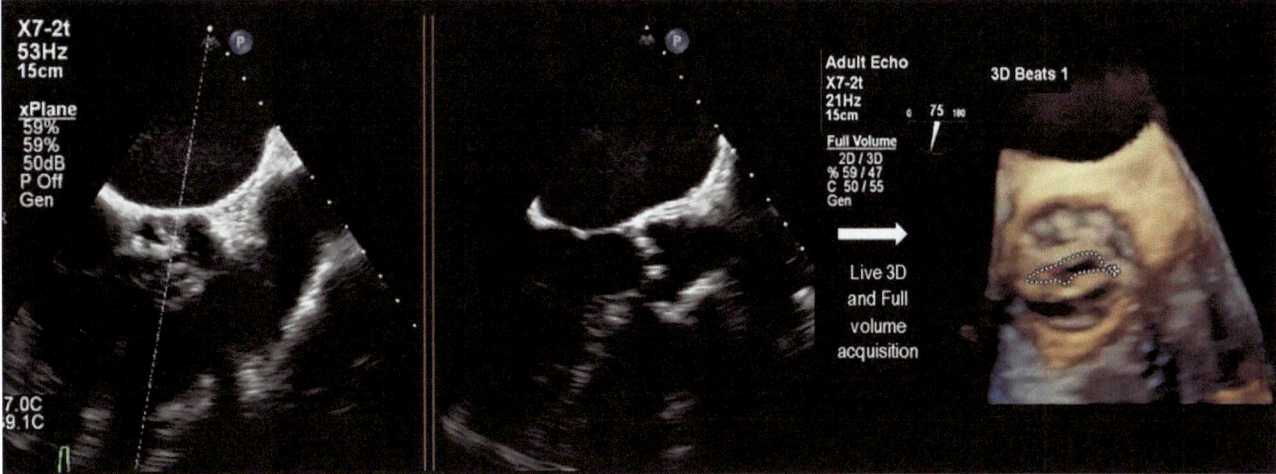

Fig. 4.3 Evaluation of valve morphology and planimetry. Left and medial panels show aortic valve centred in the acquisition boxes in two orthogonal views: ME SAX and ME LAX; then, live 3D mode should be used to optimize gain settings and full volume acquisition is per-formed. The cusp adjacent to the inter-atrial septum is the non-coronary cusp, the most anterior cusp is the right coronary cusp, and the other is the left coronary

3D-TEE for aortic evaluation is obtained from ME-SAX aortic valve view, first **using bi-plane** view at beginning to be sure to be at the centre of AV, with reduced gain of 2D TEE, then **live 3D mode** should be used to optimize gain settings and **full-volume acquisition** shows the volume acquired with sufficient frame rate; for visualization of AV, one should clockwise rotate the images 90 grades around Y axis, so that aortic valve is presented from ascending aorta view with right coronary cusp (RCC) at 6 o'clock position. After image acquisition, 3D-cropping could be done either before (during) or after data acquisition (Fig. 4.3).

3DTEE allows real time immediate and comprehensive visualization of AV morphology and root and their movements in cardiac cycle. Cutting the image in ME-AV-LAX on a plane that is orthogonal to direction of LVOT and AV flow is crucial to quantitate without geometrical assumptions the cross sectional area (CSA) of LVOT, the effective orifice area (EOA) in case of aortic stenosis and the effective regurgitant orifice area (EROA) in case of AR without any geometrical assumption (Fig. 4.4).

Indeed, for quantitation of effective orifice area (EOA), the most important sources of error is LVOT diameter since is derived mathematically from this parameter. With 3DTEE quantitation, all the geometrical assumptions related to LVOT CSA and LVOT shape are abolishes. Furthermore, left ventricle stroke volume (SV) can be computed by semi-automated end diastolic end systolic volumes computation, other than flow time-integral-velocity through LVOT (pulse wave Doppler at same level in which LVOT is computed, generally 5 mm below aortic annulus) [42]. 3D-TTE planimetered AVA has been reported to be feasible in 92% of patients outside intervention setting and to be more correlate to invasive measures of gradients than 2D-TEE derived AVA [43, 44].

Coronary ostia can be visualized in ME-AV- SAX views and in ME-AV-LAX. This is obtained with biplane images that allow to display on the right of image the coronary ostium into the sinus of Valsalva for evaluating the height of coronary ostium above AV annulus (crucial for trans-catheter aortic valve implantation). Abnormalities in origin of coronaries should be immediately recognised because in cases of atypical origin or course of the coronary arteries, it might be necessary to perform additional CABG in order to ensure perfusion of the atypical coronary (Fig. 4.5a–c).

Peak velocities across the LV outflow tract and AV are not usually obtained from ME views unless jets are markedly eccentric because of inadequate alignment of Doppler with flow. Two TG views of the AV (the deep TG five-chamber view and the TG LAX view) usually permit accurate assessment of transaortic flow and peak velocities (Fig. 4.6).

Table 4.3 summarized how to perform each of these views and the specific tools from a procedural standpoint.

4.2.2.2 Degree of AS in Patients Undergoing Other Procedures

After cardiac anesthesia, before cardioplegia, the degree of AS should be re-assessed in the pre-procedural evaluation. Generally, AVA is not sufficient alone to clarify the severity of AS, given to technical limits in clinical practice mainly due to shadowing of high degree calcification and high inter-observer variability. Therefore, the value of AVA needs to be integrated with functional parameters: LVEF, SV. Conceptually, the valve area in systolic phase (AVA and EOA) depends on the presence of a minimum pressure gradient across valve that allows AV opening. This gradient is further depending on: (1) left ventricle pump function;

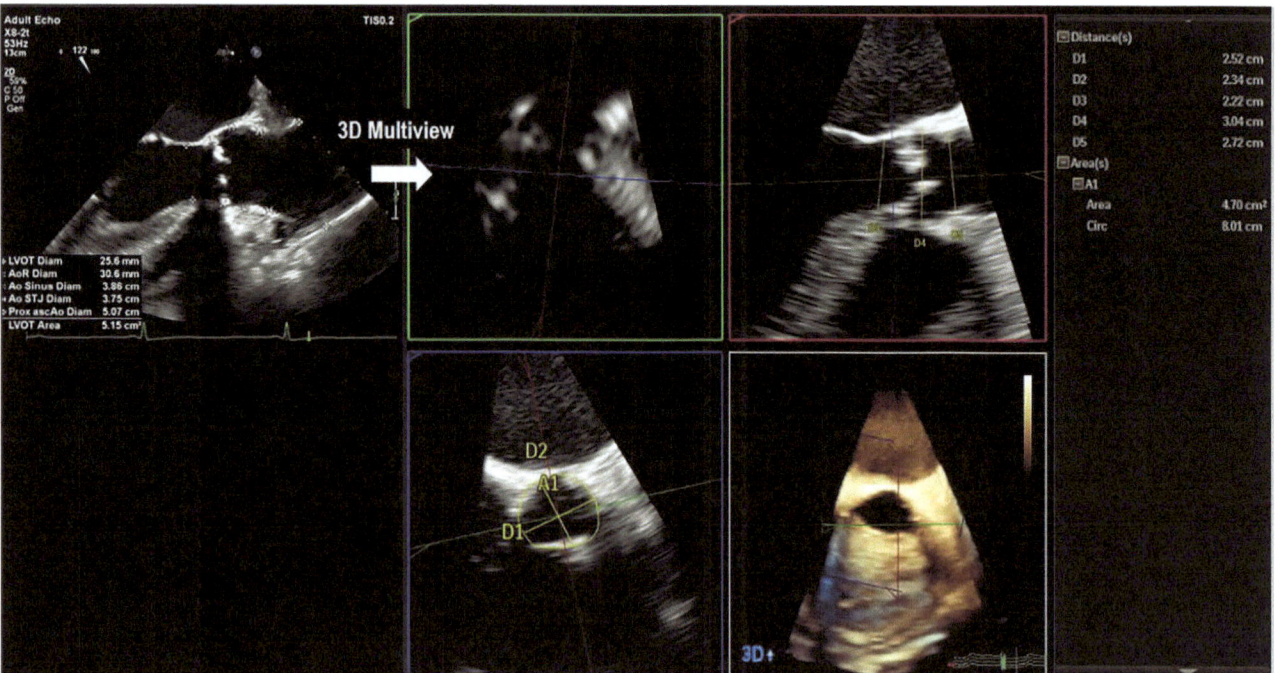

Fig. 4.4 2D measure of LVOT, aortic annulus, aortic root and ascendant aorta; LVOT area is derived from diameter assuming a circular shape. The white narrow describes how to perform the multi-planar reconstruction of aortic valve and root. These measurements allow a most accurate determination of the shape of different segments, without geometric assumption

(2) amount of effective volume inside LV that is push out into LVOT, that is the effective stroke volume index (SVi, mL/m^2); (3) peripheral resistance, that increases aortic stiffness at each systole so reducing the transaortic gradient. Combining all these factors, the grade of AS can be derived as fully explained in Table 4.3 [45–49].

After general anesthesia, peripheral resistance are usually low and constant during evaluation; the use of volume expanders and noradrenaline (by recruiting venous reserve, VR) increases the SVi; on the contrary, increased thoracic pressure in inflation phase of assisted ventilation can reduced VR so reducing SV. Finally, concomitant other valve disease can reduce or increased the effective SV. Mitral valve (MV) stenosis reduced the inflow volume in LV, MV regurgitation reduces the effective SV by increasing the amount of retrograde volume into left atrium; TR and RV dysfunction reduce the LV filling pressure and SV.

Furthermore, in the setting of non-cardiac surgery, severe aortic stenosis is a well-established risk factor for perioperative mortality and myocardial infarction. When other procedures are performed In patients with known severe AS, a careful assessment of symptoms of patients should be done. If symptoms cannot be ruled out, than valve disease should be treated before any other interventions (both SAVR or TAVI or valvuloplasty, according to surgical risk and life expectancy related to non-cardiac condition). When patient is really asymptomatic, other interventions can be performed but with more invasive haemodynamic monitoring, avoiding rapid changes in volume status an heart rhythm as far as possible [50] (Figs. 4.3 and 4.6).

4.2.2.3 Degree of AR (for Cardioplegia)

For successful surgical outcomes, protection of myocardium during ischemic cardiac arrest is essential. In patients referred for AS, LV hypertrophy makes myocardium more vulnerable to ischemic injury since it has less capillary density and vascular dilatation occurs in the sub-endocardial region [30]. Cardiac protection is even more important. In case of pure AS, where significant calcification or stenosis of the coronary ostia is detected, coronary artery bypass grafting should be performed before aortic valve replacement and cardioplegia can be given via the vein grafts.

In aortic valve surgery initial delivery of cardioplegic solution via the aortic root after cannulation (anterograde cardioplegia) is generally accepted. However, in those patients with combined AS and significant AR, this way should be avoided as it can cause significant left ventricular distension. So one of the most important aims of preoperative echocardiography in context of degenerative AV diseases is the detection of AR [51, 52].

Carefull evaluation of aortic regurgitation in preoperative echo-assessment requires multiple 2DTEE views. These include: ME-AV-SAX, ME-AV-LAX with biplane imaging for moving the cross sectional plane through all cusps and detecting even the mild commissural regurgitant jet. Measurement of aortic root and ascending aorta in 2DTEE

Fig. 4.5 (**a–c**) Evaluation of coronary ostia. For patency and anatomy it is usually sufficient to display ostia in ME-SAX-AV (anteroflexed probe from AV plane) (panel **a**). For measuring the distance of right coronary ostium to annular plane (required for transcatheter interventions) ME LAX AV is required (panel **b**). For left coronary ostium distance it is necessary to perform multiplanar reconstruction of aortic root (panel **c**)

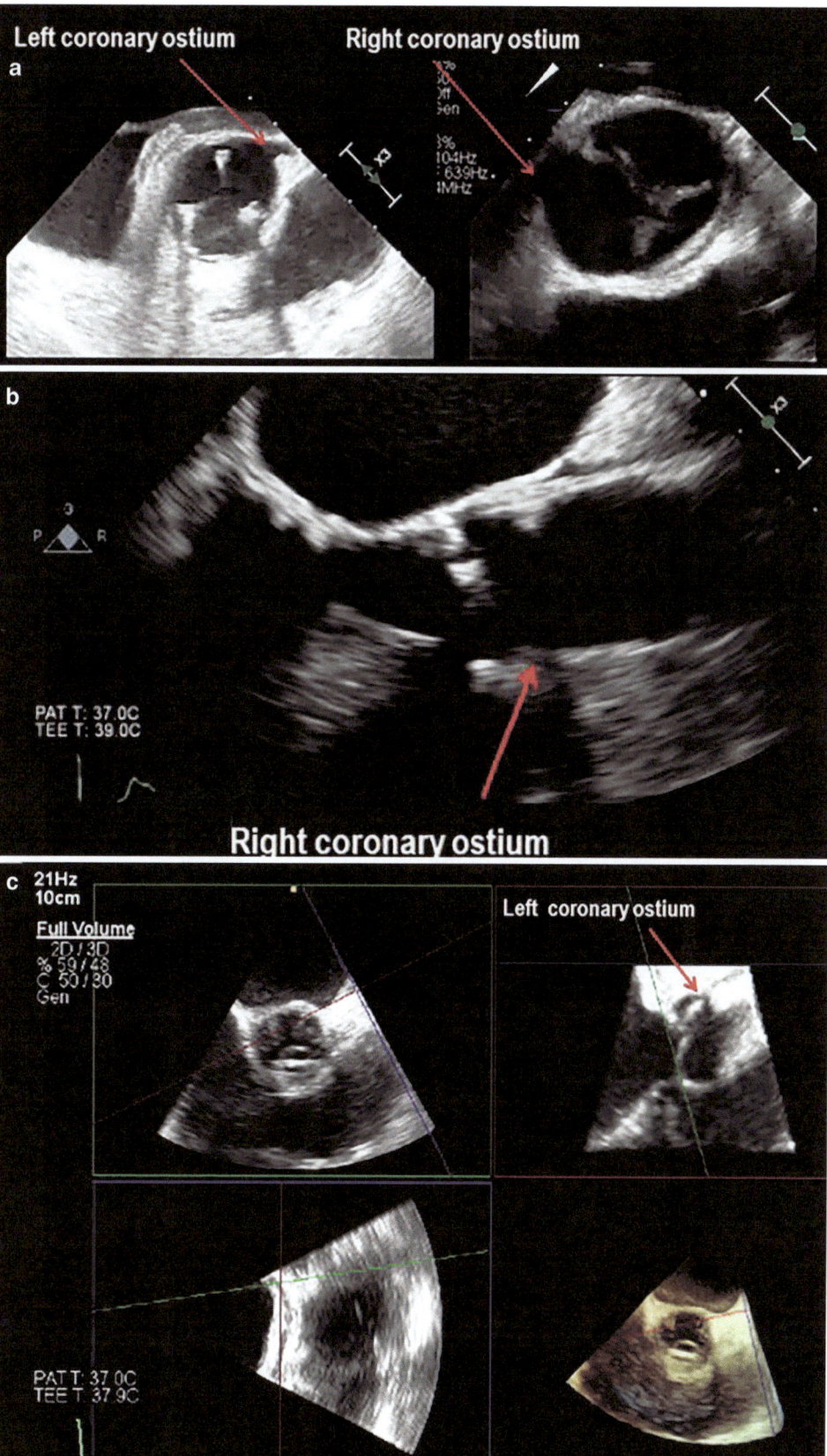

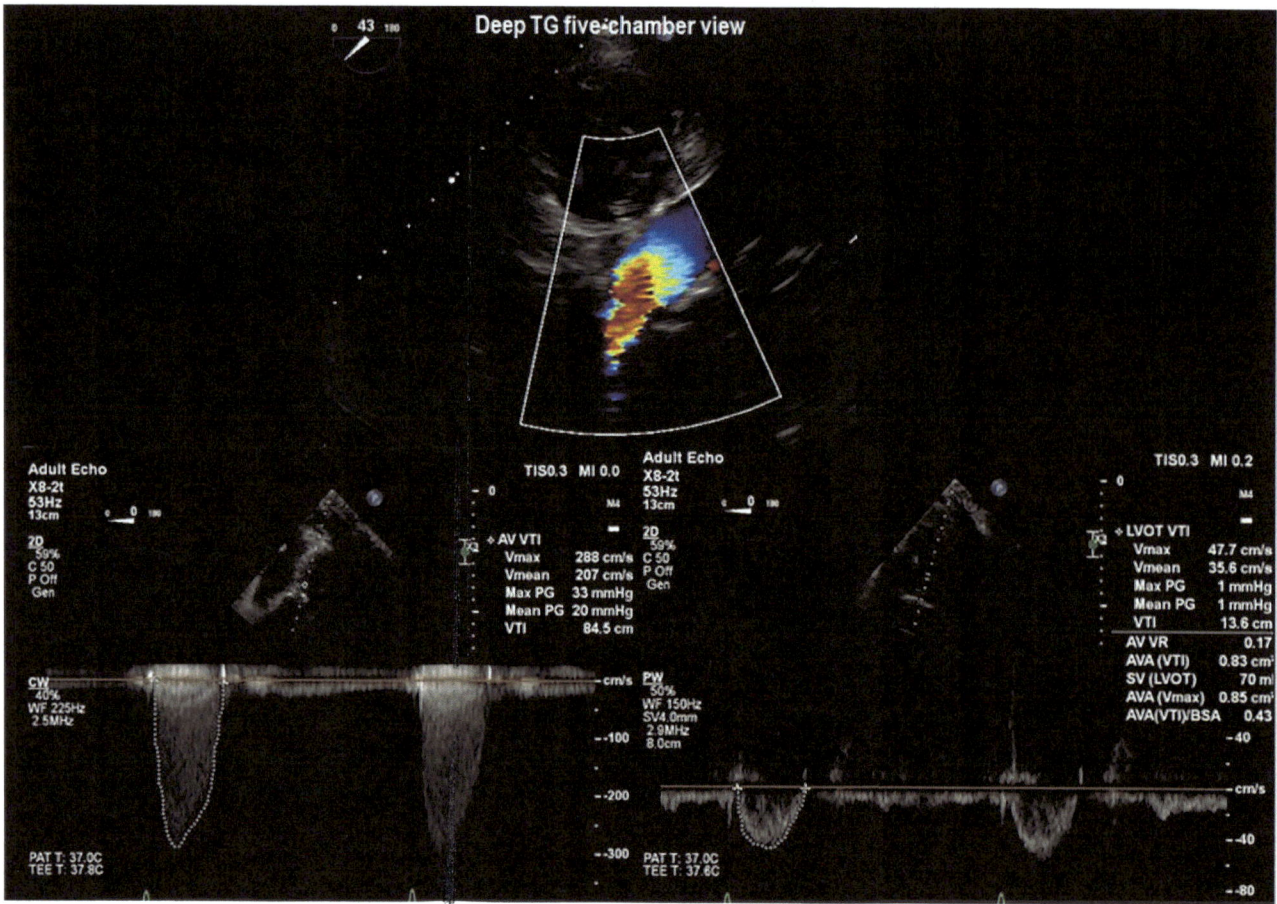

Fig. 4.6 Peak velocities across the LV outflow tract and AV are not usually obtained from ME views unless jets are markedly eccentric because of inadequate alignment of Doppler; deep TG view allows to obtain this evaluation

Table 4.3 Specific transesophageal views for AV interventions

Echocardiographic window		Probe and transducer angle movements	Cardiac structures and function aimed	Specific tools for procedural guidance and monitoring (open and transcatheter intervention)
Mid-esophageal views	Four chamber view	Advancing the probe to a depth of approximately 30–35 cm until it is immediately posterior to the left atrium. Turning the probe to the left (counterclockwise rotation of the probe) or to the right (clockwise rotation of the probe) is performed to center the mitral valve (MV) and left ventricle in the sector display. Slight retroflexion may be required to align the MV and LV apex	Right atrium, interatrial septum (IAS), left atrium, MV, tricuspid valve (TV), left ventricle, right ventricle, and interventricular septum	Monitoring of ventricular function and evaluation of pericardial effusion; evaluation of MV and TV concomitant pathologies that can affect gradient in aortic stenosis
	Two chamber view	From the ME four-chamber view, rotating the multiplane angle forward to between 80 and 100 until the right ventricle disappears from the image	Left atrium, MV, left ventricle, and left atrial appendage; coronary synus in its short axis	Monitoring of ventricular function and evaluation of pericardial effusion; evaluation of MV
	Long-Axis view (ME-AV-LAX)	From the ME two-chamber view, rotating the multiplane angle forward to between 120 and 160	LVOT and AV, SV, JST, TT, A2-P2 mitral valve; LA	**AV: anterior cusp is always right coronary cusp, posterior can be both left and non coronary cusp; X-plane can help in this distinguishing. Measures of AV annulus, LVOT, SV, STJ are performed in this view**

Table 4.3 (continued)

Echocardiographic window		Probe and transducer angle movements	Cardiac structures and function aimed	Specific tools for procedural guidance and monitoring (open and transcatheter intervention)
	ME Ascending Aortic LAX View	Withdrawing the probe from the ME LAX view allows imaging of the LAX of the ascending aorta; counterclockwise rotation results in LAX imaging of the main PA and the pulmonic valve (PV)	Right pulmonary artery (PA); ascending aorta; RVOT, CW RVOT, Pulmonic valve (PV)	Monitoring complications on aorta
	ME Ascending Aortic short axis (SAX) View	From ME ascending aortic LAX view, rotating the multiplane angle back to 20–40 images	Bifurcation of the PA, the SAX view of the ascending aorta, and the SAX view of the superior vena cava	Monitoring complications on aorta
	ME aortic valve SAX view (ME-AV-SAX)	Advancing the probe from the ME ascending aortic SAX view results in SAX imaging of the AV	Left coronary cusp should be posterior and on the right side of the image. The noncoronary cusp is adjacent to the IAS. The right coronary cusp is anterior and adjacent to the RVOT. Color flow Doppler allows to detect AR	**Allows a semiquantitation of paravalvular leak (color flow/total circumference %); is the home 2D-imaging for deriving 3D TEE of AV (full volume acquisition mode) and for coronary ostium reconstruction; transaortic wire, delivery system and transcatheter valve are visualizable in this view across the valve; cusps functioning of native and prosthetic valves is yielded**
	ME RV Inflow-Outflow View	From the ME ascending aortic SAX view, advance the probe and clockwise to center the TV in the view, multiplane angle should be rotated to between 60 and 90	Left atrium, right atrium, TV, right ventricle, PV, and proximal (main) PA	RV volume and function and TV and PV function
	ME Bicaval View	From the ME RV inflow-outflow view, the multiplane angle is rotated forward to 90–110 and the probe is turned clockwise	Right atrium, inferior vena cava, superior vena cava, left atrium, septum secundum and fossa ovalis	Used for monitoring access of extracorporeal circulation
Transgastric position	Transgastric (TG) Midpapillary SAX View	From the ME four-chamber view (at 0), the probe is advanced into the stomach and anteflexed to come in contact with the gastric wall. The multiplane angle should remain at 0; probe depth is manipulated until the posteromedial papillary muscle comes into view	Papillary muscles, mid-level left ventricle assessment motion	Useful in unstable patients; is the only view allowing simultaneous assessment of LAD, LCX, RCA territories
	TG LAX view	Turning the probe to the left (counterclockwise) then rotating the transducer angle to 120–140		Adequate alignment for measurement of peak velocities and gradients through LVOT and AV
	Deep TG five chamber view (DTG)	Advancing the probe to the deep TG level, with transducing angle of 0–20°, anteflexion and often with left flexion	LVOT, AV, SV, MV, left atrium, left ventricle	Adequate alignment for measurement of peak velocities and gradients through LVOT and AV
	Descending aorta SAX-view/LAX view	Turning the probe to the left from the ME four-chamber view until the descending thoracic aorta comes into the display. The SAX view of the aorta is obtained at a multiplane angle of 0°, using x-Plane the LAX view is displayed	Descending aorta	**Useful for monitoring endoclamping in minimally invasive surgery; aortic complications of surgery and transcatheter intervention**

are needed and quantitation of AR is performed using some recommended parameters:

(1) AV morphology: flail or coaptation defect should be assessed; width of color flow regurgitant jet relative to LVOT dimensions; density of continuous Doppler signal of regurgitant jet; enlargement of LV; (2) assessment of flow reversal in descending aorta and end diastolic velocity (AR is severe if it is >20 cm/s); (3) 2D-vena contracta (VC) diameter; (4) pressure half time (severe if <200 ms); (5) effective regurgitant orifice area (EROA, mm^2, severe if > or = 30 mm^2) and regurgitant volume (RV) (severe if > or = 60 mL); 3D VC area is another reproducible quantitative

parameter especially in case of very eccentric jets (Fig. 4.7). Using 3DE color Doppler, the cutting plane perpendicular to the flow direction of AR jet can be identified, and the area of VC can be planimetered. This has been shown to have a good correlation with aortographic grading of aortic regurgitation [53, 54]. If mild AR does not contraindicate the anterograde cardioplegia, echocardiography should be used for step by step assessment of cardiac function and distension of LV. Indeed, total volume of plegia that is required to induced asystole cannot be predicted by quantitation of LV mass [55] and should be given in an empiric method. The use of TEE allows to monitor LV distention, which is common.

4.2.2.4 Degree of FMR in Patients with AS

Clinical studies have shown that FMR associated with aortic valve disease is a strong marker of increased risk even after a successful aortic valve replacement [56, 57].

From an etiological standpoint LV remodelling secondary or concomitant to aortic valve disease can generate different pathogenetic mechanism leading to functional mitral regurgitation (FMR) [58].

Beyond the well known mechanism of leaflets tenting that affects MV in patients with impaired LV function and enlarged LVs, other pathogenic mechanisms can hit MV in patients with hypertrophic LV of normal size and preserved ejection fraction (EF). First of all intraventricular systolic pressures inside hypertrophic heart is higher and it can gen-

erate abnormal tension on MV leaflet in systole causing enlargement of annulus and degeneration of all component of MV apparatus. Even If the relation between LV pressure and FMR has been questioned, high filling pressure can lead to impaired longitudinal subclinical function in patients with hypertrophic hearts, that reduces the closure forces of MV [56]. Another mechanism that is usually superimposed is the reduced coronary flow reserve in long standing aortic disease. Asymmetric and marked hypertrophy of basal interventricular septum (IVS) can generate pull phenomena similar to that identified in hypertrophic cardiomyopathy, that lead to systolic anterior motion of mitral valve, especially when mitro-aortic continuity and/or anterior mitral annulus are stiffened and calcified summarizes these mechanisms (Fig. 4.8). Echocardiographic evaluation of MR associated to AS should aim all these factors. Main objective of 2D and 3D assessment of MR should give a comprehensive diagnosis of MV pathology for understanding if the main mechanism is functional or organic.

It has to be highlighted that the **jet area is determined** by causes other than regurgitant volume [59]. Indeed peak velocity of regurgitation is high in patients with AS. Therefore, beyond the mechanism and morphological evaluation of MR, guidelines has recommended that **jet area assessment** should be abandoned and replaced by determination of the EROA or 3D-Vena contracta area by 3DTEE. The more is AS influencing grade of MR, the more is the peak of velocity and smaller is EROA and VC despite RV is increased.

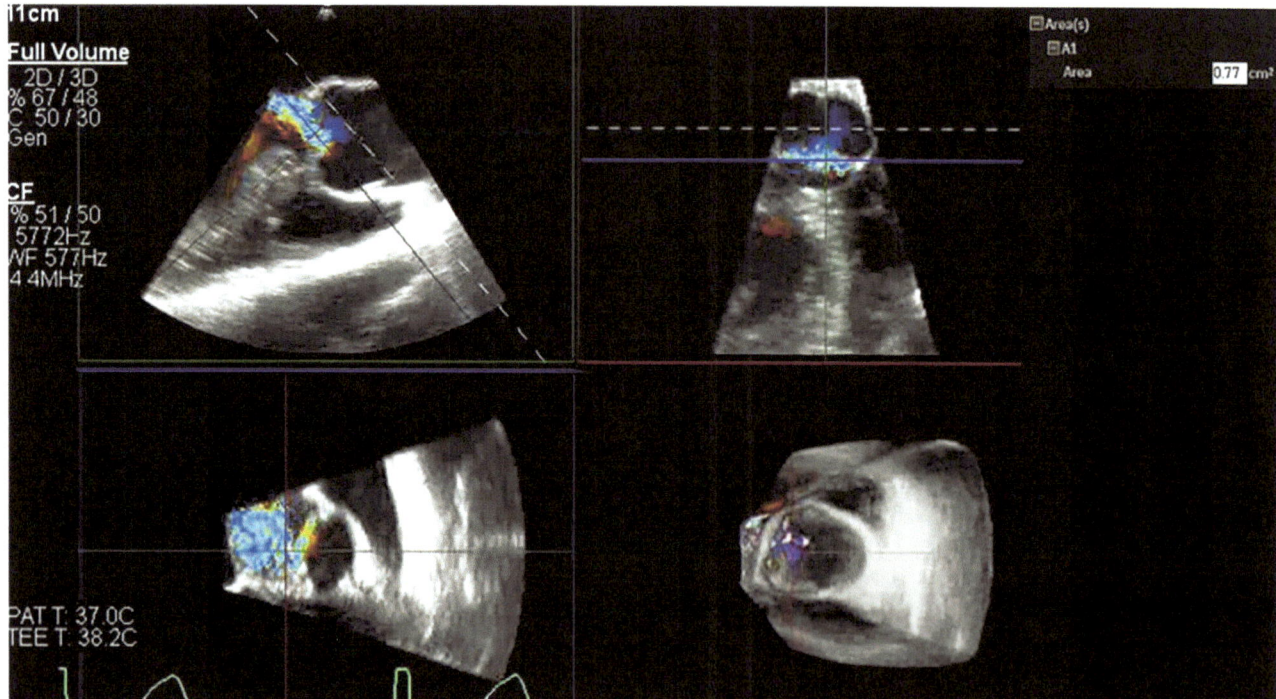

Fig. 4.7 AR quantitation in case of very eccentric jet should be performed using multi-plane reconstruction for allowing quantitation of 3D VC area

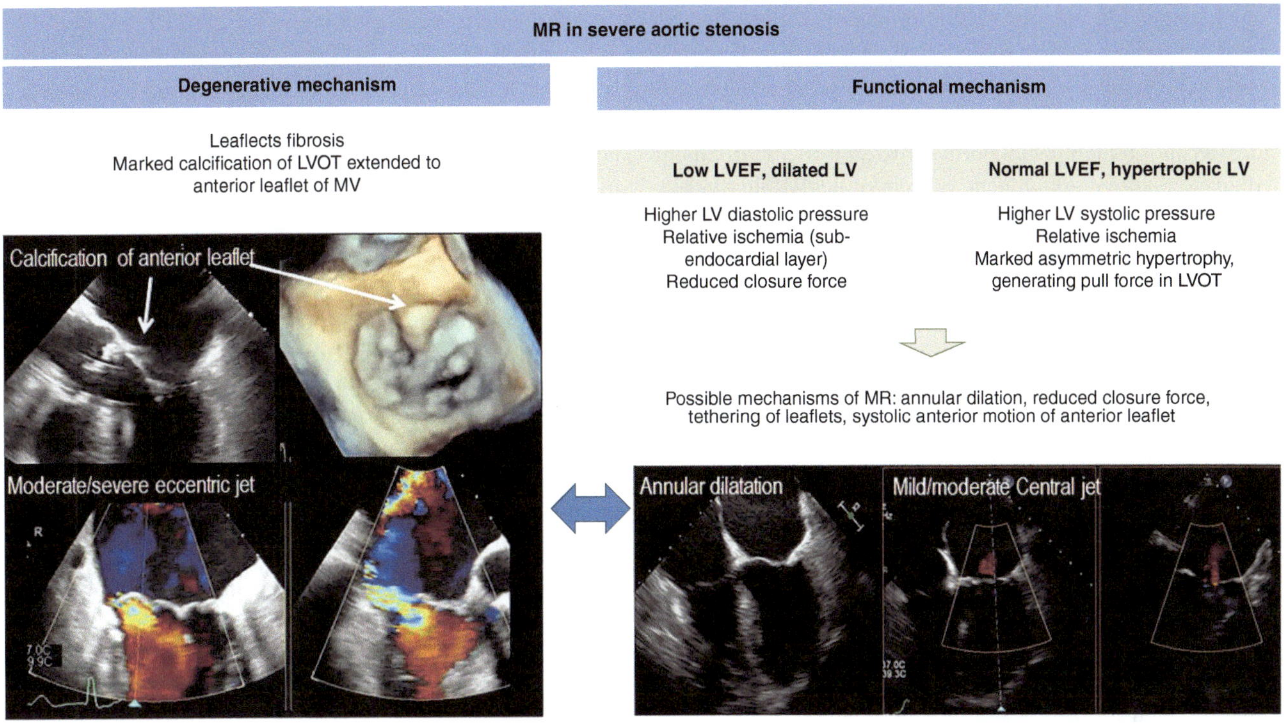

Fig. 4.8 Phenotypes of functional MR in AS. Accurate echocardiographic evaluation of mitral valve morphology and function allows to distinguish the two components of mitral regurgitation. Generally if the leaflets are normal, the annulus is dilated, jet is central and not severe, the probability of recovery of MV function after treatment of AS is more high than in case of concomitant valve degeneration

In the setting of intraoperative echocardiography the following steps are useful. 2DTEE comprehensive display of mitral valve using ME MV 4CH (0–20° of transducer angle), 2CH (80–90%), and inter-commissural view (60–70°) for identifying morphological abnormalities, calcification amount and localization, leaflets movement and integrity (Carpentier mechanism); 3D TEE allows Simultaneous Multiplane Mode for real time visualization of different scallops, zoom mode permits a focused, wide-sector view of the mitral valve apparatus from the annulus to the papillary muscle tips in a surgical view; Color flow 2D TEE and 3D color flow full volume TEE for identifying the number and origin of jets; in FMR when reduced EF usually jet Is central or centro-medial; very eccentric jets are less likely due to functional mechanism so a cleft or focal pathology should be searched (Fig. 4.8).

Three-dimensional morphologic analysis of mitral annulus that can be dilated and also assume a more circular and fatter configuration; MV annulus quantification workflow with specific software is available for last generation echo-machines, so it can be performed in intraoperative setting (Philips Medical Systems, Andover, MA) [58, 60, 61].

4.2.2.5 LV Function and Loading Condition Assessment

The determination of global LV systolic function is one of the most common indications of a basic pre-operative TEE,

since it affects outcome of intervention irrespective to underlying AV pathology.

Afterload and preload should be assessed in the setting of intraprocedural TEE because they affect all the LV performance analysis. Currently, LV performance in the setting of intraoperative monitoring is quantitated by using either ejection phase indices (LVEF, SVi, fractional shortening and fractional area changes of LV) and load independent indices (systolic index of contractility, systolic tissue Doppler velocities and speckle tracking imaging). For all these evaluations, the current validations have been completed on TTE datasets, so application of these rules to TEE is still a source of adaptation.

For LV dimensions and ejection fraction, it has been demonstrated that measurements from TTE are nearly identical to those from TEE [62, 63]. When a fast examination of global function is needed, TG- mid-papillary SAX view may suffice and has been shown to have prognostic importance [13, 34, 64].

LV-LAX view (obtained with simultaneous multiplane imaging of the TG mid-papillary SAX view, for allowing better perpendicular position and best gain resolution for lateral wall and endocardial surface) is the recommended view for obtaining M-Mode for diameters of LV. A mild difference with TTE quantitation is supposed since measurements are made closer to the mid left ventricle for TEE and closer to the MV leaflet tips for TTE [65]. For monitoring of global and regional LV function, ME four-chamber, two-chamber and LAX views should be acquired. Regional wall motion analysis using a 17-segment wall motion score described in the American and European guidelines can be performed identifying segments with normal-hyperkinetic, hypokinetic (reduced thickening), akinetic (absent or negligible thickening, e.g., scar), dyskinetic (systolic thinning or stretching, e.g., aneurysm) motion [66].

Quantitation of LVEF using 2D-TEE must be computed after optimization to identify endocardium and LV must be wholly displayed; sometimes this requires adjusting the depth, manipulating the ante-flexion and retro-flexion of the probe tip to avoid foreshortening the ventricle that can result in underestimation of ventricular volumes. The purpose of **3D imaging of the left ventricle** is to provide volume and ejection fraction measurements independent of geometric assumptions. The reproducibility of LV volume and function measurements by 3D echocardiography has been assessed in multiple studies and less variation is reported than with 2D echocardiography [67–69].

All standard acquisition views for 2D TEE are useful for 3D acquisition even if the ideal and generally the preferred approach for the acquisition of a full-volume LV data set is the apical one. The landmarks used for the quantitation process are the mitral annulus and LV apex, which are used to initiate edge detection by semi-automated quantification software. LV trabeculae and papillary muscles should be included within the LV cavity for the calculation of LV volumes. One single beat acquisition is better for having best temporal resolution. Real time full Volume acquisition has pivotal role for demonstration of structural abnormalities (thrombi, masses and septal defects) but has limited value for the quantification of LV function (Fig. 4.9 Panel a and b).

Ejection fraction has the limit to be load dependent. Another used parameters can be systolic index of contractility (dP/dt): the maximal rate of pressure increase during isovolumic phase of systole; a continuous Doppler trace of a regurgitant mitral jet is obtained and the time from 1 to 3 m/s is measured; then the index is computed as ratio between 32,000 mmHg and this time period. 32,000 mmHg of

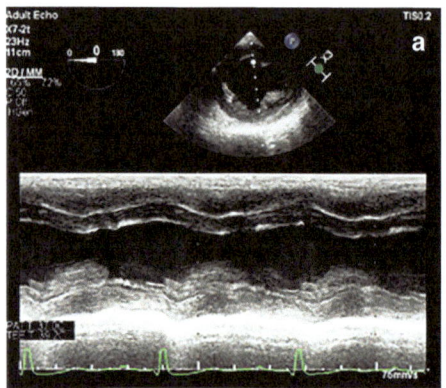

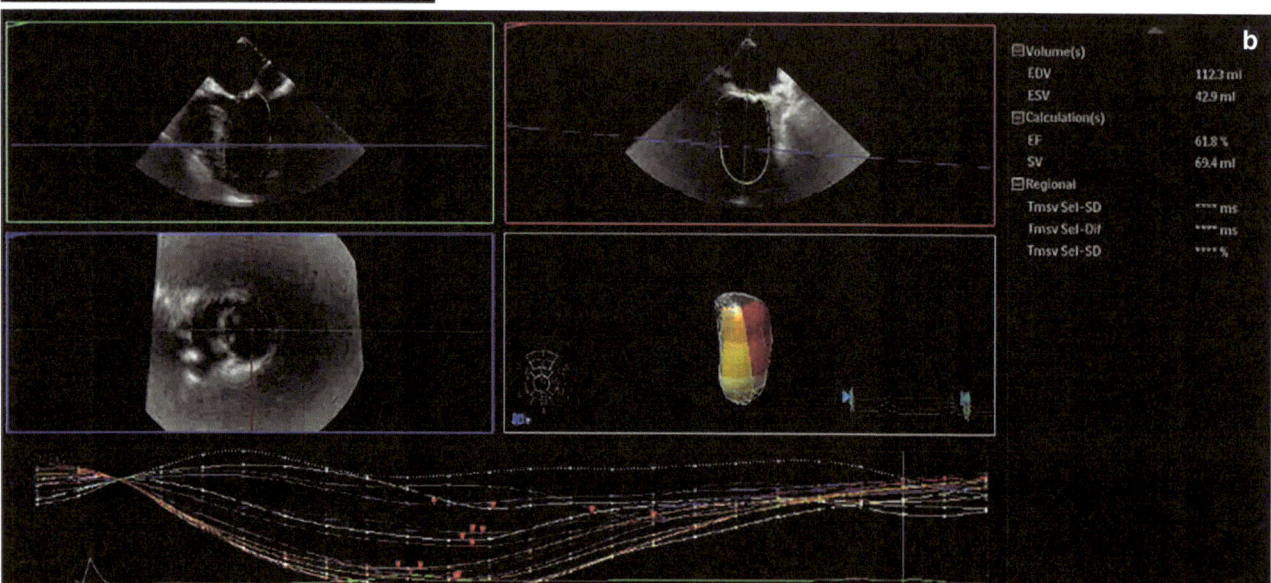

Fig. 4.9 Quantification of LV function with TEE. M-Mode can be performed by TG view (**a**). Semi-automated computation of stroke volume, left ventricle systolic and diastolic volumes, ejection fraction is performed after a 3D full volume acquisition of LV in 4CH view (**b**)

increased gradient correspond to 2 m/s of increased velocity (Bernoully simplified equation). The same index could be derived as systolic elastance of LV (EaS), that is the systolic pressure/volume slope and it is used even in case when CW on mitral regurgitation cannot be displayed (absence of MR) [70]. In the context of perioperative assessment, **evaluation of loading condition** should be always done, recording the following parameters: (1) **telediastolic area of LV: is the more accurate method to assess pre-load state** but in the setting of AS; (2) transmitral diastolic flow velocities and diastolic evaluation; low filling pressure can be depicted by a low protodiastolic flow velocity, high telediastolic flow velocity and low protodiastolic tissue Doppler velocity on mitral annulus; (3) pulmonary venous flow; the four components of the curve should be identified for having the hemodynamic correlation: early systole, late systole (often they are jointed), diastole and atrial reversal [71, 72].

4.2.2.6 Other (Thrombi in Ascending Aorta, Resection in HOCM, etc)

Ascending aorta (AA) is visualized using ME-AA SAX and ME-AA LAX (respectively 0° and 90° of transducer angle); then, when the probe is withdrawn in upper oesophageal position (UE), aortic arch can be visualized bot in short and long axis view in (UR AA SAX and UE AA LAX respectively 90° and 0° of transducer angle). Finally, by rotating the TEE probe to the left and posterior wall of oesophagus, entire descending aorta and upper abdominal aorta can be examined. The following measures should be always acquired: sinus of Valsalva (SV) diameter by MELAX view and simultaneous imaging display for asymmetric dilatation of sinus; STJ; tubular tract (TT), proximal aortic arch, distal aortic arch, descendent aorta.

Because of lack of internal anatomic landmarks, it is difficult to describe anatomical localization of abnormalities in descending thoracic aorta; one approach is to describe the location of the defect as a distance from the origin of the left subclavian artery and its location on the vessel wall relative to the position of an adjacent structure, such as the LA or the base of the LV, may also designate a level within the descending aorta.

Simultaneous multiplane acquisition by 3DTEE is useful in aorta dimension assessment. The depth should be adjust to adequate the image quality and the size of aorta displayed; transducer frequency is increased [13, 34]. With multiplane imaging is possible to check the wall for identifying the presence of aortic atheromasia and its complications such as penetrating ulcera, chronic dissections, mobile thrombosis. This pathologies should be recognise before open heart surgery and transcatheter intervention [73, 74]. Surpisingly, mobile thrombi in the aorta of patients without diffuse atherosclerosis mostly located at the aortic arch have been reported since the regular use of TOE in patients with cerebral or peripheral

emboli. The pathophysiology of these lesions is unclear, sometimes including paradoxical embolism via an open foramen ovale [74].

After AVR, there is a fall in the end systolic LVOT pressure following relief of downstream obstruction (previously due to AS). This leads to apposition of narrowed LVOT walls during systole and unmasks a dynamic "latent" obstruction as LV end-systolic pressure (LVESP) falls [75]. When some anatomical factors coexist with a dramatic fall in LVESP, systolic anterior motion (SAM) of mitral valve can happen, mainly due to a "pull" phenomenon of anterior leaflet inside LVOT.

In some patients hypertrophy of the bulbo-spiralis muscle in the left ventricular outflow tract can lead to additional significant left ventricular outflow tract obstruction. Another site of sub-aortic dynamic obstruction could be mid-ventricular in case of high degree of cardiac hypertrophy [76, 77].

The presence of significant LVOT obstruction after intervention affects immediately the surgical outcome and survival of patients and it could be very deleterious for the patients can lead to immediate post operative pulmonary oedema and crush. Echocardiographic evaluation should clarify the site of outflow tract obstruction before intervention (aliasing zone with color Doppler could be LVOT or mid-ventricular), and the presence of SAM and associated MR [78] (Figs. 4.6, 4.8, and 4.10).

Other superimposed factors like filling state, contractility (use of catecholamine), systemic vascular resistance can contribute and increase this mechanism. Some echocardiographic predictors have been associated to risk of LVOT obstruction in previous studies: small LV dimensions, high

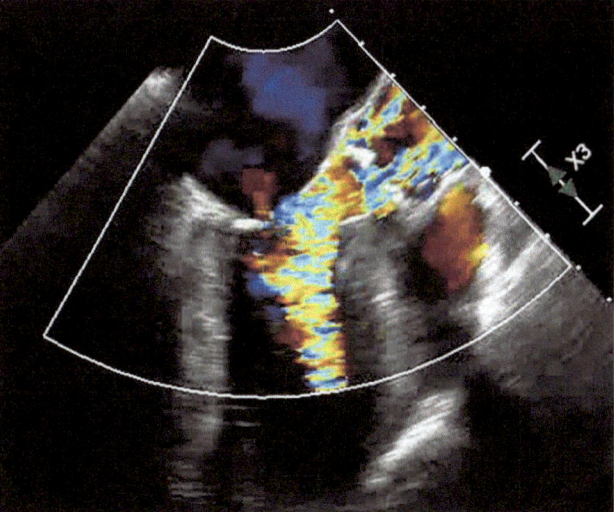

Fig. 4.10 Abnormal mid-ventricular gradient due to severe left ventricle hypertrophy. This patient was candidate to concomitant myectomy

transvalvular gradient, good LV contractility, asymmetric hypertrophy, sigmoid shaped septum and narrow LVOT.

When such factors are identified, prophylactic treatment of post-SAVR-LVOT obstruction have to be considered. Immediately after intervention, LVOTO should be detected and mechanism should be clarified; medical treatment should reduce myocardial hyper-contractility and increase afterload and filling pressure: volume, beta blockers and vasoconstrictors (phenylephrine mainly) are useful in this setting; on contrary inotrope and intraaortic balloon pump or other mechanical supports should be avoided. When hemodynamic instability persists during intraoperative monitoring period or when anatomic factors generate high risk situation enlargement of the subvalvular part is indicated, through a minimal myectomy, conceptually similar to that described by Bigelow or Morrow for hypertrophic cardiomyopathy [33].

4.2.2.7 Epicardial Echo

Ten years before the introduction of TEE epicardial echocardiography (ECE) was already in use as a diagnostic imaging modality to assist cardiac surgeons. When a TEE probe cannot be inserted or when probe placement is contraindicate, a comprehensive ECE examination can be performed efficiently and safely; moreover, it can provide better image resolution using higher frequency probes rather than TEE (Table 4.4). Epicardial imaging requires direct access to the anterior surface of the heart, and consequently can be performed only after a sternotomy [14, 15]. Epicardial echocardiography may be superior to TEE because it can provide optimal image resolution using high frequency probe and it allows to image anterior cardiac structures including the

Table 4.4 Contraindications to TEE

Main contraindications to TEE
Absolute contraindications
Perforated gastrointestinal tract
Esophageal stricture
Esophageal tumor
Esophageal perforation, laceration
Esophageal diverticulum
Active gastrointestinal bleeding
Relative contraindication
History of radiation to neck and mediastinum
History of GI surgery
Recent upper GI bleeding
Barret disease
Dysphagia
Restriction in mobility of neck (cervical arthritis, atlantoaxial joint disease)
Symtomatic Hiatal Hernia
Esophageal varices
Coagulopathy, thrombocytopenia
Active esophagitis
Active peptic ulcer disease

aorta, aortic valve (AV), pulmonic valve, and pulmonary arteries [79, 80]. Seven epicardial echocardiographic imaging planes are consistent with the ASE recommendations for transthoracic echocardiography (TTE) nomenclature [81].

Epicardial AV Short-axis View and LAX view and Epicardial LV LAX View are the most important position to obtain information about AV and coronary arteries morphology and function. Epicardial AV Short-axis View (TTE Parasternal AV Short-axis Equivalent): the transducer is placed on the aortic root above the AV annulus, with the ultrasound beam directed toward the AV in a short-axis (SAX) orientation to obtain the epicardial AV SAX view. Aortic cusps are in the same placement than in TTE view and coronary ostia can be visualized by slowing motion. **Epicardial LV LAX View (TTE Parasternal LAX Equivalent):** from the epicardial LV mid-SAX view, the ultrasound beam is angled superiorly and rotated toward the patient's right shoulder; in this position inferolateral and anteroseptal walls of the LV and the RV, left atrium (LA), LVOT, AV, and MV are yielded; color Doppler measures of MV, TV, LVOT obstruction, SAM of MV can be detected.

4.2.3 Intraoperative Monitoring with TEE

4.2.3.1 Introduction

Nowadays conventional SAVR requires general anesthesia and the use of extracorporeal circulation. Invasive blood pressure monitoring as well as central venous catheters and transesophageal echocardiography are standard monitoring modalities. Currently partial sternotomy incisions such as inverted-T or inverted-L sternotomies have been shown to increase postoperative thoracic wall stability and can be used for uncomplicated aortic valve interventions while complex or combined operations are generally performed using the standard median sternotomy [30].

After full heparinization the ascending aorta and right atrium (or superior and inferior cava individually) are dissected and cannulated for extracorporeal circulation. Prior to cannulation it is important to have precise information about presence and extension of calcium plaques in ascending aorta to avoid these. In case of extensive aorta pathology, alternative cannulation sites should be used (brachiocephalic trunk, proximal aortic arch, as well as the distal right subclavian artery).

These interventions are performed in normothermia (35 °C) or mild hypothermia (30–32 °C). Electrically induced ventricular fibrillation is performed before clamping the ascending aorta.

When heart-lung machine is working, intraoperative monitoring with TEE is no longer needed until the end of procedure. Therefore, since in aortic interventions anterograde cardioplegia is allowed, intraoperative monitoring during cardioplegic solution input allows to quantify ventricular function until the cardiac arrest is reached.

Intraoperative TEE allows to detect acute complications after cannulation of aorta and right atrium (or cava veins) for extracorporeal circulation (ECC). Moreover, if respiratory function is not stable with mechanical ventilation, immediate visualization of **pleural effusion** can be obtained turning the probe onto the right and left from ME views. **During the time of intervention organ functions are monitoring with a mean if invasive and non-invasive tools:** invasive arterial pressure; central venous pressure; diuresis; lactate concentration; central venous oxygen saturation and mixed venous oxygen saturation; cardiac index and pulmonary capillary wedge pressure; electrocardiogram.

4.2.3.2 Ruling Out Complications

4.2.3.2.1 Introduction
TEE monitoring during AV intervention allows immediate detection of complication to perform appropriate and prompt treatments.

Source of complications could be all the phases of open heart surgery:

- Induction of anesthesia can be complicated in case of cardiac insufficiency and pulmonary stasis of pleural effusion;
- Central cannulation should be monitored for the risk of injury on venous and arterial structures;
- Aortic valve and aortic root integrity should be monitored immediately after intervention for excluding acute dysfunction;
- Local complications on coronary arteries and mitral valve apparatus should be ruled out;
- LV restoring should be assess after cardioplegic solution has been washed out

4.2.3.2.2 Local: Coronary Occlusion, Mitral Valve Lesions, Root Hematomas
During AV surgery complications against surrounded tissue and nearby structures can occur and they must be ruled out by TEE evaluation post intervention to allow prompt therapy. **Decalcification** of a degenerate AV is usually the first step before aortic valve excision; this can be a complex process and protection of surrounded structure and tissues must be guarantee.

Coronary occlusion. Preoperative TEE can assess the normal position, course and the calcification of coronary ostia. In cases of atypical origin or course of the coronary arteries, it might be necessary to perform additional CABG in order to ensure perfusion of the atypical coronary. Visualization of coronary arteries is yielded by ME AV SAX view and LAX view (biplane displayment) for right coronary ostium and left main ostium. 3D TEE multiplanar reconstruction allows better quantitation of distance between annulus and ostia, but this tool is mostly relevant in transcatheter intervention than in open heart surgery. Evaluation of LV function and regional motion allow to suspect traumatic injury on coronaries during valve surgery. Coronary angiography remains the most important diagnostic tool in case of intraoperative suspect of this complication. Both surgical view, TEE view, coronary angiography can differentiate three entities in this setting: (1) **intrinsecal occlusion**, generally due to emolization during AV decalcification or thrombosis during low flow condition in patients with known coronary artery disease; (2) **estrinsecal stenosis** due to enlargement of coronary arteries ostia in suture or deformation in presence of adjacent tissue tearing. Once diagnosed, this last one complication require immediate surgical correction; risk factors can be: low height of coronary ostium, large prosthesis size, small sinus of Valsalva diameters. Therefore this estrinsecal stenosis occur more frequently during valve sparing surgery for AR (external annuloplasty, aortic root remodelling techniques, Yacoub or David procedures); (3) **dynamic stenosis:** coronary artery spasm has been recognized as a possible cause of hemodynamic and arrhythmic instability after aortic valve replacement [82–85].

Mitral valve lesions. Anatomical continuity between aortic and mitral tissue is represented by aortomitral fibrosa/curtain, that is a fibrous structure between the aortic and mitral valves where the anterior mitral leaflet becomes continuous with the non-coronary cusp of the aortic valve. It is an avascular structure so it is prone to infection and injury after aortic valve replacement, causing late complications such as pseudoaneurysm formation [86]. Perforation of AML is a very rare acute complication occurring after AV surgery and coronary surgery. In a large cohort of patients subjected to AV sparing procedures, MV perforation occurred in 2/475 cases. Similarly few cases of aortic valve perforation during MV surgery have been reported [87]. This complication has been related to the surgical removal of speckle of calcium from AV, MV and MA continuity in case of high degree calcification. Intraoperative TEE allows immediate diagnosis, identifying a severe MR with a convergence flow over the 'hole' and a jet direction that is depending on the part of the leaflet that is damaged (basal-free margin) and the scallop involved. Another type of local complications that can occur during or immediately after AV surgery includes the aortic complications. These can be local complications (annulus or aortic wall perforation or intramural hematoma) or more extended (progression of hematoma or aortic dissection). Since aortic complications can occur at all phases of intervention, TEE evaluation should aim to careful evaluate aortic wall integrity at main time-points.

Aortic complications. Intraoperative complications that may emerge during decalcification phase can be annulus or aortic wall perforation; they can be immediately recognize by surgeon and directly treated by closing the defect with a Teflon pledget or pericardium-reinforced suture, or even with a pericardial patch.

Sometimes, minimal perforation can remain undetected during intervention and are identified late, after pressure loading of the aorta leads to an enlarging sub-epicardial hematoma. In these cases, opening of the aortotomy and closure of the defect from the inside is highly recommended. These micro-traumatic injuries can occur not only during AV replacement but also in aortic root surgery, around proximal and distal anastomosis of a vascular graft. These last one are more frequent during aortic valve sparing procedures.

Intramural hematoma (IMH) is a life-threatening aortic disease included within acute aortic syndrome. This is a contained aortic wall hematoma with bleeding within the media but without initial intimal flap formation. The most common initial event leading to IMH formation is a traumatic injury on aortic wall, causing microvascular rupture inside media (intra-medial) of the aortic wall, which results in weakening of the aortic wall that is seen as a circumferentially oriented space without intimal discontinuation. Its natural history is variable: it may be reabsorbed without any intervention, or it may progress to classic aortic dissection. Similar to acute aortic dissection, it is classified as Stanford type A (ascending aorta) or B (exclusive involvement of the descending aorta). Haemorrhagic pericardial effusion occurs more frequently in IMH than in acute aortic dissection and can be fatal unless treated on an emergency basis [88, 89].

The echocardiographic criteria diagnostic of IMH include a wall thickness >7 mm and an echolucent zone in the aortic wall, which leads to compression of the aortic lume [90, 91]. The appearance and continuity of the intima and the presence of an intimal flap may help distinguish acute aortic dissection from IMH and PAU. Therefore TEE evaluation does not allow a definite diagnosis: echolucency is not present in all patients with IMH, a thrombosed false lumen of acute aortic dissection, with intimal calcification or atherosclerotic plaque in the aortic wall, can be difficult to differentiate from IMH, reverberations and other artifacts can cause linear densities and shadows within the aortic lumen, mimicking IMH or acute aortic dissection. When IMH is suspected, conservative strategy should be start including careful monitoring of arterial pressure and coagulation factors; then, magnetic resonance is the gold standard for certain diagnosis.

4.2.3.2.3 Aortic Dissection

Incidental findings can significantly influence the surgical procedure and outcome, for example in case of aortic dissection, in which mortality rate is halved when diagnosis is made intraoperatively rather than post operatively [38, 92, 93]. Fragility of the aortic wall, aortic regurgitation, and aortic wall thinning were identified as independent risk factors for dissection after surgery; conversely, previous aortic cross-clamping or cannulation or type of prosthesis were not associated factors [94]. Type I aortic dissection after SAVR occurs in approximately 0.6% of patients within 1 month to 16 years after surgery, with a poor outcome in 50% of cases [38]. Proximity of the oesophagus and the thoracic aorta permits high-resolution images from higher-frequency TEE. Availability of multiplane imaging permits improved incremental assessment of the aorta from its root to the descending aorta (Fig. 4.11).The most important transoesophageal views of the ascending aorta, aortic root and aortic valve are the UE LAX (at 120°–150°) and UE SAX (at 30°–60°). The descending aorta is easily visualized in short-axis (0°) and long-axis (90°) views from the coeliac trunk to the left subclavian artery. Withdrawal of the probe shows the aortic arch and, in the distal part of the arch the origin of the subclavian artery is easily visualized. The diagnosis of aortic dissection in the context of perioperative monitoring is based on TEE and requires the presence of an intimal flap that divides the aorta into two, true and false, lumina. In most cases, false lumen flow is detectable by colour Doppler but may be absent in totally thrombosed and retrograde dissections. Several studies have demonstrated the accuracy of TOE in the diagnosis of aortic dissection with sensitivity of 86–100%, specificity 90–100%, and a negative predictive value of 86–100% [95, 96]. TEE permits assessment of the main anatomical and functional aspects of interest for the management of aortic dis

1. *Intimal tear location*. Intimal tear appears as a discontinuity of the intimal flap; usually, the main intimal tear has a diameter over 5 mm and is located in the proximal part of the ascending aorta in type A dissections and immediately below the origin of the left subclavian artery in type B dissections; it is important distinguishing multiple small communications between the two lumina that can be detected with color Doppler to the main intimal tear.

2. *Identification of the true lumen*. The surgeon needs to know whether the supra-aortic vessels or other visceral arterial vessel originate from the false lumen or true lumen. Echocardiographic findings can differentiate the true from the false lumen: (1) true lumen is generally smaller, has systolic expansion, and systolic antegrade flow; in systolic phase the flow goes from true to false lumen; false lumen is the largest, has systolic compression, no systolic anterograde flow is detected (sometimes retrograde).

3. *Involvement of the main collateral vessels* of the aorta is important as it permits selection of an appropriate therapeutic strategy. When aortic dissection is detected in the

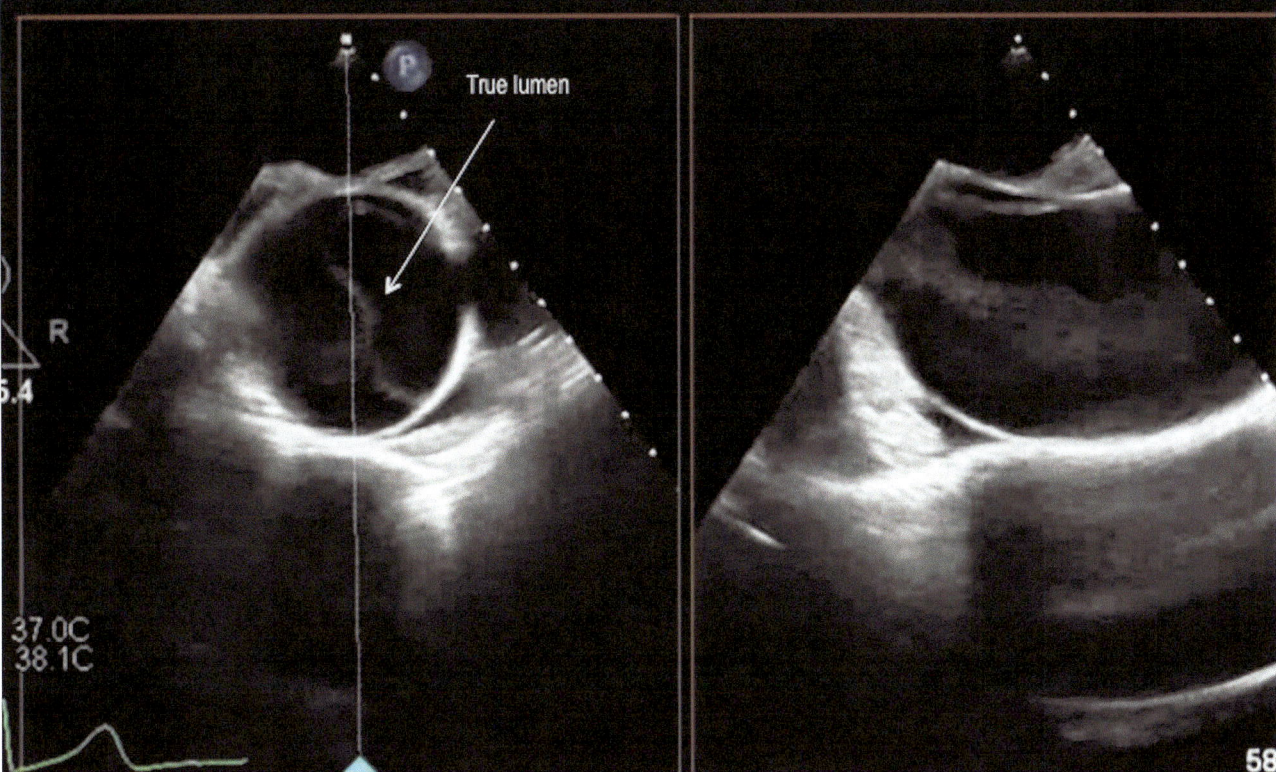

Fig. 4.11 Type A aortic dissection (true lumen—white arrow)

context of cardiac surgery for AV the strategy option can be: (1) conservative management when Type B dissection occur: monitoring arterial pressure, adequate coagulation control and serial CT assessment can be required until stabilization occur and false lumen is spontaneous excluded by thrombosis; (2) surgical strategy when type A aortic dissection is detected.

4.2.3.3 Anesthesia and Cardiac Protection Management

4.2.3.3.1 Introduction
Currently, AV surgery requires: general anesthesia, full extracorporeal circulation for peripheral organ function maintenance, cardioplegia for myocardial protection, venting in LV and ascending aorta for avoiding LV distension and obtaining a bloodless operatory field.

The induction of anesthesia in patients with impaired left-ventricular pump function or coronary heart disease is more dangerous than in healthy patients [30]. Accordingly, special care has to be taken to maintain sufficient perfusion pressure in patients with coronary artery disease. Perfusion pressure should be augmented with α-adrenergic drugs like norepinephrine during intervention. Furthermore, the heart-lung machine implies hemodilution and hypothermia can impair

autoregulation of local blood flow, increasing the risk of hypoperfusion. Immediately after the intervention has stopped, reperfusion damage must be avoided through application of a normothermic substrate-enriched blood cardioplegia mostly via the coronary sinus. In AV interventions all these mechanisms can be even more dangerous because of the presence of significant LV hypertrophy in AS or LV dilatation in AR. The purpose of **extracorporeal circulation** is to maintain peripheral perfusion and gas exchange during open heart surgery. Central cannulation of the heart and/or the adjacent large vessels offers the best drainage and consequently provides the best cardiopulmonary support. Peripheral access with a single venous cannula usually does not permit total bypass: Only 80% of blood volume can be drained via peripheral cannulas, whereas 20% of blood volume passes the lung.

According to the planned procedure, the arterial cannula can be either inserted into the ascending aorta, the aortic arch, or brachiocephalic trunk. A more distal cannulation, especially in the aortic arch, reduces the risk for cerebral embolism.

All aortic cannulas are introduced after a 5 mm stab incision and during a mean arterial pressure of 60–80 mmHg. They are fixed with purse-string sutures in the adventitial layer, which can be reinforced by pledgets. The size of the aortic cannula is kept small to avoid extensive laceration of the aortic wall. Transmural stitches are avoided as they would increase the risk of subadventitial hematomas and continuous bleeding. During cannula placement, it is important to verify that the tip is readily inserted into the aortic lumen and directed toward the aortic arch. Extrathoracic cannulas are inserted in the same manner as any other peripheral cannula. However, the tip of the cannula is the narrowest part, where pressure drops and jets and turbulences develop which can injure the aortic wall from inside.

Possible complications include vessel wall tearing and dissection (aortic dissection <1%), dislodgement of atheromas, and thrombi, with subsequent neurological complications. A screening for endovascular complicated atheromas can be performed by echocardiography in the context of periintervention evaluation. After pump is started and cannulae are functioning, aortic cross-clamp is performed to separate the systemic circulation (supported by heart and lung machine of ECC) from the outflow of the heart. Then cardioplegia is given and LV venting is placed.

4.2.3.3.2 Endoclamping in MICS

For the set up of cardiopulmonary by pass in minimally invasive cardiac surgery (MICS) peripheral cannulation and clamping of aorta should be performed. In this setting, the external aortic clamp (EAC) is still used [30]. It is introduced through a separate skin incision in the same or one intercostal space above the initial minithoracotomy in the anterior axillary line and can be positioned around the ascending aorta under direct view or videoscopic guidance. Cardioplegia and aortic-root venting are delivered through a needle-vent catheter in the aortic root.

The other available method is the endo-aortic balloon (EAB) (EndoClamp or its successor, IntraClude, Edwards Lifesciences, Irvine, CA, USA). The EAB is a triple lumen catheter with a balloon at the tip and a large central lumen for cardioplegia delivery and aortic-root venting. The other two lumens are for pressure monitoring in the aortic root and for inflation and deflation of the balloon. It is introduced via common femoral artery and is inflated in the ascending aorta under transoesophageal echocardiography (TOE) guidance in order to achieve occlusion. For this aim, TEE should assess and evaluate baseline aortic integrity, aorta tortuosity, atheromasic plaque, aortic pre-existing flaps, aortic diameters. During insertion of EAB, TEE should monitoring direction and inflation, avoiding traumatic injuries on aortic wall.

4.2.3.3.3 Cardioplegia and LV Venting

The aim of myocardial protection is to maintain myocardial integrity and function while a surgical procedure is ongoing. The heart is protected with a combination of hypothermia and cardioplegia.

Cardioplegia in AV interventions can be given either retrograde or anterograde.

Anterograde cardioplegia consists into direct introduction of solution into aortic bulb, between aortic clamping site and AV; this type of cardioplegia is elective for pure AS, but it cannot be used in case of AR because of the risk of LV reflux and LV enlargement. In this condition, anterograde cardioplegia is given through coronay ostia if significant coronaric disease has been ruled out. In patients with previous aortocoronaric by pass, myocardial protection should be ensured by coronary artery bypass grafting before aortic valve. If coronary artery disease is present, then retrograde cardioplegia is chosen, trough coronary sinus.

When a full extracorporeal circulation is ongoing, arterial blood is pushed into aortic arch (arterial cannula) and venous flow is drainaged through venous cannulation. However, bronchial and Thebesian veins drain into the left atrium and ventricle even with total bypass, so that the left ventricle can be distended, and blood can fill operative filed. During AV intervention (and during surgery on LV) a vent should be placed for maintain operative filed bloodless. Standard approach for Vent placement is the right superior pulmonary vein. Alternatively, especially in emergency situations, vent placement can occur via the left ventricular apex after a stab incision. Insertion of the vent into the pulmonary artery trunk is also possible. For coronary artery bypass surgery a vent is placed into the aortic root, often as a combined cannula for antegrade cardioplegia delivery.

For monitoring these preoperative phase, TEE evaluation should assess mostly: presence of AR, left ventricle function and dimension, abnormalities of coronary sinus and coronary ostia, correct placement of LV venting.

4.2.3.4 Post-procedural Intraoperative Monitoring

4.2.3.4.1 Introduction

At the end of interventions, when cardioplegia has been stopped and the heart beats, immediate evaluation of outcome of intervention and complications is performed. Gradual input of volume (blood from heart and lung machine) is administered, heart starts to beat and the vent is still visible until all cannulae have been removed from heart and aorta. The postoperative cardiac physiology is modified depending on preoperative cardiac anatomy and physiology and the type of intervention. The goal of postoperative cardiovascular care should be to guarantee a sufficient tissue perfusion. Optimal ranges for postoperative cardiovascular parameter were found to be: mean arterial pressure (MAP) of >65 mmHg, central venous pressure (CVP) of 8–12 mmHg (in dependence on the ventilation), diuresis of >0.5 mL/kg/h, lactate concentration of <3 mmol/L, central venous oxygen saturation (ScvO$_2$) of >70% and mixed venous oxygen saturation (SvO$_2$) >65%, cardiac index of >2.0 L/min/m^2, pulmonary capillary wedge pressure (PCWP) of

12–15 mmHg, left ventricular end-diastolic area index (LVEDAI) of 6–9 cm^2/m^2 [97].

TEE at the end of procedure has the crucial role to: (1) assess the specific outcome of intervention that in case of aortic valve surgery is the outcome of AV repair or SAVR; (2) evaluating systolic function, diastolic function, pericardial integrity, volume loading condition, aorta integrity; (3) identify complications for prompt treatment.

Hypovolemia is the more common cause of early hemodynamic instability in the immediate perioperative period. Echocardiographic parameters that can assess this hemodynamic condition are: LV end-diastolic diameter and LV end-diastolic area obtained in the TG midpapillary SAX view. The same measurements can be used for monitoring response to fluid therapy [98] and they can be a better index of LV preload compared with PA catheterization [99, 100].

Pericardial tamponade in early post operative phase can epiphenomenon of other severe complications such as: incompetency of surgical sutures with acute dehiscence of valve prosthesis or vascular graft, aortic iatrogenic damage and type A dissection; in this phase it can be triggered mainly by coagulopathies and heparin administration. Pericardial effusion can be immediately quantified after intervention as trivial (seen only in systole), small (20 mm), or very large (>25 mm).

Echocardiographic criteria to diagnose tamponade on the basis of mitral inflow patterns during inspiration and expiration period are usually not interpretable during positive-pressure ventilation, since **during positive pressure ventilation there is only minimal respiratory variation** [101, 102].

4.2.3.4.2 LV Function

In the immediate post operative phase, LV function can be unstable and is still influenced by loading conditions. Cardiac anesthesia is still ongoing and can reduce LV performance index by negative inotropic effect and reducing venous return; mechanical ventilation modifies intrathoracic pressure affecting right ventricle filling and cardiac output. LV failure is one of the major complications after cardiac surgery and cardioprotection techniques aim to reduce the incidence of such negative complication. The main cause of the left heart failure in this setting is an excessive myocardial **pressure and/or volume overload combined with global or regional ischemia, that can results into a condition of "myocardial stunning" after ECC have been stopped. These condition are mostly completely** reversible after adequate diagnosis, support and etiological treatment. Predisposing factors that cannot be modified are: advanced age, severity of underlying heart disease, Hb levels, malnutrition, diabetes, time of diagnosis and pre-existing reduction of LVEF; previous cardiac surgery, urgency of intervention, peripheral vascular disease. Factors that can be modifiable

are: cross clamp time, the quality of myocardial protection, and the degree of success obtained. Low-cardiac-output syndrome (LCOS) is the worst manifestation of LV failure after surgery and it can occur in immediate post operative period or some hour later, in intensive units. It is associated with increased morbidity and mortality [103–105]. The use of inotropic agents or mechanical circulatory support always is required to improve patient hemodynamics. Intraoperative TEE is useful to identify the specific cause. The most common causes of postoperative LCOS are: rhythm disturbances, pericardial tamponade, myocardial infarction, left or right heart failure, vasoplegic syndrome, cardiovascular arrest. Continuous monitoring of mean invasive arterial pressure, central venous pressure, diuresis, lactate concentration, central venous oxygen saturation and mixed venous oxygen saturation, cardiac index, pulmonary capillary wedge pressure, electrocardiogram are needed until hemodynamic stability is reached and cause is treated.

4.2.3.4.3 Assessment of Valve Function

After AV repair or replacement, the function of repaired AV or new prosthesis should be immediately assessed. Before ECC has been stopped, a first macroscopic evaluation of continence of the valve in the setting of AV repair might be performed by excluding retrograde flow signal in left ventricle from cannula of cardioplegic solution. If this retrograde flow is detected at this first direct surgical evaluation, then a surgical revision is necessary, so requiring to come back to extracorporeal circulation.

The most important aims of intraoperative post procedural evaluation (and of early in-hospital pre-discharge re-evaluation) should be: (1) evaluation of site and movement of leaflets of biological valve and mobile elements of mechanical valves; (2) assessment of intra-valvular pathological regurgitation, distinguishing from physiological regurgitation due to Aranzio node excision in biological prosthesis and to "washing jets" in mechanical prosthesis (that are multiple trivial jets inside the sewing ring, where the closed leaflets meet the housing, and centrally, where the closed bileaflets meet each others); (3) evaluation of suture of prosthetic valve with host native tissue, assessing the presence and quantitation of paravalvular leak; (4) valuation of anastomosis of vascular prosthesis when performed (both proximal and distal anastomosis); (5) LV and RV function and filling pressures, other correlates (Table 4.5).

The following parameters have been recommended for assessing normal functioning of aortic prosthesis: peak velocity (>4 m/s suggests stenosis), mean gradient (<35 mmHg suggests stenosis), Doppler velocity index (LVOT velocity/AV velocity < 0.25 suggests stenosis), EOA (<0.8 cm^2 suggests stenosis), acceleration time (>100 ms suggests stenosis) and contour of jet (rounded and symmetrical suggests stenosis). Table 4.6 summarized these parame-

Table 4.5 Imaging tools in open heart surgery for AV interventions

Preoperative assessment (after general anesthesia, before extracorporeal circulation)

Procedural concerns	Echocardiographic evaluations needed	Other monitoring tools
Functional assessment	Valve main vitium: aortic stenosis or aortic regurgitation or both; LVOT diameter and, whenever possible, LVOT area	
Coronary assessment	Coronary abnormalities (abnormal origin of coronaries should be detected before any type of AV intervention)	
Aortic valve repair or replacement?	Valve anatomy, number of cusps, tissue characterization and integrity, amount of calcification and distribution;	
Aortic root surgery?	Aortic root anatomy, atheromasic disease	
	Careful sizing for aortic root surgery in valve sparing procedures it should be define the following points: (1) dilation of sinotubular junction; (2) dilation of aortic annulus; (3) aortic root shape, symmetric or asymmetric dilation; (4) distal extension of aortic dilation	
Other concomitant interventions/modulation of medical therapy after intervention in intensive care unit	Biventricular function concomitant secondary/primary valve disease (mitral valve regurgitation); abnormalities in left ventricle outflow tract: assessing gradient and site of obstruction when present; establishing the wall thickness of LV for eventual myectomy and predicting the post-procedural medical treatment (more volume overload and less inotropic support)	
Cardioplegia trough aortic valve	Quantitation of concomitant aortic regurgitation	
Safely clamping	Amount and extension of aortic plaque and calcification	
Venting placement	Assessing the right placement (retrograde or anterograde)	

Intraoperative assessment (general anesthesia, extracorporeal circulation, cardioplegia)

Procedural concerns	Echocardiographic evaluations needed	Other monitoring tools
On pump	During anterograde cardioplegia assessment of LV distension and asystole during cadioplegic solution input, to avoid excessive distension; assessment of right position of extracorporeal circulation and venting cannulae	Mean invasive arterial pressure, central venous pressure; diuresis; lactate concentration; central venous oxygen saturation and mixed venous oxygen saturation; cardiac index and pulmonary capillary wedge pressure; electrocardiogram

Post-operative assessment (general anesthesia, as soon as extracorporeal circulation and cardioplegia have been stopped)

Procedural concerns	Echocardiographic evaluations needed	Other monitoring tools
Bioprosthesis function	Bioprosthesis function: position, cusps movement; transprosthetic gradients	Mean invasive arterial pressure, central venous pressure; diuresis; lactate concentration; central venous oxygen saturation and mixed venous oxygen saturation; cardiac index and pulmonary capillary wedge pressure; electrocardiogram
Correlates and complications assessment	Paravalvular leak or intraprosthetic regurgitation	
	EOA and PPM	
	LV function and filling state	
	Color flow acceleration through LV (LVOT or mid-ventricle obstruction), assessment of grade, mechanism, site and concomitant SAM or MR	
	RV function	
	Pericardial integrity	
	Aortic integrity: exclude aortic dissection, hematoma, thrombosis	

ters. Using all these parameters, one should take into account a methodological trouble: Bernoulli equation is validated for native valves and simplified the formula by neglecting V1 velocity in LVOT; in case of prosthetic valve, we are not dealing with narrow orifice so inertial component is not negligible at all and "V2", downstream velocity is very low (usually <2 m/s), that results in a overestimation of trans-prosthesis gradient. Furthermore, the first evaluation of the repaired or replaced AV is routinely performed intraoperatively, when some troubles in accurate measures can occur (Fig. 4.12). In this phase hemodynamic is highly unstable and a relatively high output state occurs immedi-

ately after intervention (either for anaemia and reduction of LV afterload); these can affect transprosthetic gradients (Fig. 4.13), as well as the hemodynamic alterations due to general anesthesia and mechanical ventilation ongoing since the beginning of intervention. Furthermore, especially in the context of AS, global LV function can be more unstable immediately after aortic valve replacement because of LV hypertrophy and stiffness that make its function more sensitive to acute changes in loading condition. Perivalvular tissues are oedematous for the surgical injury and this can further reduce the EOA. Finally, **a degree of overestimation of AV gradient is accepted** and the intraoperative values of

Table 4.6 Prosthetic aortic valve evaluation

Prosthetic aortic valve stenosis

	Normal	Mild stenosis	Moderate/severe
Quantitative parameters			
Peak velocity (m/s)	<3	3–4	>4
Mean gradient (mmHg)	<20	20–40	>40
Qualitative parameters (flow independent)			
Doppler velocity index (DVI)	>0.35	0.35–0.25	<0.25
Effective orifice area (if BSA > 1.6 m²), cm²	>1.1	1.1–0.8	
Effective orifice area index (if BSA < 1.6 cm²), cm²	>0.9	0.9–0.6	<0.6 cm²
Prosthesis-patient mismatch (PPM)			
Indexed effective orifice area (if BMI < 30 kg/m²), cm²/m²	>0.85	0.85–0.65	<0.65
Indexed effective orifice area (if BMI > 30 kg/m²), cm²/m²	>0.70	0.9–0.6	<0.6
Prosthetic aortic paravalvular regurgitation			
Qualitative parameters	Mild	Moderate	Severe
Structure and motion abnormalities of mechanical or biological valve	Usually not degenerated	Abnormal	Abnormal
LV size	Normal	Normal of mildly dilated	Dilated
Semi-quantitative parameters			
Circumferential extent of paraprosthesis color doppler regurgitation (% of annulus)	<10	10–20	>20
Diastolic flow reversal in descending aorta (PW doppler)	Absent or early diastolic	Intermediate	Prominent holodiastolic
Jet width in central jets (%LVOT diameter): color doppler	<26%	26–64%	>64%
Jet density CW doppler	Incomplete	Dense	Dense
Jet deceleration rate (PHT, ms), CW doppler	>500	200–500	<200
LVOT flow vs pulmonary flow: PW doppler	Slightly increased	Intermediate	Greatly increased
Quantitative parameters			
Regurgitant volume (mL/beat)	<30	30–59	>60
Regurgitant fraction (%)	<30	30–50	>50

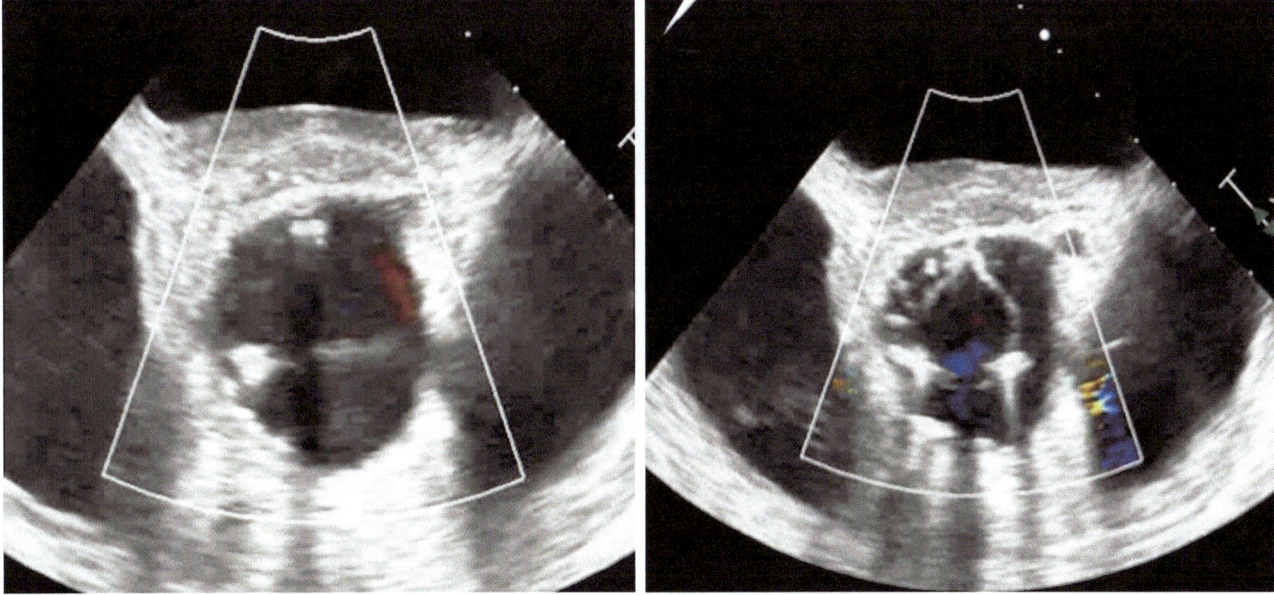

Fig. 4.12 Assessment of a surgical valve function: short axis view of aortic prosthesis with color allows exclusion of para-valvular leak

peak velocity and mean gradients don't have to be considered the baseline values for further follow up evaluations. The optimal timing of quantitative baseline assessment of valve function should be between the third and the fourth month after surgery. The normal reference values for gradients across aortic prostheses are largely variable because of the fact that different prostheses show different haemodynamics [106, 107].

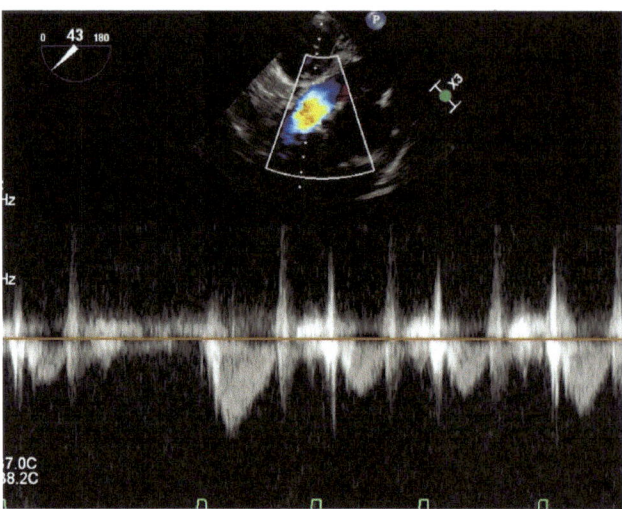

Fig. 4.13 Transgastric assessment of trans-prosthetic gradient is performed routinely but it is influenced by low pre-load of post-operative phase and acute changes in hemodynamic through LVOT

Pathologic regurgitation can be central (more frequently with biological prosthesis) or paravalvular, that is usually seen in either types of prosthesis and is more frequent when calcium debridement was difficult, in redo surgery and in older patients with smaller but stiffened tissues around AV annulus. Assessment of paravalvular leak (PVL) is usually more difficult than native valve regurgitation due to image distortion, eccentricity of jets and acoustic shadowing for presence of prosthesis (especially when it is mechanical). The use of colour Doppler is necessary to confirm the presence of the PVL and usually it is necessary to display off-axis images and multiplane mode with 3DTEE. Furthermore with 3D TEE full volume modality the frame rates are too slower for having good temporal resolution and good color 3D-Full volume display; mild jets and fine structures cannot be visualized. The incidence of mild PVL immediately after intervention ranges between 5 and 20% and the majority of these leaks are clinically not significant; they don't increase the risk of infective endocarditis but they can cause chronic haemolytic phenomena [108, 109].

Quantitation of PVL is not different from the quantitation of native aortic regurgitation, but it is more challenging: Jet diameter/LVO diameter <25% in ME-AV-LAX view; pressure Half Time <200 ms (TG LAX view for better alignment with Doppler beam), holodiastolic flow reversal in descending aorta. The extension of color flow in ME-AV-SAX view relatively to sewing ring is another recommended evaluation (<10% of sewing ring is mild; 10–20% moderate; >20% severe; 40% rocking motion). 3D-Full volume color imaging is used when feasible for computation of VC area by post-acquisition processing and cropping.

A special mechanism of PVL occurs when size of prosthesis is too small relatively to native aortic root dimension; this is called "**geometrical mismatch**" **and** happens more frequently with stentless valves.

Irrespective to the mechanism, postoperatively, any regurgitation that is at least moderate would indicate surgical correction immediately prior to leaving the operating room.

Intraoperative TEE at the end of procedure should assess the presence of "**patient-prosthesis-mismatch**" **(PPM)**. This complication was refers to situation in which EOA of the prosthesis is smaller than that of the normal aortic valve for the given body size, causing low regression in cardiac hypertrophy, more cardiac events and less survival [110, 111]. Simple calculation has been proposed by Pibarot for preventing PPM by obtaining the minimum size of prosthesis to be implanted: calculating the patient's body surface area (m²) than multiplying BSA by 0.85 cm²/m² the value obtained is the minimum EOA to avoid PPM. When at the end, despite this preventive model a PPM appears it should be quantified according to calculated EOA. Therapeutic options for PPM could be: to implant another type of prosthesis with a larger EOA such as a stentless prosthesis or mechanical prosthesis; to enlarge the aortic root to accommodate a larger prosthesis of the same type; to accept PPM according to global clinical condition of patient [112–115].

4.2.3.4.4 Coronary Artery Flow

Intraoperative Electrocardiography monitoring allows identification of acute coronary obstruction at the end of intervention, typically with ST elevation or cardiac arrhythmia and can be immediately compared with TEE findings. By a mean of accurate analysis of coronary anatomy and myocardial regional function, intraoperative TEE allows examination of coronary arteries integrity at the end of interventions. As previously described coronary artery flow can be reduced in case of coronary embolism, coronary thrombosis due to transitory low flow in patients with LV dysfunction, suture-related tearing of coronary ostia that can be distorced, coronary spasm.

When concomitant AV and CABG are performed transit-time flow measurement (TTFM) is the most common intraoperative method for assessment of the function of the graft.

4.3   Intraprocedural Imaging for Guidance and Monitoring in TAVR

4.3.1   Intro

Since the first-in-human transcatheter aortic valve implantation (TAVI) performed by Alain Cribier in 2002 [116]. The number of trans-catheter heart valve (THV) implantations has growing because of different factors: (1) aging of population, (2) better treatment of comorbidity that reduces fragility of older patients and (3) indications for trans-catheter aortic valve replacement (TAVR) expanding to lower risk patients [117, 118]. The last one factor is the most important one leading to continuous improvement of technologies and research for assessing the durability of THV. Current guidelines for aortic stenosis recommend TAVR for patients that are symptomatic and high risk for surgery (class I A and IB respectively in American and European guidelines) and patients who are at intermediate risk for SAVR (class IIA and IB respectively in American and European guidelines). Percutaneous balloon aortic valvuloplasty has still a role, mostly as bridge to other treatments (SAVR and TAVR). Table 4.7 summarized the current recommendation of American Heart Association/American College of Cardiology and European Society of Cardiology (ESC)/European Association for Cardio-Thoracic Surgery (EACTS). Device currently approved for clinical use in TAVR are summarized in Table 4.8 with their main characteristics. Importantly,

Table 4.7 Current recommendation for TAVR

Recommendation of American Heart Association/American College of Cardiology guidelines for transcatheter aortic valve replacement (TAVR)	Class	Level
TAVR is recommended for symptomatic patients with severe AS (Stage D) and a prohibitive risk for surgical AVR who have a predicted post-TAVR survival greater than 12 months	I	A
TAVR is a reasonable alternative to surgical AVR for symptomatic patients with severe AS (Stage D) and an intermediate surgical risk, depending on patient-specific procedural risks, values, and preferences	II	A
Percutaneous aortic balloon dilation may be considered as a bridge to surgical AVR or TAVR for symptomatic patients with severe AS	IIb	C
III B: No Benefit B TAVR is not recommended in patients in whom existing comorbidities would preclude the expected benefit from correction of AS	III	B
Recommendations of European Society of Cardiology (ESC) and the European Association for Cardio-Thoracic Surgery (EACTS) for transcatheter aortic valve replacement (TAVR)		
TAVI is recommended in patients who are not suitable for SAVR as assessed by the Heart Team [91, 94]	I	B
In patients who are at increased surgical risk (STS or EuroSCORE II ≥ 4% or logistic EuroSCORE I ≥ 10% or other risk factors not included in these scores such as frailty, porcelain aorta, sequelae of chest radiation), the decision between SAVR and TAVI should be made by the Heart Team according to the individual patient characteristics (see this table), with TAVI being favoured in elderly patients suitable for transfemoral access [91, 94–102]	I	B
Balloon aortic valvotomy may be considered as a bridge to SAVR or TAVI in haemodynamically unstable patients or in patients with symptomatic severe aortic stenosis who require urgent major non-cardiac surgery	IIb	C
Balloon aortic valvotomy may be considered as a diagnostic means in patients with severe aortic stenosis or other potential causes for symptoms (i.e. lung disease) and in patients with severe myocardial dysfunction, pre-renal insufficiency or other organ dysfunction that may be reversible with balloon aortic valvotomy when performed in centres that can escalate to TAVI	IIb	C
Intervention should not be performed in patients with severe comorbidities when the intervention is unlikely to improve quality of life or survival	III	C

they have been divided according to the mechanism of deployment into: balloon-expandable (SAPIEN 3), self-expandable (Evolut R, Portico, ACURATE neo, Allegra), and mechanically expandable (LOTUS). From a procedural standpoint, self-expandable valve have been associated to higher risk of paravalvular leak but less risk of annulus and aortic root ruptures. A careful assessment with imaging before procedures is needed for predicting the risk of complications and influencing the choice of specific valve [119–124].

4.3.1.1 Procedural Aspects and More Recent Perspectives

Transfemoral access is the preferable whenever possible, since it has been found to lead to shorter procedure times, superior outcomes and faster patient recovery. This type of approach allows a minimalist approach to TAVR. Other access sites could be transapical or transaortic. In these cases general anaesthesia is usually required. Other access routes options can be the trans-subclavian and trans-axillary approaches for patients with anatomy that is unsuitable for the other traditional techniques [125].

Transcatheter valves are positioned prior to deployment with the aid of aortography, fluoroscopy and, in some cases, TEE guidance. Balloon expandable valves require rapid ventricular pacing (180–220 beats per minute [bpm]) for deployment to reduce cardiac output and avoid inaccurate valve implantation. A temporary pacing wire is positioned in the right ventricle via the jugular or femoral vein.

TAVR bioprostheses are typically oversized by 5–30% relative to the aortic valve annulus diameter. This make radial force between the prosthetic valve and aortic valvar complex to be sufficient for anchoring and sealing the device. For Corevalve is recommended an oversizing of 7–30% and for Edwards of 4–27%.

After valve deployment, careful assessment of intraprocedural results is needed and complications have to be rule out. This phase is generally guided by a mean of combination of invasive hemodynamic assessment, fluoroscopy and when necessary, echocardiography (TTE or TEE in case of procedures performed with general anaesthesia).

Bicuspid aortic valves (BAV) has a lower prevalence in the elderly and accounts for 20% in surgical case of >80 years of age. Earlier experience with TAVI in BAV had poor outcomes for anatomical characteristics: more oval annulus shape, unequal leaflet size and the presence of calcified raphes. An higher incidence of THV malposition (7.2%), moderate or severe paravalvular regurgitation (PVR) in 15.9% was found and these complications occurred more frequently in patients with a calcified raphe in a Type 1 bicuspid valve. Currently BAV is a relatively contraindication to TAVR, but this option has not to be denied immediately; a careful heart team discussion should be made taking into account aortic root and valve calcification [126, 127].

Table 4.8 Available devices for TAVR

Device	Release	Valve size (mm)	Sheath access route	Repositionable?	Retrievable?	PVL* (>2)	PPM (30 days)*	Specific advantages
CoreValve Evolut R	SE	23, 26, 29, 31	14 Fr, TF, TS	Yes	No	3.4–5.7%	8.3–11.7%	Resheatable up to 80% deployment; current RCT in low risk population
SAPIEN 3	BE	20, 23, 26, 29	14 Fr, TF, TA	No	No	1.8–4.8%	8.2–10.1%	External Skirt for reducing PVL, current trial on low risk population
Portico	SE	23, 25	18 Fr, TF, TS	Yes	No	4%	9.7%	Lowest profile; resheatable up to 85% deployment; preserve coronary artery access for future interventions
ACURATE neo™	SE	23, 25, 27	18Fr, TF	No	No	0%	6.7%	Low pace-maker required
CENTERA	SE	23, 26, 29	14 Fr, TF	Yes	No	8%	27%	
Direct Flow Medical	IR	23, 25, 27, 29	18 Fr, TF	Yes	Yes	1–2.6%	13–17%	
JenaValve	SE	23, 25, 27	Sheathless 32 Fr, TA	Yes	No	0%	12.1%	Useful in AR
Engager	SE	23, 26	30 Fr, TA	Yes	No	0%	28.5%	
Lotus™ Valve	M	23, 25, 27	18 Fr, TF	Yes	Yes	1–4%	23.4–28.6%	

PVL Paravalvular leak

Transcatheter valve-in-valve (ViV) implantation has emerged as a less invasive therapy for failed bioprosthetic surgical valves [128]. The self-expanding CoreValve® (Medtronic, Minneapolis, MN, USA) and the balloon-expandable SAPIEN XT and SAPIEN 3 valves (Edwards Lifesciences, Irvine, CA, USA) have been approved for this used. Recently, outcomes of these procedures have been published and growing experience has shown that ViV TAVI-specific complications can often be prevented with accurate screening and some technical expedients [129].

It has to be noted that, compared with procedure on native valve, ViV leads less frequent to PVL and new pacemakers but more frequent to residual patient-prosthesis mismatch and coronary occlusion (0.3% in TAVR on native valves and 4–5% in ViV procedure). Higher implantation of either annular or supra-annular THVs has been shown to partially mitigate this phenomenon; iatrogenic bioprosthetic valve fracture (BVF) and coronary cusps fracture (BASILICA) have been started for reducing these two complications. For reducing patients distress due to long lasting pacing and procedures, general anesthesia is still usually performed; TEE guidance is usually still required. For BVF TEE allows to detect immediately complication that are more frequent than in other TAVR: surgical valve leaflet injury/severe regurgitation, mitral chord rupture/mitral regurgitation, ventricular septal defect, coronary obstruction, pericardial effusion, conduction abnormality, para-valvular leak [130, 131].

Coronary obstruction is more frequently seen when the TAVR is performed in a stented bioprostheses with externally mounted leaflets or stentless bioprostheses than in the more commonly encountered stented bioprostheses with internally mounted leaflets and the risk is predictable on the basis of a score calculated with MSCT: The virtual transcatheter heart valve to coronary distance (VTC). This is

CT-obtained parameter that takes into account: coronary height, sinus width, and transcatheter heart valve size, and also accounts for bioprosthetic valve tilt in the annulus. It has been shown that a short VTC distance predicts coronary obstruction, with an optimal cut-off level of <4 mm best identifying those patients at risk with high sensitivity and specificity [132, 133].

4.3.1.2 Multimodality Imaging Assessment

Imaging has a central role for preoperative evaluation and suitability to TAVR, intraoperative guidance and monitoring and for troubleshooting. The first important aim of imaging should be evaluation of feasibility of TAVR, prediction of complications and planning of procedure (annular sizing, access route). This is obtained integrating morphological and functional parameters.

4.3.1.3 Aortic Stenosis Severity

Assess of severity of AS and quantitation of associated AR and left ventricle function, contractility reserve and concomitant other valve pathologies is carried out by preoperative TTE and, whenever needed, TEE. Table 4.9 summarized the recommended echocardiographic criteria for grading valve dysfunction. Beyond gradients, LV function and structure should be assessed clearly with TTE and quantitation of both LVEF (%) and SVi (mL/m^2) is needed. When AV is highly calcified and AVA is poor opening but gradients are less than severe, this could be due to LV systolic dysfunction or presence of small ventricles (typically seen in older patients and long lasting AS). In the first case dobutamine stress echocardiography allows the differential diagnosis between true severe AS and pseudo-severe AS. If the peak velocity jet increased (over 4 m/s) and AVA remains <1.0 cm^2, then there is truly severely stenotic: low/low low gradient AS. If the

Table 4.9 Integrative approach to aortic stenosis assessment

	Aortic valve area	Mean gradient	LVEF	Stroke volume index (SVi)	Hemodynamical conditions that can affect this status
High gradient AS	<1 cm²	>40 mmHg	Any SV	Any EF	Volume changing can reflect directly on cardiac function; **high flow status** must be excluded; if high flow status is not reversible, diagnosis is confirmed (AV fistula, sepsis, anemia, significant **concomitant AR**)
LFLG-REF-AS	<1 cm²	<40 mmHg	<35 mL/m²	<50%	**Catecholamine and pacing can identify contractile reserve**; other significant valvular disease should be excluded: **MS, MV, TR**. Coronary artery disease should be treated
LFLG-NEF-AS	<1 cm²	<40 mmHg	<35 mL/m²	>50%	LV stiffness is more increased, LV is sensible to volume load; decreased in effective blood volume can cause immediate hemodynamic crash in these patients

cause of AV stenosis is low EF, then increasing SV with dobutamine, could increase AVA and reduce the gradients. This last one is pseudo-stenosis. Patients with low flow/low gradient AS benefit from AVR, but usually they are referred for TAVR since the surgical risk is high [134].

In most cases TTE is not sufficient to estimate the severity of AS, so TEE is needed and particularly for the assessment of aortic valve planimetry. As alternative, time-velocity integral ratio, between LVOT and aortic valve, expresses the size of the valvular EOA, with severe stenosis is assessed by a velocity ratio less than 0.25. Invasive measurements can assess with the best accuracy the trans-aortic gradient and are always collected when coronary angiography is available before TAVR.

Cardiac magnetic resonance being expensive and less available, is currently not recommended for routine assessment before TAVR. Therefore, it has a role in quantifying the severity of AS when some doubts derive from discrepancy between clinical and echocardiographic examinations.

Morphological assessment of AV, computation of AVA by planimetry, accurate quantitation of AR and other valve pathologies, LV dimension and function are well assessed with CMR [135, 136].

4.3.1.4 Coronary Arteries, Cusps and Aortic Root Morphology

TTE and TEE should preoperatively assess the number of cusps, thickness, and calcification. MSCT clearly integrates the information of TTE and TTE in pre-procedural assessment for TAVR, especially in patients with poor acoustic window by TTE or with high degree of AV calcifications. Three main issue should be clarified before TAVR.

1. Aortic annulus dimensions (major and orthogonal minor diameters, perimeter and area) and measurements of sinus of Valsalva (SV) diameters and sinotubular junction (STJ) should be assessed for evaluating the candidacy of patients to TAVR; annulus size less than 18 mm or more than 29 mm are contraindication.
2. Height of the coronary ostia from the aortic annulus and risk for coronary obstruction due to native cusps is assessed before procedure. With 2DTEE is possible to

assess the height of right ostium (ME AV LAX view 120–130%), but for height of left main ostium 3D TEE with multiplanar reconstruction of coronal axis is required (Fig. 4.5). When native cusps length is >2 mm longer than the height of left coronary, then the diameter of sinus of Valsalva is measured: if diameter is <30 mm the risk for coronary occlusion is significant (Fig. 4.14). Ascending and descending aorta diameters and shape can modify the outcome of TAVR; either the presence of aortic root aneurysmal dilatation and a SV wide less than 27 mm are contraindications to CoreValve implantations; horizontal aorta can be better crossed with Portico Valve.

3. The amount of calcification and its distribution (bulky calcifications) are pivotal issue.

Indeed, they determine procedural outcomes for the following mechanisms:

- degree of calcification predicts the risk for paravalvular leak after TAVR by a mean of residual space between native AV annulus and prosthesis annulus, more frequently when a self expandable prosthesis is chosen;
- asymmetrical calcifications and speckle of calcium can increase the risk of aortic annulus rupture and pericardial tamponade, more frequently when balloon expandable prosthesis is chosen;
- bulky calcifications can generate abnormal tension–force across the valve, which can cause asymmetric deployment of the prosthesis and increase the risk of compression of the coronary arteries ostium;
- calcification at the end of the cusps can increase furthermore the risk of coronary occlusion and embolization;
- calcification at STJ can generate a pushing phenomenon of the valve inside LVOT causing displacement during deployment [6, 7].

4.3.1.5 Annular Measurements Assessment

As for open heart surgery, annular dimension can be assessed easily with TTE and TEE (see Figs. 4.3 and 4.4 and Sect. 4.2.2.1).

Fig. 4.14 Evaluation of risk of coronary obstruction

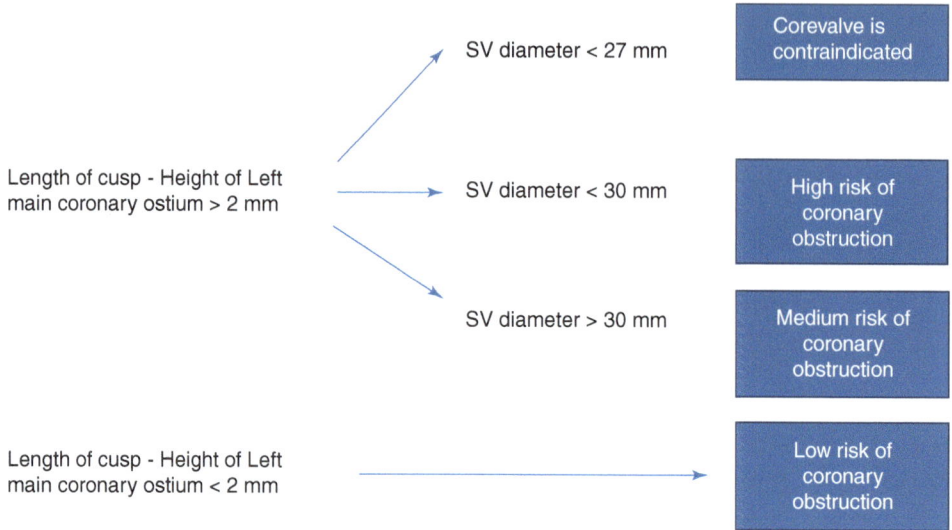

TTE slightly underestimates aortic annular size. LVOT and aortic annulus diameter should be measure in systole, zooming in the LV outflow tract, at the point of insertion of the aortic valve cusps, from tissue–blood interface to blood–tissue interface.

Before 3D TEE acquisition, a 2D image of the aortic valve at either the 45–60° ME-AV-SAX view or the 120° ME-AV-LAX view should be obtained. Both 2D TTE and 2D TEE assume the LVOT to be a circular orifice, so a geometrical simplification is introduced in a parameter that is the most important in affecting the EOA. 3D TEE with multiplane reconstruction of LVOT area and MSCT allow the best quantitative assessment of LVOT. All 3D acquisition modes can be used although '3D Zoom' and 'Live' mode are the most conventionally used, giving priority to frame rate and imaging resolution. The 3D echocardiography multiplanar reconstruction (MPR) software provides tools for 3D volume segmentation along the three axes (x, y, z) either real-time or post-processing. With MPR the perfect orthogonal alignment of the LVOT and aortic annulus can be obtained. With 2D TEE it is possible to determine the right coronary annular–ostial distance, but the left coronary annular–ostial distance can only be measured from the coronal plane, so requiring 3D TEE multiplanar reconstruction (Fig. 4.5) or MSCT.

4.3.1.6 Mitral Regurgitation and LVOT Dinamic Obstruction Risk

Mitral regurgitation can significantly change after TAVI because of (1) reduce afterload; (2) calcification in mitro-aortic continuity is pushed by TAVR and it reinforces the calcium on anterior leaflet of MV resulting in a reduction of mitral annulus height that contribute to reduce MR. MV anatomy and pathology should be assessed before procedures because of the risk of abnormality motion of anterior leaflet after TAVR.

LVOT dimension, its relation to septal thickness, to the length of anterior leaflet can predispose to dynamic obstruction of LVOT after TAVI.

4.3.1.7 Intraprocedural Guidance

An ideal image tool for guiding TAVI should have some requirements: (1) the imaging modality should be portable and compatible with sedation even in case not allowing general anesthesia; (2) should be capable of displaying any step of the procedure by uninterrupted monitoring to help with manoeuvring of catheters and devices, so an ideal tool should not interfere with fluoroscopic or angiographic imaging or with the devices needed for the TAVI procedure itself; (3) has to be safe for the patient. These ideal conditions are currently satisfied only by a mean of combination of different tools: invasive hemodynamic measurements, fluoroscopy, TEE when general anaesthesia is performed for surgical access routes, fusion imaging and ICE.

The following paragraphs detail these tools in different procedural phases.

4.3.2 Access

4.3.2.1 Echo

Ultrasound techniques used in access evaluation are: TEE that is routinely used for transapical approach and vascular ultrasound for femoral access. The use of TEE during TAVI requires the use of a general anaesthetic but leads to some advantages including the assessment of aortic root morphology and valve leaflet behaviour during balloon valvuloplasty, more precise prosthesis positioning during deployment and immediate detection/monitoring of complications. Also, the use of TEE rather than angiography during valve prosthesis positioning would reduce the use of contrast media and its use in TAVR has been associated with same early and mid term results when compared with fully angiography-guided procedures, with less incidence of acute kidney injury contrast related (AKI) [137]. A transapical approach requires a horizontal incision (left anterolateral minithoracotomy) along the fifth or sixth intercostal space to insert the delivery system directly into the apex of the heart to access LVOT and aortic valve. The location of the apex for having the best surgical access is first identified by palpation and transthoracic echocardiography (TTE). Subsequently, the pericardium is opened near the left ventricular (LV) apex, a sheath is inserted directly into the LV cavity, and a guide wire is used to cross the aortic valve under fluoroscopic and TEE guidance; this allows to avoid entanglement in the mitral valve apparatus. LV thrombus is a contraindication to transapical access and it should be excluded before procedure, as well as a complete assessment of left ventricle function and MR should be done. Some important complications can occur early after access and can be immediately diagnosed with TEE guidance: puncture bleeding, myocardial tears, entanglement and damage of mitral valve apparatus.

Ultrasound evaluation of access site can significantly reduce the incidence of vascular complication. When cardiac pacing cannot be positioned by subclavian approach, femoral vein is used for pacing positioning. Bilateral arterial accessed are required for retrograde transfemoral approach and for more complex procedure, especially in case of presence of significant LV dysfunction or when the risk of complications is judged to be high, an additive peripheral vascular access can be used for having a rapid access to hemodynamic supports in case of complications occur.

4.3.2.2 Angiography

If the peripheral vasculature is suitable, then the transfemoral vascular approach has a number of advantages. It is nowadays the default access site with new smaller sheaths. Other access sites should be considered when the transfemoral route is not thought to be suitable (e.g., minimal luminal diameter <5.5 mm, excessive tortuosity and/or calcifications).

When the transfemoral route is adopted, the crossover technique is usually performed to protect the artery in case of femoral vessel injuries. The crossover technique involves a pigtail placed in the contralateral artery (until the femoral head) to allow delivery of a balloon or stent to treat the access vessel in case of complication.

A baseline angio to check the pigtail at the right side can be done. A RAO projection may help discriminate the femoral bifurcation (for the left side LAO projection). The puncture can be done under fluoroscopic guidance (Fig. 4.15). The wire is advanced for a 6F sheath (the pigtail is removed) and preclosure systems are installed. Meanwhile, a temporary pacing wire is positioned in the right ventricle via the jugular or femoral vein (Fig. 4.16). It will be used during balloon aortic valvuloplasty, the implantation of the TAVI

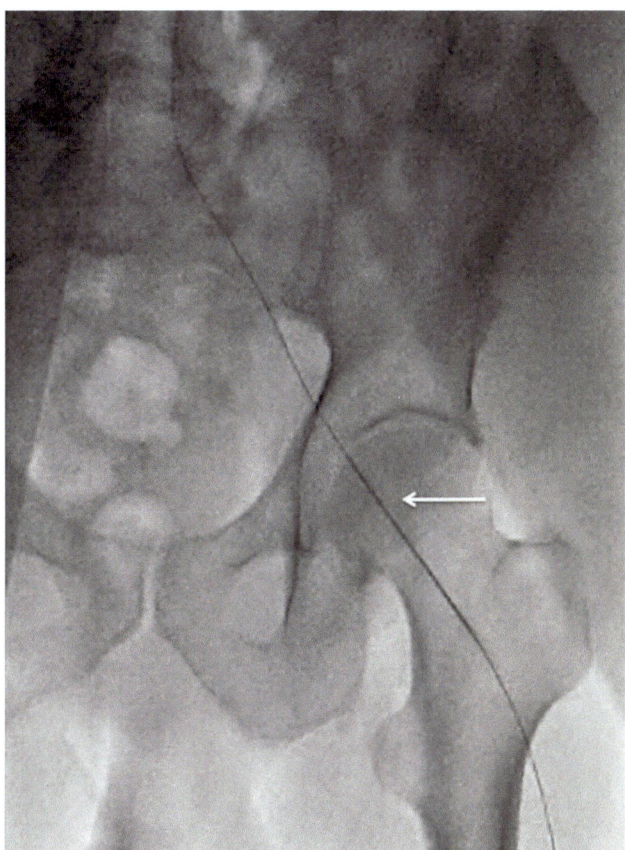

Fig. 4.15 Angiographic frame showing a left transfemoral puncture at the level of the femoral head (arrow), using a standard wire

prosthesis and during the post-dilatation, if needed. The aortic valve is usually crossed with a Judkins right 4 (JR4) or Amplatz left 1 (AL1) diagnostic catheter and a soft straight-tipped wire (Fig. 4.16).

4.3.2.3 CT Fusion Imaging

Cases of use of computed tomography (CTA)-Fluoro fusion technology have been described to identify and puncture vascular accesses. The CTA segmentation of the vessels and the overlay on fluoroscopy of the ilio-femoral vascular anatomy should make access easier, limiting the use of ionizing radiation and the use of cross-over as well as contrast medium [138]. Despite this, the application of fusion imaging is not routine in this context and offers no particular advantages except in very selected cases.

4.3.3 Delivery

4.3.3.1 Introduction

The time of insertion of the device is a key step, not to be underestimated. Once the sheath has been correctly inserted, it is necessary to follow the TAVI under fluoroscopy, while it goes up retrograde along the descending aorta. Some devices

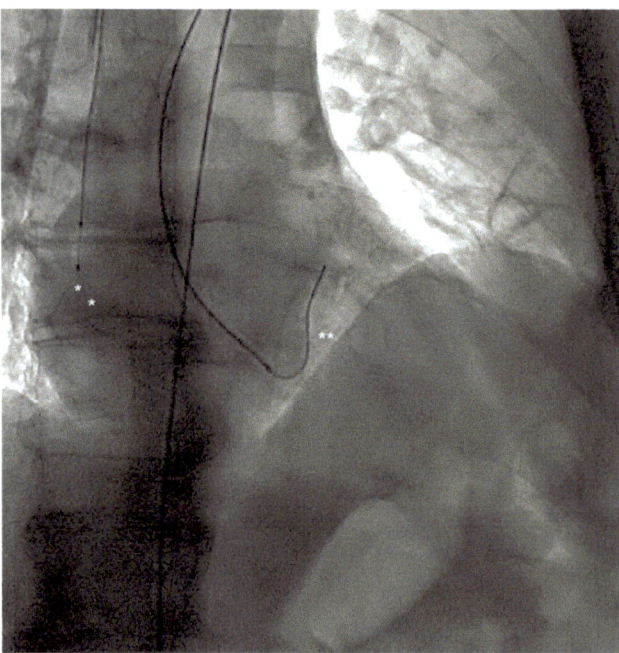

Fig. 4.16 Angiographic frame showing on the left a transjugula temporary pacemaker (white asterisk—which will go at the level of the right ventricular apex). On the right a soft wire is introduced in the left ventricle through a AL 1 catheter (two white asterisks), after having crossed the valve

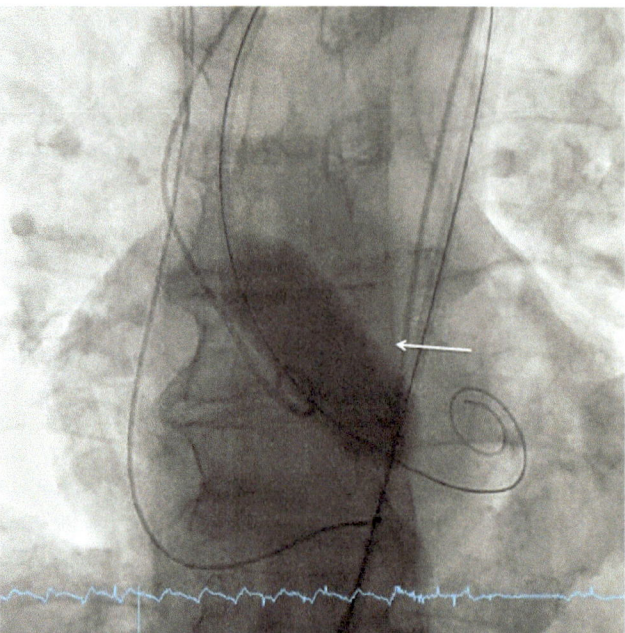

Fig. 4.17 Angiographic frame showing a non-compliant balloon (True-lumen, arrow) during balloon aortic valvuloplasty under rapid pacing. The stiff guidewire in the left ventricle is a pre-shaped Safari guidewire. The pigtail catheter serves as repere in the non-coronary cusp of the aortic valve

require a stop in the descending aorta at the thoracic level, to allow coupling of the valve with the balloon. Another key passage is the bending of the delivery system before crossing the aortic arch. Some TAVI "sheatless" technologies do not require the prior bending of the delivery system, being built in a very flexible way. We will now follow the main methods of imaging to ensure a perfect delivery.

4.3.3.2 Angiography, Fluoroscopy

Once the aortic valve is crossed, the soft wire is then exchanged for a stiffer wire taking care to ensure that this is free of the mitral valve apparatus. Pre-shaped wires (e.g., the Safari™ pre-shaped TAVI guidewire; Boston Scientific) have recently been developed to further minimize the risk of ventricular injury. Stiffer wires, including the Lunderquist Extra Stiff wire (Cook Medical, Bloomington, IN, USA) or the Back-up Meier™ guidewire (Boston Scientific), may be used when greater support is required to deliver the TAVI device. Balloon aortic valvuloplasty (BAV) is performed prior to valve implantation to facilitate device delivery and valve expansion, according to the devices used (Fig. 4.17). A non-compliant balloon (i.e. True Dilatation) or a sandglass-shaped balloon (like the V-8) is usually used to predilate. The size of the balloon should never exceed the size of the sino-tubular junction, especially in the presence of heavy calcifications. Under rapid pacing stimulation, predilatation is performed.

It is advisable to maintain strict fluoroscopic surveillance of the guidewire in the left ventricle during valve deploy-

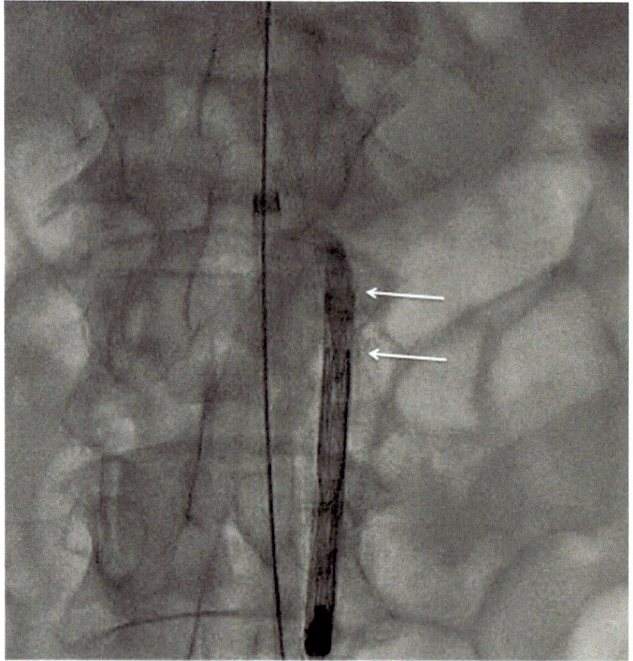

Fig. 4.18 Angiographic frame showing the control of the TAVI self-expandable prosthesis under fluoroscopy, to check the symmetric loading of the valve (longitudinal alignment of the crimped cells and perpedicularity of the end of the valve in respect to the nose cone, arrows)

ment. Before performing BAV, the loaded valve delivery system is inspected under fluoroscopy (high resolution cine at 30 frames/s) to ensure that it's properly loaded (self-expandable prostheses) (Fig. 4.18).

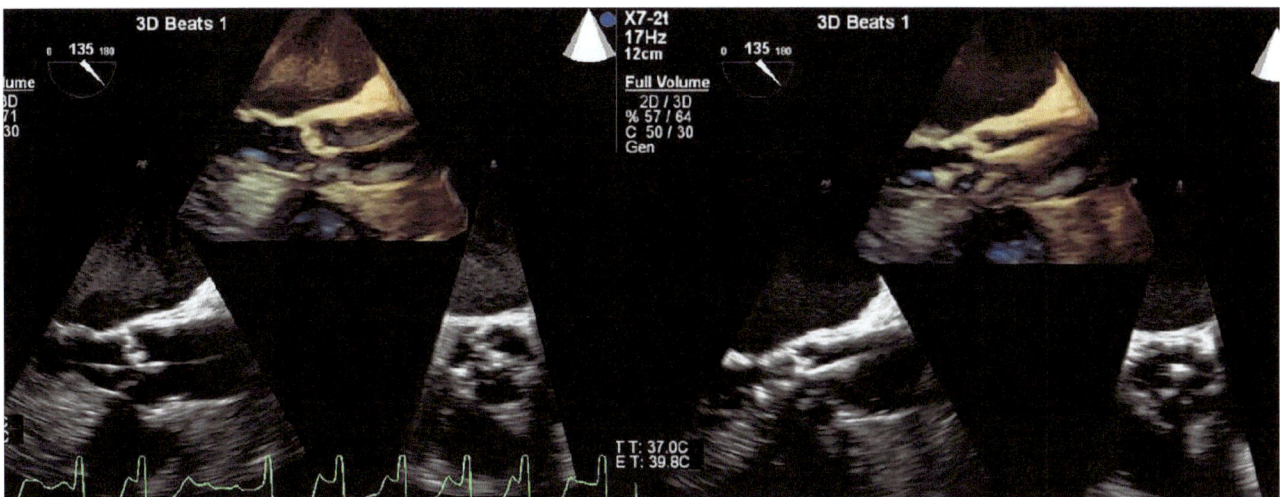

Fig. 4.19 TEE guidance during advance of wire reduces the risk of acute complication (aortic damage, left ventricle perforation when transapical access is performed) (**a**). Delivery system is advanced after the wire (**b**). When DS reaches the annulus plane (by a retrograde transfemoral access in the figure), 2D TEE ME AV LAX and ME AV SAX views allow visualization of direction and position of DS and its coaxially position with the main axis of LVOT-AV. 3DTEE can be more helpful for appreciating the anatomical relations with surrounding structures

4.3.3.3 TEE

When delivery system (DS) comes into LVOT position the hinge point of the anterior mitral valve leaflet could be used to guide the positioning of a transcatheter aortic valve [139].

When DS reaches the annulus plane, 2D TEE ME AV LAX and ME AV SAX views allow visualization of direction and position of DS and its coaxially position with the main axis of LVOT-AV (Fig. 4.19). 3DTEE can be more helpful for appreciating the anatomical relations with surrounding structures. 3D TEE imaging should be performed at the highest possible frequency while 2D TEE gain should be the less is possible. Adequate positioning of DS before deployment of AV prosthesis is needed because if the valve is deployed too low, embolization of the prosthesis into the left ventricle and paravalvular regurgitation may occur; also damage of anterior mitral valve leaflet can occur during diastole. On the contrary, if the valve is deployed too high, this may result in paravalvular regurgitation, coronary obstruction and device embolization.

4.3.3.4 Fusion Imaging

Also in the delivery of the valve, CT-Fluoro fusion does not find an important clinical application of particular interest.

4.3.4 Implant

4.3.4.1 Introduction

The time of implant of the TAVI valve (expansion) is a key step, probably the decisive one. Care should be taken to follow the TAVI mainly with fluoroscopy and targeted contrast medium injections, while positioning it along the aortic ring and then expanding the valve under rapid pacing. The implantation methods can be very different, as the valves are constructed in a different way (balloon vs. self expanding). We will now follow the main imaging methods to ensure perfect implantation, with inferences on the use of ultrasound and fusion imaging.

4.3.4.2 Angiography, Fluoroscopy

The valve delivery system is loaded onto the guidewire and the system is advanced to the aortic annulus, under fluoroscopic guidance. The system usually orients itself to the anatomy as it is advanced. Care should be taken that the capsule and the nose cone must always be monitored during advancement of the system, to achieve a safe passage through the anatomy. The valve position is monitored under fluoroscopy throughout deployment, and the position adjusted as necessary until annular contact is achieved (self-expandable prosthesis) (Fig. 4.20). The capsule has a flare feature that enables the valve to self center as it deploys. In patients with aortic regurgitation, hypertension or large annuli, controlled pacing (90–130 beats/min) is considered during deployment. For a balloon-expandable prosthesis, care should be taken to coalign the fluoro view on the aortic annulus, rather than on the prosthesis itself, like it happens with the self expandable ones.

If the operator is satisfied with the valve position at annular contact, valve is continually deployed until just before the point of no recapture (Fig. 4.21). Once blood pressure has recovered, approaching 80% deployment, the angiographic imaging projection should be adjusted to remove the parallax in valve inflow to determine valve position. Once satisfied with valve positioning and performance, a bit of tension in the system is released, just before final deployment of the prosthesis (Fig. 4.22).

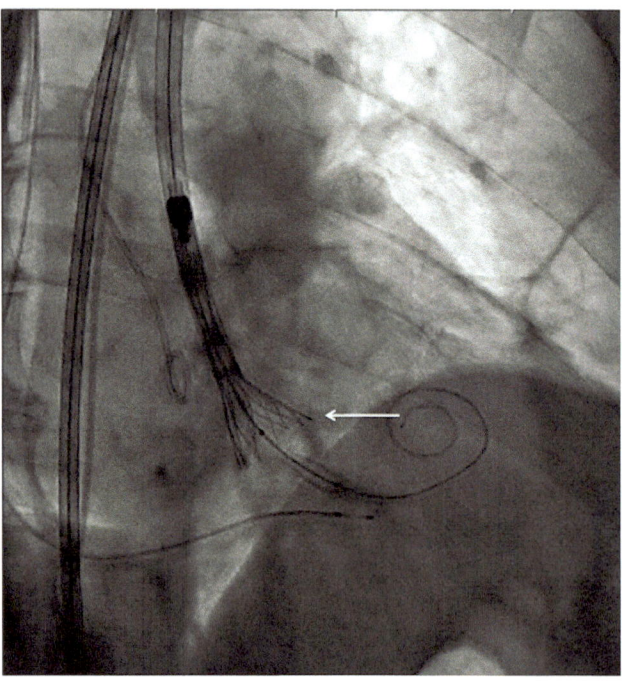

Fig. 4.20 Angiographic frame showing the initial phase of a TAVI self expandable deployment, with the proximal flare already partially opened just below the annular plane (arrow)

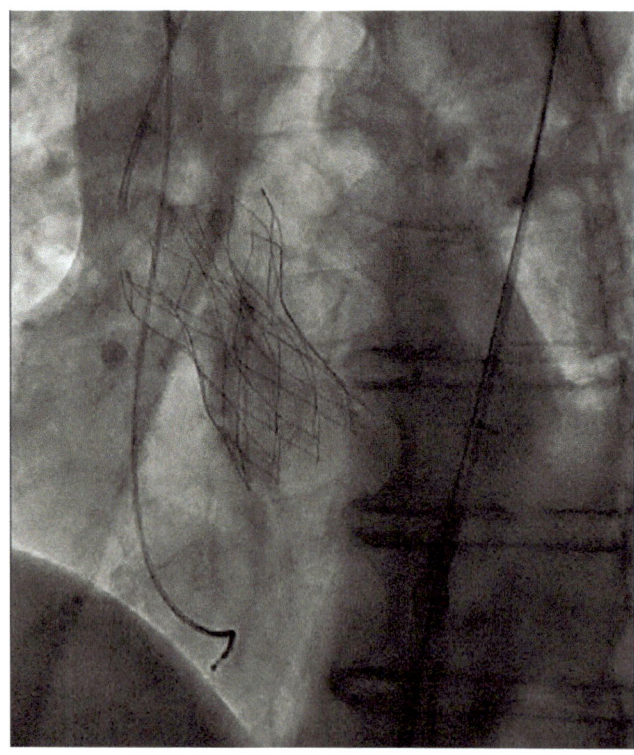

Fig. 4.22 Angiographic frame showing the final result of a TAVI self expandable implantation, with perfect prosthetic cells' opening

4.3.4.3 TEE

One important aim of TEE during implant phase is monitoring balloon aortic valvuloplasty (BAV). For the balloon-expandable valve, most operators use a balloon aortic valvuloplasty (BAV) for increasing valve opening and improve precise positioning. Of more interest, BAV is also used as adjunctive imaging for valve sizing and for predicting the risk for coronary occlusion by looking at the final position of the native cusps after TAVR [140–142].

Simultaneous longitudinal and transverse images (biplane imaging) of the aortic valve, aortic root, and LV outflow tract are required in this phase (Fig. 4.23). TEE allows to appreciate significant AR immediately after BAV and to estimate the grade of fitting of balloon size into the valve annulus, that is useful in case of overlap between different manufacturer suggested sizes for intermediate values of aortic annulus, when generally the first attempted is done with the smaller prosthesis (Fig. 4.23). Imaging the balloon into the native valve and root permits to understand if there is enough space for the leaflets to fit into the sinuses.

Occlusion of the coronary ostia can occur if they are low (close to the annulus), the leaflets are long, and the sinuses are small (Figs. 4.14 and 4.24). The coronary ostia can be imaged during the balloon valvuloplasty and if coronary occlusion occurs it is likely to happen post-valve implant and this may be an indication to abandon the procedure [137, 143].

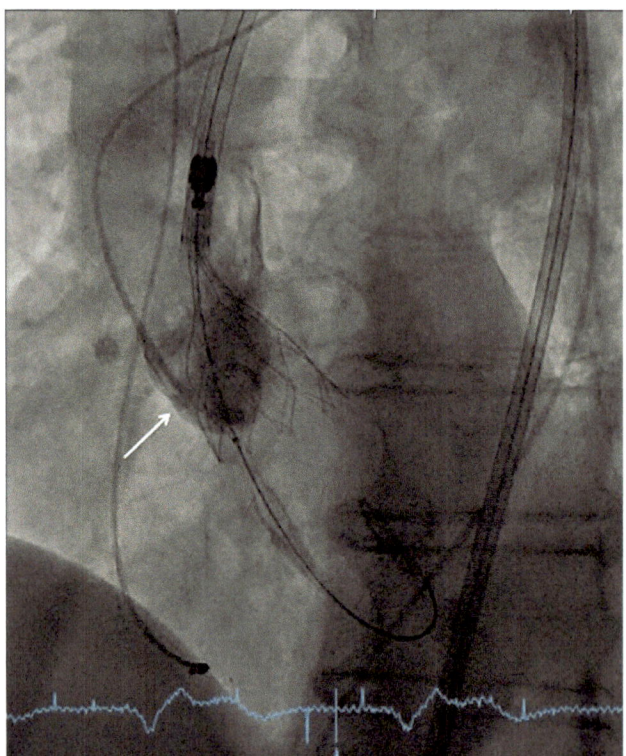

Fig. 4.21 Angiographic frame showing the central phase of a TAVI self expandable deployment, injecting contrast in the non-coronary cusp through the pigtail catheter, to check if the height of implantation is acceptable in respect to the annular plane

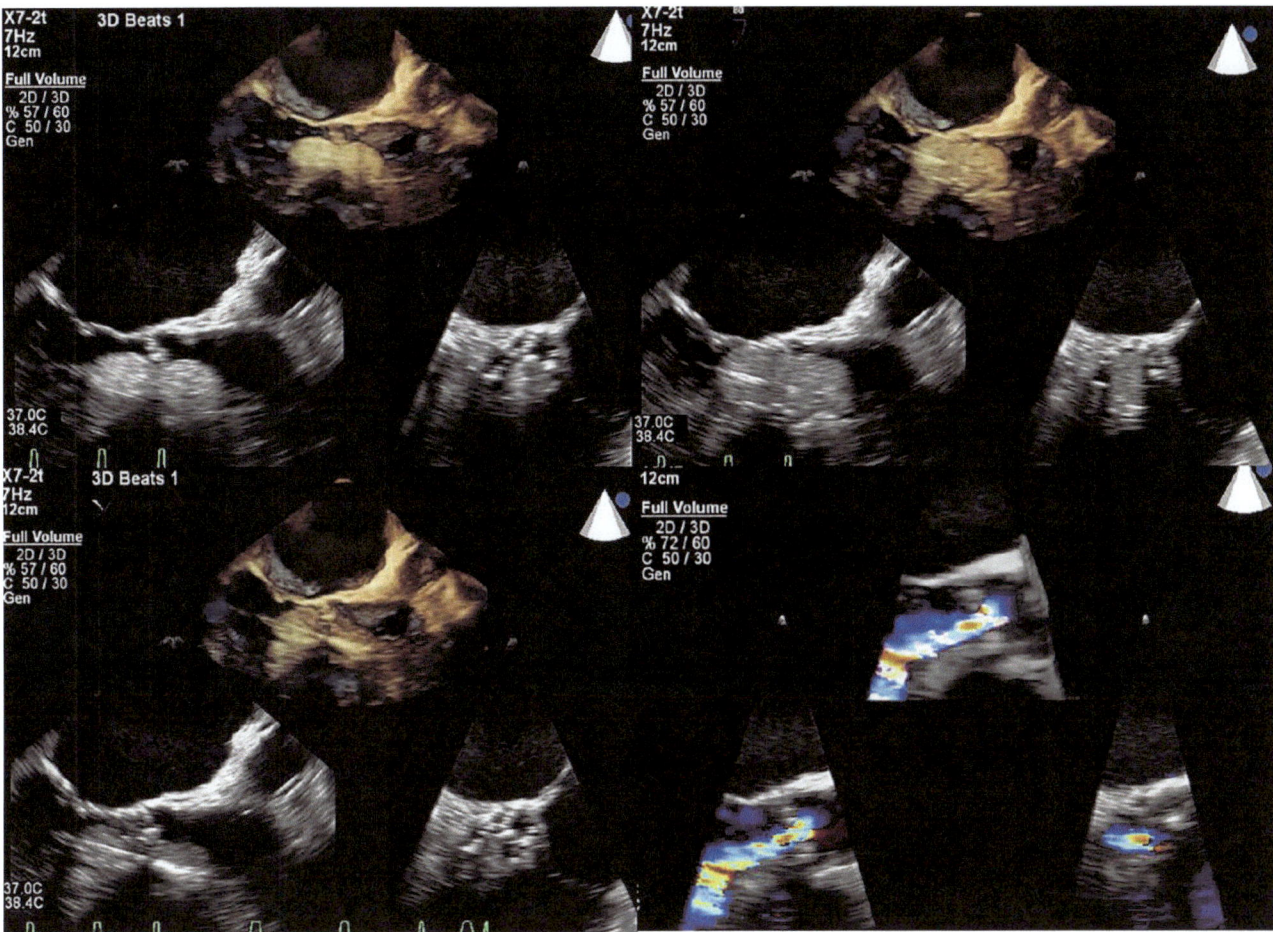

Fig. 4.23 Echo Imaging during Balloon aortic valvuloplasty

4.3.4.3.1 During Valve Deployment

During valve deployment, TEE imaging should be concentrate on the top of the valve, especially when dealing with balloon expandable prosthesis. This is because it is needed to assess to be positioned above the native aortic valve leaflets, for avoiding too low implant. The 2D TEE ME AV LAX view allows this aim but when the valve is crimped on balloon 3DTEE can help more by facilitating appreciation of crimping process of balloon onto the valve and valve into native AV (Fig. 4.24). Either the upper and lower margins of the crimped valve should be visualized in the 3D volume cut. Finally, Live 3-D mode, or equivalent, provides an essential real-time visualization with acceptable temporal and spatial resolution.

Finally, prior to deployment, rotating 3D image can ensure the coaxial position into native annulus and LVOT [144, 145].

It has to be highlight that severe calcifications of the aortic valve and annulus may reduce the quality of echocardiographic visualization of the prosthetic valve, which may limit the performance of TEE for the guidance of valve positioning; in such cases, as well as in case of contraindications to TEE, ICE can be used.

During valve deployment it has to be taken into account that **operator independent movement and shortening** can occur and they can be recognised by using TEE guidance; this is mostly seen with balloon expandable valves. Significant septal hypertrophy can lead to a dynamic reduction of LVOT diameter after valve deployment, causing a pull effect during the deployment of the valve; this Venturi effect is an important risk for low implant. The shortening of the valve during pacing is mainly due to the combination of a systolic forward motion and annulus and aortic sinus calcification in smaller sinus volume. Some echocardiographic considerations have been concluded by reanalysis of imaging compendium of PARTNER trial and should be considered during valve deployment to avoid malpositioning. First of all: during non-paced beats the diastolic valve position is ~50% above and below the annulus and during paced beats the valve should be 30–40% (~5–6 mm) below the annulus. The final optimal positioning should be ~10–20% (~2–3 mm) below the **hinge-points** of the aortic cusps on ventricular side. Superior (aortic edge) of the stented valve should be imaged to ensure that native calcified cusps are covered for 1–2 mm by the prosthesis, remaining inferior to STJ. When this last one aim could not be reached and a over-

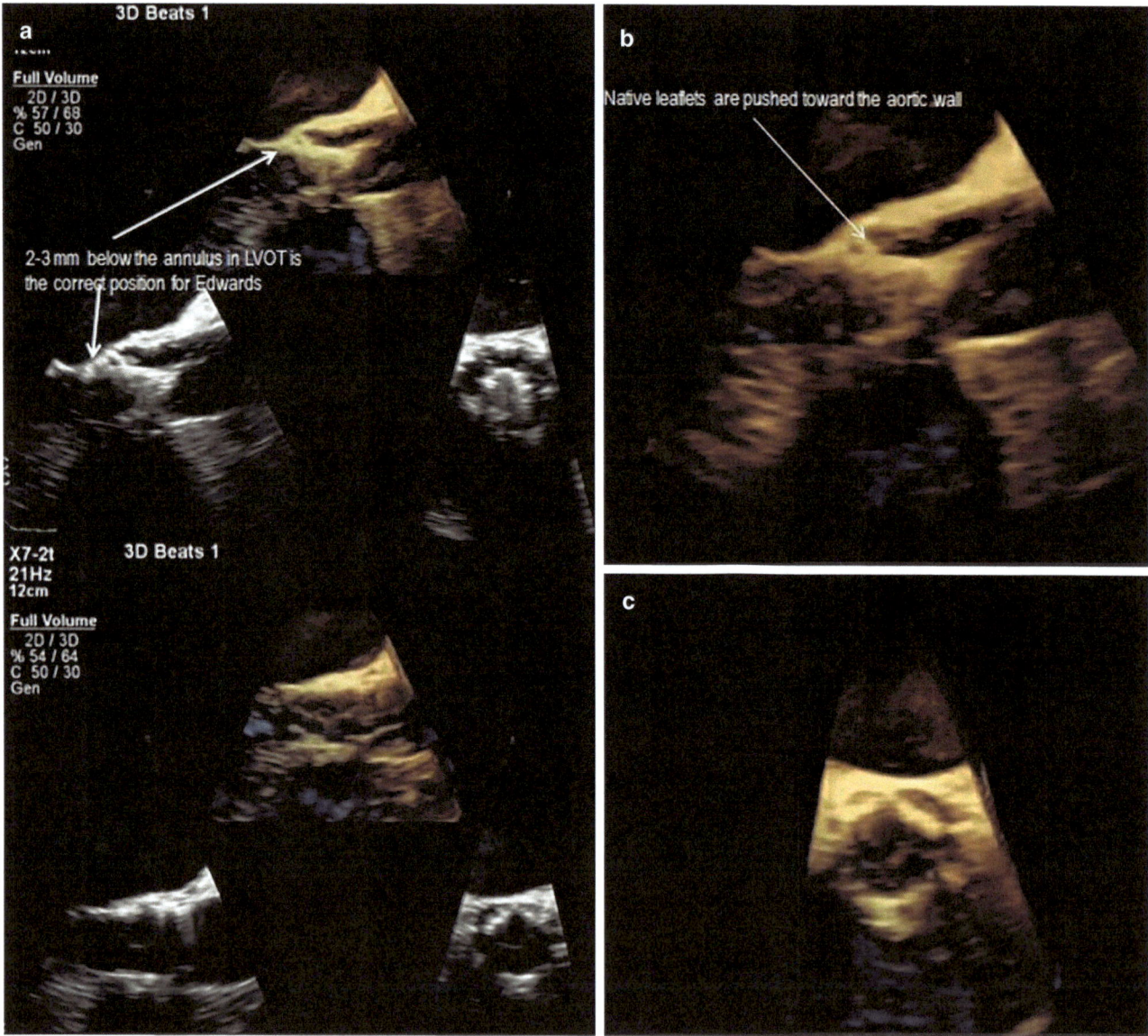

Fig. 4.24 Echo Valve deployment. The ventricular aspect of the valve is opening in Fig. 4.18 (**a**) and the right panel (**b**) shows the native leaflets into the narrow space between the expanding valve and the native Valsalva sinus. In figure (**c**) It is represented the final deployment of aortic valve bioprosthesis

hang of a small amount of native leaflet occurs, these native leaflets can cause acute or delayed migration of valve into the ventricle. Therefore, TEE should diagnose the overhang of native leaflets for allowing procedural decision making [146, 147]. Figure 4.24 summarized the echocardiographic findings during deployment.

4.3.4.4 ICE

When TEE is contraindicated or general anaesthesia cannot be performed or optimal visualization of aortic valve cannot be obtained especially for trans-catheter AV interventions, intra-cardiac echocardiography (ICE) can be used. This method was initially explored by Seward et al. and Valdez-Cruz et al. and the method was improved in early 2000 mainly for guidance of atrial septal defect closures and trans-septal puncture in electrophysiological procedures [16, 147–150].

The most important advantages of ICE are defined in guiding structural intervention on interatrial septum, tricuspid valve, pulmonary valve, interventricular septum. In AV interventions it can be complemental to TEE. There are two categories of ICE catheters available for commercial use. The first is rotational ICE devices, such as the UltraICEw catheter (Boston Scientific, Natick, Massachusetts) and the FORESIGHT ICE system (Conavi Medical, Toronto, Ontario, Canada) are not steerable and allow only near-field imaging so are used mainly for IAS procedures; these catheters are less expensive than the phased array devices.

Other category is phased-array ICE catheters, that are steerable and offer far-field imaging being so the imaging catheters of choice to guide SHD interventions. For TAVI monitoring, the steerable ICE catheter is introduced into the femoral vein and advanced through the inferior vena cava and the right atrium (RA). Utilization of a 45-cm-long 9 F or 10 F access sheath is recommended. While in the RA, 'Home View' is yielded; in addition to the 'Home View' (the Low RA position), three other standard cut planes have been defined for adequate monitoring and guidance during TAVI: longitudinal, short-axis, and transventricular views. The longitudinal view is considered the main ICE view and it is obtained from the cavo-atrial junction tilting the tip of catheter towards the adjacent ascending aorta. Placement of wires, catheters, and the valve mounted on a delivery balloon catheter can be precisely monitored.

4.3.4.5 Fusion Imaging

In most centres, preprocedural screening includes—besides echocardiography—investigations necessitating application of contrast media (coronary angiography, aortic root angiography, peripheral angiography, computed tomography). Increased risk of acute kidney injury (AKI) following TAVI is associated with poor outcomes and presence of CKD increases the incidence of kidney disorders after TAVI up to 30%. Efforts to reduce the amount of contrast before or during the procedure appear therefore beneficial. More, TAVI requires an X-ray angle where the aortic valve (AV) sinuses are aligned such that the virtual annulus is perpendicular to the fluoroscopy plane and hence to the TAVI device (coplanar view). This warrants accurate sitting of the valve prosthesis. Contrast is essential for aortic root angiography and prior multislice computed tomography (MSCT) is used to determine this coplanar view. To avoid this, the AV plane can be identified with echo-fluoro fusion and three fiducial markers can be placed in correspondence of the nadir of the three cusps (Figs. 4.25, 4.26, and 4.27), using the X-plane 2D view. The advantage is that by superimposing the echo images, the AV and the root become visible on the fluoroscopic screen and the angulation of C-arm can be gradually adjusted to obtain the correct view, coaligning the three markers on one plane. In high-risk patients with chronic kidney disease, measures to minimize the risk of acute disease during TAVI appear desirable, and the use of echo-fluoro fusion help to overcome this limitation (Fig. 4.28) [151].

4.3.5 Assessment

4.3.5.1 Introduction

After valve deployment, immediate assessment should be aimed to evaluate procedural success that means normal prosthetic valve position and function with no complications. This evaluation is performed combining information from different tools: angiography, fluoroscopy, cardiac catheterism, TTE, TEE, ICE [152, 153].

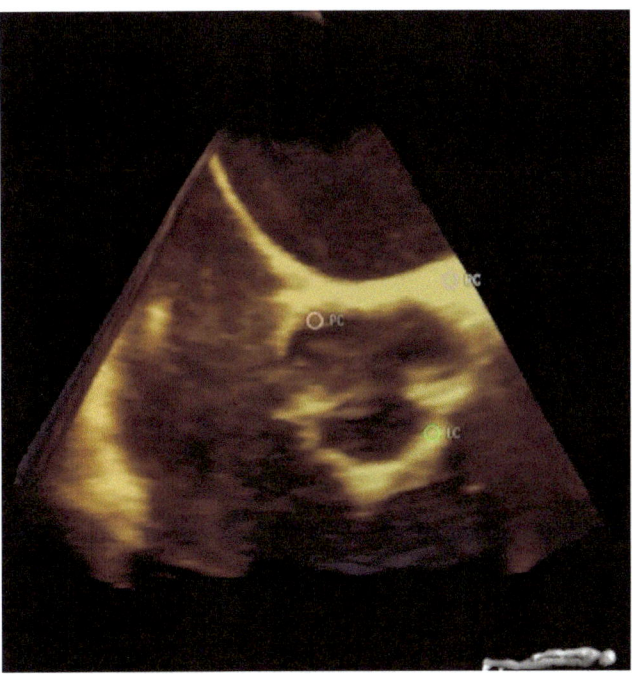
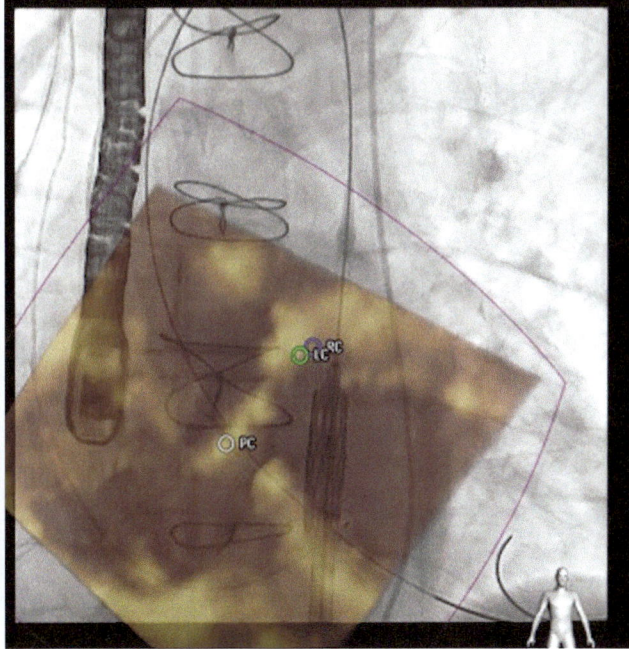

Fig. 4.25 Echo 3D-fluoro fusion imaging during a TAVI procedure. The delivery through the guidewire is performed retrogradely from the femoral vessel and the aorta, where the TAVI prosthesis is advanced towards the aortic annulus (echo overlayed on fluoro) through a Backup Meier guidewire

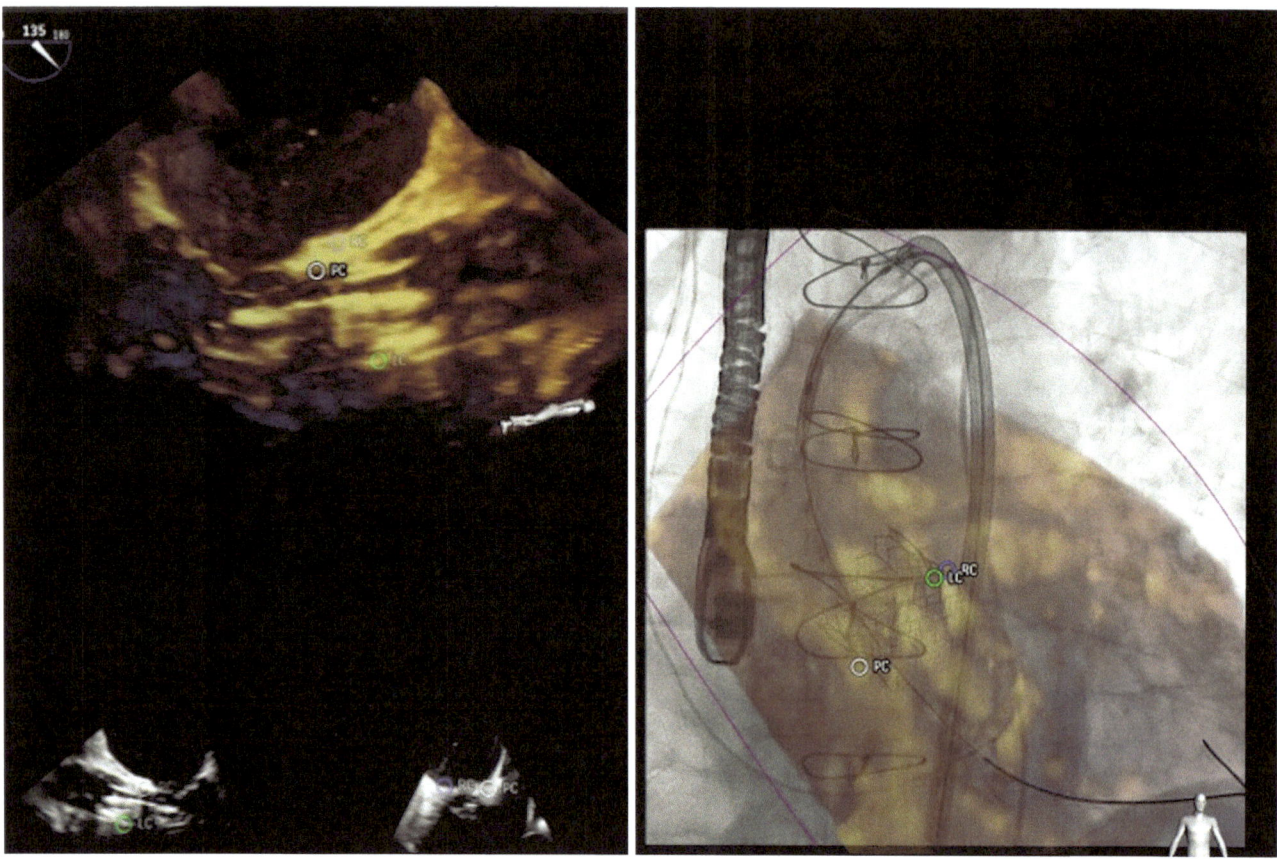

Fig. 4.26 Echo-fluoro fusion imaging during a TAVI procedure. The delivery through the wire is the next step, following the crossing of the valve

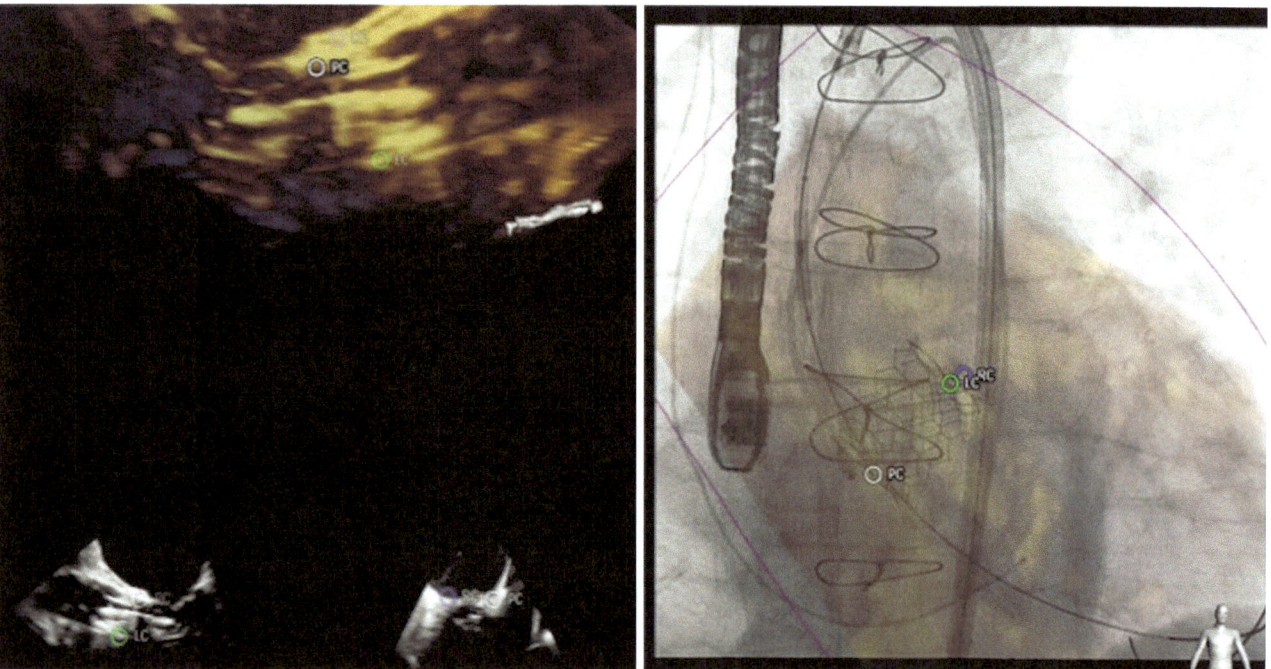

Fig. 4.27 Echo 3D-fluoro fusion imaging during a TAVI procedure. Final implantation of the transcatheter prosthesis, with a reduced degree of transparency of the 3D echo overlay on the fluoroscopy, to appreciate at its best the alignment of the prosthesis on the annulus

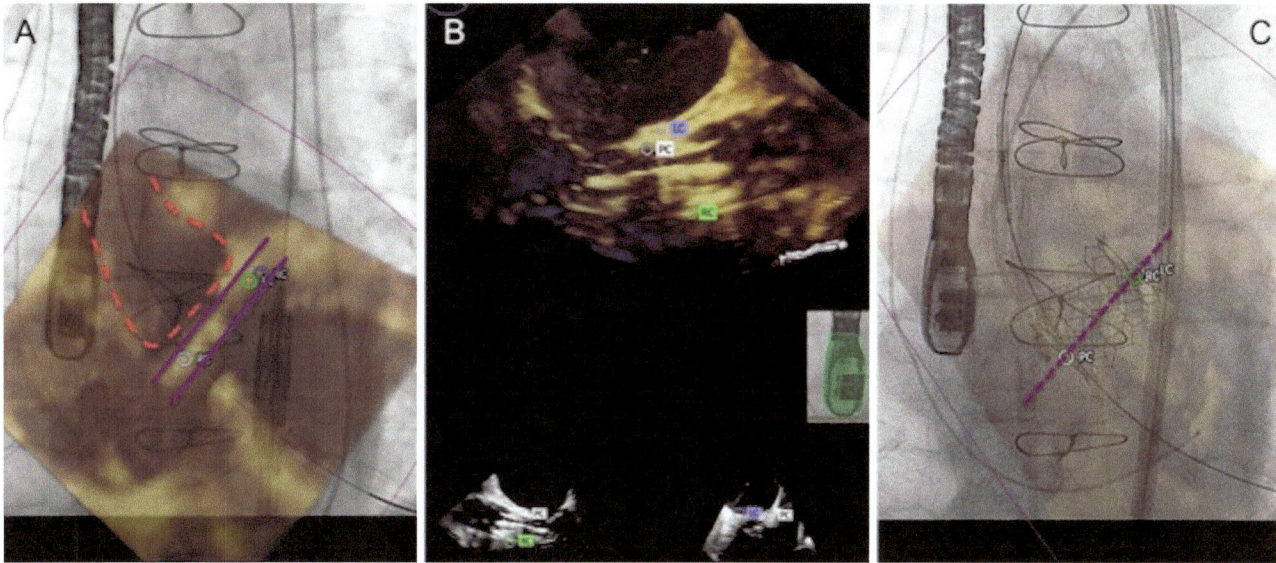

Fig. 4.28 Echo 3D-fluoro fusion imaging after TAVI implantation. The procedure was guided by fluoro and echo, without any need of contrast media. The contours of the aortic root (dotted red line, panel **a**) and of the aortic valve plane (violet line, panel **a** and **c**) are outlined to mark the structures of interest

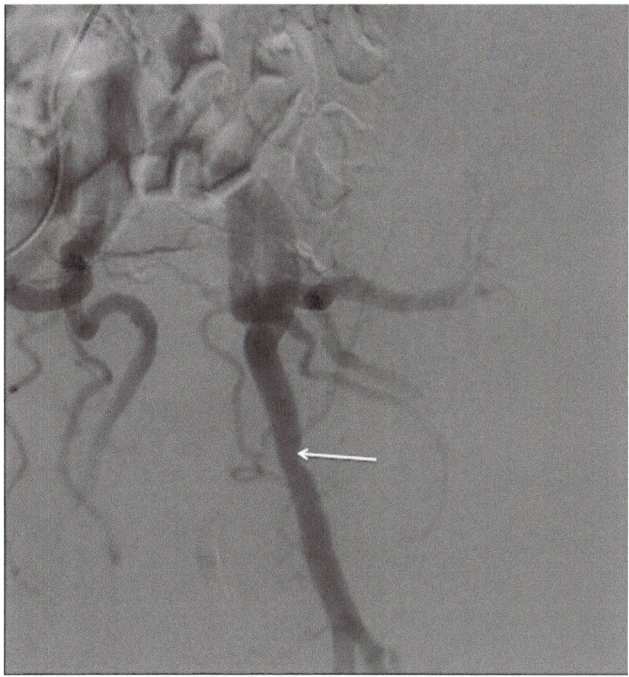

Fig. 4.29 Digital subtraction angiography showing no active bleeding from the left femoral artery access (arrow), after having used pre-closing systems

4.3.5.2 Angiography, Fluoroscopy, Catheterism

In case of incomplete expansion or PVL graded more than mild, post-dilatation is typically performed, usually with the same balloon used for pre-dilatation (size of the balloon should never be bigger than the nominal diameter of the native annulus). A 14F Sheath can be used to perform the post-dilation. Following removal of the delivery system, percutaneous closure with the previously implanted Proglides is

performed, checking with a contrast injection the final result (Fig. 4.29). An Angio Seal device may also be used in instances where residual femoral oozing is encountered following Proglides stitching.

4.3.5.3 TEE

Optimal position for the Edwards valve is with the ventricular side of the prosthesis positioned 2–4 mm below the annulus in the LVOT. CoreValve has a different structure so that the ventricular edge of the prosthesis should be placed 5–10 mm below the aortic valve annular plane. When the prosthesis is positioned too low, it may impinge on the mitral valve apparatus or it may embolize because of instability due to marked sub-aortic septal hypertrophy; on the other side, at the top of the prosthesis the native cusps are not completely included into the frame of prosthetic valve, so they can prejudge its functioning.

If the prosthesis is implanted too high, it may obstruct the coronary ostia, migrate up the aorta, or be associated with significant PVR. The 3DTEE is most useful immediately following valve deployment when the echocardiographer must rapidly and accurately assess the position and function of the valve including identifying the presence/severity of aortic regurgitation (Fig. 4.30).

Physiological mild valvular regurgitation may be transiently observed and usually occurs because the prosthetic valve is crossed by wire and delivery system and in case of balloon expandable valve it is crimped; so the cusps may not coapt completely immediately after deployment for a sort of "stunning" of the leaflets.

Transgastric TEE views with continuous-wave, pulsed-wave, and colour Doppler should be used to confirm satisfactory prosthetic functioning before the probe is finally

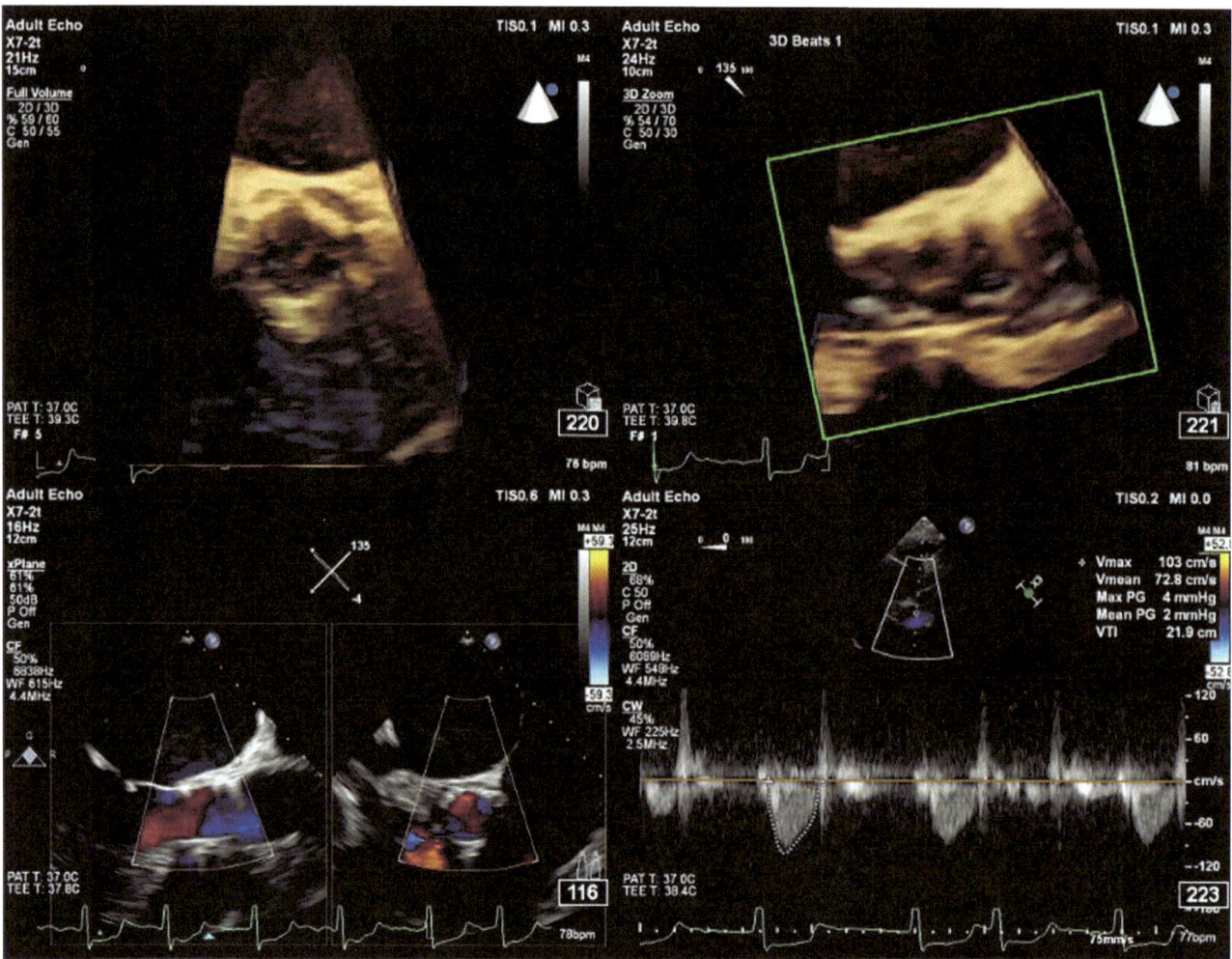

Fig. 4.30 Final echo assessment of a TAVI procedure

removed. Slatentization of LVOT obstruction can be detect and abnormal valve opening should be immediately recognized as well as the PVL.

PVL in TAVR is not infrequently with multiple jets and is commonly observed after TAVI because of the fact that a degenerate and calcified valve is hosting a new valve without any tissue removal or decalcification such in SAVR.

Conversely, severe aortic regurgitation may occur as a consequence of incomplete expansion or incorrect positioning of the device, or inappropriate prosthetic size. Severe asymmetric calcification of the native aortic valve have been related to incidence of severe PVL. In the setting of the immediate post-implantation assessment, conventional criteria including using colour jet dimensions, vena contracta, pressure half-time, and quantitative Doppler are helpful Three-dimensional TEE is an additional tool to define the severity and precise location of paravalvular and/or central regurgitation. Significant regurgitation may be an indication for repeat balloon inflation to attempt maximal expansion of the valve. Quantification of PVL after prosthetic valves has already been described in Sect. 4.2.3 for

evaluation after SAVR; it is applicable to TAVR too (Fig. 4.30).

4.3.5.4 TTE

Most cases of TAVR are currently performed using femoral access so that general anesthesia is not performed and TEE is not available immediately for procedural guidance and post procedural assessing of valve function. In these cases, TTE should be always immediately available for assessing outcomes when some troubles occur and are detected with aortic angiography. When complications is suspected because of aortography detection of severe AR, or arterial hypotension occur, immediate TTE can confirm or exclude the aetiology. Acoustic window in the context of immediate post deployment assessment can be not achievable easily, but TTE yields basic assessment for ruling out pericardial tamponade, LV dysfunction and regional motion, MR severity and acute mitral valve complication, severe aortic regurgitation.

Accurate evaluations are usually not allowed but a severe PVL is detected by a mean of different combined methods for rapid evaluations: high invasive differential aortic pressure, holo-diastolic flow reversal with pulsed Doppler in descending aorta, large color jet of AR, early severe diastolic flow during aortography. These methods facilitate a rapid assessment and help decide whether post-dilatation of the prosthesis is necessary to improve the fit of the valve into the aortic annulus.

4.3.5.5 ICE

After THV deployment, from the home view (low RA position) the short-axis view is obtained with the catheter in the RA and the tip tilted by 90° towards the aortic annulus to rule out annulus dissection and to check for transvalvular and paravalvular leak and quantification by color Doppler by the same semi-quantitative measurement according ratio between total circumferential extent of regurgitant flow and circumference of the left ventricular outflow tract. Tilting the tip towards TV and advance the catheter into the right ventricle (RV) until "RV outflow position", long-axis view of the left ventricle (which is similar to a parasternal long-axis TTE view) allows to image mitral valve, the valvular apparatus, left ventricular cavity, and left ventricular outflow tract (Fig. 4.5).

4.3.5.6 Fusion Imaging

According to a recent study, fusion imaging of pre- and post-TAVI CTA can be used to allow an exact evaluation of TAVI prosthesis position in relation to the native annulus plane. A low TAVI position as assessed by fusion imaging is therefore associated with the development of new conduction disturbances post-TAVI [154].

4.3.6 Troubleshooting

4.3.6.1 Intro (Differential Diagnosis in Case of Hypertension)

The value of intra-procedural TEE is predicted to diminish in the future, since minimalist approach is nowadays used in many centres, consisting of a mild sedation, local anaesthesia, peripheral access (mainly femoral). In this context, positioning of intra-oesophageal probe is not possible, and it is used only when a transapical access is planned. However is desirable that sites using this minimalist approach should be only higher procedural volumes. Otherwise, mortality after TAVR can be higher despite a lower risk population is included, making this approach having no clinical sense [155, 156].

An echocardiographic analysis of complications during TAVR from PARTNER trials including 527 patients has been published and has revealed a total prevalence of 9% of complications.

They included access site complications, aortic root trauma, coronary obstruction, malpositioning of the prosthetic valve and PVL, ventricular septal or mitral leaflet perforation; these complications can evolve immediately in emergency like pericardial tamponade and cardiogenic shock.

The advent of **severe hypotension** following valve deployment is a life-threatening condition and the prompt and accurate diagnosis of the underlying problem has a pivotal role. After aortic TAVR, the differential diagnosis that must be pointed out in case of hemodynamic collapse are: acute severe valve dysfunction (mainly AR), aortic rupture or dissection, coronary obstruction, LV dysfunction.

Beyond etiological cause, when these complications cause acute haemodynamic crash, an immediate stabilization can be reached using urgent pericardiocentesis in case of pericardial tamponade and supporting circulatory function with extracorporeal life support (ECLS, Extracorporeal membrane oxygenation, ECMO). In this case immediate venous and arterial access should be needed. So, when risk of complications at pre-procedural assessment is definite as high, preventive measures should be adopted: TEE guided procedures and predisposed additive vascular accessed to be used in case of complications.

When acute collapse occurs, TTE can be immediately used to assess presence of pericardial effusion (Fig. 4.31 Panel a and b), acute LV severe impairment (global or regional); diagnosis of acute prosthetic valve severe dysfunction, acute damage of mitral valve (severe MR, chordae or papillary muscle rupture, leaflet perforation), ventricular septal defect, acute aortic rupture can be sometimes reached with early TTE, but usually required TEE.

While the TTE is performed and hemodynamic support is maintained, TEE probe is positioned and allows accurate diagnosis of complications. When TEE is available, immediate assessment of biventricular function, aortic root integrity, coronary patency, pericardial effusion, interventricular septum, valvular (mitral, prosthetic, tricuspid, and pulmonic) morphology/function must be ruled out.

Hypovolemia can be diagnosed easily by comparing ventricular size with baseline imaging when available; if they are not available, venous collapse and protodiastolic transmitral Doppler velocity can be useful.

While hypovolemia, mainly due to bleeding, can occur at different procedural phase, for all the other complications, **the specific time-point of procedure** in which the complication occurs can be an important tool for suspecting a specific diagnosis.

1. **Wire Location.** When acute respiratory failure or hemodynamic collapse occurs in this phase, the most common cause to be excluded are:
   - entanglement in mitral apparatus
   - perforation of left ventricle, interventricular septum;
   - right ventricle perforation when pace maker lead is placed

Fig. 4.31 Pericardial tamponade by TTE in subcostal view (**a**) and TEE in transgastric view (**b**)

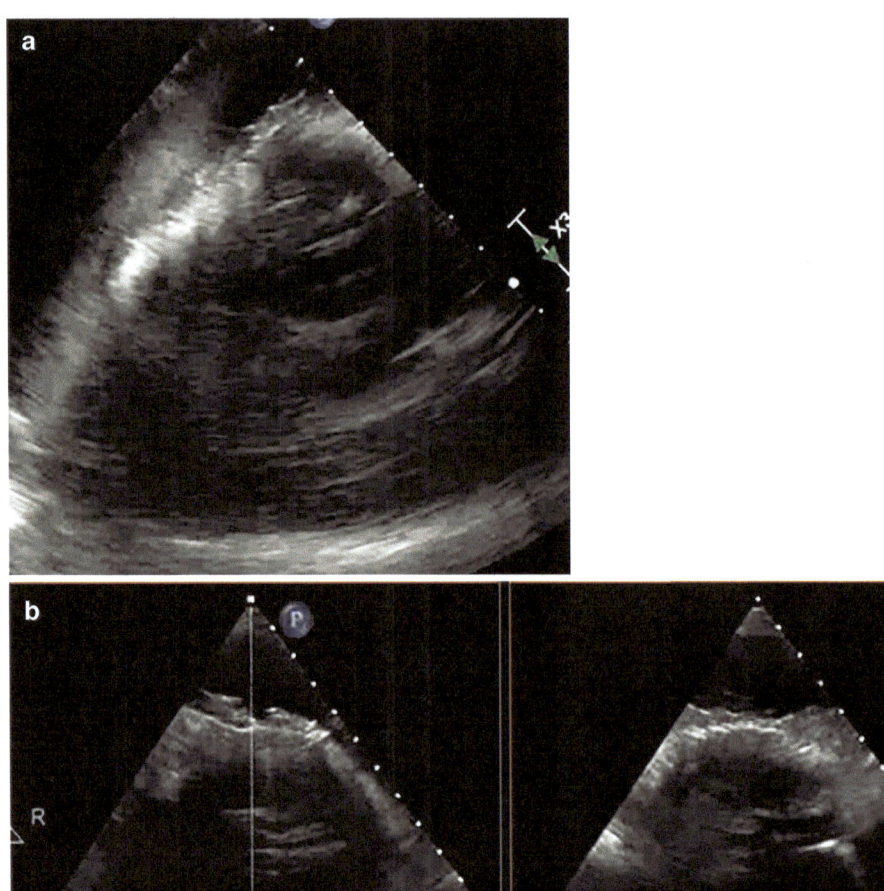

– During trans-apical approach, acute myocardial infarction can occur for direct compromise of distal coronary flow [157–159].

2. **Balloon valvuloplasty**. Complications In this phase can be:

– Torrential acute aortic regurgitation due to avulsion of native valve (irreversible), displacement of cusps and stunning of one or more cusps that are pushed onto the aortic sinus wall (reversible usually spontaneously). An immediate deployment of the THV is usually indicated.

– Aortic annulus and root complicacies. The cusps crimped toward aortic root, especially when this last one is very calcified can increase the risk for aortic injury, hematoma and rupture.

– Under-deployment of valve due to balloon rupture; this is caused by speckles of calcium and leads to acute aortic regurgitation and high risk of acute embolization.

– Coronary occlusion: the mechanism is direct obstruction by the calcified left coronary cusp; the risk has been associated with female sex, small aortic root (sinus diameter 27.8 ± 2.0 mm), and height of the left main coronary above the annulus [160].

– In patients with significantly reduced baseline left or right ventricular function, the 5–10 s of low forward flow due to rapid pacing may be sufficient to cause significant global or regional ischemia, leading to cardiac arrest/pulseless electrical activity; prolonging the time between BAV and TAVR is a good strategy for prevention of this complication.

3. **Valve deployment**

– Aortic annulus and root complicacy. More frequently this is seen after BAV that make the first injury to aortic wall.

– Malposition and failure to implant. Evidence suggest that this is the most frequently reported reason for emergent bailout surgery (41% of interventions). Malposition of device can cause paravalvular aortic regurgitation (PAR), mitral valve compromise, and conduction defects, with hemodynamic instability. The risk factors for malposition are: marked septal hypertrophy (narrow anatomic LVOT), transfemoral access (less control on movements).

– Coronary occlusion by native leaflets can occur in this phase if BAV is not performed before [161, 162].

Table 4.10 summarized the most important complication occurring during TAVR, risk factors and management.

Table 4.10 Imaging aims for Procedural Guidance (TEE, fluoroscopy, fusion imaging and ICE)

Procedural steps	
Access and delivery	In all type of access, evaluation of LV wire movements for avoiding entanglement in the mitral valve apparatus
	For transapical approach: exclusion of LV thrombus, guiding the correct positioning of access into LV apex
Valvuloplasty	Appreciation of balloon size fits into the valve annulus fitting
	Determination and live visualization of space within the sinuses to accommodate calcified leaflets during valvuloplasty
	Imaging of coronary ostia to determine risk of obstruction
	Detection of severe regurgitation post-valvuloplasty
Valve deployment	3D appears better than 2D TEE for visualizing balloon-expandable valves
	Ensure that the top of a balloon-expandable valve cage is high enough to just cover the native valve leaflets (1–2 mm over the end of cusps); overhang of native leaflet must be diagnosed and quantified for predicting risk of acute and delay migration of valve
	Monitoring the operator independent movements due to LVOT dynamic narrowing during deployment (especially for self-expandable valves)
	Coaxiality assessment between prosthesis and native AV
Post deployment assessment	
	Aortic regurgitation intraprosthesis
	Prosthesis malpositioning
	Paravalvar regurgitation
Complications	Myocardial ischaemia
	Coronary occlusion
	Mitral regurgitation: damage to the valve leaflets or subvalvar apparatus
	Pericardial effusion
	LV or RV perforation
	Unmasked LV dynamic obstruction
	Aortic dissection or root rupture

4.3.6.2 Pericardial Tamponade

4.3.6.2.1 Intro

Cardiac tamponade has been reported in 1.8–4.3% of patients after TAVI, depending on population characteristics, type of implanted prosthesis and procedural aspects. According to VARC criteria, pericardial tamponade could be considered a "surrogate" of procedural complications, since its impact on mortality (all cause and cardiovascular cause) has been related to the specific aetiology determining the pericardial effusion [152].

Indeed, the most frequent cause has been found to be RV perforation due to pacemaker leads; this complication can be treated with pericardiocentesis with good results, without increasing procedural mortality. RV perforation occurs more frequently in case of screw-in lead pacing rather than passive lead.

Other causes of tamponade can be the perforations in the arterial side: annular/supra-annular ruptures and LV perforations; in these cases open surgery is usually needed and mortality has been reported around 50%. In a single center experience with TAVR, pericardial tamponade after TAVI has been related to patient-related and technical-procedural aspects [163].

With regard to patient risk factors (unavoidable), annular size, annular calcification, commissural calcification must all be thoroughly evaluated before the procedure because they have been associated to more incidence of tamponade causing annular tear.

Annular tear can occur during BAV (balloon expandable valves) or during valve post-dilatation (all types of valves); post-hoc analysis of preoperative CT revealed that annular tear is related to annular size and distribution of calcifications (mainly in case of speckle calcification of commissures). In case of hemodynamic collapse with TTE or TEE revealing pericardial tamponade, aortography shows extravasation of contrast around the aortic annulus when annular tear is the cause.

LV perforation (including perforation of papillary muscles and interventricular septum) can be the result of excessive wire stiffening in case of small LV size, marked LV hypertrophy, and concomitant myocardial ischemia/scar tissue. A method for reducing this complication has been described and consists into covering the distal part of wire with a pig-tail catheter to make it less aggressive ("cushioned stiff").

Aortic dissection/aortic hematoma can be caused by the same mechanism of LV perforation, when the stiffened wire is advanced especially in case of aortic atheromasia and increased vascular stiffness (Figs. 4.11 and 4.32). Pericardial tamponade can occur in case of aortic acute injury and it has a poor prognostic significance.

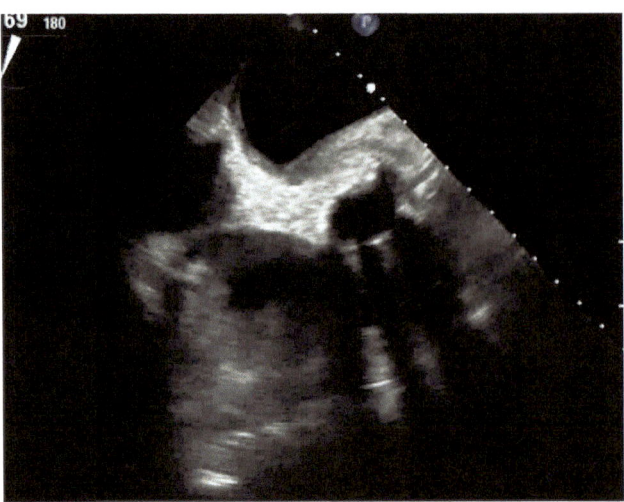

Fig. 4.32 Type A aortic root hematoma (posterior thickening of aortic wall >7 mm, with compression of lumen)

From therapeutic standpoint, when a cardiac chamber is perforated by a wire, if possible, the perforating catheter should not be removed until the fluid is drained and the pericardial sac is secured with another catheter in case the perforation can cause increased bleeding into the pericardium [164].

Depending on the type, size, and location of the cardiac lesion, if percutaneous puncture and drainage are successful, the perforating catheter can be withdrawn and surgery avoided by prompt drainage and auto-transfusion of pericardial blood. However, if the patient is still unstable, surgical repair should not be further deferred.

4.3.6.2.2 TEE
The TEE can be of help in the diagnosis of pericardial tamponade only and exclusively to evaluate and quantify the posterior (rare) effusions. Usually the organized formations (fibrin with clotted blood) near the left atrium and/or posterior to the right atrium can benefit from this more invasive methodic

4.3.6.2.3 TTE
Pericardial effusion is diagnosed as a collection of fluid within pericardial sac, with clinical manifestations depending on timing of accumulation and amount of fluid. Pericardial tamponade is the worst complication of pericardial effusion and it happens when the fluid compromise RV filling by a mean of equalisation of intra-pericardial pressures with right chambers pressure (typically around 15–20 mmHg); this cause cardiogenic shock and is a life treating condition.

Of most importance, diagnosis of pericardial tamponade is clinical. When hemodynamic instability occurs during TAVR, echocardiographic evaluation is needed and the

first approach when TEE is not available (minimalist procedure setting, without TEE) should be TTE (Fig. 4.31 Panel a and b).

Specific findings are: large pericardial effusion (>20 mm, >500 mL) occasionally with some clots inside (hemopericardium), RV systolic collapse and diastolic collapse, reciprocal respiratory changes in RV and LV volumes only during spontaneous ventilation (pulsus paradoxus): fall in arterial pressure during inspiration due to increased filling of RV, shift of interventricular septum and reduced LV filling (transmitral doppler echocardiographic finding can confirm this hemodynamic behaviour); plethora of inferior vena cava (IVC); these last two findings are not yielded by TTE or TEE when mechanical ventilation is ongoing [165].

As soon as possible, TEE is needed for detecting cause and starting appropriate treatment. First of all ME views of LV or TG views can detect RV or LV perforation. Then, aortic annulus tear and aortic dissection should be excluded. If RV is perforated, percutaneous drainage is usually sufficient to allow stabilization; when LV is perforated or aortic annulus is fractured, surgical approach should be undertaken.

In all these conditions, because of instability of haemodynamic, an emergent procedure is mandatory [166, 167].

Right ventricular perforation from the pacing wire may be undetected until removal of the wire. At that time, rapid but focal accumulation of pericardial blood is seen at intraprocedural imaging.

Perforation of the left ventricle is typically seen immediately, with accumulation of relatively echo-dense pericardial effusion (blood). It could appear during stiffed wire navigation into LV or after cardiopulmonary resuscitation if the wire and the BAV catheter are crushed up onto LV wall. **Echocardiographic or angiographic detection** of arterial/LV perforation is needed because aortic dissection and perforation of LV free wall (arterial side perforation) are indications for urgent surgical drainage that should not be delayed in any way by pericardiocentesis (percutaneous drainage of pericardial effusion) [168].

4.3.6.2.4 Pericardial Puncture Guidance
Pericardiocentesis is the first useful therapeutic procedure for the early management or diagnosis of large, symptomatic pericardial effusion and cardiac tamponade. The effect of pericardiocentesis is immediate: increase in stroke volume, reduction of intrapericardial and atrial pressures, and separation between right and left filling pressures [166].

The techniques recommended for a safe and successful pericardiocentesis have changed considerably, particularly with the introduction of fluoroscopic, electrocardiographic and, finally, echocardiographic guidance and with the description of approaches other than the substernal: apical and parasternal [167].

The aimed location for pericardiocentesis is the one closest to the largest amount of the effusion. Therefore TTE or TEE can better identify the most suitable approach, that in most cases is subxiphoid or apical. Indeed, the most serious complications of pericardiocentesis are the laceration and perforation of the myocardium and the coronary vessels, that occur rarely in echoguided procedure (1.5% in subxifoideal approach). In order to prevent laceration, no lateral movements of the needle should be made while approaching the effusion [169].

Guidelines recommend that echocardiography is mandatory to guide pericardiocentesis and select the approach (intercostal vs. subxiphoid), except in case of life-threatening tamponade.

However, when clinical conditions are rapidly worsening **in the context of acute complication after TAVR,** if TTE or TEE is not immediately available, fluoroscopy can be considered for early diagnosis and rescue pericardiocentesis in iatrogenic effusions. The fluoroscopic approach is performed through the subxiphoid approach with a needle containing a contrast medium, directed toward the left shoulder at an angle of 30° to the skin. The contrast agent medium injection, can immediately confirm position in the pericardial space: the appearance of a layering of the contrast inferiorly indicates the correct position; then a soft guidewire can be introduced; then, it is essential to check the guidewire position in at least two angiographic projections (lateral view and anterior-posterior view) [164].

An echocardiographic examination to assess the distribution of pericardial effusion should always precede the fluoroscopy-guided procedure, whenever possible. If not possible, TTE and TEE, however, should be promptly obtained for monitoring complications during the manoeuvre. This type of urgent pericardiocentesis is called "Echo-assisted" (in contrast with "Echo-guided"): the phase of insertion of the needle it is not directly monitored by TTE/TEE but they are used for ruling out any peri-procedural complications. Moreover, visualisation of the needle within the pericardial space allows confirmation of reaching the space, avoiding repeated punctures when the needle is inserted in hemorrhagic pericardial sac. Indeed, in 20–40% of cases of haemorrhagic effusion, no fluid can be seen, because of rapid formation of clots, which impede aspiration of blood [170].

4.3.6.3 LV Dysfunction

4.3.6.3.1 Intro

LV dysfunction is often present before TAVR. This is due to a combination of valvular and ischemic aetiology. Especially in case of ischaemic aetiology, the risk of a marked decline in the pump function of LV should be taken into account before procedure and should lead to take care in phase of rapid pacing and BAV, in which **imbalance between demand and supply of oxygen is unavoidable.** This "myocardial stunning" is a reversible condition than can last some minutes and required inotropic support. Ventricular arrhythmia can occur and are promptly treated with defibrillation.

Moreover, at each time LV dysfunction can occur as result of **direct injury** of wire and catheters to the LV wall at each level. Intra-**cardiac abnormal communication** can be created after perforation of the cardiac tissue at the proximal or distal border of the THV. They are mostly related to significant offending calcific protrusion near the edge of the stent. Indeed, more frequently, septal defect in membranous part occurs at the proximal ventricular edge of the bioprosthesis when calcium extends into the LVOT from the right coronary cusp or commissure between the right coronary cusp and the non-coronary cusp. Often, rupture of the septum in this region results in malapposition of the edge of the THV, so PVL may accompany this complication.

Rare **cases of muscular ventricular septal defects have** also been reported after transapical implantation of the THV [99, 100]. This complication is **due to direct perforation** by the apical cannula and is avoidable with imaging of the cannulation site before apical puncture.

Intraprocedural treatment of this complications is limited given the proximity to the new bioprosthesis, so surgery is required. An immediate stabilization can be reached using mechanical circulatory device (Extracorporeal membrane oxygenation, ECMO) [171, 172].

4.3.6.3.2 TEE

LV function should be immediately assessed in case of hypotension, after having excluded hypovolemic status (bleeding). Visual assessment of LV function compared with baseline images available is a rapid method and should always be combined with ECG findings and derived functional Doppler parameters.

The best view for having a rapid assessment of global LV function using TEE are TG views at basal and medial level; for regional motion, ME views are needed. Computation of SV can be rapidly assessed by pulsed Doppler through LVOT.

When intracardiac perforation occurs and a interventricular defects happens, spectral Doppler flow profiles may have prominent diastolic flow, as well as typical systolic flow. The diastolic flow is a result of PVL that usually accompany this situation after TAVR: flow from the aorta crosses the ventricular septal defect; the systolic flow is a result of the typical ventricular left-to-right flow.

4.3.6.4 Aortic Dissection

4.3.6.4.1 Intro

Aortic complications can occur as a result of the TAVR procedure, including aortic dissections, thoracic aorta perforation with resulting hemorrhage, and aortic annular rupture. **All these complication** may occur immediately (intraprocedural) or become evident later and they can be mainly due to the traumatic injury of the procedure itself: during BAV, introducing catheter, deployment of the valve, post dilatation or displacement of speckles of calcium during procedure.

4.3.6.4.2 TEE

When **acute aortic dissection** extends into the sinuses of Valsalva, it can lead to acute tamponade necessitating open repair but often with a poor outcome (Fig. 4.11). Some dissections may be undiagnosed at the time of implantation, suggesting a more benign complication. Especially when the dissection flap extended to the sinotubular junction but not into the sinuses, a conservative approach can be attempted.

Echocardiographic detection of aortic flap is needed for diagnosis; extension should be immediately clarified (Fig. 4.11): ME and UE aortic views with 2DTEE and 3DTEE real time modality are useful (Table 4.3).

Rupture of the AV annulus is a rare complication of TAVR (<1% of cases) and it is manifested with pericardial tamponade [173, 174].

In these cases, urgent surgery is necessary. Rarely, the injury is limited, no hemodynamic instability occurs and there is no evidence of pericardial tamponade but only local effusion; in such cases a conservative approach may be attempted. Correct any coagulopathy and closely monitor the patient with serial imaging (usually CT) [175, 176].

TEE before intervention and peri-intervention should assess presence of the most important risk factors for aortic annular rupture: moderate/severe LVOT/sub-annular calcifications; simultaneous multiplane imaging allows an accurate assessment of this factor. In such condition of risk, careful prosthesis sizing and avoidance of oversizing >20% are important modifiable factors to be considered. Of more interest, it has to be pointed out that this issue is still a challenge because usually the presence of subannular calcifications leads itself to increased prosthesis malapposition and PVL, that can be fixed with balloon postdilation. For risk of annular rupture, a risk/benefit analysis should be performed when assessing the possible effectiveness of re-ballooning [177].

Periaortic hematoma is a complication with a reported single-site incidence of 1.6% can be managed medically if recognized early. **Microrupture of the external layers of aortic wall is detected as a tissue-density mass around the outside of the aortic root. Usually it is associated with annular overdistension and pericardial effusion.**

Periaortic hematoma must be diagnosed for modulating medical management (periinterventional administration of protamine, continued intubation with restricted activity, and meticulous blood pressure control), **in order to avoid complications in the same site of aortic injury**.

More unfavourable complication is **intramural hematoma (IMH)**, which is a contained aortic wall hematoma with bleeding within the media but without initial intimal flap formation. It is detected as local thickening within aortic wall and, similar to acute aortic dissection, it is classified as Stanford type A (ascending aorta) or B (exclusive involvement of the descending aorta).

Natural history of IMH is variable; it may be reabsorbed without any intervention, or it may progress to classic aortic dissection, with outward aortic rupture observed in 15–20% of patients. IMH converts to acute aortic dissection in 3–14% of patients with involvement of the descending aorta and in 88% of those with involvement of the ascending aorta. As in case of aortic dissection, it is generally recommended that patients with type A IMH undergo early surgery, whereas patients with type B IMH can be managed conservatively in the absence of complications [88].

4.3.6.5 Coronary Occlusion

4.3.6.5.1 Intro

As previously detailed, pre-procedural risk assessment for coronary obstruction is yielded mainly by evaluation of calcium amount and extension, aortic dimensions, relation between coronary ostia height and leaflet length (Figs. 4.5, 4.14, and 4.24). Evidence suggest an incidence of coronary occlusion ranging from 0.0 to 4.1%. When the risk is not low, BAV can be used for assessment this occurrence before valve deployment.

Acute manifestations can be: LV failure, LV regional abnormal motion, ECG changes (ST-segment elevation and ventricular arrhythmias).

In the context of TAVR, coronary obstruction can occur immediately after valve implantation (83.3%) or, rarely in the first few hours after the procedure (8.3%), or within the first 2 days after the procedure (8.3%).

Coronary obstruction occurs more frequently in the left coronary artery (LCA) (reported incidence of 83.3%) and can be successfully treated with percutaneous coronary intervention.

The main cause of coronary obstruction in acute context is the displacement of calcified cusps into the coronary ostium. The aetiologies of delayed coronary occlusion are theoretical. Late embolization of calcium or low flow with thrombus formation seem plausible. Aortic root complications can result in coronary artery distortion and low flow with increased thrombosis risk [178].

4.3.6.5.2 TEE

Characterizing "at-risk" anatomy is of paramount importance in avoiding the complication of coronary occlusion.

This is aimed before intervention by a combination of MSCT evaluation and TEE. When TEE is available for procedural guidance, 2D modality is able to define the annular-ostial distance for the right coronary and 3DTEE with multiplanar reconstruction of coronal plane allows evaluation of Left main coronary ostium. Immediate post-TAVR imaging of coronary occlusion by using 2D echocardiography and color Doppler with associated regional wall motion abnormalities may prompt confirmation with coronary angiography.

4.3.6.6 Acute Valve Dysfunction

4.3.6.6.1 Intro

Valve Academic Research Consortium-2 recommends to use echocardiography as the primary imaging modality for the assessment of prosthetic valve function. This should include the valve position, morphology, function, and evaluation of the left ventricle (LV) and right ventricle (RV) size and function.

Proposed criteria by Valve Academic Research Consortium (VARC) to evaluate impaired prosthetic valve performance are: (1) prosthetic valve haemodynamics assessed by echocardiography and (2) associated clinical findings. Serial echocardiography evaluations after surgical AVR and TAVI should be performed at baseline, soon after the index procedure (ideally within 24–48 h), at 1 month (especially for TAVI), 12 months, and yearly thereafter. In addition to echocardiography, during follow up multi-slice computed tomography may also provide useful insights on pathobiological mechanisms of device malfunction such as valve subclinical thrombosis and deterioration.

Recent guidelines for evaluation of prosthetic valve function recommend different echocardiographic measurements to assess prosthetic dysfunction. Table 4.6 summarized the main parameters that should be evaluated.

Aortic Regurgitation

It is important to distinguish between post-TAVR paravalvular leak (PVL) and central aortic regurgitation since the approach to treatment of these two entities are different.

Paravalvular Aortic Regurgitation/leak (PVL) is associated to increased late mortality. Factors associated to significant PVL have been found to be: (1) undersizing of the annulus; (2) severity of aortic calcification; (3) implantation depth [120, 179, 180].

Management of PVL depends mainly on the severity of the jet but also on other findings that should be carefully assessed by TEE evaluation after TAVR.

If PVL is greater than mild and the cause is malposition, then other complications should be detected by TEE, such as perforation of surrounding structures (annulus and membranous septum). Fully retrievable prosthesis should be chosen in case of high risk for malposition (calcification, anatomy of LVOT).

If the prosthesis is normal positioned but it is under-expanded, then in the setting of low-risk "landing zone" (i.e., no bulky calcium in the LVOT or annulus), a post-dilation or a valve-in-valve procedure may then be warranted. If there is a significant risk of rupture or the risk of central regurgitation from overexpansion is high, then no further intervention may be warranted (Fig. 4.33) summarize these steps.

Central aortic regurgitation following TAVR may occur. Recent evidence suggest that it may be due to leaflet malfunction in 54% of cases, malpositioning in 41% of cases, and unknown causes in 5% of cases. If significant, it requires placement of a second valve or a valve in valve procedure.

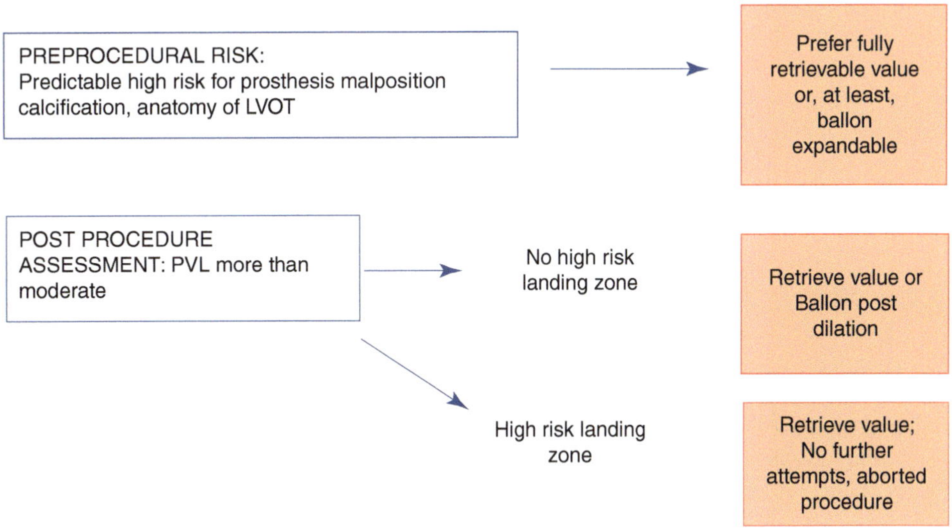

Fig. 4.33 Acute management of PVL

Native leaflet overhanging, calcium speckles protrusion into prosthetic frame, tilted native valve are possible causes of significant central AR. Prosthetic leaflet traumatism occurs usually when the wire is across the valve and this stunning of leaflets can be solved by removing wire and leaving time to restore motion. When leaflet eversion is detected, the placement of a pigtail catheter in each of the sinuses of the prosthetic valve may help in ameliorating the central insufficiency. When valve-in-valve is performed in the setting of PAR, the etiology was most commonly malpositioning [181].

Aortic gradient has been rarely found after TAVR implantation and usually it is associated to paravalvular leak. Patient prosthesis mismatch can be immediately detected when it is severe and it should require immediate intervention.

4.3.6.6.2 Gradient

Intro

Abnormal gradient can be found after TAVR implantation, since different from surgical AVR, here the native valve is left outside the prosthetic valve. Indeed, degeneration of prosthetic valve have been carefully assessed and described at follow up.

Normally, in acute phase immediately after implantation transvalvular gradient is affected by hemodynamic conditions (LV function and load), and concomitant PVL regurgitant volume when present. Indeed, the most important causes of high gradients after TAVI could be malpositioning and under-expansion and they cause concomitant severe AR. Hemodynamic assessment can be useful in this intraprocedural phase for confirming abnormal gradient; fluoroscopy can identify the underexpanded valves and echocardiographic findings should aim to understand underlying mechanisms of abnormal gradients.

Therefore, a specific condition can be immediately detected: patient prosthesis mismatch, that occurs when prosthetic size is relatively small for that patient.

Echo

Doppler echocardiography is the cornerstone of noninvasive hemodynamic assessment of any valvular prosthesis. Similar to surgically implanted bioprostheses, quantitative hemodynamic assessment relies on flow-dependent and flow-independent parameters, but different from surgical bioprosthesis, for transcatheter valves a specific characteristic should be taken into account: in-stent flow acceleration occurs at two levels (subvalvular and post-cusp). Therefore, LVOT diameter and flow should be measured at the inferior edge of the stent.

Furthermore, final hemodynamic performance depends on the type/size of prosthesis, native valvular anatomy, and procedural variables. In this context, establishing a "normal range" is challenging, and comparisons to the baseline hemodynamic characteristics of the TAV become paramount in determining valve function. As with any other aortic valve Doppler assessment, peak aortic velocity and mean AV gradient should be measured; for TEE assessment, TG view are often needed. EOA and DVI are then calculated according to the standard guidelines [153, 182, 183].

Suggested normal values for optimal outcome after TAVR are AVA >1.1 cm^2, and DVI >0.35; however, these values may need adjustment in the case of extreme body sizes.

By a mean of the combination of different parameters we can differentiate different states:

– AV obstruction: High gradient and reduced DVI and EOA/EOAi; in this case abnormal cusps motion need to be detected.
– High flow condition: High gradient and normal DVI and EOA/EOAi
– Patient-prosthesis mismatch: High gradient, normal DVI, normal EOA, but reduced EOAi.

Prosthesis-patient mismatch is s present when the effective orifice area of the inserted prosthetic valve is too small in relation to body size. Indexed EOA is the only parameter that has been found to consistently correlate with postoperative gradient. It has been related to poor early and long-term outcomes, mainly due to higher cardiovascular mortality and less regression of LV hypertrophy [184].

ICE

When aortic valve obstruction is suspected after TAVR, ICE can be used to clarify the mechanism involved. The most important view is the low RA position with catheter tilted toward aortic annulus, that allow short axis of aortic valve to be yielded. In this position, perfect visualization of prosthetic cusps allow to identify: morphological abnormalities and reduced movements.

4.3.6.6.3 Regurgitation

Intro

Appropriate quantitation of the severity of PVL and thus appropriate intra-procedural treatment remains challenging. Recent guidelines suggest numerous qualitative and semi-quantitative parameters for assessing surgical prosthetic leaks [185, 186].

Irregular shape, and the number of paravalvular jets seen after TAVR makes assessment using these traditional methods poor reliable. Indeed, the most important semiquantitative parameter suggested for evaluation of PVL is circumferential extent of the jet, but it has been poor validated after TAVR. Indeed, the updated VARC-2 (Valve Academic Research Consortium) consensus document **uses different**

cut-offs for this parameter: no PAR (no regurgitant color flow), a trace (pinpoint jet in AV short axis view), mild (jet arc length is <10% of the AV annulus short axis view circumference), moderate (jet arc length is 10–30% of the AV annulus short axis view circumference), and severe (jet arc length is >30% of the AV annulus short axis view circumference) [153].

Recent studies using cardiac magnetic resonance (CMR) confirm the limitations of echocardiographic methods mainly due to high interobserver variability of AR and risk of echocardiographic underestimation of PVL entity using multiparametric approach (by one grade in 59.5% and by two grades in 2.4% of evaluations), and overestimation of PVL entity using semiquantitative approach in 38% of cases.

Echo

The qualitative, semiquantitative and quantitative haemodynamic assessment of AR severity should be performed with Doppler echocardiography according to the guidelines. All prosthetic aortic valve regurgitation criteria should be assessed by the following measurements: (1) valve structure and motion and LV function (this last one is more important for chronic follow up of prosthetic valve); (2) qualitative evaluation of amount of color jet and location. 2DTEE in ME SAX VIEW and TTE in parasternal SAX view are the most useful for localization. 3DTEE color flow images, when optimization of display is possible through adjustment of gain and framerate, are useful for evaluating width of 3D vena contracta by multiplanar reconstruction; however, these parameters are not validated as for native valve assessment; (3) Colour Doppler evaluation.

It should be performed just below the valve stent for paravalvular jets, and at the coaptation point of the leaflets for central regurgitation. Although all imaging windows should be used, the parasternal long and short-axis view for TTE and ME AV SAX and LAX view for TEE are critical in assessing the number and severity of paravalvular jets. Semiquantitative parameters are: Jet width (%LVOT diameter) (evaluable only for central jets), continuous wave (CW) Doppler density, deceleration rate (PHT, ms), ratio between PW aortic and pulmonary, descending aorta diastolic flow reversal, circumferential extent of paraprosthetic AR (% of circumference). Whenever possible, the quantification of the prosthetic regurgitant volume, effective regurgitant orifice area, and regurgitant fraction should be performed. The regurgitant volume may be calculated as the difference between the stroke volume across any non-regurgitant orifice (RVOT or mitral valve) and the stroke volume across the LVOT (Table 4.6).

ICE

In the context of intraprocedural evaluation, sometimes it is not possible to assess by a multiparametric way the grade of AR associated to central jet or PVL. Therefore, ICE can be used. From home view (low RA position) the aortic short-axis view is obtained with the catheter tilted by 90° towards the aortic annulus, allowing to evaluate presence and quantification of PVL using the semi-quantitative proposed approach. Then, tilting the tip towards TV and advance the catheter into the right ventricle (RV) untill "RV outflow position", long-axis view of the left ventricle and left ventricular outflow tract are yielded, allowing evaluation of jets origin and amount of jets area.

4.3.6.6.4 Mitral Valve Regurgitation and Functional Narrowing of LVOT

Mitral Valve Regurgitation

Recent evidence suggest that after TAVR, moderate to severe MR had improved in 57%, unchanged in 36% and worsened in 5.8%.

Worsening MR after TAVR can be detected immediately and can cause hemodynamic instability and intraoperative pulmonary edema.

Mitral valve entitlement during catheters navigation in LV is uncommon but severe situation that can cause chordae rupture resulting in flail leaflets, and mitral leaflet perforation. This complication is more common in transapical approach as the catheter might trap the subvalvular apparatus when passing through the LV towards the outflow tract. Moreover, MR worsening may occur due to right ventricular pacing (LV asynchrony and ischemia in rapid pacing), or as consequence of prosthetic misplacement with abnormal pressure exerted on the anterior leaflet from ventricular edge of prosthesis. Careful echocardiographic monitoring of the mitral valve during and after implantation can help avoid this complication [187].

LVOT Dynamic Narrowing

Immediately after TAVR, a slight fall in end systolic LVOT pressure that can lead to systolic apposition of LVOT, especially when the following risk factors are present: small LV dimensions, high transvalvular gradient, good LV contractility, asymmetric hypertrophy, sigmoid shaped septum and narrow LVOT.

This dynamic narrowing of LVOT during systole can cause persistence of abnormal gradient during systolic phase and, by Venturi mechanism, it can cause a pull phenomenon on anterior leaflet of mitral valve inside LVOT (systolic anterior motion).

This condition must be immediately recognized because after TAVR it can cause circulatory collapse, pulmonary oedema and death. Temporary superimposed factors like filling state, contractility (use of catecholamine), systemic vascular resistance must be rule out for appropriate diagnosis because they can contribute to this dynamic narrowing. Conservative treatment should be attempted and it aims to reduce myocardial hyper-contractility and increase afterload and filling pressure (increasing volume and venous retourn with noradrenaline and stop diuretic and inotropic support, even when pulmonary congestion and arterial hypotension occur). When hemodynamic instability persists, surgical approach can be necessary.

References

1. Patel DK, Green KD, Fudim M, Harrell FE, Wang TJ, Robbins MA. Racial differences in the prevalence of severe aortic stenosis. J Am Heart Assoc. 2014;3(3):e000879.
2. Iung B, Baron G, Butchart EG, Delahaye F, Gohlke-Barwolf C, Levang OW, et al. A prospective survey of patients with valvular heart disease in Europe: the Euro Heart Survey on Valvular Heart Disease. Eur Heart J. 2003;24(13):1231–43.
3. Ye J, Cheung A, Yamashita M, Wood D, Peng D, Gao M, et al. Transcatheter aortic and mitral valve-in-valve implantation for failed surgical bioprosthetic valves: an 8-year single-center experience. JACC Cardiovasc Interv. 2015;8(13):1735–44.
4. Odim J, Laks H, Allada V, Child J, Wilson S, Gjertson D. Results of aortic valve-sparing and restoration with autologous pericardial leaflet extensions in congenital heart disease. Ann Thorac Surg. 2005;80(2):647–53; discussion 53–4.
5. Cawley PJ, Maki JH, Otto CM. Cardiovascular magnetic resonance imaging for valvular heart disease: technique and validation. Circulation. 2009;119(3):468–78.
6. Schultz CJ, Tzikas A, Moelker A, Rossi A, Nuis RJ, Geleijnse MM, et al. Correlates on MSCT of paravalvular aortic regurgitation after transcatheter aortic valve implantation using the Medtronic CoreValve prosthesis. Catheter Cardiovasc Interv. 2011;78(3):446–55.
7. Gurvitch R, Wood DA, Leipsic J, Tay E, Johnson M, Ye J, et al. Multislice computed tomography for prediction of optimal angiographic deployment projections during transcatheter aortic valve implantation. JACC Cardiovasc Interv. 2010;3(11):1157–65.
8. Nishimura RA, Otto CM, Bonow RO, Carabello BA, Erwin JP 3rd, Fleisher LA, et al. 2017 AHA/ACC focused update of the 2014 AHA/ACC guideline for the management of patients with valvular heart disease: a report of the American College of Cardiology/American Heart Association Task Force on Clinical Practice Guidelines. J Am Coll Cardiol. 2017;70(2):252–89.
9. Matsumoto M, Oka Y, Strom J, Frishman W, Kadish A, Becker RM, et al. Application of transesophageal echocardiography to continuous intraoperative monitoring of left ventricular performance. Am J Cardiol. 1980;46(1):95–105.
10. Practice guidelines for perioperative transesophageal echocardiography. A report by the American Society of Anesthesiologists and the Society of Cardiovascular Anesthesiologists Task Force on Transesophageal Echocardiography. Anesthesiology. 1996;84(4):986–1006.
11. Cahalan MK, Stewart W, Pearlman A, Goldman M, Sears-Rogan P, Abel M, et al. American Society of Echocardiography and Society of Cardiovascular Anesthesiologists task force guidelines for training in perioperative echocardiography. J Am Soc Echocardiogr. 2002;15(6):647–52.
12. Practice guidelines for perioperative transesophageal echocardiography. An updated report by the American Society of Anesthesiologists and the Society of Cardiovascular Anesthesiologists Task Force on Transesophageal Echocardiography. Anesthesiology. 2010;112(5):1084–96.
13. Reeves ST, Finley AC, Skubas NJ, Swaminathan M, Whitley WS, Glas KE, et al. Basic perioperative transesophageal echocardiography examination: a consensus statement of the American Society of Echocardiography and the Society of Cardiovascular Anesthesiologists. J Am Soc Echocardiogr. 2013;26(5):443–56.
14. Eltzschig HK, Kallmeyer IJ, Mihaljevic T, Alapati S, Shernan SK. A practical approach to a comprehensive epicardial and epiaortic echocardiographic examination. J Cardiothorac Vasc Anesth. 2003;17(4):422–9.
15. Klein AL, Stewart WC, Cosgrove DM, Salcedo EE. Intraoperative epicardial echocardiography: technique and imaging planes. Echocardiography (Mount Kisco, NY). 1990;7(3):241–51.
16. Alkhouli M, Hijazi ZM, Holmes DR Jr, Rihal CS, Wiegers SE. Intracardiac echocardiography in structural heart disease interventions. JACC Cardiovasc Interv. 2018;11(21):2133–47.
17. Hijazi ZM, Shivkumar K, Sahn DJ. Intracardiac echocardiography during interventional and electrophysiological cardiac catheterization. Circulation. 2009;119(4):587–96.
18. Dill KE, George E, Abbara S, Cummings K, Francois CJ, Gerhard-Herman MD, et al. ACR appropriateness criteria imaging for transcatheter aortic valve replacement. J Am Coll Radiol. 2013;10(12):957–65.
19. Osnabrugge RL, Mylotte D, Head SJ, Van Mieghem NM, Nkomo VT, LeReun CM, et al. Aortic stenosis in the elderly: disease prevalence and number of candidates for transcatheter aortic valve replacement: a meta-analysis and modeling study. J Am Coll Cardiol. 2013;62(11):1002–12.
20. Coffey S, Cox B, Williams MJ. The prevalence, incidence, progression, and risks of aortic valve sclerosis: a systematic review and meta-analysis. J Am Coll Cardiol. 2014;63(25 Pt A):2852–61.
21. Rahimtoola SH, Frye RL. Valvular heart disease. Circulation. 2000;102(20 Suppl 4):Iv24–33.
22. Probst V, Le Scouarnec S, Legendre A, Jousseaume V, Jaafar P, Nguyen JM, et al. Familial aggregation of calcific aortic valve stenosis in the western part of France. Circulation. 2006;113(6):856–60.
23. Nishimura RA, Otto CM, Bonow RO, Carabello BA, Erwin JP 3rd, Guyton RA, et al. 2014 AHA/ACC guideline for the management of patients with valvular heart disease: a report of the American College of Cardiology/American Heart Association Task Force on Practice Guidelines. J Thorac Cardiovasc Surg. 2014;148(1):e1–e132.
24. Baumgartner H, Falk V, Bax JJ, De Bonis M, Hamm C, Holm PJ, et al. 2017 ESC/EACTS Guidelines for the management of valvular heart disease. Eur Heart J. 2017;38(36):2739–91.
25. Jasinski MJ, Gocol R, Malinowski M, Hudziak D, Duraj P, Deja MA. Predictors of early and medium-term outcome of 200 consecutive aortic valve and root repairs. J Thorac Cardiovasc Surg. 2015;149(1):123–9.
26. Bentall H, De Bono A. A technique for complete replacement of the ascending aorta. Thorax. 1968;23(4):338–9.
27. Hagl C, Strauch JT, Spielvogel D, Galla JD, Lansman SL, Squitieri R, et al. Is the Bentall procedure for ascending aorta or aortic valve replacement the best approach for long-term event-free survival? Ann Thorac Surg. 2003;76(3):698–703; discussion 703.
28. Urbanski PP, Diegeler A, Siebel A, Zacher M, Hacker RW. Valved stentless composite graft: clinical outcomes and hemodynamic characteristics. Ann Thorac Surg. 2003;75(2):467–71.
29. Houel R, Soustelle C, Kirsch M, Hillion ML, Renaut C, Loisance DY. Long-term results of the bentall operation versus separate replacement of the ascending aorta and aortic valve. J Heart Valve Dis. 2002;11(4):485–91.
30. Ziemer G, Haverich A. Operations on the heart and great vessels in adults and children. In: Cardiac surgery. (Misfeld MCE, Sievers HH). Springer-Verlag Berlin Heidelberg 2017; p. 759–94.

31. David TE, Feindel CM. An aortic valve-sparing operation for patients with aortic incompetence and aneurysm of the ascending aorta. J Thorac Cardiovasc Surg. 1992;103(4):617–21; discussion 22.

32. Yacoub MH, Gehle P, Chandrasekaran V, Birks EJ, Child A, Radley-Smith R. Late results of a valve-preserving operation in patients with aneurysms of the ascending aorta and root. J Thorac Cardiovasc Surg. 1998;115(5):1080–90.

33. Morrow AG, Reitz BA, Epstein SE, Henry WL, Conkle DM, Itscoitz SB, et al. Operative treatment in hypertrophic subaortic stenosis. Techniques, and the results of pre and postoperative assessments in 83 patients. Circulation. 1975;52(1):88–102.

34. Hahn RT, Abraham T, Adams MS, Bruce CJ, Glas KE, Lang RM, et al. Guidelines for performing a comprehensive transesophageal echocardiographic examination: recommendations from the American Society of Echocardiography and the Society of Cardiovascular Anesthesiologists. J Am Soc Echocardiogr. 2013;26(9):921–64.

35. Kallmeyer IJ, Collard CD, Fox JA, Body SC, Shernan SK. The safety of intraoperative transesophageal echocardiography: a case series of 7200 cardiac surgical patients. Anesth Analg. 2001;92(5):1126–30.

36. Click RL, Abel MD, Schaff HV. Intraoperative transesophageal echocardiography: 5-year prospective review of impact on surgical management. Mayo Clin Proc. 2000;75(3):241–7.

37. Mishra M, Chauhan R, Sharma KK, Dhar A, Bhise M, Dhole S, et al. Real-time intraoperative transesophageal echocardiography—how useful? Experience of 5,016 cases. J Cardiothorac Vasc Anesth. 1998;12(6):625–32.

38. Eltzschig HK, Rosenberger P, Loffler M, Fox JA, Aranki SF, Shernan SK. Impact of intraoperative transesophageal echocardiography on surgical decisions in 12,566 patients undergoing cardiac surgery. Ann Thorac Surg. 2008;85(3):845–52.

39. Leye M, Brochet E, Lepage L, Cueff C, Boutron I, Detaint D, et al. Size-adjusted left ventricular outflow tract diameter reference values: a safeguard for the evaluation of the severity of aortic stenosis. J Am Soc Echocardiogr. 2009;22(5):445–51.

40. Shiran A, Adawi S, Ganaeem M, Asmer E. Accuracy and reproducibility of left ventricular outflow tract diameter measurement using transthoracic when compared with transesophageal echocardiography in systole and diastole. Eur J Echocardiogr. 2009;10(2):319–24.

41. Messika-Zeitoun D, Serfaty JM, Brochet E, Ducrocq G, Lepage L, Detaint D, et al. Multimodal assessment of the aortic annulus diameter: implications for transcatheter aortic valve implantation. J Am Coll Cardiol. 2010;55(3):186–94.

42. Altiok E, Koos R, Schroder J, Brehmer K, Hamada S, Becker M, et al. Comparison of two-dimensional and three-dimensional imaging techniques for measurement of aortic annulus diameters before transcatheter aortic valve implantation. Heart. 2011;97(19):1578–84.

43. Gutierrez-Chico JL, Zamorano JL, Prieto-Moriche E, Hernandez-Antolin RA, Bravo-Amaro M, Perez de Isla L, et al. Real-time three-dimensional echocardiography in aortic stenosis: a novel, simple, and reliable method to improve accuracy in area calculation. Eur Heart J. 2008;29(10):1296–306.

44. Poh KK, Levine RA, Solis J, Shen L, Flaherty M, Kang YJ, et al. Assessing aortic valve area in aortic stenosis by continuity equation: a novel approach using real-time three-dimensional echocardiography. Eur Heart J. 2008;29(20):2526–35.

45. Monin JL, Quere JP, Monchi M, Petit H, Baleynaud S, Chauvel C, et al. Low-gradient aortic stenosis: operative risk stratification and predictors for long-term outcome: a multicenter study using dobutamine stress hemodynamics. Circulation. 2003;108(3):319–24.

46. Cueff C, Serfaty JM, Cimadevilla C, Laissy JP, Himbert D, Tubach F, et al. Measurement of aortic valve calcification using multislice computed tomography: correlation with haemodynamic severity of aortic stenosis and clinical implication for patients with low ejection fraction. Heart. 2011;97(9):721–6.

47. Clavel MA, Messika-Zeitoun D, Pibarot P, Aggarwal SR, Malouf J, Araoz PA, et al. The complex nature of discordant severe calcified aortic valve disease grading: new insights from combined Doppler echocardiographic and computed tomographic study. J Am Coll Cardiol. 2013;62(24):2329–38.

48. Hachicha Z, Dumesnil JG, Bogaty P, Pibarot P. Paradoxical low-flow, low-gradient severe aortic stenosis despite preserved ejection fraction is associated with higher afterload and reduced survival. Circulation. 2007;115(22):2856–64.

49. Clavel MA, Dumesnil JG, Capoulade R, Mathieu P, Senechal M, Pibarot P. Outcome of patients with aortic stenosis, small valve area, and low-flow, low-gradient despite preserved left ventricular ejection fraction. J Am Coll Cardiol. 2012;60(14):1259–67.

50. Kristensen SD, Knuuti J, Saraste A, Anker S, Botker HE, De Hert S, et al. 2014 ESC/ESA Guidelines on non-cardiac surgery: cardiovascular assessment and management: the Joint Task Force on non-cardiac surgery: cardiovascular assessment and management of the European Society of Cardiology (ESC) and the European Society of Anaesthesiology (ESA). Eur J Anaesthesiol. 2014;31(10):517–73.

51. Buckberg GD. Update on current techniques of myocardial protection. Ann Thorac Surg. 1995;60(3):805–14.

52. Menasche P, Subayi JB, Piwnica A. Retrograde coronary sinus cardioplegia for aortic valve operations: a clinical report on 500 patients. Ann Thorac Surg. 1990;49(4):556–63; discussion 63–4.

53. Rajappan K, Rimoldi OE, Dutka DP, Ariff B, Pennell DJ, Sheridan DJ, et al. Mechanisms of coronary microcirculatory dysfunction in patients with aortic stenosis and angiographically normal coronary arteries. Circulation. 2002;105(4):470–6.

54. Fang L, Hsiung MC, Miller AP, Nanda NC, Yin WH, Young MS, et al. Assessment of aortic regurgitation by live three-dimensional transthoracic echocardiographic measurements of vena contracta area: usefulness and validation. Echocardiography. 2005;22(9):775–81.

55. Canty DJ, Joshi P, Royse CF, McMillan J, Tayeh S, Smith JA. Transesophageal echocardiography guidance of antegrade cardioplegia delivery for cardiac surgery. J Cardiothorac Vasc Anesth. 2015;29(6):1498–503.

56. Barreiro CJ, Patel ND, Fitton TP, Williams JA, Bonde PN, Chan V, et al. Aortic valve replacement and concomitant mitral valve regurgitation in the elderly: impact on survival and functional outcome. Circulation. 2005;112(9 Suppl):I443–7.

57. Vanden Eynden F, Bouchard D, El-Hamamsy I, Butnaru A, Demers P, Carrier M, et al. Effect of aortic valve replacement for aortic stenosis on severity of mitral regurgitation. Ann Thorac Surg. 2007;83(4):1279–84.

58. Unger P, Dedobbeleer C, Van Camp G, Plein D, Cosyns B, Lancellotti P. Mitral regurgitation in patients with aortic stenosis undergoing valve replacement. Heart. 2010;96(1):9–14.

59. Adams PB, Otto CM. Lack of improvement in coexisting mitral regurgitation after relief of valvular aortic stenosis. Am J Cardiol. 1990;66(1):105–7.

60. Grayburn PA, Carabello B, Hung J, Gillam LD, Liang D, Mack MJ, et al. Defining "severe" secondary mitral regurgitation: emphasizing an integrated approach. J Am Coll Cardiol. 2014;64(25):2792–801.

61. Rossi A, Dandale R, Nistri S, Faggiano P, Cicoira M, Benfari G, et al. Functional mitral regurgitation in patients with aortic stenosis: prevalence, clinical correlates and pathophysiological determinants: a quantitative prospective study. Eur Heart J Cardiovasc Imaging. 2014;15(6):631–6.

62. Hozumi T, Shakudo M, Shah PM. Quantitation of left ventricular volumes and ejection fraction by biplane transesophageal echocardiography. Am J Cardiol. 1993;72(3):356–9.

63. Colombo PC, Municino A, Brofferio A, Kholdarova L, Nanna M, Ilercil A, et al. Cross-sectional multiplane transesophageal echocardiographic measurements: comparison with standard transthoracic values obtained in the same setting. Echocardiography. 2002;19(5):383–90.

64. Reichert CL, Visser CA, van den Brink RB, Koolen JJ, van Wezel HB, Moulijn AC, et al. Prognostic value of biventricular function in hypotensive patients after cardiac surgery as assessed by transesophageal echocardiography. J Cardiothorac Vasc Anesth. 1992;6(4):429–32.

65. Stoddard MF, Liddell NE, Vogel RL, Longaker RA, Dawkins PR. Comparison of cardiac dimensions by transesophageal and transthoracic echocardiography. Am Heart J. 1992;124(3):675–8.

66. Voigt JU, Lindenmeier G, Exner B, Regenfus M, Werner D, Reulbach U, et al. Incidence and characteristics of segmental post-systolic longitudinal shortening in normal, acutely ischemic, and scarred myocardium. J Am Soc Echocardiogr. 2003;16(5):415–23.

67. Jenkins C, Bricknell K, Hanekom L, Marwick TH. Reproducibility and accuracy of echocardiographic measurements of left ventricular parameters using real-time three-dimensional echocardiography. J Am Coll Cardiol. 2004;44(4):878–86.

68. Muraru D, Badano LP, Piccoli G, Gianfagna P, Del Mestre L, Ermacora D, et al. Validation of a novel automated border-detection algorithm for rapid and accurate quantitation of left ventricular volumes based on three-dimensional echocardiography. Eur J Echocardiogr. 2010;11(4):359–68.

69. Jenkins C, Chan J, Hanekom L, Marwick TH. Accuracy and feasibility of online 3-dimensional echocardiography for measurement of left ventricular parameters. J Am Soc Echocardiogr. 2006;19(9):1119–28.

70. Kolias TJ, Aaronson KD, Armstrong WF. Doppler-derived dP/dt and -dP/dt predict survival in congestive heart failure. J Am Coll Cardiol. 2000;36(5):1594–9.

71. Chen CH, Fetics B, Nevo E, Rochitte CE, Chiou KR, Ding PA, et al. Noninvasive single-beat determination of left ventricular end-systolic elastance in humans. J Am Coll Cardiol. 2001;38(7):2028–34.

72. Lang RM, Badano LP, Mor-Avi V, Afilalo J, Armstrong A, Ernande L, et al. Recommendations for cardiac chamber quantification by echocardiography in adults: an update from the American Society of Echocardiography and the European Association of Cardiovascular Imaging. J Am Soc Echocardiogr. 2015;28(1):1–39.e14.

73. Hager A, Kanz S, Kaemmerer H, Schreiber C, Hess J. Coarctation Long-term Assessment (COALA): significance of arterial hypertension in a cohort of 404 patients up to 27 years after surgical repair of isolated coarctation of the aorta, even in the absence of restenosis and prosthetic material. J Thorac Cardiovasc Surg. 2007;134(3):738–45.

74. Laperche T, Laurian C, Roudaut R, Steg PG. Mobile thromboses of the aortic arch without aortic debris. A transesophageal echocardiographic finding associated with unexplained arterial embolism. The Filiale Echocardiographie de la Societe Francaise de Cardiologie. Circulation. 1997;96(1):288–94.

75. Bach DS. Subvalvular left ventricular outflow obstruction for patients undergoing aortic valve replacement for aortic stenosis: echocardiographic recognition and identification of patients at risk. J Am Soc Echocardiogr. 2005;18(11):1155–62.

76. Routledge T, Nashef SA. Severe mitral systolic anterior motion complicating aortic valve replacement. Interact Cardiovasc Thorac Surg. 2005;4(5):486–7.

77. Kerut EK, Hanawalt C, Dearstine M, Frank R, Everson C. Mitral systolic anterior motion (SAM) with dynamic left ventricular outflow obstruction following aortic valve replacement. Echocardiography. 2007;24(6):658–60.

78. Gupta R, Sewani A, Ahmad M. Dynamic systolic left ventricular gradients: differential diagnosis and management. Echocardiography. 2006;23(2):168–71.

79. Frenk VE, Shernan SK, Eltzschig HK. Epicardial echocardiography: diagnostic utility for evaluating aortic valve disease during coronary surgery. J Clin Anesth. 2003;15(4):271–4.

80. Edrich T, Shernan SK, Smith B, Eltzschig HK. Usefulness of intraoperative epiaortic echocardiography to resolve discrepancy between transthoracic and transesophageal measurements of aortic valve gradient—a case report. Can J Anaesth. 2003;50(3):293–6.

81. Cerqueira MD, Weissman NJ, Dilsizian V, Jacobs AK, Kaul S, Laskey WK, et al. Standardized myocardial segmentation and nomenclature for tomographic imaging of the heart. A statement for healthcare professionals from the Cardiac Imaging Committee of the Council on Clinical Cardiology of the American Heart Association. Circulation. 2002;105(4):539–42.

82. Marino M, Cellini C, Tsiopoulos V, Pavone N, Zamparelli R, Corrado M, et al. A case of myocardial infarction effectively treated by emergency coronary stenting soon after a Bentall-De Bono aortic surgery. Cardiovasc Revasc Med. 2010;11(4):263. e5–9.

83. Thomopoulou S, Sfirakis P, Spargias K. Angioplasty, stenting and thrombectomy to correct left main coronary stem obstruction by a bioprosthetic aortic valve. J Invasive Cardiol. 2008;20(4):E124–5.

84. Ziakas AG, Economou FI, Charokopos NA, Pitsis AA, Parharidou DG, Papadopoulos TI, et al. Coronary ostial stenosis after aortic valve replacement: successful treatment of 2 patients with drug-eluting stents. Tex Heart Inst J. 2010;37(4):465–8.

85. Pragliola C, Altamura L, Niccoli G, Siviglia M, De Paulis S, Possati GF. Postoperative coronary artery spasm complicating aortic valve replacement: implications for identification and treatment. Ann Thorac Surg. 2007;83(2):670–2.

86. Sudhakar S, Sewani A, Agrawal M, Uretsky BF. Pseudoaneurysm of the mitral-aortic intervalvular fibrosa (MAIVF): a comprehensive review. J Am Soc Echocardiogr. 2010;23(10):1009–18; quiz 112.

87. Kolakalapudi P, Chaudhry S, Omar B. Iatrogenic aortic insufficiency following mitral valve replacement: case report and review of the literature. J Clin Med Res. 2015;7(6):485–9.

88. Harris KM, Braverman AC, Eagle KA, Woznicki EM, Pyeritz RE, Myrmel T, et al. Acute aortic intramural hematoma: an analysis from the International Registry of Acute Aortic Dissection. Circulation. 2012;126(11 Suppl 1):S91–6.

89. Coady MA, Rizzo JA, Elefteriades JA. Pathologic variants of thoracic aortic dissections. Penetrating atherosclerotic ulcers and intramural hematomas. Cardiol Clin. 1999;17(4):637–57.

90. Pelzel JM, Braverman AC, Hirsch AT, Harris KM. International heterogeneity in diagnostic frequency and clinical outcomes of ascending aortic intramural hematoma. J Am Soc Echocardiogr. 2007;20(11):1260–8.

91. Hiratzka LF, Creager MA, Isselbacher EM, Svensson LG, Nishimura RA, Bonow RO, et al. Surgery for aortic dilatation in patients with bicuspid aortic valves: a statement of clarification from the American College of Cardiology/American Heart Association Task Force on Clinical Practice Guidelines. Circulation. 2016;133(7):680–6.

92. Bodenhamer RM, Johnson RG, Randolph JD, Pohost G, Boucher C, Okada R, et al. The effect of adding mannitol or albumin to a crystalloid cardioplegic solution: a prospective, randomized clinical study. Ann Thorac Surg. 1985;40(4):374–9.

93. Troianos CA, Savino JS, Weiss RL. Transesophageal echocardiographic diagnosis of aortic dissection during cardiac surgery. Anesthesiology. 1991;75(1):149–53.

94. Russo CF, Mazzetti S, Garatti A, Ribera E, Milazzo A, Bruschi G, et al. Aortic complications after bicuspid aortic valve replacement:

long-term results. Ann Thorac Surg. 2002;74(5):S1773–6; discussion S92–9.

95. Pepi M, Campodonico J, Galli C, Tamborini G, Barbier P, Doria E, et al. Rapid diagnosis and management of thoracic aortic dissection and intramural haematoma: a prospective study of advantages of multiplane vs. biplane transoesophageal echocardiography. Eur J Echocardiogr. 2000;1(1):72–9.

96. Meredith EL, Masani ND. Echocardiography in the emergency assessment of acute aortic syndromes. Eur J Echocardiogr. 2009;10(1):i31–9.

97. Carl M, Alms A, Braun J, Dongas A, Erb J, Goetz A, et al. S3 guidelines for intensive care in cardiac surgery patients: hemodynamic monitoring and cardiocirculary system. Ger Med Sci. 2010;8:Doc12.

98. Swenson JD, Harkin C, Pace NL, Astle K, Bailey P. Transesophageal echocardiography: an objective tool in defining maximum ventricular response to intravenous fluid therapy. Anesth Analg. 1996;83(6):1149–53.

99. Thys DM, Hillel Z, Goldman ME, Mindich BP, Kaplan JA. A comparison of hemodynamic indices derived by invasive monitoring and two-dimensional echocardiography. Anesthesiology. 1987;67(5):630–4.

100. Girard F, Couture P, Boudreault D, Normandin L, Denault A, Girard D. Estimation of the pulmonary capillary wedge pressure from transesophageal pulsed Doppler echocardiography of pulmonary venous flow: influence of the respiratory cycle during mechanical ventilation. J Cardiothorac Vasc Anesth. 1998;12(1):16–21.

101. Faehnrich JA, Noone RB Jr, White WD, Leone BJ, Hilton AK, Sreeram GM, et al. Effects of positive-pressure ventilation, pericardial effusion, and cardiac tamponade on respiratory variation in transmitral flow velocities. J Cardiothorac Vasc Anesth. 2003;17(1):45–50.

102. Klein AL, Abbara S, Agler DA, Appleton CP, Asher CR, Hoit B, et al. American Society of Echocardiography clinical recommendations for multimodality cardiovascular imaging of patients with pericardial disease: endorsed by the Society for Cardiovascular Magnetic Resonance and Society of Cardiovascular Computed Tomography. J Am Soc Echocardiogr. 2013;26(9):965–1012.e15.

103. Maganti MD, Rao V, Borger MA, Ivanov J, David TE. Predictors of low cardiac output syndrome after isolated aortic valve surgery. Circulation. 2005;112(9 Suppl):I448–52.

104. Lomivorotov VV, Efremov SM, Boboshko VA, Nikolaev DA, Vedernikov PE, Lomivorotov VN, et al. Evaluation of nutritional screening tools for patients scheduled for cardiac surgery. Nutrition. 2013;29(2):436–42.

105. Nozohoor S, Nilsson J, Luhrs C, Roijer A, Algotsson L, Sjogren J. B-type natriuretic peptide as a predictor of postoperative heart failure after aortic valve replacement. J Cardiothorac Vasc Anesth. 2009;23(2):161–5.

106. Rosenhek R, Binder T, Maurer G, Baumgartner H. Normal values for Doppler echocardiographic assessment of heart valve prostheses. J Am Soc Echocardiogr. 2003;16(11):1116–27.

107. Seiler C. Management and follow up of prosthetic heart valves. Heart. 2004;90(7):818–24.

108. Kliger C, Eiros R, Isasti G, Einhorn B, Jelnin V, Cohen H, et al. Review of surgical prosthetic paravalvular leaks: diagnosis and catheter-based closure. Eur Heart J. 2013;34(9):638–49.

109. Ionescu A, Fraser AG, Butchart EG. Prevalence and clinical significance of incidental paraprosthetic valvar regurgitation: a prospective study using transoesophageal echocardiography. Heart. 2003;89(11):1316–21.

110. Blais C, Dumesnil JG, Baillot R, Simard S, Doyle D, Pibarot P. Impact of valve prosthesis-patient mismatch on short-term mortality after aortic valve replacement. Circulation. 2003;108(8):983–8.

111. Hanayama N, Christakis GT, Mallidi HR, Joyner CD, Fremes SE, Morgan CD, et al. Patient prosthesis mismatch is rare after aortic valve replacement: valve size may be irrelevant. Ann Thorac Surg. 2002;73(6):1822–9; discussion 9.

112. Pibarot P, Dumesnil JG. Hemodynamic and clinical impact of prosthesis-patient mismatch in the aortic valve position and its prevention. J Am Coll Cardiol. 2000;36(4):1131–41.

113. Pibarot P, Dumesnil JG, Cartier PC, Metras J, Lemieux MD. Patient-prosthesis mismatch can be predicted at the time of operation. Ann Thorac Surg. 2001;71(5 Suppl):S265–8.

114. Rahimtoola SH, Murphy E. Valve prosthesis—patient mismatch. A long-term sequela. Br Heart J. 1981;45(3):331–5.

115. Mohty D, Dumesnil JG, Echahidi N, Mathieu P, Dagenais F, Voisine P, et al. Impact of prosthesis-patient mismatch on long-term survival after aortic valve replacement: influence of age, obesity, and left ventricular dysfunction. J Am Coll Cardiol. 2009;53(1):39–47.

116. Cribier A, Eltchaninoff H, Bash A, Borenstein N, Tron C, Bauer F, et al. Percutaneous transcatheter implantation of an aortic valve prosthesis for calcific aortic stenosis: first human case description. Circulation. 2002;106(24):3006–8.

117. Capodanno D, Leon MB. Upcoming TAVI trials: rationale, design and impact on clinical practice. EuroIntervention. 2016;12(Y):Y51–5.

118. Grover FL, Vemulapalli S, Carroll JD, Edwards FH, Mack MJ, Thourani VH, et al. 2016 Annual report of the Society of Thoracic Surgeons/American College of Cardiology Transcatheter Valve Therapy Registry. J Am Coll Cardiol. 2017;69(10):1215–30.

119. Leon MB, Smith CR, Mack M, Miller DC, Moses JW, Svensson LG, et al. Transcatheter aortic-valve implantation for aortic stenosis in patients who cannot undergo surgery. N Engl J Med. 2010;363(17):1597–607.

120. Athappan G, Patvardhan E, Tuzcu EM, Svensson LG, Lemos PA, Fraccaro C, et al. Incidence, predictors, and outcomes of aortic regurgitation after transcatheter aortic valve replacement: meta-analysis and systematic review of literature. J Am Coll Cardiol. 2013;61(15):1585–95.

121. Chieffo A, Buchanan GL, Van Mieghem NM, Tchetche D, Dumonteil N, Latib A, et al. Transcatheter aortic valve implantation with the Edwards SAPIEN versus the Medtronic CoreValve Revalving system devices: a multicenter collaborative study: the PRAGMATIC Plus Initiative (Pooled-RotterdAm-Milano-Toulouse In Collaboration). J Am Coll Cardiol. 2013;61(8):830–6.

122. Nombela-Franco L, Ruel M, Radhakrishnan S, Webb JG, Hansen M, Labinaz M, et al. Comparison of hemodynamic performance of self-expandable CoreValve versus balloon-expandable Edwards SAPIEN aortic valves inserted by catheter for aortic stenosis. Am J Cardiol. 2013;111(7):1026–33.

123. Abdel-Wahab M, Comberg T, Buttner HJ, El-Mawardy M, Chatani K, Gick M, et al. Aortic regurgitation after transcatheter aortic valve implantation with balloon- and self-expandable prostheses: a pooled analysis from a 2-center experience. JACC Cardiovasc Interv. 2014;7(3):284–92.

124. Abdel-Wahab M, Zahn R, Horack M, Gerckens U, Schuler G, Sievert H, et al. Aortic regurgitation after transcatheter aortic valve implantation: incidence and early outcome. Results from the German transcatheter aortic valve interventions registry. Heart. 2011;97(11):899–906.

125. Wiegerinck EM, Boerlage-van Dijk K, Koch KT, Yong ZY, Vis MM, Planken RN, et al. Towards minimally invasiveness: transcatheter aortic valve implantation under local analgesia exclusively. Int J Cardiol. 2014;176(3):1050–2.

126. Mylotte D, Lefevre T, Sondergaard L, Watanabe Y, Modine T, Dvir D, et al. Transcatheter aortic valve replacement in bicuspid aortic valve disease. J Am Coll Cardiol. 2014;64(22):2330–9.

127. Yoon SH, Bleiziffer S, De Backer O, Delgado V, Arai T, Ziegelmueller J, et al. Outcomes in transcatheter aortic valve replacement for bicuspid versus tricuspid aortic valve stenosis. J Am Coll Cardiol. 2017;69(21):2579–89.

128. Dvir D, Webb JG, Bleiziffer S, Pasic M, Waksman R, Kodali S, et al. Transcatheter aortic valve implantation in failed bioprosthetic surgical valves. JAMA. 2014;312(2):162–70.

129. Webb JG, Mack MJ, White JM, Dvir D, Blanke P, Herrmann HC, et al. Transcatheter aortic valve implantation within degenerated aortic surgical bioprostheses: PARTNER 2 valve-in-valve registry. J Am Coll Cardiol. 2017;69(18):2253–62.

130. Deeb GM, Chetcuti SJ, Reardon MJ, Patel HJ, Grossman PM, Schreiber T, et al. 1-year results in patients undergoing transcatheter aortic valve replacement with failed surgical bioprostheses. JACC Cardiovasc Interv. 2017;10(10):1034–44.

131. Dvir D, Khan J, Kornowski R, Komatsu I, Chatriwalla A, Mackenson GB, et al. Novel strategies in aortic valve-in-valve therapy including bioprosthetic valve fracture and BASILICA. EuroIntervention. 2018;14(Ab):Ab74–82.

132. Dvir D, Leipsic J, Blanke P, Ribeiro HB, Kornowski R, Pichard A, et al. Coronary obstruction in transcatheter aortic valve-in-valve implantation: preprocedural evaluation, device selection, protection, and treatment. Circ Cardiovasc Interv. 2015;8(1):e002079.

133. Blanke P, Soon J, Dvir D, Park JK, Naoum C, Kueh SH, et al. Computed tomography assessment for transcatheter aortic valve in valve implantation: the vancouver approach to predict anatomical risk for coronary obstruction and other considerations. J Cardiovasc Comput Tomogr. 2016;10(6):491–9.

134. Herrmann HC, Pibarot P, Hueter I, Gertz ZM, Stewart WJ, Kapadia S, et al. Predictors of mortality and outcomes of therapy in low-flow severe aortic stenosis: a Placement of Aortic Transcatheter Valves (PARTNER) trial analysis. Circulation. 2013;127(23):2316–26.

135. Baumgartner H, Hung J, Bermejo J, Chambers JB, Evangelista A, Griffin BP, et al. Echocardiographic assessment of valve stenosis: EAE/ASE recommendations for clinical practice. J Am Soc Echocardiogr. 2009;22(1):1–23; quiz 101–2.

136. Jabbour A, Ismail TF, Moat N, Gulati A, Roussin I, Alpendurada F, et al. Multimodality imaging in transcatheter aortic valve implantation and post-procedural aortic regurgitation: comparison among cardiovascular magnetic resonance, cardiac computed tomography, and echocardiography. J Am Coll Cardiol. 2011;58(21):2165–73.

137. Bagur R, Rodes-Cabau J, Doyle D, De Larochelliere R, Villeneuve J, Lemieux J, et al. Usefulness of TEE as the primary imaging technique to guide transcatheter transapical aortic valve implantation. JACC Cardiovasc Imaging. 2011;4(2):115–24.

138. Schulz CJ, Schmitt M, Bockler D, Geisbusch P. Feasibility and accuracy of fusion imaging during thoracic endovascular aortic repair. J Vasc Surg. 2016;63(2):314–22.

139. Dumont E, Lemieux J, Doyle D, Rodes-Cabau J. Feasibility of transapical aortic valve implantation fully guided by transesophageal echocardiography. J Thorac Cardiovasc Surg. 2009;138(4):1022–4.

140. Kasel AM, Cassese S, Bleiziffer S, Amaki M, Hahn RT, Kastrati A, et al. Standardized imaging for aortic annular sizing: implications for transcatheter valve selection. JACC Cardiovasc Imaging. 2013;6(2):249–62.

141. Babaliaros VC, Liff D, Chen EP, Rogers JH, Brown RA, Thourani VH, et al. Can balloon aortic valvuloplasty help determine appropriate transcatheter aortic valve size? JACC Cardiovasc Interv. 2008;1(5):580–6.

142. Patsalis PC, Al-Rashid F, Neumann T, Plicht B, Hildebrandt HA, Wendt D, et al. Preparatory balloon aortic valvuloplasty during transcatheter aortic valve implantation for improved valve sizing. JACC Cardiovasc Interv. 2013;6(9):965–71.

143. Smith LA, Monaghan MJ. Monitoring of procedures: peri-interventional echo assessment for transcatheter aortic valve implantation. Eur Heart J Cardiovasc Imaging. 2013;14(9):840–50.

144. Toggweiler S, Leipsic J, Binder RK, Freeman M, Barbanti M, Heijmen RH, et al. Management of vascular access in transcatheter aortic valve replacement: part 1: basic anatomy, imaging, sheaths, wires, and access routes. JACC Cardiovasc Interv. 2013;6(7):643–53.

145. Smith LA, Dworakowski R, Bhan A, Delithanasis I, Hancock J, Maccarthy PA, et al. Real-time three-dimensional transesophageal echocardiography adds value to transcatheter aortic valve implantation. J Am Soc Echocardiogr. 2013;26(4):359–69.

146. Hahn RT, Kodali S, Tuzcu EM, Leon MB, Kapadia S, Gopal D, et al. Echocardiographic imaging of procedural complications during balloon-expandable transcatheter aortic valve replacement. JACC Cardiovasc Imaging. 2015;8(3):288–318.

147. Dvir D, Lavi I, Eltchaninoff H, Himbert D, Almagor Y, Descoutures F, et al. Multicenter evaluation of Edwards SAPIEN positioning during transcatheter aortic valve implantation with correlates for device movement during final deployment. JACC Cardiovasc Interv. 2012;5(5):563–70.

148. Seward JB, Packer DL, Chan RC, Curley M, Tajik AJ. Ultrasound cardioscopy: embarking on a new journey. Mayo Clin Proc. 1996;71(7):629–35.

149. Valdes-Cruz LM, Sideris E, Sahn DJ, Murillo-Olivas A, Knudson O, Omoto R, et al. Transvascular intracardiac applications of a miniaturized phased-array ultrasonic endoscope. Initial experience with intracardiac imaging in piglets. Circulation. 1991;83(3):1023–7.

150. Alqahtani F, Bhirud A, Aljohani S, Mills J, Kawsara A, Runkana A, et al. Intracardiac versus transesophageal echocardiography to guide transcatheter closure of interatrial communications: Nationwide trend and comparative analysis. J Interv Cardiol. 2017;30(3):234–41.

151. Pozzoli A, Taramasso M, Kuwata S, Zuber M, Nietlispach F, Maisano F. Echo-fluoro fusion imaging guidance for no contrast transfemoral aortic valve implantation. Eur Heart J Cardiovasc Imaging. 2018;19(6):710–1.

152. Leon MB, Piazza N, Nikolsky E, Blackstone EH, Cutlip DE, Kappetein AP, et al. Standardized endpoint definitions for transcatheter aortic valve implantation clinical trials: a consensus report from the Valve Academic Research Consortium. Eur Heart J. 2011;32(2):205–17.

153. Kappetein AP, Head SJ, Genereux P, Piazza N, van Mieghem NM, Blackstone EH, et al. Updated standardized endpoint definitions for transcatheter aortic valve implantation: the Valve Academic Research Consortium-2 consensus document. J Am Coll Cardiol. 2012;60(15):1438–54.

154. Ruile P, Pache G, Minners J, Hein M, Neumann FJ, Breitbart P. Fusion imaging of pre- and post-procedural computed tomography angiography in transcatheter aortic valve implantation patients: evaluation of prosthesis position and its influence on new conduction disturbances. Eur Heart J Cardiovasc Imaging. 2019;20(7):781–8.

155. Greif M, Lange P, Nabauer M, Schwarz F, Becker C, Schmitz C, et al. Transcutaneous aortic valve replacement with the Edwards SAPIEN XT and Medtronic CoreValve prosthesis under fluoroscopic guidance and local anaesthesia only. Heart. 2014;100(9):691–5.

156. Motloch LJ, Rottlaender D, Reda S, Larbig R, Bruns M, Muller-Ehmsen J, et al. Local versus general anesthesia for transfemoral aortic valve implantation. Clin Res Cardiol. 2012;101(1):45–53.

157. Rahnavardi M, Santibanez J, Sian K, Yan TD. A systematic review of transapical aortic valve implantation. Ann Cardiothorac Surg. 2012;1(2):116–28.

158. Ye J, Cheung A, Lichtenstein SV, Nietlispach F, Albugami S, Masson JB, et al. Transapical transcatheter aortic valve implantation: follow-up to 3 years. J Thorac Cardiovasc Surg. 2010;139(5):1107–13, 13.e1.

159. Dvir D, Assali A, Porat E, Kornowski R. Distal left anterior descending coronary artery obstruction: a rare complication of transapical aortic valve implantation. J Invasive Cardiol. 2011;23(12):E281–3.

160. Ben-Dor I, Pichard AD, Satler LF, Goldstein SA, Syed AI, Gaglia MA Jr, et al. Complications and outcome of balloon aortic valvuloplasty in high-risk or inoperable patients. JACC Cardiovasc Interv. 2010;3(11):1150–6.

161. Schultz CJ, Weustink A, Piazza N, Otten A, Mollet N, Krestin G, et al. Geometry and degree of apposition of the CoreValve ReValving system with multislice computed tomography after implantation in patients with aortic stenosis. J Am Coll Cardiol. 2009;54(10):911–8.

162. Saia F, Lemos PA, Bordoni B, Cervi E, Boriani G, Ciuca C, et al. Transcatheter aortic valve implantation with a self-expanding nitinol bioprosthesis: prediction of the need for permanent pacemaker using simple baseline and procedural characteristics. Catheter Cardiovasc Interv. 2012;79(5):712–9.

163. Rezq A, Basavarajaiah S, Latib A, Takagi K, Hasegawa T, Figini F, et al. Incidence, management, and outcomes of cardiac tamponade during transcatheter aortic valve implantation: a single-center study. JACC Cardiovasc Interv. 2012;5(12):1264–72.

164. Maisch B, Ristic AD, Seferovic PM, Tsang TSM. Interventional Pericardiology: Pericardiocentesis, Pericardioscopy, Pericardial Biopsy, Balloon Pericardiotomy, and Intrapericardial Therapy. 2011 Springer-Verlag Berlin Heidelberg. ISBN 978-3-642-11335-2. DOI 10.1007/978-3-642-11335-2.

165. Roy CL, Minor MA, Brookhart MA, Choudhry NK. Does this patient with a pericardial effusion have cardiac tamponade? JAMA. 2007;297(16):1810–8.

166. Adler Y, Charron P, Imazio M, Badano L, Baron-Esquivias G, Bogaert J, et al. 2015 ESC Guidelines for the diagnosis and management of pericardial diseases: the Task Force for the Diagnosis and Management of Pericardial Diseases of the European Society of Cardiology (ESC) Endorsed by: the European Association for Cardio-Thoracic Surgery (EACTS). Eur Heart J. 2015;36(42):2921–64.

167. Tsang TS, Freeman WK, Sinak LJ, Seward JB. Echocardiographically guided pericardiocentesis: evolution and state-of-the-art technique. Mayo Clin Proc. 1998;73(7):647–52.

168. Maisch B, Seferovic PM, Ristic AD, Erbel R, Rienmuller R, Adler Y, et al. Guidelines on the diagnosis and management of pericardial diseases executive summary; The Task force on the diagnosis and management of pericardial diseases of the European society of cardiology. Eur Heart J. 2004;25(7):587–610.

169. Tsang TS, Enriquez-Sarano M, Freeman WK, Barnes ME, Sinak LJ, Gersh BJ, et al. Consecutive 1127 therapeutic echocardiographically guided pericardiocenteses: clinical profile, practice patterns, and outcomes spanning 21 years. Mayo Clin Proc. 2002;77(5):429–36.

170. Sugg WL, Rea WJ, Ecker RR, Webb WR, Rose EF, Shaw RR. Penetrating wounds of the heart. An analysis of 459 cases. J Thorac Cardiovasc Surg. 1968;56(4):531–45.

171. Al-Attar N, Ghodbane W, Himbert D, Rau C, Raffoul R, Messika-Zeitoun D, et al. Unexpected complications of transapical aortic valve implantation. Ann Thorac Surg. 2009;88(1):90–4.

172. Massabuau P, Dumonteil N, Berthoumieu P, Marcheix B, Duterque D, Fournial G, et al. Left-to-right interventricular shunt as a late complication of transapical aortic valve implantation. JACC Cardiovasc Interv. 2011;4(6):710–2.

173. Pasic M, Unbehaun A, Buz S, Drews T, Hetzer R. Annular rupture during transcatheter aortic valve replacement: classification, pathophysiology, diagnostics, treatment approaches, and prevention. JACC Cardiovasc Interv. 2015;8(1 Pt A):1–9.

174. Lange R, Bleiziffer S, Piazza N, Mazzitelli D, Hutter A, Tassani-Prell P, et al. Incidence and treatment of procedural cardiovascular complications associated with trans-arterial and trans-apical interventional aortic valve implantation in 412 consecutive patients. Eur J Cardiothorac Surg. 2011;40(5):1105–13.

175. Aminian A, Lalmand J, Dolatabadi D. Late contained aortic root rupture and ventricular septal defect after transcatheter aortic valve implantation. Catheter Cardiovasc Interv. 2013;81(1):E72–5.

176. Genereux P, Reiss GR, Kodali SK, Williams MR, Hahn RT. Periaortic hematoma after transcatheter aortic valve replacement: description of a new complication. Catheter Cardiovasc Interv. 2012;79(5):766–76.

177. Barbanti M, Yang TH, Rodes Cabau J, Tamburino C, Wood DA, Jilaihawi H, et al. Anatomical and procedural features associated with aortic root rupture during balloon-expandable transcatheter aortic valve replacement. Circulation. 2013;128(3):244–53.

178. Kukucka M, Pasic M, Dreysse S, Hetzer R. Delayed subtotal coronary obstruction after transapical aortic valve implantation. Interact Cardiovasc Thorac Surg. 2011;12(1):57–60.

179. Unbehaun A, Pasic M, Dreysse S, Drews T, Kukucka M, Mladenow A, et al. Transapical aortic valve implantation: incidence and predictors of paravalvular leakage and transvalvular regurgitation in a series of 358 patients. J Am Coll Cardiol. 2012;59(3):211–21.

180. Detaint D, Lepage L, Himbert D, Brochet E, Messika-Zeitoun D, Iung B, et al. Determinants of significant paravalvular regurgitation after transcatheter aortic valve: implantation impact of device and annulus discongruence. JACC Cardiovasc Interv. 2009;2(9):821–7.

181. Makkar RR, Jilaihawi H, Chakravarty T, Fontana GP, Kapadia S, Babaliaros V, et al. Determinants and outcomes of acute transcatheter valve-in-valve therapy or embolization: a study of multiple valve implants in the U.S. PARTNER trial (Placement of AoRTic TraNscathetER Valve Trial Edwards SAPIEN Transcatheter Heart Valve). J Am Coll Cardiol. 2013;62(5):418–30.

182. Burstow DJ, Nishimura RA, Bailey KR, Reeder GS, Holmes DR Jr, Seward JB, et al. Continuous wave Doppler echocardiographic measurement of prosthetic valve gradients. A simultaneous Doppler-catheter correlative study. Circulation. 1989;80(3):504–14.

183. Shames S, Koczo A, Hahn R, Jin Z, Picard MH, Gillam LD. Flow characteristics of the SAPIEN aortic valve: the importance of recognizing in-stent flow acceleration for the echocardiographic assessment of valve function. J Am Soc Echocardiogr. 2012;25(6):603–9.

184. Pibarot P, Dumesnil JG. Prosthesis-patient mismatch: definition, clinical impact, and prevention. Heart. 2006;92(8):1022–9.

185. Zoghbi WA, Chambers JB, Dumesnil JG, Foster E, Gottdiener JS, Grayburn PA, et al. Recommendations for evaluation of prosthetic valves with echocardiography and doppler ultrasound: a report From the American Society of Echocardiography's Guidelines and Standards Committee and the Task Force on Prosthetic Valves, developed in conjunction with the American College of Cardiology Cardiovascular Imaging Committee, Cardiac Imaging Committee of the American Heart Association, the European Association of Echocardiography, a registered branch of the European Society of Cardiology, the Japanese Society of Echocardiography and the Canadian Society of Echocardiography, endorsed by the American College of Cardiology Foundation, American Heart Association, European Association of Echocardiography, a registered branch of the European Society of Cardiology, the Japanese Society of Echocardiography, and Canadian Society of Echocardiography. J Am Soc Echocardiogr. 2009;22(9):975–1014; quiz 82–4.

186. Zoghbi WA, Enriquez-Sarano M, Foster E, Grayburn PA, Kraft CD, Levine RA, et al. Recommendations for evaluation of the severity of native valvular regurgitation with two-dimensional and Doppler echocardiography. J Am Soc Echocardiogr. 2003;16(7):777–802.

187. Barbanti M, Webb JG, Hahn RT, Feldman T, Boone RH, Smith CR, et al. Impact of preoperative moderate/severe mitral regurgitation on 2-year outcome after transcatheter and surgical aortic valve replacement: insight from the Placement of Aortic Transcatheter Valve (PARTNER) Trial Cohort A. Circulation. 2013;128(25):2776–84.

Assessment and Follow-Up

5

Edwin Ho, Alberto Pozzoli, Mizuki Miura, Shehab Anwer,
Frederic Baumann, Tim Sebastian, Zoran Rancic,
Ricarda Hinzpeter, Gilbert Puippe, Philipp Haager,
Hans Rickli, Mara Gavazzoni, Nils Kucher, Buechel Ronny,
Philipp Kaufmann, Hatem Alkadhi, Francesco Maisano,
Felix Tanner, and Michel Zuber

5.1 Introduction

After aortic valve intervention, either through surgical or transcatheter techniques, ongoing follow up is essential to optimize patient outcomes. In addition to performing a detailed clinical assessment and physical examination, imaging is often performed for both routine evaluation as well as targeted evaluation when there is a suspected problem. This chapter will outline the utility of multimodality imaging in the follow up assessment of patients after aortic valve itnervention.

5.2 Prosthetic Valve Performance

5.2.1 Introduction

The evaluation of the performance of prosthetic valves is described in this chapter. Both surgical aortic valve replacement (SAVR) and trans-catheter aortic valve replacement (TAVR) will be included.

5.2.2 Residual Aortic Gradient or Regurgitation

5.2.2.1 Introduction

Ideally, a prosthetic aortic valve should have minimal to no transvalvular gradient nor have any valvular regurgitation. In reality, no prosthetic devices perform identically to a normal native aortic valve and therefore have an expected gradient range. There may also be a trace degree of regurgitation, either intravalvular or paravalvular, especially in the setting of TAVR. The following sections will discuss the evaluation of prosthetic aortic valve function with particular emphasis on TAVR.

5.2.2.2 Stent Creep

Stent creep is one of the causes of bioprosthetic structural dysfunction induced by altered mechanical stress on the leaflets when stent posts are internally deflected or deformed due to continuous mechanical stress or complicating improper implantation/deployment of the SAVR or TAVR bioprosthesis [1–4].

E. Ho
Heart Center, Zurich University Hospital, Zurich, Switzerland

Division of Cardiology, St. Michael's Hospital, Toronto, ON, Canada

Division of Cardiology, Montefiore Medical Center, Bronx, NY, USA
e-mail: edwin.ho@unityhealth.to

A. Pozzoli · F. Maisano
Heart Surgery Unit, Zurich University Hospital, Zurich, Switzerland
e-mail: alberto.pozzoli@usz.ch; francesco.maisano@usz.ch

M. Miura · S. Anwer · M. Gavazzoni
Heart Center, Zurich University Hospital, Zurich, Switzerland
e-mail: mizuki.miura@usz.ch; shehab.anwer@usz.ch; mara.gavazzoni@usz.ch

F. Baumann · T. Sebastian · N. Kucher
Angiology Unit, Zurich University Hospital, Zurich, Switzerland
e-mail: frederic.baumann@usz.ch; tim.sebastian@usz.ch; nils.kucher@usz.ch

Z. Rancic
Vascular Surgery Unit, Zurich University Hospital, Zurich, Switzerland
e-mail: zoran.rancic@usz.ch

R. Hinzpeter · G. Puippe · H. Alkadhi
Radiology Unit, Zurich University Hospital, Zurich, Switzerland
e-mail: ricarda.hinzpeter@usz.ch; gilbert.puippe@usz.ch; hatem.alkadhi@usz.ch

P. Haager · H. Rickli
Cardiology Unit, Kantonsspital St. Gallen, St. Gallen, Switzerland
e-mail: philipp.haager@usz.ch; hans.rickli@kssg.ch

B. Ronny · P. Kaufmann
Nuclear Medicine Unit, Zurich University Hospital, Zurich, Switzerland
e-mail: buechel.ronny@usz.ch; pak@usz.ch

F. Tanner · M. Zuber (✉)
Cardiology Unit, Zurich University Hospital, Zurich, Switzerland
e-mail: felix.tanner@usz.ch; michel.zuber@usz.ch

© Springer Nature Switzerland AG 2020
F. Maisano et al. (eds.), *Multimodality Imaging for Cardiac Valvular Interventions, Volume 1 Aortic Valve*,
https://doi.org/10.1007/978-3-030-27584-6_5

Older generations of SAVR bioprostheses were more prone to stent creep due to mal-suturing around stent posts which impedes leaflet motion. If not corrected, such prostheses were more liable to tears and calcification upon implantation. However, this has become rare in newer generations of SAVR bioprostheses whose stent tips are pre-sutured to prevent prosthesis deformation until successful implantation has been performed. Another cause for creep is the polypropylene-based ultrastructure of some SAVR bioprostheses [2, 3, 5].

Stent creep can lead to TAVR structural dysfunction through similar mechanisms that lead to SAVR stent deformation and improper orientation. Furthermore, reduced stent-tip deflection during implantation in TAVR can also cause this form of structural deterorioration [4, 6]. Although it is difficult to properly visualize this abnormality, it is usually included in the differential diagnosis of prosthetic valve dysfunction presenting with a change in hemodynamic function [6–8] (Figs. 5.1 and 5.2).

5.2.2.3 Pannus

Identification of masses on prosthetic aortic valves implanted by conventional surgery (SAVR) or a trans-catheter approach (TAVR) has been reported widely [8–12]. In SAVR, pannus formation has been documented more often as compared to TAVR, but this may be related to reporting of much longer follow-up durations in SAVR patients [8, 11–16].

Pannus formation on a prosthetic valve can be non-obstructive or obstructive and thus may or may not cause clinical manifestations or events [17–20]. Echocardiography can provide useful information on the presence of pannus, but it can be difficult to differentiate from other massess including thrombus or vegetation, particularly when artifacts caused by the prosthesis interfere with image quality. A thorough 2-dimensional and 3-dimensional echocardiographic investigation in combination with a detailed clinical and laboratory profile is required in such situations to avoid erroneous diagnosis of thrombosis or endocarditis of the prosthesis [8–13]. In some cases, differentiation between these entities is only possible by observing changes over time (including mass size/volume and prosthesis function) with antithrombotic or antibiotic treatment.

Transoesophageal (TOE) rather than transthoracic echocardiography (TTE) may also be required for optimal visualization of valve leaflets, masses and pannus. In general, pannus takes more time to develop and appears of higher echo density when compared to thrombus or vegetation, due to its fibrotic tissue nature. For the same reason, pannus is usually less mobile than thrombus or vegetation. Prosthetic leaflet motion can be restricted due to the pannus, but this is not observed in all cases. Pannus can be rather diffuse, or even circular, and is therefore more likely than a thrombus or a vegetation if a dysfunctional prosthesis demonstrates apparent normal leaflet mobility and absence of a clearly identifiable discrete mass by TOE [8, 13, 21, 22]. When it can be visualised, pannus usually appears as an immobile mass. This is an important feature that can distinguish it from thrombus or vegetation, which more commonly appears as one or multiple discrete and independently mobile masses [23].

Computed tomography (CT) may be helpful when pannus is suspected or difficult to differentiate from thrombus or vegetation. Increased attenuation, usually more than that of the myocardium for comparison, raises suspicion of pannus formation [22–25]. Furthermore, pannus is usually more diffuse and extensive than thrombus or vegetation, extending on the leaflets as well as across the sewing ring to the seating site. Both attenuation and extension of pannus can be examined by CT, therefore, multimodality imaging can indeed be very helpful in reaching a definitive diagnosis when pannus is considered in the differential diagnosis [11, 12, 26].

5.2.2.4 Calcification

Similar to surgically replaced prosthetic valves, transcatheter aortic valves (TAV) may demonstrate functional deterioration and certain features specific to TAVR prostheses may contribute to this [8, 13, 27]. Recent studies have reported severe leaflet calcification as a cause of structural dysfunction in addition to cusp damage or rupture [8, 13, 27, 28]. The underlying culprit mechanisms leading to leaflet matrix degeneration and tissue calcification have not yet been identified. It is postulated that chronic mechanical stress on native and bio prosthetic TAVR valve leaflets may lead to the initiation of degenerative processes that eventually result in tissue calcification [29]. This can primarily be explained mechanically as a mismatch between implantation site geometry and the TAVR implant, which can cause deformation of prosthesis, especially in the presence of heavily calcified native aortic valves. Therefore, implanting the TAVR in such landing zones can lead to high shear stress regions on some areas of the TAVR leaflets more than others in addition to recurrent dynamic changes in load and pressure. Explants from patients who suffered from degenerative calcification of

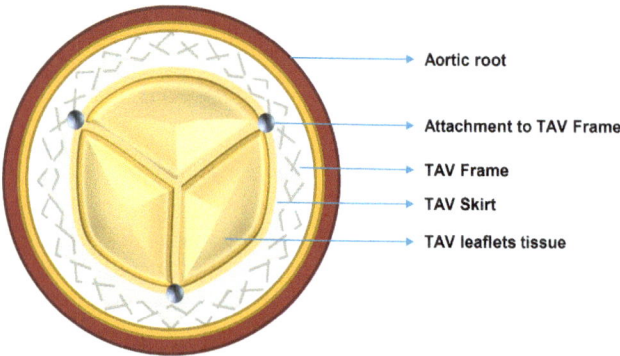

Fig. 5.1 TAVR prosthesis structure overview (normal)

Aortic root

Attachment to TAV Frame

TAV Frame

TAV Skirt

TAV leaflets tissue

Fig. 5.2 Stent creep and the effect on valve function

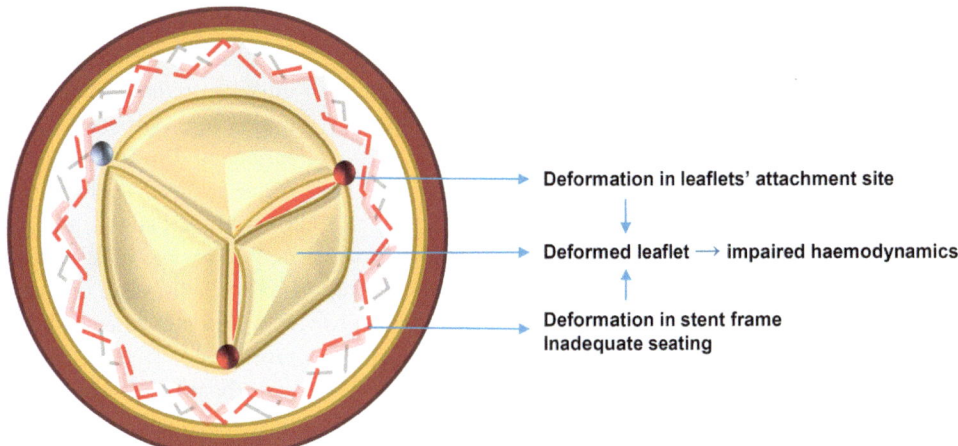

Deformation in leaflets' attachment site

Deformed leaflet → impaired haemodynamics

Deformation in stent frame
Inadequate seating

TAVR prostheses exhibited severe leaflet calcification, tissue degeneration, and thrombus formation. These reports were documented within a 5-year follow-up period [30].

As a result, regular and dedicated imaging follow-up after valve replacement using TTE, TOE, and possibly CT is recommended to understand any changes in prosthetic valve function, define the natural history of such valves, and correlate this to information to valve pathology [8, 13]. The application of TAVR has been expanding widely over the past few years and reports covering longer duration of post-TAVR follow-up are expected in the near future [31]. Unfortunately, we still lack detailed knowledge on the biological in-vivo processes underlying prosthesis degeneration and calcification, therefore research in this area should be intensified.

5.2.2.5 Structure Deformation, Underexpansion, Fracture

Transcatheter aortic valve (TAV) dysfunction or failure can be associated with suboptimal deployment or occur as a result of stent structure abnormalities, chronic mechanical fatigue, and the sequalae of bio prosthesis leaflet tearing, degeneration, and calcification. Intra- and immediate post-procedural echocardiographic assessment of the TAV provides a baseline from which the prosthesis can be compared to during follow-up with respect to morphology and function. This can increase the sensitivity for detecting prosthesis related structural problems and improve differentiation from other complications such as thrombosis or endocarditis, although it should be noted that structural and non-structural complications often progress in parallel and may cause more pronounced dysfunction in combination with each other. When compared to surgically replaced aortic bio prostheses, some mechanisms of structural dysfunction are unique to TAV prostheses and may have an impact on their long term durability. Structure related factors may indeed provide important clues for the development and progression of TAV dysfunction [4, 8, 13, 32, 33].

TAV leaflets are thinner than those of SAVR bioprostheses to allow prosthesis crimping required for achieving the small diameters necessary for transcatheter vascular delivery. Studies using electron microscopy have shown that this crimping process can play a role in structural deformation and promote accelerated calcification and thrombosis. The smaller the diameter is, the higher the chances are for such problems. However, long-term clinical outcomes associated with extensive mechanical crimping have yet to be investigated [4, 13, 34]. Implantation site calcification can have a major impact on the expansion of the TAV stent, since baseline anatomy and inflexibility of the implantation site may cause inadequate and asymmetric TAV frame expansion. Such situations can lead to stent deformation, especially if additional efforts are made to fully expand the stent, and may also lead to stent fracture. As a later consequence, TAV functional deterioration may occur related to stent damage directly or due to functional alterations secondary to stent damage. The mechanical stress between the stent and the leaflets of TAV prostheses is also higher than that of SAVR bioprostheses, especially at the commissures and site of leaflet attachment to the stent [4, 6, 35–37].

In addition to inducing stent deformation and fracture, the underlying anatomy and degree of compliance of the implantation site may simply lead to underexpansion of the TAV prosthesis. This does not allow the valve to function as intended, leading to increased mechanical stress and decreased haemodynamic function of TAV leaflets, especially in cases where underexpansion occurs in an asymmetric manner. Finally, the implantation site may also modulate the biological properties of the TAV prosthesis due to inflammatory processes occurring in the native valve, which may then have a long term impact on the mechanics of prosthetic valve leaflets [1, 6, 37, 38].

Accordingly, these aforementioned mechanisms may result in decreased TAV prosthesis durability in comparison to SAVR bioprostheses [7, 39–42]. Although the first studies on long-term durability show promising results, early structural failure has also been reported in the first years after TAVR [43–45]. More studies on how valve deployment methods and the stent structure may impact long term TAV durability are therefore of great importance (Fig. 5.2).

5.2.2.6 Patient Prosthesis Mismatch

Patient prosthesis mismatch (PPM) is a condition where the effective orifice area (EOA) of the implanted valve is not sufficient for the patient's hemodynamic demand in relation to body surface area. PPM is diagnosed when the indexed EOA is less than 0.85 cm^2/m^2 and it is considered severe when indexed EOA is less than 0.65 cm^2/m^2 [8, 13]. These cut off values, however, are controversial because there is the possibility of overdiagnosis of PPM in a systematic manner if there is underestimation of EOA by echocardiography due to incorrect and underestimated stroke volume calculations (required for calculation of EOA using the continuity equation). The left ventricular outflow tract is oval shape in most patients, but this geometry is ignored by routine echocardiographic calculations of EOA (a circular shape of the outflow tract is used when calculating the area). Furthermore, it may not be correct to index the EOA to body surface area in obese patients. Accordingly, the VARC-2 consensus document recommends lower indexed EOA cut-off values for obese patients with body mass indexes above 30 kg/m^2, under 0.7 cm^2/m^2 for diagnosing PPM and less than 0.6 cm^2/m^2 for severe PPM [46].

Different factors can increase the probability and predict the development of severe PPM. Procedure related factors include valves with a diameter ≤23 mm or valve-in-valve TAVR. Other factors are patient related, such as body surface area, female sex, young age, or non-white and Hispanic origin. Cardiac conditions can predict PPM in TAVR patients as well since patients with reduced ejection fraction, atrial fibrillation, and severe mitral or tricuspid regurgitation have an increased risk of PPM. Studies report that the incidence of PPM is lower among TAVR patients in comparison to those who underwent SAVR, particularly among patients with a small aortic annulus, as reported by a review of the PARTNER trials [47–51].

Severe PPM has been associated with worse outcomes after both SAVR and TAVR. The "Transcatheter Valve Therapy Registry of the Society of Thoracic Surgeons and American College of Cardiology" includes 62,125 TAVR patients, 12% of whom meet criteria for severe PPM and 25% for moderate PPM. In patients with severe PPM, 1-year mortality and rehospitalization for heart failure were significantly higher as compared to patients without PPM. No reports on long-term outcomes associated with PPM in TAVR patients are available thus far [8, 13, 52].

5.2.2.7 Endocarditis

Both SAVR and TAVR patients are at increased of endocarditis due to the presence of prosthetic materials. Keeping an eye on suggestive signs and symptoms is crucial during their follow-up. Preventive measures must be considered and performed as well, such as antimicrobial prophylaxis, especially when these patients are undergoing procedures or interventions known to be associated with bacteremia [53].

Prosthetic valve endocarditis (PVE) can occur within the first 2 months after implantation and is then known as early prosthetic valve endocarditis, within the first year (intermediate prosthetic valve endocarditis), or after the first year (late prosthetic valve endocarditis), and its incidence may reach up to 3% in TAVR patients per year. Staphylococci and enterococci are the most common causative organisms. Cardiac imaging modalities and intravenous antibiotic therapy are the main pillars of PVE management [27, 53–56].

Endocarditis can lead to serious complications. Echocardiography and multidetector computed tomography (MDCT) play an important role in assessing valvular structure and function as well as endocarditis related complications, such as abscesses and fistulas, embolisation of vegetations, or destruction of valve leaflets and valve structures resulting in intravalvular and/or paravalvular regurgitation [53].

Endocarditis of the aortic valve can cause problems other than just prosthetic valve dysfunction. Heart failure is common among endocarditis patients, and spread of the infection to nearby structures, such as the mitral valve, occurs frequently. Mitral valve involvement is caused by local spread of infection along a contiguous tissue plane, seeding by a regurgitant jet (jet lesion), or due to low-seated TAV prosthesis [27, 54]. Other manifestations of endocarditis are systemic and include embolisation events, such as cerebrovascular events, remote abscess formation, immunologic phenomena, mycotic aneurysms as well as systemic sepsis [27, 53–56]. In-hospital mortality can reach up to 47% in TAVR patients with PVE [56].

Similar to SAVR patients with PVE, management of prosthetic valve endocarditis in TAVR patients is prolonged antibiotic therapy, either with or without additional surgical management of the infected valve. However, risk evaluation of such patients before surgical management is crucial to avoid even worse outcomes if the risk of repeat surgery is prohibitively high [27, 53, 54] (Fig. 5.3).

5.2.2.8 Thrombosis and Leaflet Motion Abnormalities

It is not common for TAVR patients to experience prosthesis failure with haemodynamic and clinical impact due to thrombosis based on currently available data. Studies documented clinically significant TAV thrombosis in less than 1% of

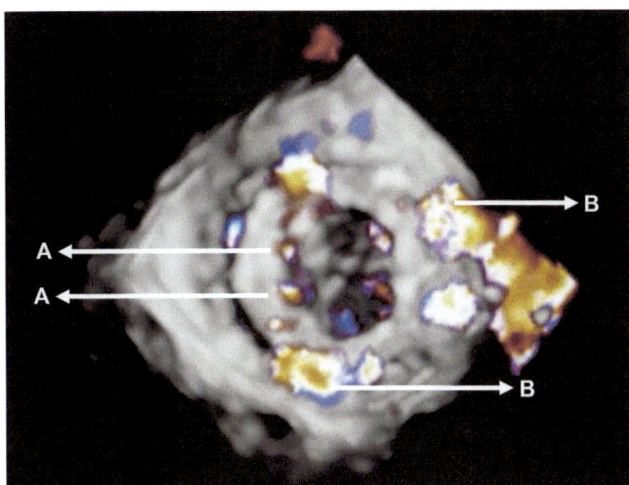

Fig. 5.3 3-dimensional transesophageal echocardiographic view of a bileaflet mechanical prosthetic aortic valve with expected intra-valvular washing jets (A) and abnormal paravalvular regurgitation jets due to endocarditis (B)

TAVR patients, yet the true incidence is still a matter of debate due to possible underdiagnosis [8, 13, 33, 57–61].

Prosthetic valve thrombosis is suspected when there is onset and progression of cardiac symptoms in follow up, such as exertional dyspnoea, and/or when there is an elevated transvalvular pressure gradient by echocardiographic examination. It is not always possible to visualize a thrombus by transthoracic (TTE) or even transoesophageal echocardiography (TOE). Multimodality imaging using multidetector computed tomography (MDCT) can therefore be helpful in such situations.

The significance of subclinical leaflet thrombosis is an unresolved but very important question, as it may affect long-term outcomes both in TAVR and SAVR. Subclinical leaflet thrombosis is an imaging finding and is not detected due to clinical symptoms or signs x. In subclinical cases, it is usually less extensive than a clinically evident thrombosis and thus even more difficult to visualise using transthoracic or transoesophageal echocardiography. MDCT should be used in such patients to make the diagnosis [61, 62].

Post-TAVR hemodynamic deterioration is defined as an increase in mean transvalvular pressure gradient by more than 10 mmHg at the latest follow-up in comparison to the immediate post-TAVR echocardiogram [39]. Studies have reported several independent predictors of bioprosthetic valve hemodynamic deterioration due to thrombosis including prior thromboembolic events, subtherapeutic anticoagulation, atrial fibrillation, and presence of various cardiovascular risk factors. Other factors associated with thrombosis of bio-prostheses include cusp thickness and

cusp motion abnormalities [63]. Empirical anti-coagulation is recommended to try to decrease transvalvular gradients when a clinical or subclinical bioprosthetic valve thrombosis is suspected [59].

Echocardiographic assessment should focus on increased or altered cusp thickness, reduced or abnormal cusp motion, other signs of bioprosthesis degeneration, and include evaluation for intracardiac thrombus. Spontaneous echocardiographic contrast may also suggest low flow, but is not specific with modern harmonic imaging and may be gain dependent. Increased cusp thickness and/or reduced cusp mobility with more than 50% increase in transvalvular gradient compared to baseline should raise the possibility of thrombosis [8, 64]. If a thrombus is suspected, TOE should performed as well since its sensitivity for thrombus identification is higher than that of TTE. This is particularly true regarding thromboses of prosthetic valve leaflets [8, 65]. Furthermore, multimodality imaging with MDCT may again be very helpful in such situations.

MDCT has demonstrated good efficacy in detecting and defining TAV thrombosis. Subclinical thrombosis by MDCT is defined as the presence of restricted or reduced leaflet motion in the presence of hypoattenuating prosthesis lesions [39, 62]. In a study performing a four-dimensional computed tomography (4D-CT) imaging protocol to detect the development of subclinical thrombosis in patients with bioprosthetic valves who underwent TAVR or SAVR, subclinical leaflet thrombosis was identified in 4% of SAVR patients and 13% of TAVR patients. Patients with subclinical thrombosis presented with trans-prosthesis mean pressure gradients higher than 20 mmHg or had a 10 mmHg or more increase in their gradients from baseline. Subclinical bioprosthesis thrombosis was also associated with higher rates of transient ischaemic attacks. Patients on any type of anticoagulant therapy were less prone to subclinical thrombosis in comparison to those on dual antiplatelet therapy (4% versus 15%), while those on direct oral anticoagulants (DOACs) were similar to those on warfarin (3 versus 4%) [39].

Hypoattenuating leaflet thickening with or without reduced motion detected by MDCT seems to occur and can change over time during follow-up [66]. Currently, the clinical impact of these findings is still unclear. Further investigations are in progress in an attempt to report the true incidence, identify the clinical impact, and help define the management goals for subclinical thrombosis [67] (Fig. 5.4).

5.2.2.9 Malposition

Prosthesis malpositioning is a complication that can be detected intra-procedurally or shortly post-TAVR with a total incidence around 1%. Intra-procedural imaging allows

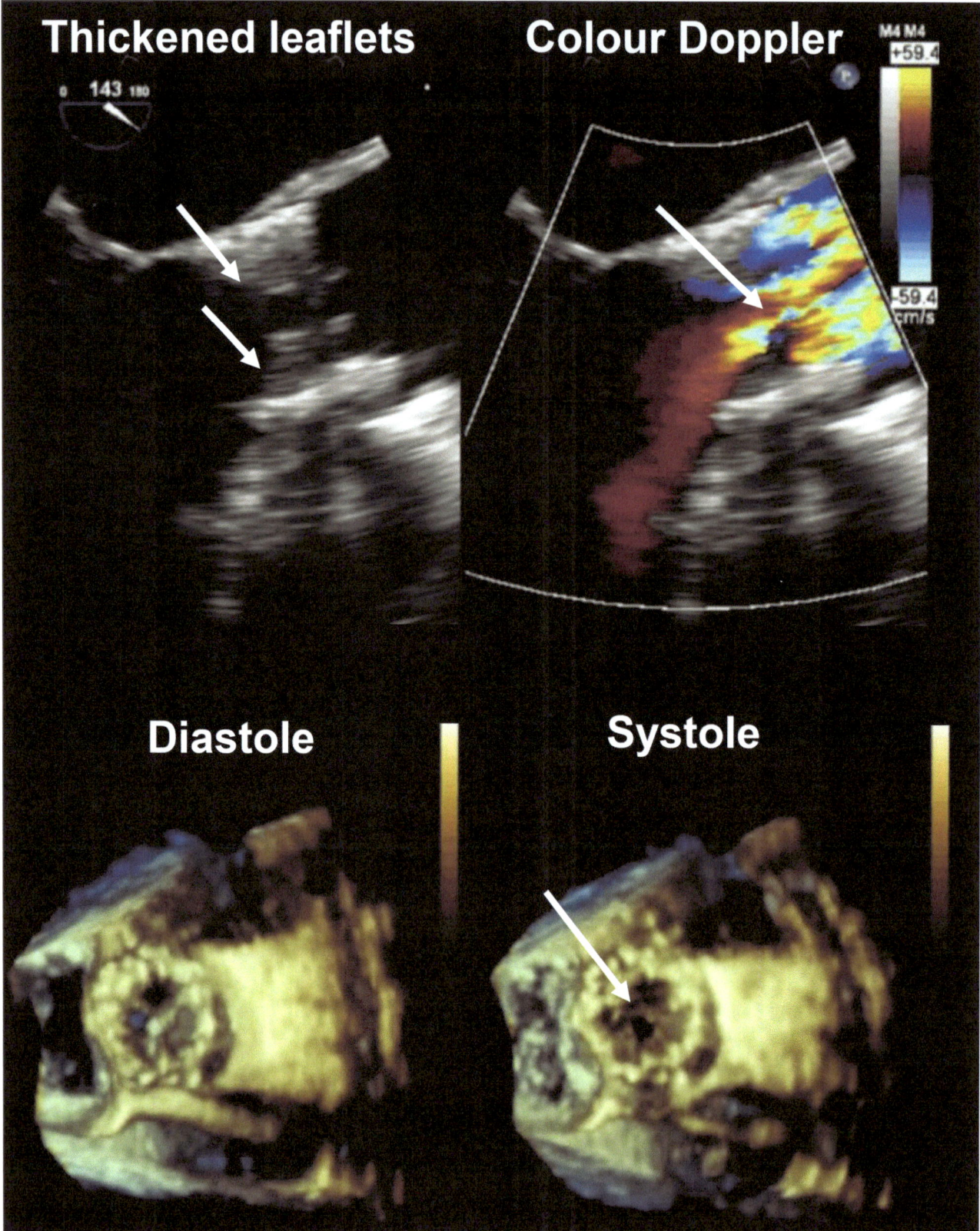

Fig. 5.4 Post-TAVR leaflet thrombosis represented by TAV stenosis. Arrows mark reduced leaflet opening and flow turbulence during systole (Arrows)

guidance during implantation and early detection of malpositioning [4, 8, 13, 32]. Cases of delayed malpositioning due to prosthesis migration have also been reported.

Factors related to patient anatomy, valve mechanics, and operator experience have been recognised as the main causes leading to TAV malpositioning. These include inaccurate assessment of the aortic annulus, improper implantation of the prosthetic valve, inadequate or premature cessation of rapid ventricular pacing, the presence of severe mitral annular calcification, or the presence of a mitral valve prosthesis. If suspected, aortography and/or TOE are used for assessment of TAV position and confirmation of the diagnosis [4, 8, 13, 32, 33, 68].

In order to position the TAV properly, the procedure can be guided by TOE, fluoroscopy, and aortography. TOE mid-oesophageal views can be performed when the patient is in their native rhythm, during rapid ventricular pacing, and after TAV implantation when pacing has been stopped. The recommended TAV position is device specific and it is therefore important to understand the manufacturer specific instructions for each prosthesis. Typically, the ventricular edge of the stent should be located 2–4 mm below the aortic annulus for balloon-expandable valves, 4–6 mm below the aortic annulus for first generation self-expanding valves, and 3–5 mm for second generation self-expanding valves. The position of the coronary ostia or focal calcifications may occasionally require modification of the implantation depth. An ideally positioned TAV prosthesis should neither lead to coronary artery ostial obstruction nor impingement of the anterior mitral leaflet [8, 13, 32].

Delayed TAV migration has been reported. Usually, the prosthesis migrates towards the left ventricular outflow tract and left ventricular cavity, resulting in paravalvular regurgitation, recurrence of native aortic stenosis, or disturbance of mitral valve function. It should be suspected when there are clinical manifestations or echocardiographic signs of haemodynamic impairment during follow-up. These patients may suffer from recurrent aortic stenosis, paravalvular aortic regurgitation, conduction abnormalities, and disturbances in mitral valve function resulting from impingement or tear of mitral valve leaflets [8, 13, 15, 27, 32, 33, 42, 68–76] (Figs. 5.5 and 5.6).

5.2.2.10 Leaflet Malfunction

Leaflet malfunction can significantly impact TAV prostheses function, causing leaflet thickening and/or restriction, and is associated with prosthesis degeneration and/or thrombosis [8, 13, 50, 57, 62, 77–79]. These alterations can occur with normal or increased systolic pressure gradients, but should be followed-up closely in any case because they may negatively impact long-term outcomes [62, 78, 79].

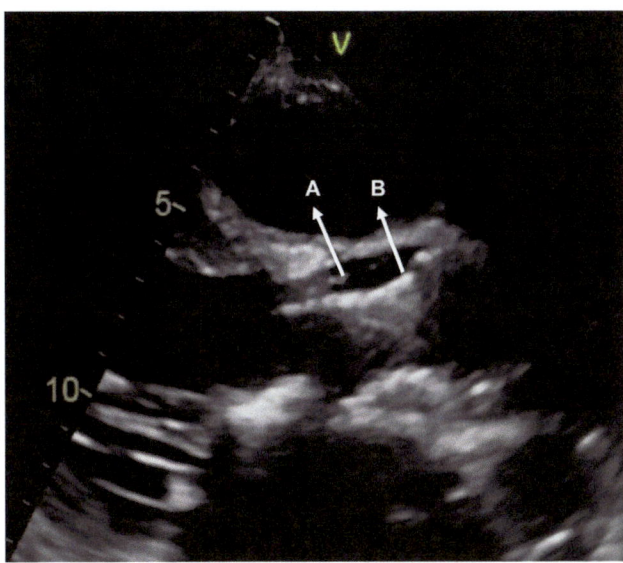

Fig. 5.5 Malposition: high implantation position. (A) Aortic root and Native Aortic Valve leaflet. (B) Malposition of TAV

According to different TAVR registries, thrombosis as a reason for leaflet malfunction has a cumulative incidence of almost 3% [57, 77]. TAV thrombosis usually manifests as worsening clinical status and increased transvalvular pressure gradient. On echocardiography or MDCT, it appears as thickening or thrombotic mass on the leaflets. Both leaflet thickening and leaflet restriction can occur in asymptomatic patients with normal transvalvular pressure gradients or may lead to symptoms of aortic stenosis with increased systolic pressure gradients [8, 13, 62, 78–80].

Although TTE is a key tool in TAV assessment, it may not present adequate information regarding the aforementioned leaflet malfunction, because the alterations of the leaflets may be subtle and present with normal systolic pressure gradients. For such reasons, leaflet malfunction may be under-recognized in clinical practice and underreported in the literature. TOE is more sensitive for identification of restricted leaflet motion; however, it may still be difficult to provide a definitive diagnosis of leaflet malfunction in patients with normal pressure gradients and no other findings supporting the interpretation of leaflet malfunction [8, 13, 39, 80].

Visualization of leaflets with restricted motion and detection of subclinical thrombosis using dynamic 4D CT imaging can provide useful data complementary to the echocardiographic examination [13, 39]. CT indeed detects early subclinical thrombosis whereas echocardiography detects the late consequences of thrombosis i.e. leaflet malfunction and valvular stenosis [57, 80]. However, in spite of the ability of dynamic 4D CT scans in detecting subclinical

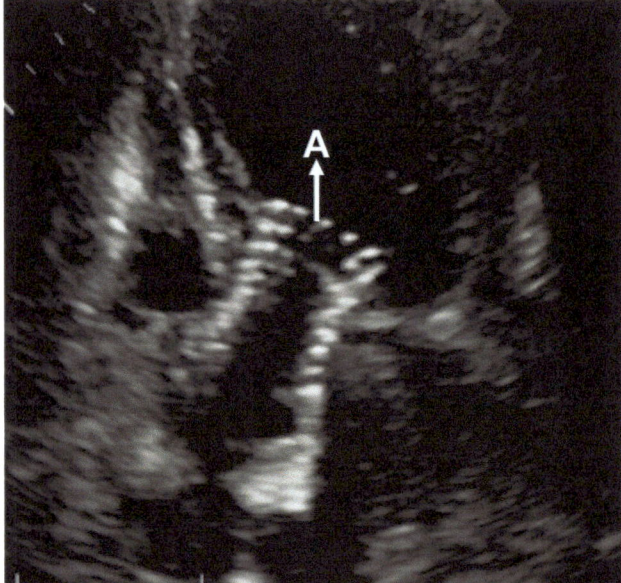

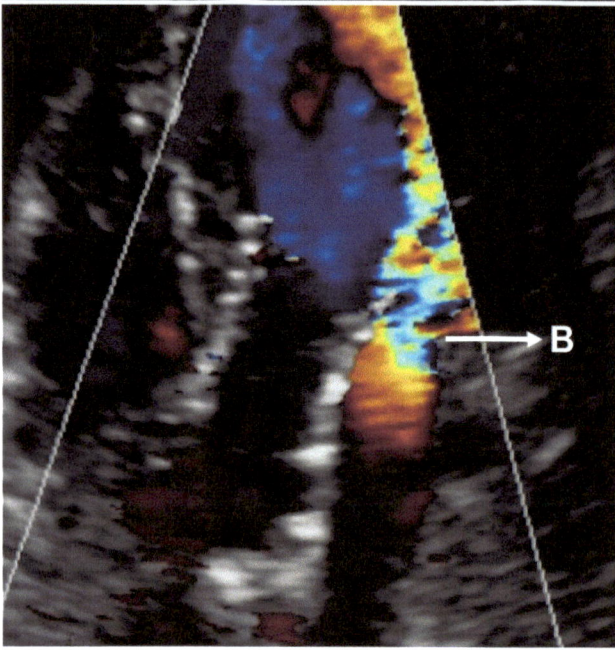

Fig. 5.6 Malposition: Low implantation position. (A) Malpositioned TAV (seated too low). (B) Mitral valve stenosis due to restricted opening of the anterior mitral leaflet by the malpositioned TAV

detected in patients who are not anti-coagulated, leaflet malfunction usually resolves upon initiation of anticoagulation. This observation suggests that leaflet dysfunction may be an early indicator of TAV thrombosis [39, 80–83]. Thus, an integrative approach using TTE, TOE, and MDCT is recommended whenever leaflet dysfunction is suspected [13, 39].

5.2.2.11 Paravalvular Regurgitation

Regurgitation of aortic valve prostheses can be physiologic or pathologic. Physiologic prosthetic valve regurgitation is usually minimal and is determined by valve design and/or anatomic orientation of the implanted valve relative to the native aortic valve tissue. Potentially physiologic prosthetic valve regurgitation is transvalvular in case of surgical mechanical valves and paravalvular in case of TAVR prostheses. Pathologic prosthetic valve regurgitation may have different causes including valve malposition, leaflet degeneration or prolapse, leaflet destruction or perforation by endocarditis, or mechanical leaflet restriction from pannus, thrombus, or vegetations. Most of these causes are shared between SAVR and TAVR [8, 9, 11–13].

Physiologic regurgitation jets are common and occur in all mechanical prosthesis to some degree. These jets are attributed to backward blood flow during leaflet closure and function as "washing jet" in that they may contribute to prevention of thrombus formation. Normal bioprosthetic valves as well as heterografts exhibit this phenomenon to a much lower extent and usually only a very small central jet or no jet is detectable. In contrast to surgical mechanical or biological prostheses, TAVR prostheses may exhibit a minimal or mild paravalvular regurgitation as an expected and clinically acceptable phenomenon due to the fact that they are mounted on a stent which is pressed against a very heterogenous surface in the landing zone. Physiologic regurgitation jets of prostheses in the aortic position are often more easily detected by colour Doppler TTE as compared to TOE due to shadowing of the prosthesis in midesophageal TOE views, although this problem can largely be avoided in the transgastric TOE views.

Trivial paravalvular prosthetic valve regurgitation can be detected just after SAVR or TAVR due to seating and positioning of the valve, and follow-up examinations are required to document stability or detect any progression [8, 11–13]. If paravalvular regurgitation develops later in SAVR patients, it is mostly due to suture dehiscence on top of poor valve ring seating, or as a sign of endocarditis. In SAVR, severe paravalvular regurgitation can occur when there is a partial dehiscence of the sewing ring. The echocardiographic appearance is a rocking valve with pulsatile blood flow during the cardiac cycle, as well as potentially floating masses nearby representing sutures or vegetations. Such findings are mainly suggestive of prosthetic valve endocarditis, in particular in the aortic position [11, 12].

thromboses, no solid consensus is available so far to quantify such lesions in TAV prosthesis [13, 81]. Quantification of leaflet thrombosis would be particularly helpful because not all the thromboses result in prosthetic valve degeneration and early thromboses may resolve spontaneously. Another important and still unclear factor is routine timing of MDCT scans after TAVR, since different TAV prostheses may present with a different time course and different degrees of TAV subclinical thrombosis [81, 82].

In anti-coagulated TAVR patients, it is rare to detect subclinical thrombosis or restricted leaflet motion. Even when

During TAVR, TOE is frequently used for the detection and assessment of paravalvular regurgitation. If TOE is not available, angiography can provide diagnostic information on the presence of paravalvular regurgitation. However, its use is associated with a high variability related to operator dependence, contrast dose and volume, and fluoroscopy imaging projection. Furthermore, the increased volume of contrast agent used may lead to renal complications [59, 84]. After TAVR, paravalvular aortic regurgitation is commonly detected. Paravalvular regurgitation occurs when the prosthesis is not completely set on the aortic annulus. This can either be attributed to the problems with the prosthesis due to incomplete expansion of the prosthesis stent, or to the native valve due to heavy (especially asymmetric) calcification preventing adequate seating. Hence, the interaction of the TAVR prosthesis with its landing zone is the main reason for development of paravalvular aortic regurgitation after TAVR [8, 13, 42]. The variability in the incidence and severity of paravalvular regurgitation after TAVR can be attributed to differences in individual anatomy, valve generation, valve model, implantation approach, and timing as well as method of assessment after TAVR [8, 13, 14, 59, 84]. TTE is the key tool for detection of paravalvular regurgitation during follow-up, while TOE can help in intra-procedural assessment of valve placement, early detection of paravalvular regurgitation, and further assessment of prosthesis function during follow-up, especially as it has been reported to impact outcomes after TAVR [8, 11–13]. Moderate or severe paravalvular regurgitation has been reported variably with an incidence of up to 24% for patients who underwent TAVR. Unfortunately, moderate or severe paravalvular regurgitation has also been associated with a threefold increase in 30-day mortality and twofold increase in 1-year mortality after TAVR. Mild paravalvular regurgitation can occur in up to 70% of TAVR and its association with worse outcomes is controversial. Newer generations of transcatheter valves have shown lower rates of moderate or severe paravalvular regurgitation due to adaptations in the design of the prosthesis, such as the presence of a skirt along the lower aspect of the prosthesis [8, 13–16, 42, 59, 84, 85].

Different cardiac imaging modalities can be utilised to diagnose paravalvular regurgitation of aortic valve prostheses; however, Doppler echocardiography remains the most common and reliable tool for assessment of such lesions using high frame rate colour images in different views and angles around the replaced aortic valve. Recently, 3-D echocardiography has emerged as an effective tool to describe the extent of paravalvular regurgitation and assist in guidance of percutaneous device closure [11].

Grading of paravalvular regurgitation severity requires an integrative approach using echocardiography [11, 12]. After SAVR, valve dehiscence >40% of the circumference and an rocking motion usually allow to grade regurgitation as

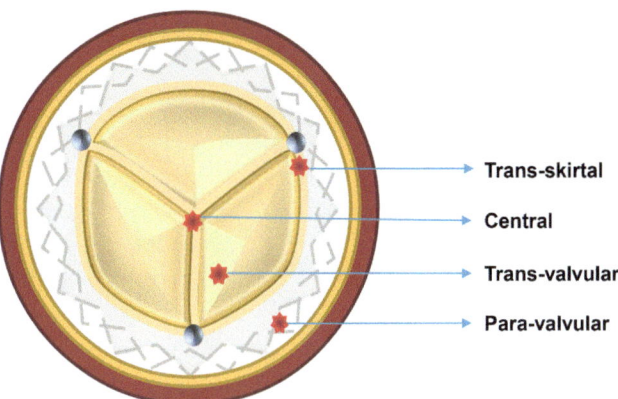

Fig. 5.7 Typical locations of post-TAVR regurgitation

severe. After TAVR, the percentage of the prosthesis circumference occupied by the regurgitant jet in the short axis view is a useful method for the defining regurgitation severity. Other measurements suggestive of severe paravalvular regurgitation are similar to those applied for grading transvalvular aortic regurgitation and include holodiastolic flow reversal in the descending aorta, spectral Doppler pressure half-time <200 ms, regurgitant volume >60 mL, and regurgitant fraction >50%. While TTE can usually detect and grade paravalvular regurgitation, TOE is recommended for further assessment and provide additional diagnostic insights, for example, to rule out aortic root abscess with endocarditis-associated regurgitation or the presence of a mass or pannus impeding disc closure in mechanical prostheses. In addition to acoustic shadowing by the prosthesis or calcification, irregular eccentric paravalvular regurgitation jets across imaging planes can make the echocardiographic assessment of paravalvular regurgitation severity more difficult [8, 11–13, 84]. When echocardiographic findings are not conclusive, cardiac magnetic resonance imaging has emerged as an alternative imaging method for the assessment of paravalvular regurgitation because of its ability to determine regurgitant volume regardless of jet shape and number [84, 85] (Figs. 5.7, 5.8, and 5.9).

5.3 Vascular Access and Surgical Access Complications

5.3.1 Introduction

In the current era of transcatheter valve devices, an increasing number of patients qualify for and desire minimally-invasive cardiovascular intervention. This requires percutaneous access, which is associated with its own set of complications. This is particularly relevant since many new transcatheter devices push the limits of percutaneous access (in terms of required sheath size). In addition, efforts

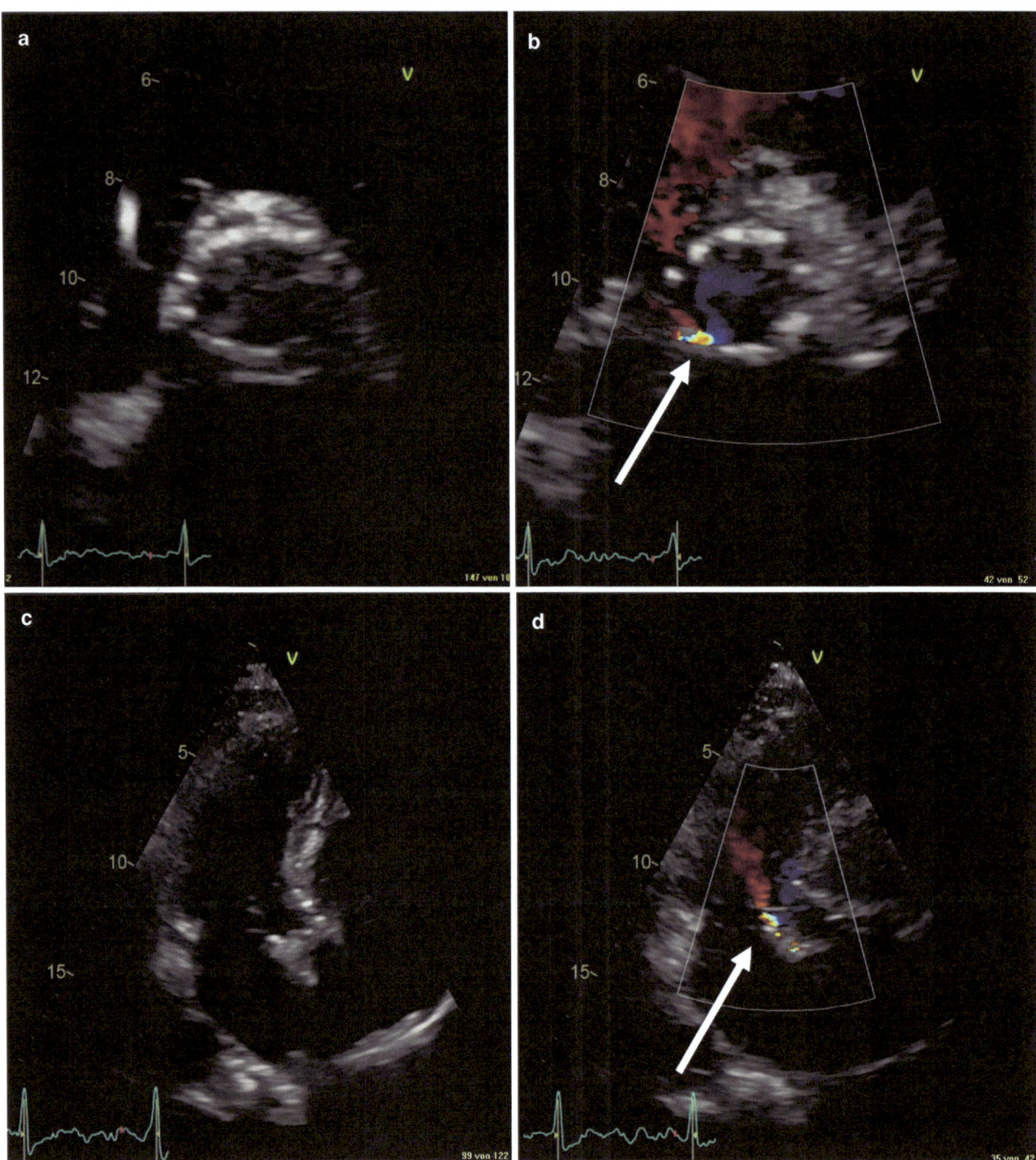

Fig. 5.8 Post-TAVR paravalvular regurgitation: (**a, b**) Parasternal short axis views, (**c, d**) Apical three-chamber view, and (**b, d**) Colour Doppler demonstrating turbulence and high velocity flow (aliasing) at site of regurgitation

to minimize length of stay require early mobilization of the patients after these procedures.

The most frequent complications following percutaneous therapy are access-related. They may be categorized as (1) bleeding, or (2) malperfusion complications.

Bleeding complications include hematoma, hemorrhage, pseudoaneurysm (=aneurysm spurium), and secondary complications derived from bleeding as a result from compression (such as sensorymotor deficits due to nerve compression).

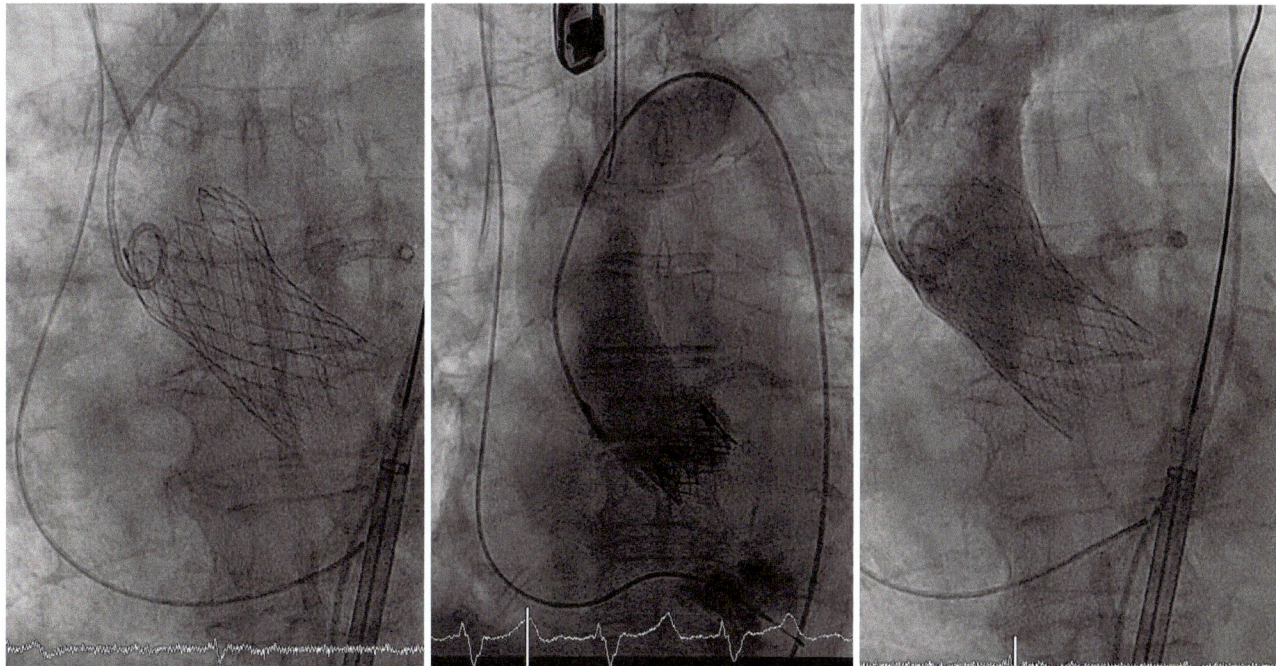

Fig. 5.9 Aortography for the initial assessment of TAV positioning and trans- or para-valvular regurgitation

Malperfusion complications usually occur in an acute manner, and are frequently attributed to an iatrogenic cause. This may include (1) dissection of the artery by puncture or wire manipulation, (2) sheath-associated thrombotic arterial occlusion, (3) acute vessel occlusion due to plaque shift, or (4) acute vessel occlusion due to a closure device.

The clinical findings of bleeding may vary. In general, non-life threatening bleeding is generally clinically relevant due to local (painful) swelling. Depending on clinical severity, the primary diagnostic approach is generally duplex ultrasound. This modality is used to obtain further information on the bleeding site including: (1) rule out/document persistent bleeding, and (2) document the size of a hematoma, if present. Based on this information, further therapeutic decisions can be made. On the other hand, bleeding may be occult, which means that it may not be clinically evident until later due to laboratory detection of decreasing hemoglobin levels, development of hypotensive shock, or secondary compression of structures adjacent to the site of bleeding (e.g. sensorymotor deficits due to nerve compression). These occult bleeding complications may require immediate diagnostic and therapeutic management, frequently requiring computed tomographic imaging (CT) to clarify the diagnosis.

5.3.2 Access Bleeding After TAVR

5.3.2.1 Introduction

Transcatheter aortic valve replacement (TAVR) is an evolving percutaneous treatment option to treat patients with aor-

tic valve diseases. TAVR requires large vascular access due to the delivery system and size of the crimped valve. In the beginning of TAVR procedures, surgical cutdown was frequently performed to obtain vascular access. Nowadays, vascular access can usually obtained percutaneously due to improved low profile sheaths and delivery systems. The newest generation valves are currently introduced through a 14–16 French (F) sheath while older valves necessitated sheath sizes up to 24 F.

TAVR significantly reduced all-cause mortality and adverse cardiovascular outcomes when compared to medical therapy and conventional surgery in some patient populations. However, vascular complications such as vessel dissection, caval-aortic fistula and access site bleeding remain a problem. The incidence of access site bleeding complications is reported up to 16.7%. The most frequent access site for TAVR is the common femoral artery. Alternative arterial access sites for TAVR include the subclavian artery or via a caval-aortic approach.

Risk factors associated with bleeding complications of the common femoral artery (CFA) are as follows: female gender, renal failure, peripheral artery disease with significant calcification at the puncture site and small arteries. A ratio >1.05 of the sheath: CFA diameter is also considered a risk factor for access site complications.

Considerations/strategies to reduce access site complications:

- Ultrasound-/digital subtraction angiography (DSA) "road map" assisted puncture

- Initial insertion of a small sheath (4 or 5 F) with secondary enlargement of sheath size
- Insertion of sheath over a stiff wire
- Consider surgical cutdown in case of severe circumferential calcification at the puncture site
- CFA puncture below the infrainguinal ligament to avoid retroperitoneal bleeding

5.3.2.2 Diagnosis

The clinical findings of bleeding complications after TAVR may vary. It may present as occult bleeding, which only becomes clinically apparent by laboratory detection of decreasing hemoglobin levels, or development of hypotensive shock. Less severe manifestations may also include a localized (usually painful) hematoma. Depending on clinical severity, the primary diagnostic approach is duplex ultrasound especially in the presence of a hematoma. Ultrasound serves as a valuable tool to detect most active arterial bleeding sites and to document the size of a hematoma. Of note, ultrasound examination is limited in detecting venous bleeding and retroperitoneal bleeding, which is frequently associated with suprainguinal puncture. In these cases, a secondary CT may be necessary. In patients with shock, a computed tomography (CT) is considered the primary diagnostic modality. In patients with adequate renal function, we recommend performing contrast enhanced CT imaging. Of note, even in patients with severely compromised renal function, a non-contrast CT can be very helpful to diagnose and estimate the extent of hematoma.

5.3.2.3 Treatment

5.3.2.3.1 Introduction

The primary goal of treatment is to gain control of the hemorrhage to prevent life-threatening hemodynamic instability. First, clinical stability must be established, by volume resuscitation, and if deemed necessary, with vasopressive agents. Second, the source of bleeding needs treatment. In cases of a groin hematoma, external (ultrasound-assisted) compression therapy should be applied. A covered stent can also be considered.

Case example

TAVR patient with primary access site from the left common femoral artery. Due to difficulties in advancing the wire and sheath from the left site, access was then obtained from the right site. After the intervention completed without further complications, the patient became hemodynamically unstable, and laboratory findings revealed a continuing decrease in hemoglobin. An ultrasound examination provided no further guidance. Therefore, a CT-angiogram was performed showing active bleeding from the proximal left external iliac

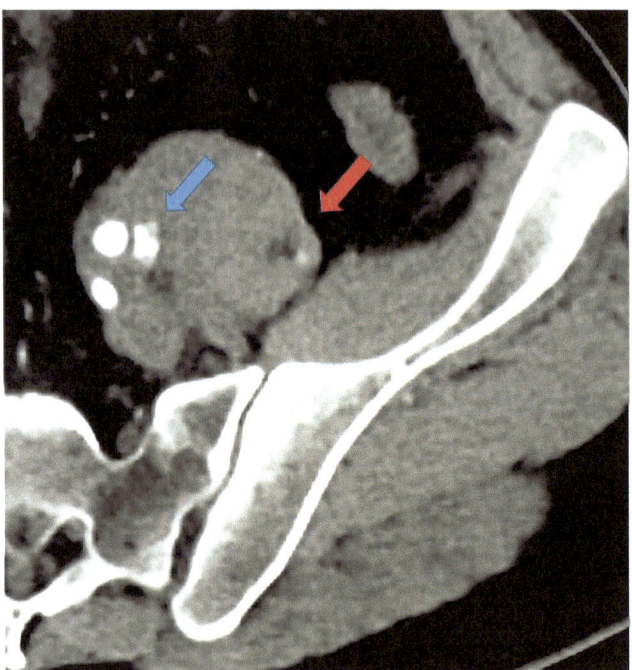

Fig. 5.10 Computer angiogram showing active bleeding originating from the proximal left external iliac artery (blue arrow) and a retroperitoneal hematoma (red arrow) along the psoas major muscle

artery (Fig. 5.10). For treatment, a covered stent graft was implanted from the left groin (Fig. 5.11).

5.3.2.3.2 Computed Tomography

Transcatheter aortic valve replacement (TAVR) is a minimally invasive surgical procedure that involves the implantation of a prosthetic valve mounted on a stent and introduced with a catheter usually through a transfemoral (TF) access site [86, 87]. Vascular complications still occur in up to 16% of all transfemoral procedures including access bleeding, typically caused by failure of the commonly used preclosure systems [88, 89]. Severe intra- or postoperative bleeding events in the less frequently used transapical (TA) approach are rare and have been reported in only 1.3–4.4% of cases [88, 90]. Access site bleeding after a TA approach might include bleeding into the pleural or pericardial cavity, possibly resulting in cardiac tamponade. Bleeding in this case usually originates from intercostal musculature or vessels [91]. The TF access approach can result in retroperitoneal or inguinal bleeding caused by injury of the aorta, the iliac or femoral vessels or small branch vessels such as the inferior epigastric artery. In patients with aortoiliac stenosis, tortuosity or severe atherosclerosis and those with smaller vessels, there is a higher rate of bleeding after TF access [92].

To provide appropriate patient selection in order to reduce vascular access complications, pre-procedural contrast-enhanced computed tomography angiography

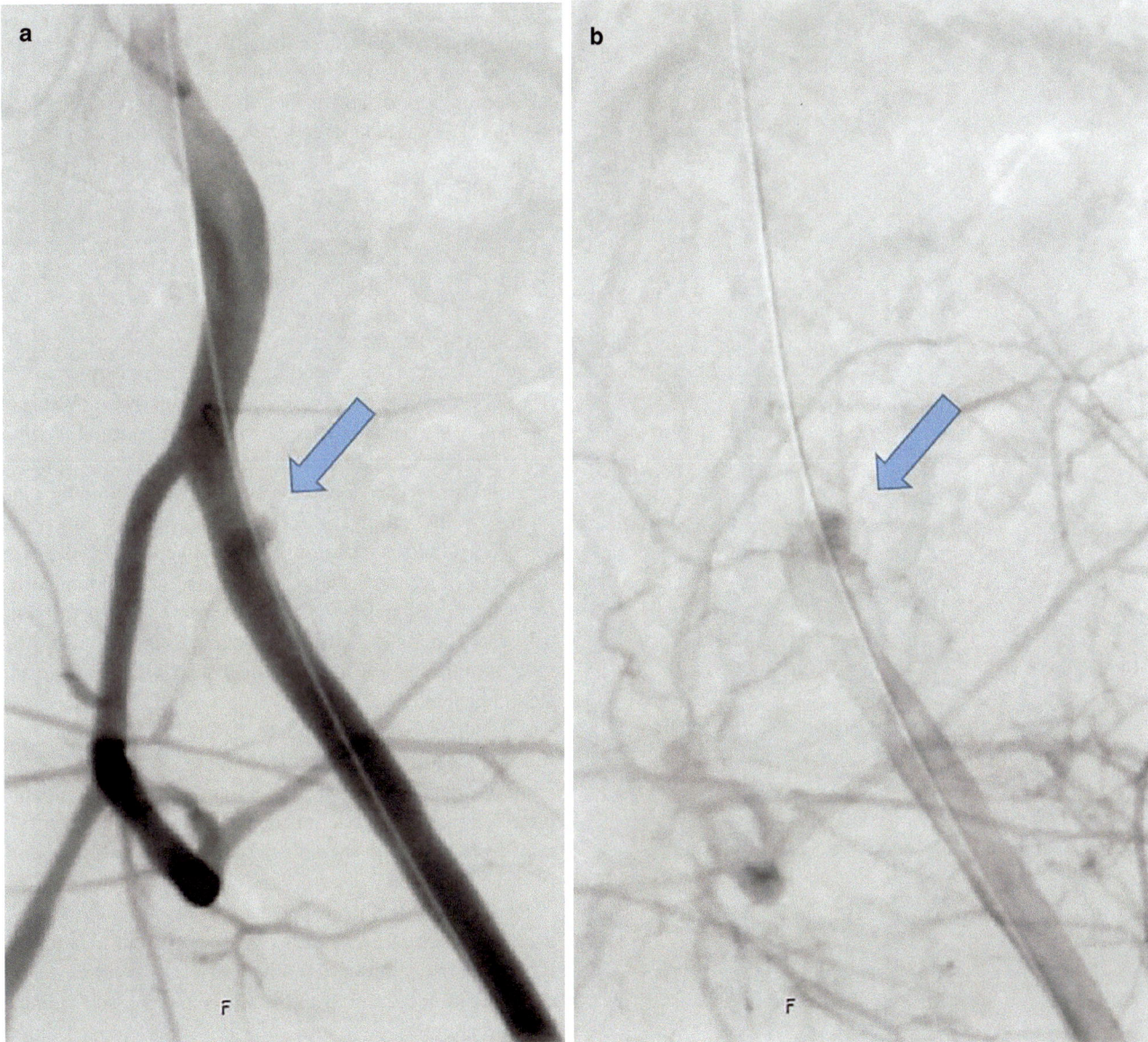

Fig. 5.11   Angiogram of the left external iliac artery from crossover showing the bleeding site (blue arrow; different phases **a/b**). Final Angiogram (same projection as illustration a) after neutralized bleeding with stent graft insertion (**c**)

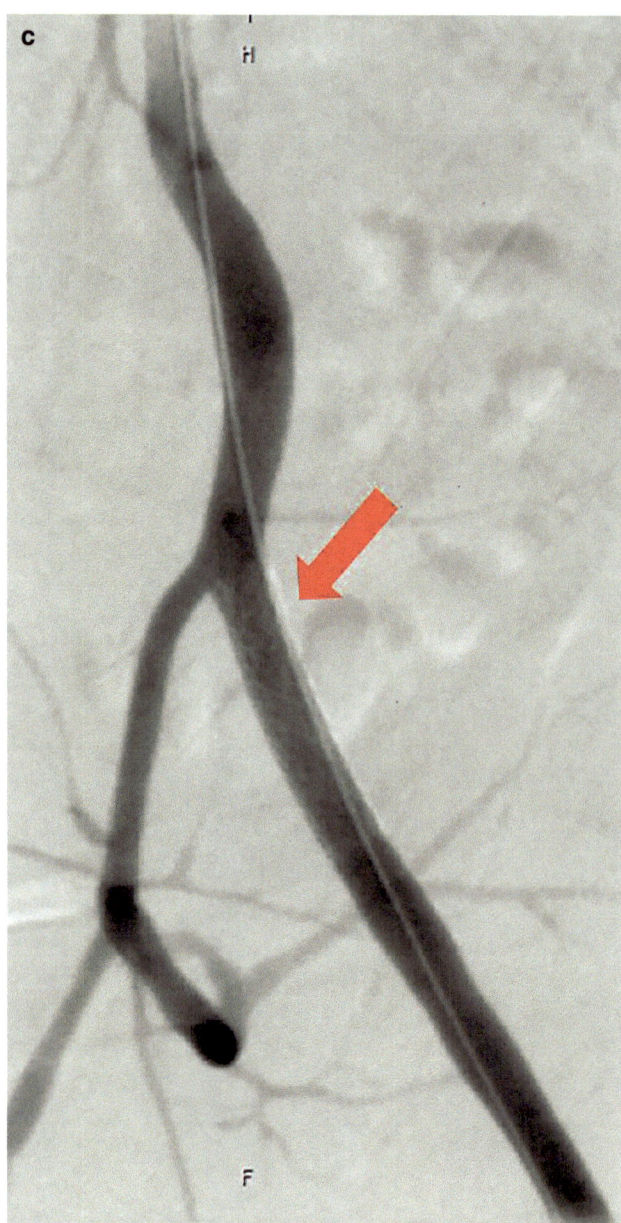

Fig. 5.11 (continued)

phases are then performed. Unenhanced CT may show a mildly hyperattenuating structure with hazy or well-defined margins in cases of formed hematoma with a potential sign of active bleeding on CTA. Active bleeding on CT is characterized by contrast media extravasation with continuous increase from the arterial to the venous phase (Fig. 5.12).

5.3.3 Pseudoaneurysm

5.3.3.1 Introduction

In general, access site bleeding after percutaneous interventions occur with (painful) swelling. A bruit heard by auscultation may also be indicative of an active pseudoaneurysm (= aneurysm spurium). In contrast to active bleeding, the pathophysiology of a pseudoaneurysm is bleeding within the outer layers of the arterial vessel, forming a false aneurysm sack (essentially a hematoma with active flow inside). This may grow, rupture, and compromise surrounding structures due to compression, such as the nerves or veins, leading to sensory motor deficits, venous congestion, or even deep vein thrombosis. For these reasons, large pseudoaneurysms should be treated.

5.3.3.2 Computed Tomography

Femoral pseudoaneurysm formation can occur with incomplete sealing of the arterial puncture site, resulting in contained bleeding into the soft tissue within a pseudocapsule [93]. The frequency of pseudoaneursym ranges from 2 to 6% [94]. The risk factors for pseudoaneurysms affecting the access site are larger sheath size, cannulation of an artery other than the common femoral artery, access artery calcification, combined arterial and venous puncture, and failure to provide appropriate compression [95]. Color-coded duplex sonography is a safe, fast and sensitive method to diagnose femoral pseudoaneurysm, however in patients with a pulsatile mass in the groin, CT is indicated to confirm the diagnosis and more precisely localize the pseudoaneurysm for interventional treatment planning. Unenhanced CT scans demonstrate a well-defined low-attenuating rounded structure with a usually smooth wall. CTA shows a contrast-filled sac adjacent to the artery that might contain non-enhancing, low attenuation areas, indicating partial thrombosis of the pseudoaneursym sac (Fig. 5.13). In distinction to active bleeding, a pseudoaneurysm shows usually no difference in contrast media extravasation between the arterial and the venous phase of enhancement.

(CTA) is necessary for a comprehensive evaluation of the ilio-femoral vessels and the thoracic anatomy.

When there is suspicion of postoperative bleeding at the access site, CT is mandatory to confirm the diagnosis and to localize and quantify the bleeding, which is of particular importance for the interventional radiologist who needs to make important treatment decisions.

After acquiring the unenhanced phase of the vascular region of interest, contrast enhanced arterial and venous

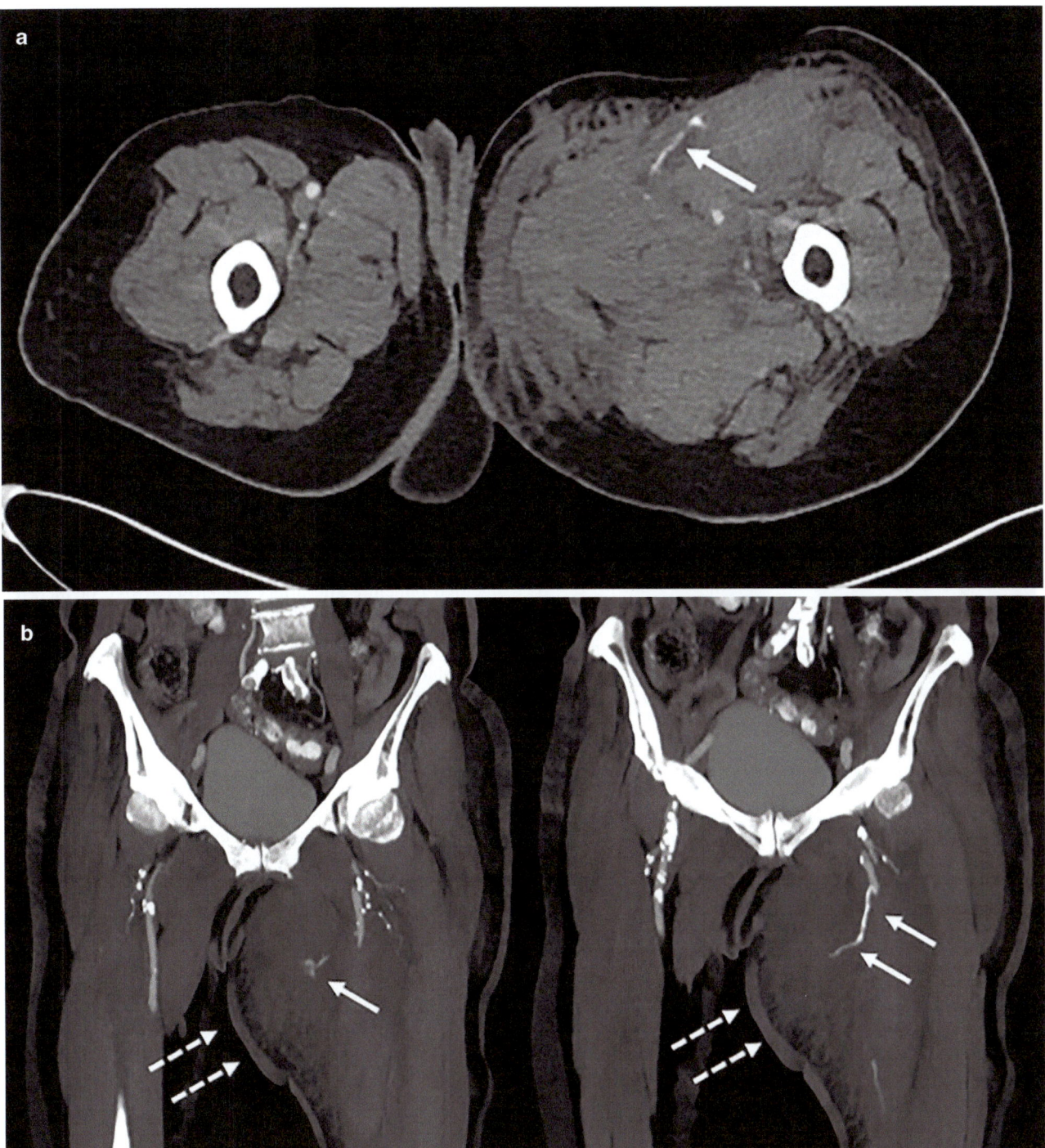

Fig. 5.12 Axial view (**a**) and coronal maximum intensity projections (**b**) of CTA of the iliofemoral arteries in a 78-year old female patient who was referred to the emergency department with massive swelling in the left groin and symptoms of hemorrhagic shock after TAVR. CTA showed active arterial bleeding at the access site from the left superficial femoral artery (SFA) (indicated by the solid white arrows) and large soft tissue hematoma in the left groin and proximal lower limb (white dashed arrows)

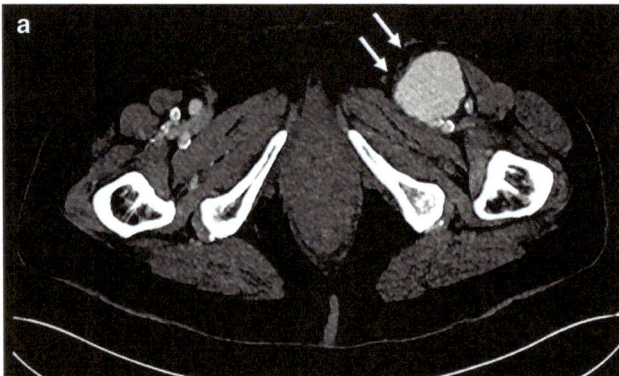

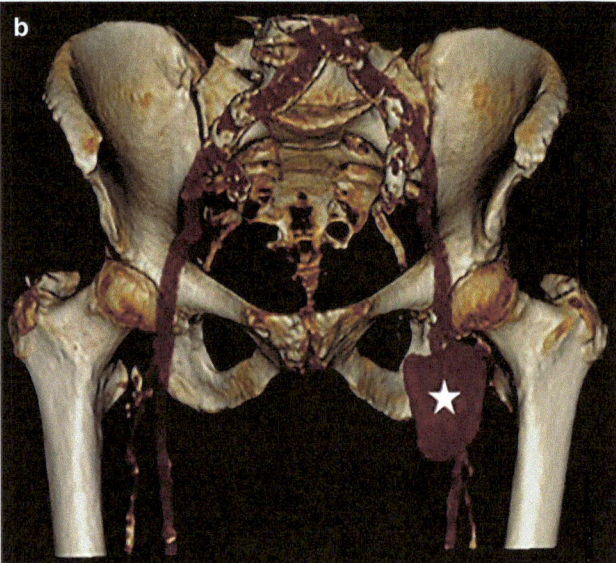

Fig. 5.13 Axial view (**a**) and volume rendering (**b**) of CTA of the ilio-femoral arteries in a 86-year old female patient who developed pulsatile swelling in the left groin after TAVR. CTA showed a large pseudoaneurysm from the left superficial femoral artery (indicated by the white arrows and white star)

5.3.3.3 Ultrasound

Ultrasound examination detects the majority of bleeding complications including active persistent bleeding or pseudoaneurysms. Depending on whether antithrombotic therapy was used, smaller pseudoaneurysms may be treated with prolonged (1) manual compression, or (2) ultrasound-assisted compression. In case of treatment failure, or large-sized pseudoaneurysms, ultrasound-assisted thrombin injection is considered as first-line treatment. Using duplex ultrasound, the width and length of the aneurysm neck may be estimated. This information is helpful for determining whether thrombin injection also requires endovascular assistance (balloon occlusion) to prevent secondary complications from "spillover", or whether a covered stent graft is necessary.

Case example

Sixty-eight year old female patient undergoing diagnostic coronary angiography from the left radial artery (radial

artery occlusion on the right). Two weeks after discharge, the patient complains about progressive swelling at the puncture site (Fig. 5.14a). Palpation revealed a pulsating mass, and auscultation a bruit. Duplex ultrasound showed a pseudoaneurysm of the distal radial artery (Fig. 5.14b). Due to the morphology and the rather narrow pseudoaneurysm neck, successful ultrasound-assisted thrombin injection (1.5 mL thrombin solution) was performed. On the next day, the pseudoaneurysm was completely occluded, and the radial artery patent (Fig. 5.14c).

5.3.3.4 Diagnosis

5.3.3.4.1 Introduction

Occlusion of the arterial puncture vessel accounts for the most frequent malperfusion complications, and is usually associated with the use of a closure device, especially when used in stenotic atherosclerotic arteries. This is attributed to either plaque shift as a result to the insertion of the closure device, or displacement of the closure device itself. This occurs more often with small vessel diameters, a severely calcified puncture site artery (atherosclerosis), or incorrect use of the closure device.

In addition, inappropriate puncture (such as subintimal lumen, puncture at the femoral bifurcation) may result in dissection of the artery. This can be avoided largely by ultrasound-guided puncture.

In the majority of patients, the clinical manifestation is an acute event of limb ischemia immediately after the intervention. These patients may present with a limb temperature difference, sensory motor deficits, and/or ischemic pain in the affected limb. Proper medical history and review of the interventional reports and images may provide important clues to the diagnosis. After completing a clinical examination and non-invasive diagnostics, duplex ultrasound is the primary diagnostic tool. Depending on the severity of malperfusion, revascularization therapy may be indicated. In this situation, ultrasound information may also provide further guidance on vascular access strategy required for revascularization (crossover/antegrade etc.).

Case example

Seventy year old female patient undergoing endovascular revascularization of a femoro-popliteal occlusion of her right leg via left femoral cross-over access. A closure device was applied at the left groin. After the intervention, the patient complained about a cold left leg. Clinical examination revealed missing pedal pulses (present pulses prior to intervention). Non-invasive diagnostics showed a critical limb perfusion of the left leg (Fig. 5.15a).

On the same day, endovascular revascularization of the left common femoral artery was performed from a cross-over access. The diagnostic angiogram showed a total

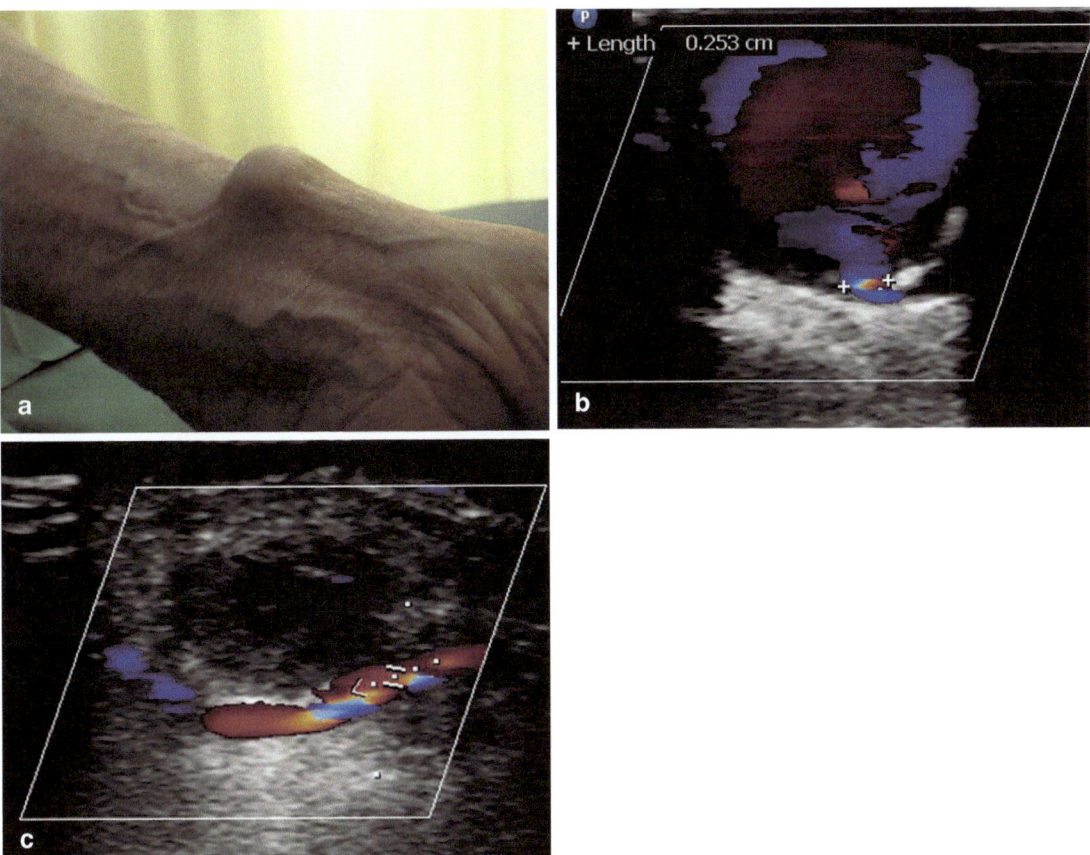

Fig. 5.14 Clinical image of a radial artery pseudoaneurysm after diagnostic coronary catheterization (**a**). Duplex ultrasound showing the perfused radial artery pseudoaneurysm (**b**). Control duplex ultrasound after thrombin injection: total occlusion of pseudoaneurysm and preserved radial artery perfusion (**c**)

Fig. 5.15 Non-invasive examination showing critical ischemia of the left leg (**a**). Angiography showing total occlusion of the left common femoral artery due to severe puncture site dissection (**b, c**). Final angiography showing perfusion of the superficial femoral artery from the false lumen (**d**)

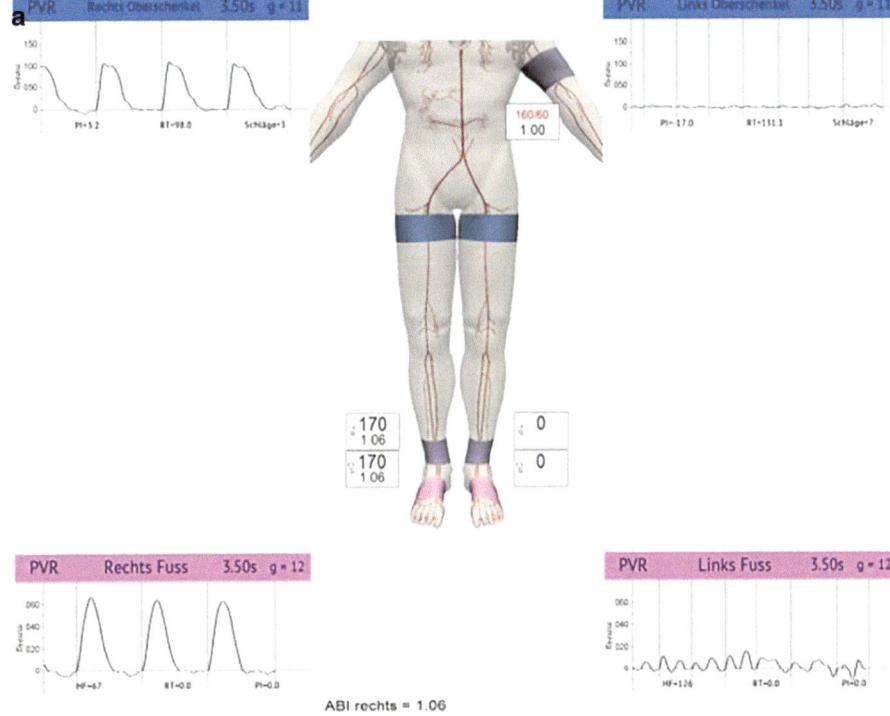

Fig. 5.15 (continued)

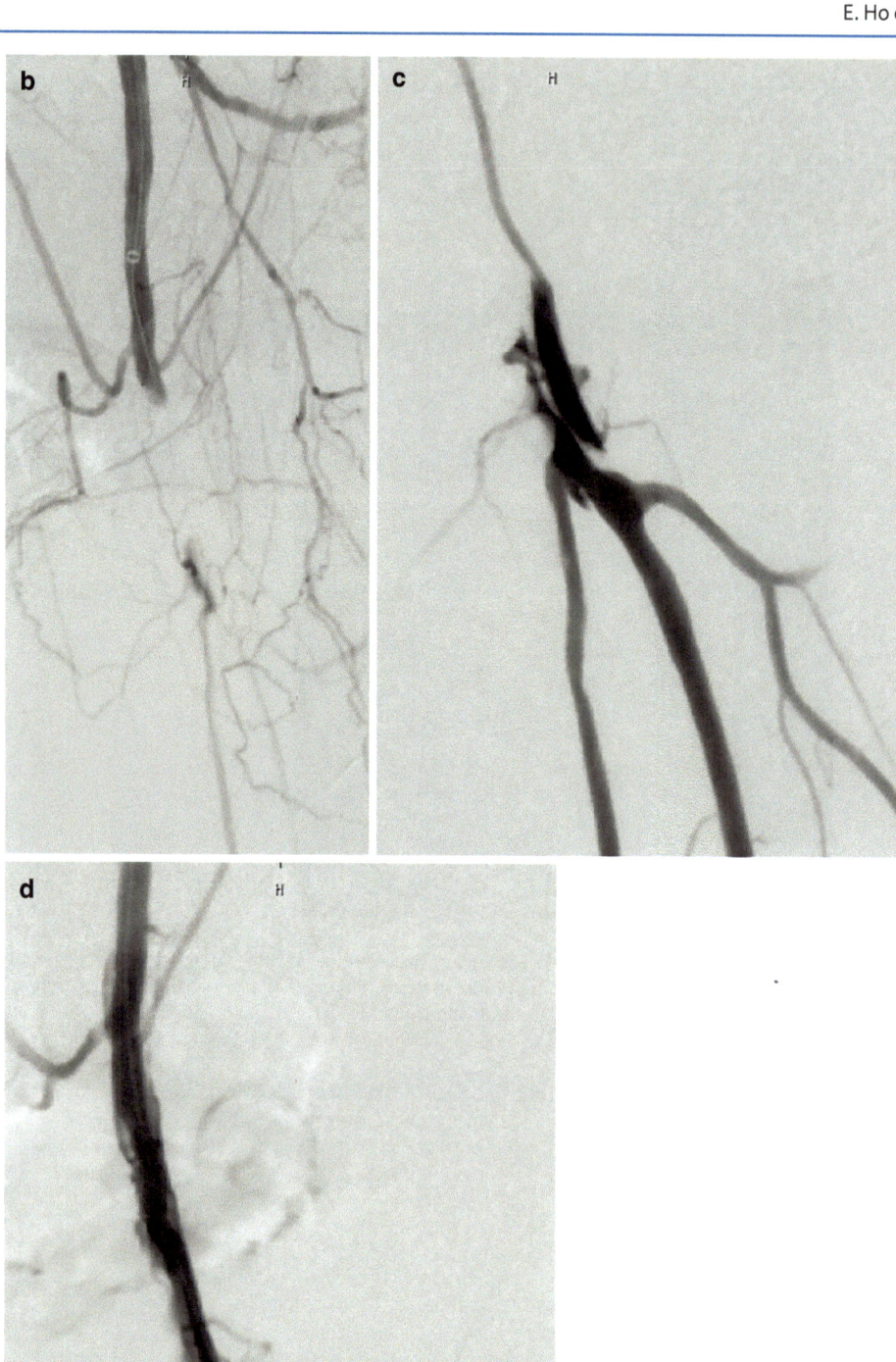

occlusion of the common femoral artery (Fig. 5.15b). This because of a severe access related dissection of the puncture vessel. The superficial femoral artery was perfused via the false lumen of the dissection (Fig. 5.15c, d), and wire passage was not possible. After catheterization of the deep femoral artery and balloon angioplasty of the common femoral artery, the symptoms resolved. For that reason, retrograde puncture of the superficial femoral artery was not performed.

5.3.3.4.2 Computed Tomography

Dissection of the ilio-femoral artery requiring further percutaneous or surgical intervention in patients undergoing transfemoral TAVI has been reported to occur in 2.0–7.4% of cases [96–98]. Dissections and vascular occlusions often occur in cases with an inadequate access vessel size. With an incidence of up to 0.14%, arteriovenous fistula (AVF) constitute a rare but important complication in patients undergoing intervention with a femoral access [99]. Kelm et al. [99] described the degree of anticoagulation as an independent risk factor in the development of AVF.

For patient selection, pre-interventional CT is mandatory to evaluate vascular conditions and potentially choose an alternative access route in order to reduce the aforementioned complications. In the event of access dissection, which mainly presents with symptoms suggestive of vessel occlusion, CTA is indicated to identify the focus and extent of the dissection or occlusion (Fig. 5.16).

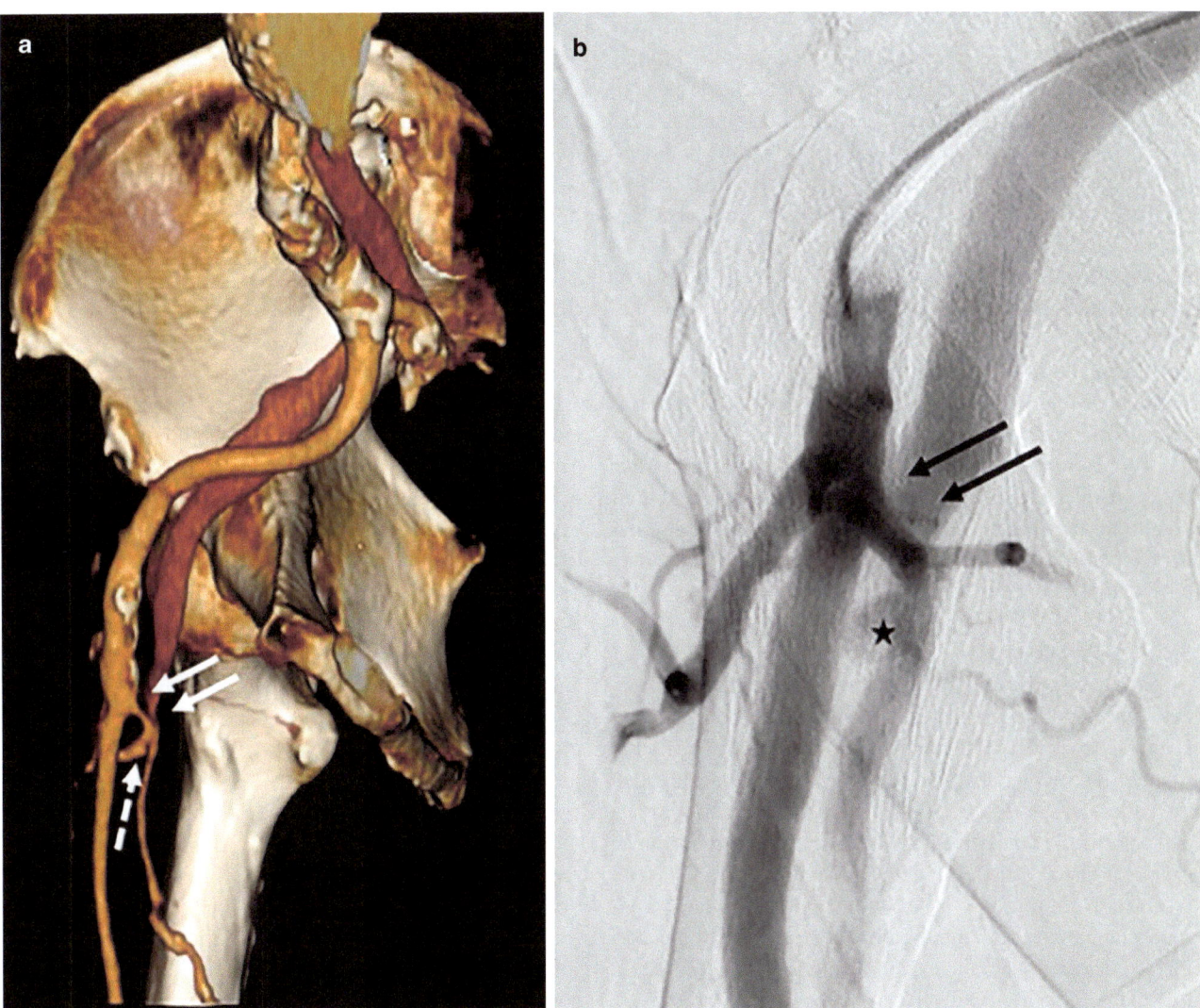

Fig. 5.16 Volume rendering of the right pelvis (**a**) CTA of the ilio-femoral arteries and corresponding fluoroscopic view (**b**) in a 75-year old male patient who developed an arterio-venous fistula between the right deep femoral artery and the femoral vein (black and white arrows) post- TAVR. CTA additionally showed a small pseudoaneurysm of the right deep femoral artery (black star and white dashed arrow)

5.3.3.5 Treatment

5.3.3.5.1 Introduction

Treatment of vascular access complications associated with transcatheter aortic valve replacement is dependent on the type and extent of injury as well as immediate clinical consequence. In general, they are managed percutaneously whenever possible [100–102].

Iliofemoral dissection can be treated conservatively with prolonged balloon inflation that allows apposition of the intimal and medial layers of the vessel if the dissection is very small. A larger dissection may require stent placement. Both the use of covered and uncovered stents have been described. The usually done using a "crossover" technique where the vasculature is accessed on the contralateral limb to facilitate wiring of the dissected artery and stent placement. If percutaneous treatment is not successful, then urgent surgery is performed. More extensive artery injury, such as rupture, may also require urgent surgical repair if bleeding cannot be controlled with balloon inflation and covered stent implantation.

Access site stenosis or occlusion can occur due to the use of percutaneous closure devices. These will often cause a mild degree of stenosis that does not have any clinical consequence. If the degree of stenosis is more severe, then dilatation of the site can also be performed. Stent placement is rarely needed. Thrombosis is a rare, but potentially devastating complication. Balloon angioplasty may be able to restore flow to the limb, but there is a risk of distal embolization and subsequent ongoing ischemia. Surgical revascularization is also an option.

Fistula formation is rare after transcatheter aortic valve replacement, but is possible if there is injury to the venous system at the time of the procedure. This complication has been reported in the literature and can be repaired percutaneously using a covered stent [103].

5.3.3.5.2 Angiography

Angiography plays an important role in the treatment of vascular access site complications. This is because it is readily available to the procedural operator in the fluoroscopic environment used for transcatheter aortic valve replacement. It also offers high resolution visualization of the vessel lumen and can easily identify stenosis, occlusion and fistulas due to excellent visualization of luminal flow pattern.

Once a complication has been identified, dedicated fluoroscopic imaging with intra-arterial contrast injection is performed to understand the extent of injury and target site for treatment. This is usually performed using a "crossover" technique where the contralateral limb is accessed for the treatment [100–102].

Prolonged balloon inflation and potential stent placement are performed under live fluoroscopy to ensure the position of the device is appropriate and the inflation is adequate. The results of the repair maneuver can then also be checked with a repeat contrast injection to ensure the dissection flap has been controlled, stenosis improved, occlusion revascularized or fistula closed.

Fusion imaging currently does not play an important role in the management of access site complications during transcatheter aortic valve replacement. This is because computed tomography data obtained prior to the procedure is fixed and may be difficult to align with the live fluoroscopic view. However, since the arterial tree and calcification pattern are seen very well by computed tomography, the ability to superimpose this data accurately on the fluoroscopic image may be helpful in improving the therapeutic plan or potentially reducing the amount of contrast use during access site repair. Further product development and studies are needed. Additionally, the workflow would need to be optimized to allow for rapid alignment of the two data sources, since this acute procedural complication generally requires prompt treatment. Fusion with ultrasound imaging will unlikely be helpful in this situation because of the limited field of view offered by vascular ultrasound and since the transducer would need to be over the vessel under evaluation, likely obscuring the fluoroscopic view (Fig. 5.17).

5.3.4 Compartment Syndrome

5.3.4.1 Introduction

Extremity acute compartment syndrome (CS) is a surgical emergency that may lead to severe disabilities, amputation, or even death, if not recognized and treated promptly. It can occur in the upper extremity (primarily forearm) or lower extremity (primarily the lower leg, foot or thigh in that order of frequency). The widespread use of transfemoral percutaneous approaches to cardiac and vascular procedures is the reason why lower extremity CS an important vascular complication to consider. There is a significant impact of vascular complications on 30-day mortality: mortality was consistently higher in those with vascular complications compared to those without (17 vs. 6.6%). The Economic impact and prolonged in-hospital length of stay in patients with major vascular complications are also important consequences.

The crucial pathophysiological mechanism is the elevated interstitial pressure within the muscle compartments that exceeds capillary blood pressure (tissue perfusion pressure). Resting pressure in a muscle compartment with healthy tissue is 6–8 mmHg, and pressure above 30 mmHg is highly confirmative for compartment syndrome.

Risk factors for CS are patient related (baseline diameter of artery) and non-patient related (proceduralist/procedure/center related). At increased risk are women with smaller arteries. Peripheral arterial disease with moderate to severe high-grade artery stenosis and complicated or calcified

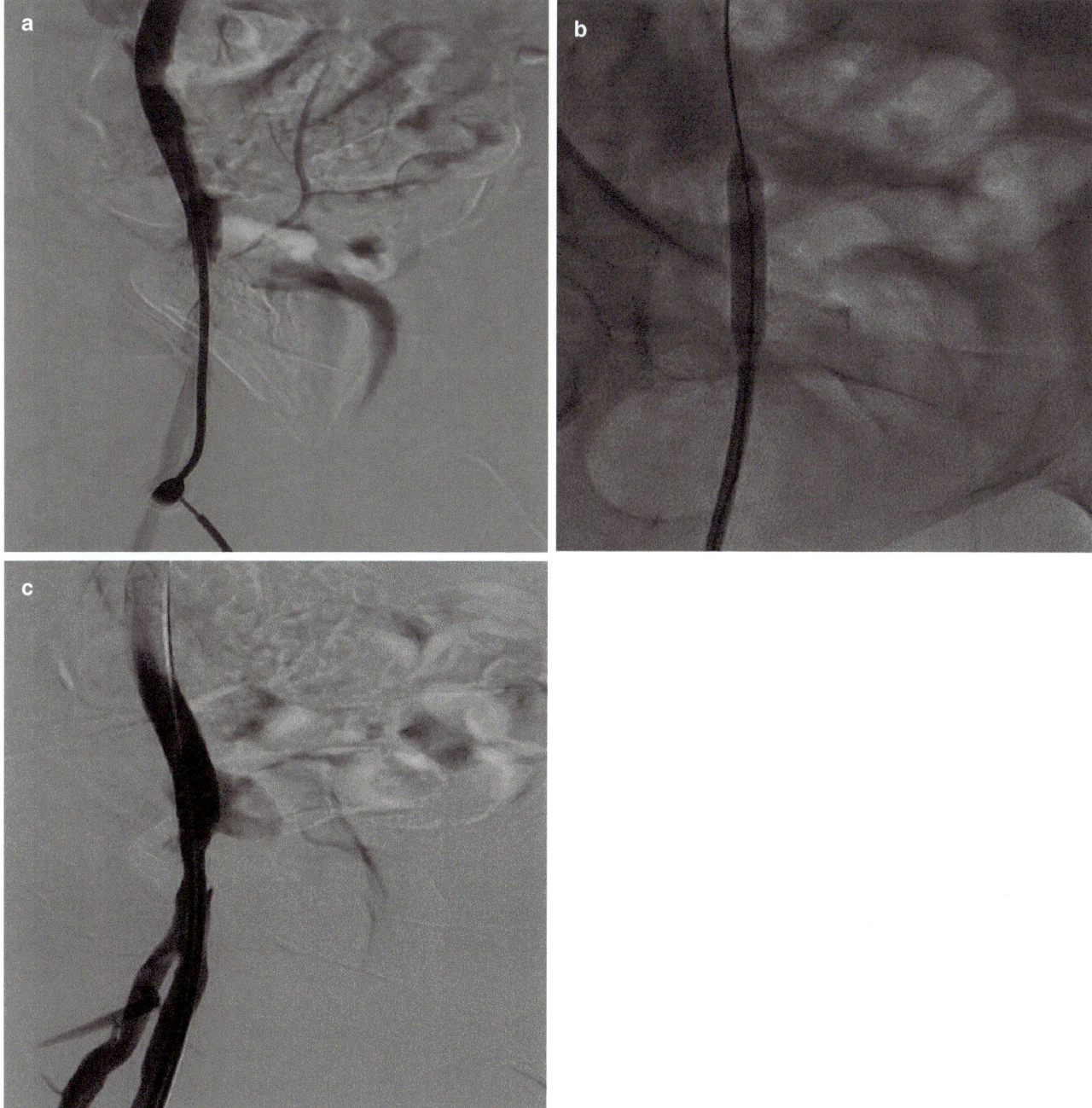

Fig. 5.17 Angiographic appearance of common femoral artery occlusion following transcatheter aortic valve replacement (**a**) treated with balloon inflation (**b**), restoring flow in the artery (**c**)

plaques will also increase the risk of limb ischemia related to the procedure. Flow obstruction with ischemia occurs if the external sheath diameter is greater than the minimal arterial diameter (one proposed risk factor for CS is a sheath to femoral arterial ratio of >1.05) and a sheath size larger than 19 Fr. Older generation Edwards Lifesciences SAPIEN and SAPIEN XT valves required up to 24 Fr and 20 Fr sheaths, respectively, while the first Medtronic CoreValve required up to a 25 Fr sheath. Newer generation valves require only

14–16 Fr sheaths due to advancement in transcatheter technologies. The importance of procedural and center experience is significant because shorter procedures performed by experienced operators minimize ischemic time and associated reperfusion injury. Adequate patient screening and selection, including the appropriate use of multimodality imaging within the heart team, can also prevent vascular complications or minimize the consequences in those who have been identified upfront at being at increased risk.

The most frequent cause of limb compartment syndrome overall is reperfusion injury after a period of ischemia. Ischemia is typically the result of distal obstruction of the access artery: common femoral, superficial femoral, or external iliac in the lower extremity and subclavian or axillary in the upper extremity. This can be due to thrombosis, embolization or vessel dissection during endovascular procedures. Intramuscular bleeding due to anticoagulation during procedures, or after thrombolysis for acute arterial thrombosis, can also result in CS.

5.3.4.2 Diagnosis

Hallmark clinical findings and clinical suspicion are crucial for diagnosis. Symptoms and signs include severe pain, hypoesthesia, and weakness of the affected limb. The accuracy of these findings is limited in an unconscious patient compared to an alert (conscious) one. Pain tends to be out of proportion to what is expected from a percutaneous procedure or physical examination findings. This includes severe pain with passive stretching of the muscle compartment, tenderness on palpation in all compartments. The anterior calf compartment (peroneal nerve), is frequently the most tender with severe pain even with light percussion. Paresthesia, hypoesthesia, paresis and pallor might be present similar to acute limb ischemia, but the pulses are typically present. Loss of pulses, paralysis and foot anesthesia are signs of advanced compartment syndrome, where recovery, if possible at all, will generally still result in permanent disabilities. It is also important to highlight the dynamic nature of CS. Over several hours, symptoms of CS could progress rapidly and result in irreversible muscle and nerve damage. This is why close observation and serial examination of patients at increased risk for CS are of great importance.

Diagnosis of CS in unconscious patient is not easy since the majority of clinical signs of CS are subjective. Diagnosis in this setting will be based on the detection of raised compartment pressure. There is no consensus on how often to measure in these cases, but a reasonable approach is to perform measurements every 4 hours for a minimum of 24 hours after the suspected reperfusion injury. Furthermore, the residual effects of procedural anesthetic drugs and postoperative sedation could delay the immediate detection of CS after a procedure. Local anesthesia with analgosedation is therefore often considered the optimal anesthetic method when there is an increased risk for CS.

Laboratory findings are unfortunately nonspecific. Myoglobinuria and elevation of the creatine kinase level often occur.

5.3.4.3 Treatment

Fasciotomy of the calf compartments is universally the definitive treatment for lower extremity CS. Four muscle compartments need decompression through two incisions (medial and lateral). Through a medial calf incision, we decompress the deep and superficial posterior muscle compartments. Through a lateral calf incision, we decompress the anterior and lateral compartments. While there are some aspects of fasciotomy that vary among surgeons, there are some aspects that are commonly agreed upon. For example, incisions should be at least 12–20 cm in length. The lateral incision should be between the fibular shaft and the anterior tibial margin. The medial incision should be 1–2 cm medial to the tibial margin. A single incision fasciotomy uses a lateral incision, and is exclusively performed for isolated anterior calf compartment syndrome. However, single incision fasciotomy may still be inadequate in these cases because of the inability to predict the evolution of muscle swelling in other compartments. Complete fasciotomy should be performed with long enough incisions to successfully decompress all four calf compartments.

Technical complications of fasciotomy are incomplete fasciotomy and neurovascular injury. The most frequent site of injury is the superficial peroneal nerve. Normally, this nerve is located anteriorly under the fascia and descends as a branch from the common peroneal nerve in the lateral compartment adjacent to the intermuscular septum of the anterior and lateral compartments. It is important to avoid injury to the great saphenous vein as well during medial incision. Sharp division of skin and subcutaneous fat reaches the fascia. The skin and subcutaneous fat is mobilized *en bloc* anteriorly and posteriorly to expose it enough to provide access to the compartments.

After fasciotomy, the wounds should stay open and dressed with moist gauze (soaked with 0.9% NaCl) to allow swelling to subside. There are also synthetic skin replacement products (e.g. *Epigard®*) for temporary wound covering and conditioning of the wound bed in preparation for definitive wound closure. In situations when the muscles are extremely swollen, the use of NWPT (negative wound pressure therapy) dressing with different foams helps facilitate the resolution of swelling and prevents the retraction of the wound. Closure of fasciotomy wounds can be primary (rarely), primary delayed (mostly after 2 weeks with vessel loops and staples) or secondary using the split-thickness skin graft. The disadvantages of latter is suboptimal cosmetic and functional outcomes. Another option at this time is a specialized dynamic wound closure system for fasciotomy wounds (*ABRA®, Canica*) that eliminates the need for skin grafting through graduate approximation of the wound edges [104, 105].

5.3.4.3.1 Angiography and Fusion

The utility of angiography in the treatment of compartment syndrome after transcatheter aortic valve replacement is limited. This is because after the diagnosis is made clinically, through direct pressure measurements, or based on radiographic evidence, it is managed surgically using a fasciotomy [106, 107].

In the setting of transcatheter aortic valve replacement, one potential relevant finding that can be seen with angiography is thrombosis or occlusion of the femoral artery used for vascular access [100]. This rare complication can cause acute limb ischemia, which can then result in compartment syndrome, especially if there was prolonged ischemia time and underlying arterial disease, resulting in significant ischemia-reperfusion injury [107].

5.3.4.4 Follow Up

5.3.4.4.1 Introduction
After successful treatment of compartment syndrome following transcatheter aortic valve replacement, the follow up consists predominantly of ensuring clinical improvement. After fasciotomy, there may be significant morbidity due to delayed closure, possible skin grafting, poor cosmesis, chronic pain, chronic muscle weakness and chronic venous insufficiency [106].

The utility of imaging techniques is predominantly to rule out any post-treatment complications and ensure the underlying etiology, such as arterial occlusion causing ischemia, has resolved.

5.3.4.4.2 Angiography
Angiography plays a limited role in the follow up of patients who were treated for the complication of compartment syndrome after transcatheter aortic valve replacement. If the initial etiology was due to access site thrombosis and occlusion, rather than transient ischemia due to occlusion from the device in a small artery, then angiography can be considered to re-evaluate the vessel lumen. However, since it is invasive and carries risk of further vascular access complications, noninvasive imaging of the vasculature is generally preferred.

5.3.5 Iatrogenic Aortic Dissection

5.3.5.1 Introduction
Aortic dissection during a transcatheter aortic valve procedure is a rare but potentially devastating complication [100]. It can also be seen rarely in the setting of surgical aortic valve replacement [108]. This most common timing of dissection is immediately following balloon valvuloplasty in preparation for device implantation, or is due to the stent edge of the prosthesis itself [109, 110]. Rare delayed cases of aortic dissection due to the prosthesis have also been described [111]. Dissections can occur in the proximal ascending aorta due to manipulation of and forces applied to the aortic root but can also be isolated to the descending aorta if injury occurred while the delivery system is being maneuvered from a femoral access site to the aortic valve [112].

The management if this complication is suspected is prompt diagnosis and treatment, utilizing all available urgent imaging modalities and tools available [100, 109, 110]. It is also important to classify the extent of dissection according to commonly used classification schemes because of the potential implication on prognosis and management strategy [113].

5.3.5.2 Diagnosis

5.3.5.2.1 Introduction
Since acute aortic dissection at the time of transcatheter aortic valve replacement can be a life threatening complication, prompt diagnosis is crucial to allow for rapid treatment. Although rare, this complication is associated with high mortality [100].

Rapid diagnosis can occur using different imaging modalities, but the most readily available modalities in the procedural lab are generally the fastest. In this section, the use of direct aortic angiography, echocardiography and computed tomography to diagnose and understand the extent of iatrogenic aortic dissection will be reviewed.

5.3.5.2.2 Angiography
Aortic dissection during transcatheter aortic valve implantation can be diagnosed immediately with angiography. With adequate contrast opacification of the aorta, a dissection will appear as a luminal filling defect that may take a variable course depending on the direction and pattern of the tear. This may cause the aorta to appear irregular along one of its curvatures or be seen as a contrast-free band [100, 109, 112]. The filling defect is seen because of the lack of contrast opacification of the false lumen and as a result, the entry point to the false lumen may be visible by angiography due to the appearance of partial contrast entry into that space.

Since angiography only provides a 2-dimensional imaging plane, the extent of dissection may need to be confirmed using additional imaging modalities such as transesophageal echocardiography or computed tomography. One of the advantages of angiography is that it is used during the transcatheter aortic valve replacement procedure and is therefore readily available immediately at the time of the suspected complication. Transesophageal echocardiography generally requires deeper sedation than the conscious sedation protocols commonly used for transcatheter replacement [114]. Additionally, angiography provides high resolution visualization of the aortic lumen. One major disadvantage of the use of aortography to assess aortic dissection is the contrast volume required, which may be significant in patients with underlying chronic renal dysfunction (Fig. 5.18).

5.3.5.2.3 Computed Tomography
Iatrogenic aortic dissection is an uncommon but potentially fatal complication of TAVR, with an incidence of up to 1.9% when a transfemoral access site is used [115]. With varying access approaches, any segment of the aorta can be involved including the ascending or descending aorta. The clinical

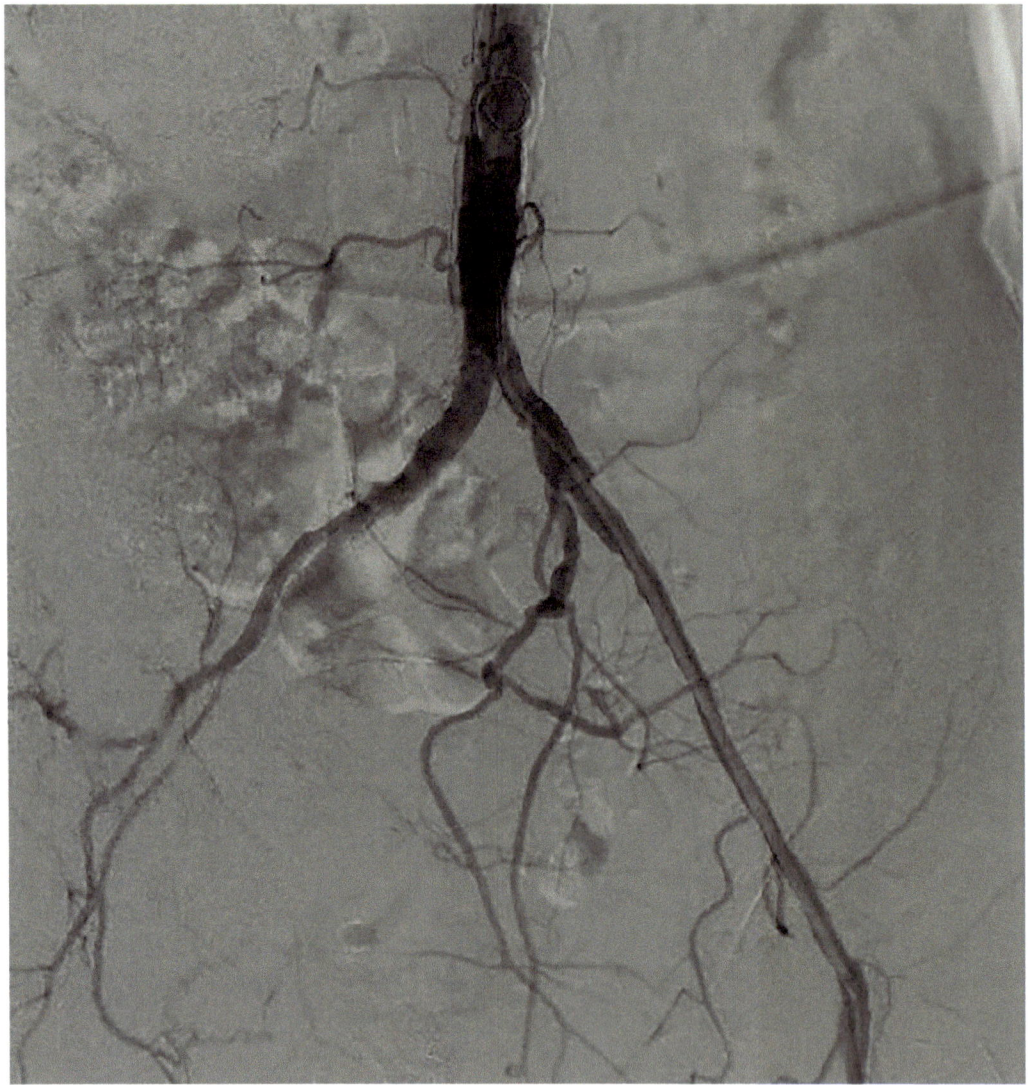

Fig. 5.18 A case of iatrogenic dissection and occlusion of right external iliac artery after transcatheter aortic valve implantation

manifestation of aortic dissection may manifest at any time during or after the procedure. If there is suspicion of iatrogenic aortic dissection, immediate CT angiography including unenhanced, arterial and venous phases should be performed in order to localize the initial site of dissection, extent and vascular compromise [94] (Fig. 5.19).

5.3.5.3 Treatment

5.3.5.3.1 Angiography
Acute aortic dissection by definition is a separation of the layers of the aortic wall due to an intimal tear. The two other different presentations of acute aortic syndrome are penetrating aortic ulcer and aortic intramural hematoma (IMH). All three conditions can affect the thoracic aorta, abdominal aorta, and in some cases, both.

Iatrogenic aortic dissection does not occur spontaneously and is result of instrumentation related to a procedure. The exact prevalence of dissection after percutaneous coronary

interventions (PCI) is unknown, because occurrences might be under reported. Iatrogenic IMH (e.g. with intra-aortic balloon pump placement, TAVR, coronary angiography) combined with trauma is responsible for 6% of cases of all IMH in one review. Focusing on PCI, iatrogenic dissection has been reported to occur in 0.02–0.07% of cases. In the systematic analysis of Shah et al., which included 86 patients, iatrogenic dissection was limited to the aortic root and the ascending aorta in about 40% in each equally, followed by the aortic arch (13%), and the descending aorta (5–7%). The cause of dissection was identified as catheter trauma in 55%, balloon inflation in 25%, contrast injection in 20%, and wire trauma in only 10%.

There are no guidelines for treating iatrogenic aortic dissection during cardiovascular procedures. Some suggestions, such as by Dunning et al., include open surgical intervention if a dissection extends more than 4 cm into the ascending aorta. However, there are patients with dissections extending even to the aortic arch who are treated non-operatively using

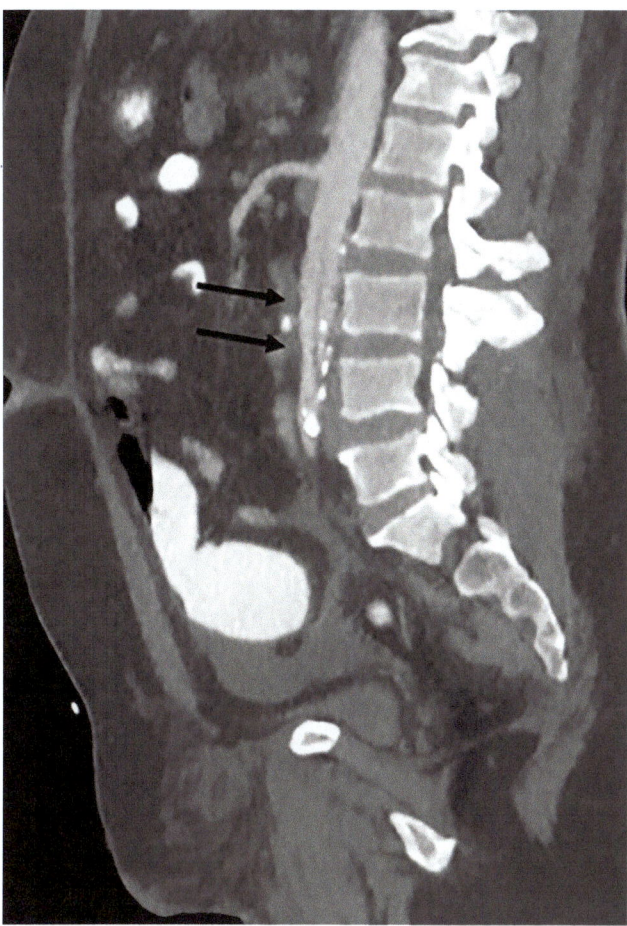

Fig. 5.19 Sagittal reconstruction of CTA of the thoraco-abdominal aorta in a 47-year old female patient who underwent TAVR. CT showed post-procedural segmental infrarenal aortic dissection (black arrows)

optimal medical therapy only. In cases of organ malperfusion, endovascular options can also be considered, including fenestration of the dissection flap, thoracic stent-graft implantation (TEVAR) or branch vessel stenting. In the case of aortic rupture, TEVAR has become the standard owing to its lower mortality compared to open surgical repair. The most important factors that guide treatment are the patient's hemodynamic stability and the practitioner's ability to rapidly stent the origin of the dissection to prevent the dissection from expanding.

Fenestration of the dissection flap is of use in situations where the blood through the entry tear pressurizes the false lumen. As a blind sac, especially in diastole, the true lumen is completely collapsed resulting in dynamic (80%) or static (20%) true lumen obstruction. The goal of the fenestration is to create a re-entry point (making an additional communication between the true and false lumen) to faciliate re-entry of blood into the true lumen to allow depressurization of the false lumen. This is performed using special re-entry devices (e.g. outback catheters) or a long puncture needle. Balloon dilatation can then also be performed, to ensure the new re-entry point is successfully allowing pressure equalization between the true and the false lumen. In patients with purely

dynamic obstruction, fenestration is usually sufficient to eliminate organ malperfusion.

The ultimate goal of thoracic stent-graft implantation (TEVAR) is to occlude the proximal entry point of the dissection so that the false lumen is no longer perfused from an antegrade fashion. Decrease in false lumen pressure will lead to the re-expansion of the true lumen and thus to the elimination of the any dynamic obstruction resulting in malperfusion. The reduced pressure in the false lumen also prevents further progression of the dissection distally and allow for thrombosis and healing of the false lumen. Anatomical requirements for successful TEVAR is presence of a non-aneurysmal nor dissected 1–2 cm proximal landing zone (depending on the prosthesis used). In situations where a TEVAR graft will obstruct the origin of the supraaortic, renal or visceral arteries, endovascular parallel grafts (chimney, periscope), extra-anatomical, transthoracic or renovisceral debranching (more frequent in subacute aortic dissection) can be performed to maintain artery patency. The complications of TEVAR should also be noted, which include retrograde type A dissection (about 1.5%), stroke (2%), spinal ischemia (3%) and the appearance of a new entry point at the distal end of the prosthesis (3%). In patients with static obstruction, the use of TEVAR needs additional stenting to restore end organ perfusion.

Branch vessel stenting is used to eliminate the static component of aortic dissection. In these cases, it is necessary to expand the true lumen of the end organ artery actively by means of a stent [116–118].

5.4 Follow-Up

5.4.1 Introduction

Follow up of patients after aortic valve intervention is important for many reasons. There may be ongoing management required in the setting of prosthetic valves, such as endocarditis prophylaxis or anticoagulation [9, 10, 119]. If there was a valve repair procedure, then durability of the repair should be assessed. Additionally, the clinical status of the patient should be followed on a regular basis to ensure there has been sustained improvement and to rule out any complications or prosthetic valve degeneration. It is important to note that after valve intervention, especially replacement, patients are not fully cured of heart disease. Rather, native valve disease has either been improved or replaced by prosthetic valve disease.

The frequency of follow up will be determined by each individual heart valve center. In many clinics, uncomplicated patients are assessed clinically on an annual basis. Imaging plays an important role in the follow up of patients after aortic valve intervention because it allows for assessment of valve morphology and hemodynamics. This includes transthoracic or transesophageal echocardiography, computed tomography and cardiac magnetic resonance imaging. Guidelines for each modality exist regarding its use in prosthetic valve evaluation as well as the application of multimodality imaging for valvular disease follow up [120].

5.4.2 Echocardiography

Echocardiographic follow up after aortic valvular intervention is well outlined by worldwide imaging guideline societies. If aortic valve repair was performed, then routine assessment of native valvular regurgitation can be performed using transthoracic echocardiography, and transesophageal echocardiography when needed [121–123]. This should be done in the post-operative period to establish a new baseline and then repeated as clinically indicated depending on the residual degree of valve disease, clinical course of the patient and their symptoms [9, 119].

In the setting of treated aortic stenosis, echocardiographic evaluation of the prosthetic valve should be performed in accordance to guideline recommendations for prosthetic valve assessment [11, 12, 124]. This should include a detailed assessment of transvalvular gradients, and if elevated, determination of prosthetic valve dysfunction exists. A prolonged acceleration time on the continuous wave spectral Doppler profile across the prosthetic valve in association with a low Doppler velocity index are suggestive of prosthetic valve dysfunction. On the other hand, a short acceleration time with higher Doppler velocity index may be due to a high flow state or patient-prosthesis mismatch. These two entities can be distinguished from one another based on the effective orifice area indexed to body surface area. Normal values for transvalvular gradients and expected effective orifice area are available from device manufacturers and in guideline publications.

Prosthetic valve regurgitation may originate from multiple areas and requires an integrative assessment to grade its severity. It should also be noted that specific criteria for grading the severity of paravalvular regurgitation following transcatheter aortic valve replacement have been established [124]. In addition to the qualitative, semi-quantitative and quantitative parameters used for the evaluation of native aortic valve regurgitation, the circumferential extent of paravalvular regurgitation is also used in this setting.

An initial follow up transthoracic echocardiogram should be done 6 weeks to 3 months after prosthetic valve implantation to establish a new baseline and evaluate valve hemodynamics. Studies can be repeated if there is a change in clinical status or symptoms. The frequency of routine echocardiography after prosthetic valve implantation is not well defined, but the guidelines suggest it is reasonable to perform this annually after 10 years even in the absence of a clinical status change due to the risk of prosthetic valve dysfunction [119]. The long-term durability of transcatheter aortic valve

replacement devices is not as well established, so frequent echocardiographic follow up even before 10 years may be reasonable. Transesophageal echocardiography can be considered as needed if better visualization of the prosthesis is needed (Figs. 5.20, 5.21, and 5.22).

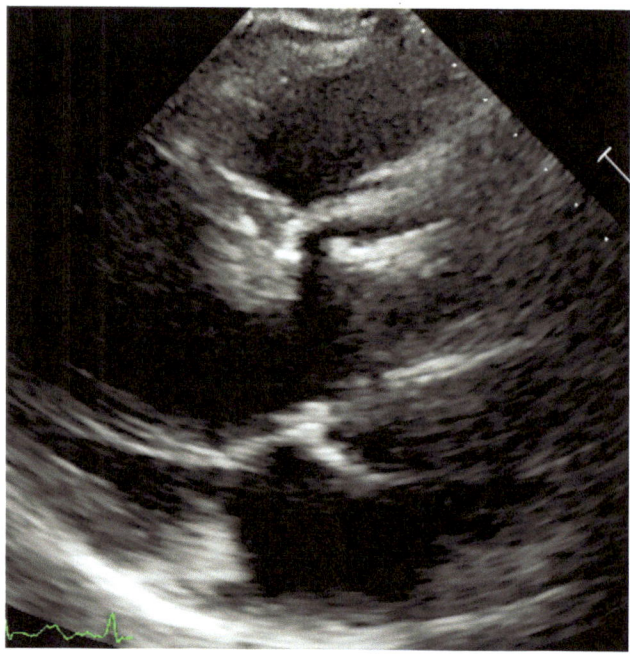

Fig. 5.20 Aortic prosthesis dehiscence seen by transthoracic echocardiography on the parasternal long axis view

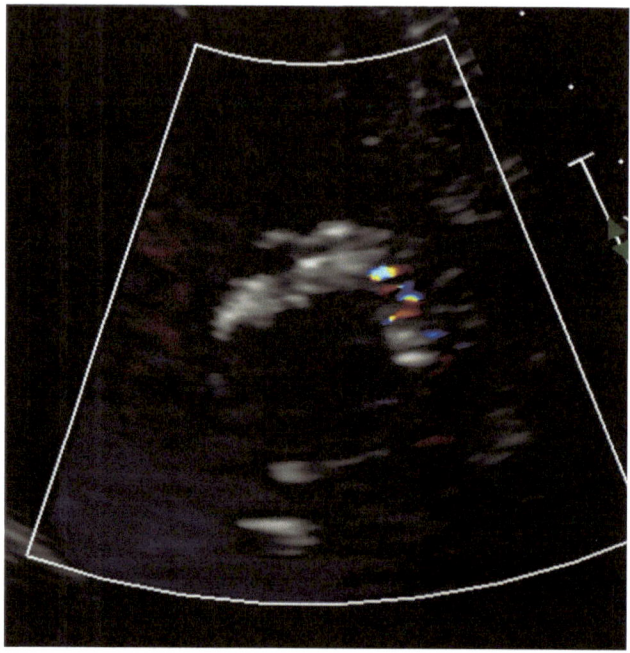

Fig. 5.21 Mild paravalvular regurgitation after transcatheter aortic valve replacement seen by transthoracic echocardiography on the short axis view of the prosthesis

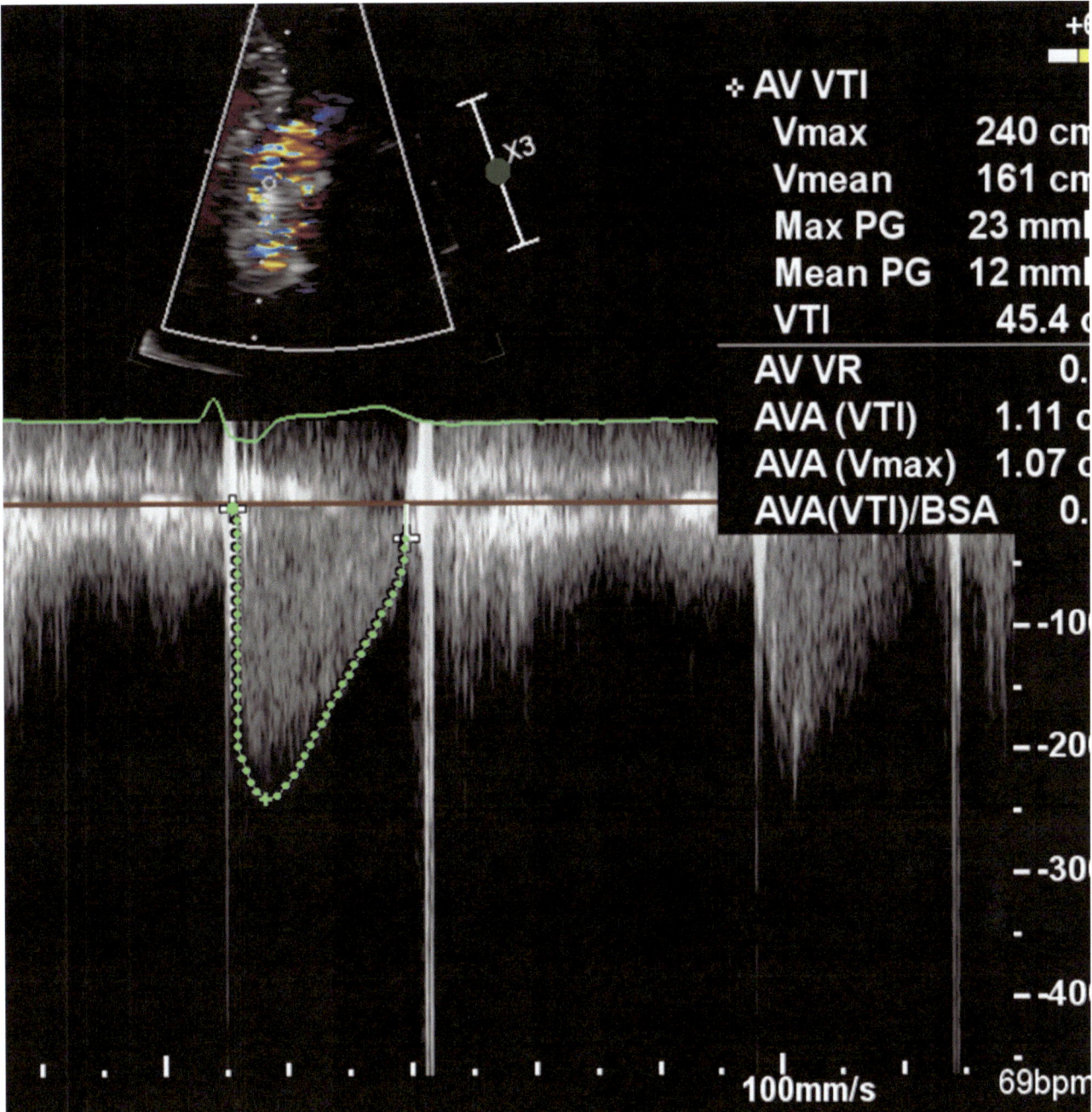

Fig. 5.22 Continuous wave spectral Doppler across a mechanical aortic valve prosthesis and measurement of the transvalvular gradients. The acceleration time, which is helpful in determining if there is prosthetic valve dysfunction, is measured as the interval between the onset of flow across the prosthesis to the peak velocity in the spectral Doppler profile

References

1. Kataruka A, Otto CM. Valve durability after transcatheter aortic valve implantation. J Thorac Dis. 2018;10(Suppl 30):S3629–s3636.
2. Butany J, Collins MJ. Analysis of prosthetic cardiac devices: a guide for the practising pathologist. J Clin Pathol. 2005;58(2): 113–24.
3. Wang M, Furnary AP, Li HF, Grunkemeier GL. Bioprosthetic aortic valve durability: a meta-regression of published studies. Ann Thorac Surg. 2017;104(3):1080–7.
4. Dasi LP, Hatoum H, Kheradvar A, Zareian R, Alavi SH, Sun W, Martin C, Pham T, Wang Q, Midha PA, Raghav V, Yoganathan AP. On the mechanics of transcatheter aortic valve replacement. Ann Biomed Eng. 2017;45(2):310–31.
5. Foroutan F, Guyatt GH, O'Brien K, Bain E, Stein M, Bhagra S, Sit D, Kamran R, Chang Y, Devji T, Mir H, Manja V, Schofield

T, Siemieniuk RA, Agoritsas T, Bagur R, Otto CM, Vandvik PO. Prognosis after surgical replacement with a bioprosthetic aortic valve in patients with severe symptomatic aortic stenosis: systematic review of observational studies. BMJ. 2016;354:i5065.

6. Martin C, Sun W. Transcatheter valve underexpansion limits leaflet durability: implications for valve-in-valve procedures. Ann Biomed Eng. 2017;45(2):394–404.

7. Martin C, Sun W. Comparison of transcatheter aortic valve and surgical bioprosthetic valve durability: a fatigue simulation study. J Biomech. 2015;48(12):3026–34.

8. Pislaru SV, Nkomo VT, Sandhu GS. Assessment of prosthetic valve function after TAVR. JACC Cardiovasc Imaging. 2016;9(2):193–206.

9. Baumgartner H, Falk V, Bax JJ, De Bonis M, Hamm C, Holm PJ, Iung B, Lancellotti P, Lansac E, Rodriguez Munoz D, Rosenhek R, Sjogren J, Tornos Mas P, Vahanian A, Walther T, Wendler O, Windecker S, Zamorano JL. 2017 ESC/EACTS Guidelines for the management of valvular heart disease. Eur Heart J. 2017;38(36):2739–91.

10. Nishimura RA, Otto CM, Bonow RO, Carabello BA, Erwin JP 3rd, Fleisher LA, Jneid H, Mack MJ, McLeod CJ, O'Gara PT, Rigolin VH, Sundt TM 3rd, Thompson A. 2017 AHA/ACC focused update of the 2014 AHA/ACC guideline for the management of patients with valvular heart disease: a report of the American College of Cardiology/American Heart Association Task Force on Clinical Practice Guidelines. Circulation. 2017;135(25):e1159–95.

11. Lancellotti P, Pibarot P, Chambers J, Edvardsen T, Delgado V, Dulgheru R, Pepi M, Cosyns B, Dweck MR, Garbi M, Magne J, Nieman K, Rosenhek R, Bernard A, Lowenstein J, Vieira ML, Rabischoffsky A, Vyhmeister RH, Zhou X, Zhang Y, Zamorano JL, Habib G. Recommendations for the imaging assessment of prosthetic heart valves: a report from the European Association of Cardiovascular Imaging endorsed by the Chinese Society of Echocardiography, the Inter-American Society of Echocardiography, and the Brazilian Department of Cardiovascular Imaging. Eur Heart J Cardiovasc Imaging. 2016;17(6):589–90.

12. Zoghbi WA, Chambers JB, Dumesnil JG, Foster E, Gottdiener JS, Grayburn PA, Khandheria BK, Levine RA, Marx GR, Miller FA Jr, Nakatani S, Quinones MA, Rakowski H, Rodriguez LL, Swaminathan M, Waggoner AD, Weissman NJ, Zabalgoitia M. Recommendations for evaluation of prosthetic valves with echocardiography and doppler ultrasound: a report From the American Society of Echocardiography's Guidelines and Standards Committee and the Task Force on Prosthetic Valves, developed in conjunction with the American College of Cardiology Cardiovascular Imaging Committee, Cardiac Imaging Committee of the American Heart Association, the European Association of Echocardiography, a registered branch of the European Society of Cardiology, the Japanese Society of Echocardiography and the Canadian Society of Echocardiography, endorsed by the American College of Cardiology Foundation, American Heart Association, European Association of Echocardiography, a registered branch of the European Society of Cardiology, the Japanese Society of Echocardiography, and Canadian Society of Echocardiography. J Am Soc Echocardiogr. 2009;22(9):975–1014; quiz 1082–4.

13. Bloomfield GS, Gillam LD, Hahn RT, Kapadia S, Leipsic J, Lerakis S, Tuzcu M, Douglas PS. A practical guide to multimodality imaging of transcatheter aortic valve replacement. JACC Cardiovasc Imaging. 2012;5(4):441–55.

14. Holmes DR Jr, Mack MJ, Kaul S, Agnihotri A, Alexander KP, Bailey SR, Calhoon JH, Carabello BA, Desai MY, Edwards FH, Francis GS, Gardner TJ, Kappetein AP, Linderbaum JA, Mukherjee C, Mukherjee D, Otto CM, Ruiz CE, Sacco RL, Smith D, Thomas JD, Harrington RA, Bhatt DL, Ferrari VA, Fisher JD, Garcia MJ, Gardner TJ, Gentile F, Gilson MF, Hernandez AF, Jacobs AK, Kaul S, Linderbaum JA, Moliterno DJ, Weitz HH. 2012 ACCF/AATS/SCAI/STS expert consensus document on transcatheter aortic valve replacement: developed in collaboration with the American Heart Association, American Society of Echocardiography, European Association for Cardio-Thoracic Surgery, Heart Failure Society of America, Mended Hearts, Society of Cardiovascular Anesthesiologists, Society of Cardiovascular Computed Tomography, and Society for Cardiovascular Magnetic Resonance. J Thorac Cardiovasc Surg. 2012;144(3):e29–84.

15. Thourani VH, Kodali S, Makkar RR, Herrmann HC, Williams M, Babaliaros V, Smalling R, Lim S, Malaisrie SC, Kapadia S, Szeto WY, Greason KL, Kereiakes D, Ailawadi G, Whisenant BK, Devireddy C, Leipsic J, Hahn RT, Pibarot P, Weissman NJ, Jaber WA, Cohen DJ, Suri R, Tuzcu EM, Svensson LG, Webb JG, Moses JW, Mack MJ, Miller DC, Smith CR, Alu MC, Parvataneni R, D'Agostino RB Jr, Leon MB. Transcatheter aortic valve replacement versus surgical valve replacement in intermediate-risk patients: a propensity score analysis. Lancet. 2016;387(10034):2218–25.

16. Leon MB, Smith CR, Mack MJ, Makkar RR, Svensson LG, Kodali SK, Thourani VH, Tuzcu EM, Miller DC, Herrmann HC, Doshi D, Cohen DJ, Pichard AD, Kapadia S, Dewey T, Babaliaros V, Szeto WY, Williams MR, Kereiakes D, Zajarias A, Greason KL, Whisenant BK, Hodson RW, Moses JW, Trento A, Brown DL, Fearon WF, Pibarot P, Hahn RT, Jaber WA, Anderson WN, Alu MC, Webb JG. Transcatheter or surgical aortic-valve replacement in intermediate-risk patients. N Engl J Med. 2016;374(17):1609–20.

17. Hammermeister KE, Sethi GK, Henderson WG, Oprian C, Kim T, Rahimtoola S. A comparison of outcomes in men 11 years after heart-valve replacement with a mechanical valve or bioprosthesis. Veterans Affairs Cooperative Study on Valvular Heart Disease. N Engl J Med. 1993;328(18):1289–96.

18. Hammermeister K, Sethi GK, Henderson WG, Grover FL, Oprian C, Rahimtoola SH. Outcomes 15 years after valve replacement with a mechanical versus a bioprosthetic valve: final report of the Veterans Affairs randomized trial. J Am Coll Cardiol. 2000;36(4):1152–8.

19. Durrleman N, Pellerin M, Bouchard D, Hebert Y, Cartier R, Perrault LP, Basmadjian A, Carrier M. Prosthetic valve thrombosis: twenty-year experience at the Montreal Heart Institute. J Thorac Cardiovasc Surg. 2004;127(5):1388–92.

20. Roudaut R, Serri K, Lafitte S. Thrombosis of prosthetic heart valves: diagnosis and therapeutic considerations. Heart. 2007;93(1):137–42.

21. Barbetseas J, Nagueh SF, Pitsavos C, Toutouzas PK, Quinones MA, Zoghbi WA. Differentiating thrombus from pannus formation in obstructed mechanical prosthetic valves: an evaluation of clinical, transthoracic and transesophageal echocardiographic parameters. J Am Coll Cardiol. 1998;32(5):1410–7.

22. Tanis W, Habets J, van den Brink RB, Symersky P, Budde RP, Chamuleau SA. Differentiation of thrombus from pannus as the cause of acquired mechanical prosthetic heart valve obstruction by non-invasive imaging: a review of the literature. Eur Heart J Cardiovasc Imaging. 2014;15(2):119–29.

23. Lin SS, Tiong IY, Asher CR, Murphy MT, Thomas JD, Griffin BP. Prediction of thrombus-related mechanical prosthetic valve dysfunction using transesophageal echocardiography. Am J Cardiol. 2000;86(10):1097–101.

24. Gunduz S, Ozkan M, Kalcik M, Gursoy OM, Astarcioglu MA, Karakoyun S, Aykan AC, Biteker M, Gokdeniz T, Kaya H, Yesin M, Duran NE, Sevinc D, Guneysu T. Sixty-four-section cardiac computed tomography in mechanical prosthetic heart valve dysfunction: thrombus or pannus. Circ Cardiovasc Imaging. 2015;8(12):e003246.

25. Ueda T, Teshima H, Fukunaga S, Aoyagi S, Tanaka H. Evaluation of prosthetic valve obstruction on electrocardiographically gated multidetector-row computed tomography—identification of sub-prosthetic pannus in the aortic position. Circ J. 2013;77(2):418–23.

26. Sucha D, Symersky P, Tanis W, Mali WP, Leiner T, van Herwerden LA, Budde RP. Multimodality imaging assessment of prosthetic heart valves. Circ Cardiovasc Imaging. 2015;8(9):e003703.

27. Mylotte D, Andalib A, Theriault-Lauzier P, Dorfmeister M, Girgis M, Alharbi W, Chetrit M, Galatas C, Mamane S, Sebag I, Buithieu J, Bilodeau L, de Varennes B, Lachapelle K, Lange R, Martucci G, Virmani R, Piazza N. Transcatheter heart valve failure: a systematic review. Eur Heart J. 2015;36(21):1306–27.

28. Ong SH, Mueller R, Iversen S. Early calcific degeneration of a CoreValve transcatheter aortic bioprosthesis. Eur Heart J. 2012;33(5):586.

29. Thubrikar MJ, Deck JD, Aouad J, Nolan SP. Role of mechanical stress in calcification of aortic bioprosthetic valves. J Thorac Cardiovasc Surg. 1983;86(1):115–25.

30. Richardt D, Hanke T, Sievers HH. Two cases of heart failure after implantation of a CoreValve prosthesis. N Engl J Med. 2015;372(11):1079–80.

31. Arsalan M, Walther T. Durability of prostheses for transcatheter aortic valve implantation. Nat Rev Cardiol. 2016;13(6):360–7.

32. Hahn RT, Kodali S, Tuzcu EM, Leon MB, Kapadia S, Gopal D, Lerakis S, Lindman BR, Wang Z, Webb J, Thourani VH, Douglas PS. Echocardiographic imaging of procedural complications during balloon-expandable transcatheter aortic valve replacement. JACC Cardiovasc Imaging. 2015;8(3):288–318.

33. Holmes DR Jr, Mack MJ, Kaul S, Agnihotri A, Alexander KP, Bailey SR, Calhoon JH, Carabello BA, Desai MY, Edwards FH, Francis GS, Gardner TJ, Kappetein AP, Linderbaum JA, Mukherjee C, Mukherjee D, Otto CM, Ruiz CE, Sacco RL, Smith D, Thomas JD. 2012 ACCF/AATS/SCAI/STS expert consensus document on transcatheter aortic valve replacement. J Am Coll Cardiol. 2012;59(13):1200–54.

34. Alavi SH, Groves EM, Kheradvar A. The effects of transcatheter valve crimping on pericardial leaflets. Ann Thorac Surg. 2014;97(4):1260–6.

35. Sun W, Li K, Sirois E. Simulated elliptical bioprosthetic valve deformation: implications for asymmetric transcatheter valve deployment. J Biomech. 2010;43(16):3085–90.

36. Martin C, Sun W. Simulation of long-term fatigue damage in bioprosthetic heart valves: effects of leaflet and stent elastic properties. Biomech Model Mechanobiol. 2014;13(4):759–70.

37. Vesely I. The influence of design on bioprosthetic valve durability. J Long-Term Eff Med Implants. 2001;11(3–4):137–49.

38. Salaun E, Zenses AS, Evin M, Collart F, Habib G, Pibarot P, Rieu R. Effect of oversizing and elliptical shape of aortic annulus on transcatheter valve hemodynamics: an in vitro study. Int J Cardiol. 2016;208:28–35.

39. Chakravarty T, Sondergaard L, Friedman J, De Backer O, Berman D, Kofoed KF, Jilaihawi H, Shiota T, Abramowitz Y, Jorgensen TH, Rami T, Israr S, Fontana G, de Knegt M, Fuchs A, Lyden P, Trento A, Bhatt DL, Leon MB, Makkar RR. Subclinical leaflet thrombosis in surgical and transcatheter bioprosthetic aortic valves: an observational study. Lancet. 2017;389(10087):2383–92.

40. Doris MK, Dweck MR. Is bioprosthetic leaflet thrombosis a trigger to valve degeneration? Heart. 2018;104(10):792–3.

41. Flameng W, Herregods MC, Vercalsteren M, Herijgers P, Bogaerts K, Meuris B. Prosthesis-patient mismatch predicts structural valve degeneration in bioprosthetic heart valves. Circulation. 2010;121(19):2123–9.

42. Genereux P, Head SJ, Hahn R, Daneault B, Kodali S, Williams MR, van Mieghem NM, Alu MC, Serruys PW, Kappetein AP, Leon MB. Paravalvular leak after transcatheter aortic valve replacement: the new Achilles' heel? A comprehensive review of the literature. J Am Coll Cardiol. 2013;61(11):1125–36.

43. Bruschi G, Botta L, Fratto P, Martinelli L. Failed valve-in-valve transcatheter mitral valve implantation. Eur J Cardiothorac Surg. 2014;45(4):e127.

44. Harbaoui B, Courand PY, Schmitt Z, Farhat F, Dauphin R, Lantelme P. Early Edwards SAPIEN valve degeneration after transcatheter aortic valve replacement. JACC Cardiovasc Interv. 2016;9(2):198–9.

45. Kiefer P, Seeburger J, Chu MW, Ender J, Vollroth M, Noack T, Mohr FW, Holzhey DM. Reoperative transapical aortic valve implantation for early structural valve deterioration of a SAPIEN XT valve. Ann Thorac Surg. 2013;95(6):2169–70.

46. Kappetein AP, Head SJ, Genereux P, Piazza N, van Mieghem NM, Blackstone EH, Brott TG, Cohen DJ, Cutlip DE, van Es GA, Hahn RT, Kirtane AJ, Krucoff MW, Kodali S, Mack MJ, Mehran R, Rodes-Cabau J, Vranckx P, Webb JG, Windecker S, Serruys PW, Leon MB. Updated standardized endpoint definitions for transcatheter aortic valve implantation: the Valve Academic Research Consortium-2 consensus document. J Am Coll Cardiol. 2012;60(15):1438–54.

47. Pibarot P, Weissman NJ, Stewart WJ, Hahn RT, Lindman BR, McAndrew T, Kodali SK, Mack MJ, Thourani VH, Miller DC, Svensson LG, Herrmann HC, Smith CR, Rodes-Cabau J, Webb J, Lim S, Xu K, Hueter I, Douglas PS, Leon MB. Incidence and sequelae of prosthesis-patient mismatch in transcatheter versus surgical valve replacement in high-risk patients with severe aortic stenosis: a PARTNER trial cohort—a analysis. J Am Coll Cardiol. 2014;64(13):1323–34.

48. Ewe SH, Muratori M, Delgado V, Pepi M, Tamborini G, Fusini L, Klautz RJ, Gripari P, Bax JJ, Fusari M, Schalij MJ, Marsan NA. Hemodynamic and clinical impact of prosthesis-patient mismatch after transcatheter aortic valve implantation. J Am Coll Cardiol. 2011;58(18):1910–8.

49. Jilaihawi H, Chin D, Spyt T, Jeilan M, Vasa-Nicotera M, Bence J, Logtens E, Kovac J. Prosthesis-patient mismatch after transcatheter aortic valve implantation with the Medtronic-Corevalve bioprosthesis. Eur Heart J. 2010;31(7):857–64.

50. Clavel MA, Webb JG, Pibarot P, Altwegg L, Dumont E, Thompson C, De Larochelliere R, Doyle D, Masson JB, Bergeron S, Bertrand OF, Rodes-Cabau J. Comparison of the hemodynamic performance of percutaneous and surgical bioprostheses for the treatment of severe aortic stenosis. J Am Coll Cardiol. 2009;53(20):1883–91.

51. Kim SJ, Samad Z, Bloomfield GS, Douglas PS. A critical review of hemodynamic changes and left ventricular remodeling after surgical aortic valve replacement and percutaneous aortic valve replacement. Am Heart J. 2014;168(2):150–9.e1–7.

52. Herrmann HC, Daneshvar SA, Fonarow GC, Stebbins A, Vemulapalli S, Desai ND, Malenka DJ, Thourani VH, Rymer J, Kosinski AS. Prosthesis-patient mismatch in patients undergoing transcatheter aortic valve replacement: from the STS/ACC TVT registry. J Am Coll Cardiol. 2018;72(22):2701–11.

53. Habib G, Lancellotti P, Antunes MJ, Bongiorni MG, Casalta JP, Del Zotti F, Dulgheru R, El Khoury G, Erba PA, Iung B, Miro JM, Mulder BJ, Plonska-Gosciniak E, Price S, Roos-Hesselink J, Snygg-Martin U, Thuny F, Tornos Mas P, Vilacosta I, Zamorano JL. ESC Guidelines for the management of infective endocarditis: the Task Force for the Management of Infective Endocarditis of the European Society of Cardiology (ESC). Endorsed by: European Association for Cardio-Thoracic Surgery (EACTS), the European Association of Nuclear Medicine (EANM). Eur Heart J. 2015;36(44):3075–128.

54. Latib A, Naim C, De Bonis M, Sinning JM, Maisano F, Barbanti M, Parolari A, Lorusso R, Testa L, Actis Dato GM, Miceli A, Sponga S, Rosato F, De Vincentiis C, Werner N, Fiorina C, Bartorelli A,

Di Gregorio O, Casilli F, Muratori M, Alamanni F, Glauber M, Livi U, Nickenig G, Tamburino C, Alfieri O, Colombo A. TAVR-associated prosthetic valve infective endocarditis: results of a large, multicenter registry. J Am Coll Cardiol. 2014;64(20):2176–8.

55. Sulzenko J, Tousek P, Linkova H. Infective endocarditis as a mid-term complication after transcatheter aortic valve implantation: case report and literature review. Catheter Cardiovasc Interv. 2014;84(2):311–5.

56. Amat-Santos IJ, Messika-Zeitoun D, Eltchaninoff H, Kapadia S, Lerakis S, Cheema AN, Gutierrez-Ibanes E, Munoz-Garcia AJ, Pan M, Webb JG, Herrmann HC, Kodali S, Nombela-Franco L, Tamburino C, Jilaihawi H, Masson JB, de Brito FS Jr, Ferreira MC, Lima VC, Mangione JA, Iung B, Vahanian A, Durand E, Tuzcu EM, Hayek SS, Angulo-Llanos R, Gomez-Doblas JJ, Castillo JC, Dvir D, Leon MB, Garcia E, Cobiella J, Vilacosta I, Barbanti M, Makkar R R, Ribeiro HB, Urena M, Dumont E, Pibarot P, Lopez J, San Roman A, Rodes-Cabau J. Infective endocarditis after transcatheter aortic valve implantation: results from a large multicenter registry. Circulation. 2015;131(18):1566–74.

57. Latib A, Naganuma T, Abdel-Wahab M, Danenberg H, Cota L, Barbanti M, Baumgartner H, Finkelstein A, Legrand V, de Lezo JS, Kefer J, Messika-Zeitoun D, Richardt G, Stabile E, Kaleschke G, Vahanian A, Laborde JC, Leon MB, Webb JG, Panoulas VF, Maisano F, Alfieri O, Colombo A. Treatment and clinical outcomes of transcatheter heart valve thrombosis. Circ Cardiovasc Interv. 2015;8(4):e001779.

58. Mylotte D, Piazza N. Transcatheter aortic valve replacement failure: deja vu ou jamais vu? Circ Cardiovasc Interv. 2015;8(4):e002531.

59. Sinning JM, Vasa-Nicotera M, Chin D, Hammerstingl C, Ghanem A, Bence J, Kovac J, Grube E, Nickenig G, Werner N. Evaluation and management of paravalvular aortic regurgitation after transcatheter aortic valve replacement. J Am Coll Cardiol. 2013;62(1):11–20.

60. Trepels T, Martens S, Doss M, Fichtlscherer S, Schachinger V. Images in cardiovascular medicine. Thrombotic restenosis after minimally invasive implantation of aortic valve stent. Circulation. 2009;120(4):e23–4.

61. De Marchena E, Mesa J, Pomenti S, Marin YKC, Marincic X, Yahagi K, Ladich E, Kutz R, Aga Y, Ragosta M, Chawla A, Ring ME, Virmani R. Thrombus formation following transcatheter aortic valve replacement. JACC Cardiovasc Interv. 2015;8(5):728–39.

62. Makkar RR, Fontana G, Jilaihawi H, Chakravarty T, Kofoed KF, De Backer O, Asch FM, Ruiz CE, Olsen NT, Trento A, Friedman J, Berman D, Cheng W, Kashif M, Jelnin V, Kliger CA, Guo H, Pichard AD, Weissman NJ, Kapadia S, Manasse E, Bhatt DL, Leon MB, Sondergaard L. Possible subclinical leaflet thrombosis in bioprosthetic aortic valves. N Engl J Med. 2015;373(21):2015–24.

63. Egbe AC, Pislaru SV, Pellikka PA, Poterucha JT, Schaff HV, Maleszewski JJ, Connolly HM. Bioprosthetic valve thrombosis versus structural failure: clinical and echocardiographic predictors. J Am Coll Cardiol. 2015;66(21):2285–94.

64. Pislaru SV, Pellikka PA, Schaff HV, Connolly HM. Bioprosthetic valve thrombosis: the eyes will not see what the mind does not know. J Thorac Cardiovasc Surg. 2015;149(6):e86–7.

65. Pislaru SV, Hussain I, Pellikka PA, Maleszewski JJ, Hanna RD, Schaff HV, Connolly HM. Misconceptions, diagnostic challenges and treatment opportunities in bioprosthetic valve thrombosis: lessons from a case series. Eur J Cardiothorac Surg. 2015;47(4):725–32.

66. Sondergaard L, Sigitas C, Chopra M, Bieliauskas G, De Backer O. Leaflet thrombosis after TAVI. Eur Heart J. 2017;38(36):2702–3.

67. Sondergaard L, De Backer O, Kofoed KF, Jilaihawi H, Fuchs A, Chakravarty T, Kashif M, Kazuno Y, Kawamori H, Maeno Y, Bieliauskas G, Guo H, Stone GW, Makkar R. Natural history of subclinical leaflet thrombosis affecting motion in bioprosthetic aortic valves. Eur Heart J. 2017;38(28):2201–7.

68. Khatri PJ, Webb JG, Rodes-Cabau J, Fremes SE, Ruel M, Lau K, Guo H, Wijeysundera HC, Ko DT. Adverse effects associated with transcatheter aortic valve implantation: a meta-analysis of contemporary studies. Ann Intern Med. 2013;158(1):35–46.

69. Pang PY, Chiam PT, Chua YL, Sin YK. A survivor of late prosthesis migration and rotation following percutaneous transcatheter aortic valve implantation. Eur J Cardiothorac Surg. 2012;41(5):1195–6.

70. Masson JB, Kovac J, Schuler G, Ye J, Cheung A, Kapadia S, Tuzcu ME, Kodali S, Leon MB, Webb JG. Transcatheter aortic valve implantation: review of the nature, management, and avoidance of procedural complications. JACC Cardiovasc Interv. 2009;2(9):811–20.

71. Latib A, Michev I, Laborde JC, Montorfano M, Colombo A. Post-implantation repositioning of the CoreValve percutaneous aortic valve. JACC Cardiovasc Interv. 2010;3(1):119–21.

72. Schultz CJ, Weustink A, Piazza N, Otten A, Mollet N, Krestin G, van Geuns RJ, de Feyter P, Serruys PW, de Jaegere P. Geometry and degree of apposition of the CoreValve ReValving system with multislice computed tomography after implantation in patients with aortic stenosis. J Am Coll Cardiol. 2009;54(10):911–8.

73. Schultz CJ, Tzikas A, Moelker A, Rossi A, Nuis RJ, Geleijnse MM, van Mieghem N, Krestin GP, de Feyter P, Serruys PW, de Jaegere PP. Correlates on MSCT of paravalvular aortic regurgitation after transcatheter aortic valve implantation using the Medtronic CoreValve prosthesis. Catheter Cardiovasc Interv. 2011;78(3):446–55.

74. Eggebrecht H, Doss M, Schmermund A, Nowak B, Krissel J, Voigtlander T. Interventional options for severe aortic regurgitation after transcatheter aortic valve implantation: balloons, snares, valve-in-valve. Clin Res Cardiol. 2012;101(6):503–7.

75. Lerakis S, Hayek SS, Douglas PS. Paravalvular aortic leak after transcatheter aortic valve replacement: current knowledge. Circulation. 2013;127(3):397–407.

76. Nkomo VT, Suri RM, Pislaru SV, Greason KL, Sinak LJ, Holmes DR, Mathew V, Rihal CS. Delayed transcatheter heart valve migration and failure. JACC Cardiovasc Imaging. 2014;7(9):960–2.

77. Jose J, Sulimov DS, El-Mawardy M, Sato T, Allali A, Holy EW, Becker B, Landt M, Kebernik J, Schwarz B, Richardt G, Abdel-Wahab M. Clinical bioprosthetic heart valve thrombosis after transcatheter aortic valve replacement: incidence, characteristics, and treatment outcomes. JACC Cardiovasc Interv. 2017;10(7):686–97.

78. Pache G, Schoechlin S, Blanke P, Dorfs S, Jander N, Arepalli CD, Gick M, Buettner HJ, Leipsic J, Langer M, Neumann FJ, Ruile P. Early hypo-attenuated leaflet thickening in balloon-expandable transcatheter aortic heart valves. Eur Heart J. 2016;37(28):2263–71.

79. Leetmaa T, Hansson NC, Leipsic J, Jensen K, Poulsen SH, Andersen HR, Jensen JM, Webb J, Blanke P, Tang M, Norgaard BL. Early aortic transcatheter heart valve thrombosis: diagnostic value of contrast-enhanced multidetector computed tomography. Circ Cardiovasc Interv. 2015;8(4):e001596.

80. Sondergaard L. Subclinical leaflet thrombosis in bioprosthetic aortic valves. JACC Cardiovasc Interv. 2017;10(2):204–5.

81. Testa L, Latib A. Assessing the risk of leaflet motion abnormality following transcatheter aortic valve implantation. Interv Cardiol. 2018;13(1):37–9.

82. Bax JJ, Stone GW. Bioprosthetic surgical and transcatheter heart valve thrombosis. Lancet. 2017;389(10087):2352–4.

83. Laschinger JC, Wu C, Ibrahim NG, Shuren JE. Reduced leaflet motion in bioprosthetic aortic valves—the FDA perspective. N Engl J Med. 2015;373(21):1996–8.

84. Pibarot P, Hahn RT, Weissman NJ, Monaghan MJ. Assessment of paravalvular regurgitation following TAVR: a proposal of unifying grading scheme. JACC Cardiovasc Imaging. 2015;8(3):340–60.

85. Ribeiro HB, Orwat S, Hayek SS, Larose E, Babaliaros V, Dahou A, Le Ven F, Pasian S, Puri R, Abdul-Jawad Altisent O, Campelo-Parada F, Clavel MA, Pibarot P, Lerakis S, Baumgartner H, Rodes-Cabau J. Cardiovascular magnetic resonance to evaluate aortic regurgitation after transcatheter aortic valve replacement. J Am Coll Cardiol. 2016;68(6):577–85.

86. Leon MB, Smith CR, Mack M, Miller DC, Moses JW, Svensson LG, Tuzcu EM, Webb JG, Fontana GP, Makkar RR, Brown DL, Block PC, Guyton RA, Pichard AD, Bavaria JE, Herrmann HC, Douglas PS, Petersen JL, Akin JJ, Anderson WN, Wang D, Pocock S. Transcatheter aortic-valve implantation for aortic stenosis in patients who cannot undergo surgery. N Engl J Med. 2010;363(17):1597–607.

87. Klein AA, Skubas NJ, Ender JJA. Controversies and complications in the perioperative management of transcatheter aortic valve replacement. Anesth Analg. 2014;119(4):784–98.

88. Hamm CW, Möllmann H, Holzhey D, Beckmann A, Veit C, Figulla H-R, Cremer J, Kuck K-H, Lange R, Zahn R. The German aortic valve registry (GARY): in-hospital outcome. Eur Heart J. 2013;35(24):1588–98.

89. Généreux P, Head SJ, Van Mieghem NM, Kodali S, Kirtane AJ, Xu K, Smith C, Serruys PW, Kappetein AP, Leon MB. Clinical outcomes after transcatheter aortic valve replacement using valve academic research consortium definitions: a weighted meta-analysis of 3,519 patients from 16 studies. J Am Coll Cardiol. 2012;59(25):2317–26.

90. Kempfert J, Rastan A, Holzhey D, Linke A, Schuler G, van Linden A, Blumenstein J, Mohr FW, Walther TJC. Transapical aortic valve implantation: analysis of risk factors and learning experience in 299 patients. 2011;124(11 Suppl):S124–9.

91. Sharma A, Arbab-Zadeh A, Dubey D, Shani J, Lazar J, Frankel R. Access site bleeding after transcatheter aortic valve implantation. J Thromb Thrombolysis. 2013;35(4):463–8.

92. Mollmann H, Kim WK, Kempfert J, Walther T, Hamm C. Complications of transcatheter aortic valve implantation (TAVI): how to avoid and treat them. Heart. 2015;101(11):900–8.

93. Tonnessen BH. Iatrogenic injury from vascular access and endovascular procedures. Perspect Vasc Surg Endovasc Ther. 2011;23(2):128–35.

94. Chaudhry MA, Sardar MR. Vascular complications of transcatheter aortic valve replacement: a concise literature review. World J Cardiol. 2017;9(7):574.

95. Stone PA, AbuRahma AF, Flaherty SK, Bates MC. Femoral pseudoaneurysms. Vasc Endovascular Surg. 2006;40(2):109–17.

96. Toggweiler S, Gurvitch R, Leipsic J, Wood DA, Willson AB, Binder RK, Cheung A, Ye J, Webb JG. Percutaneous aortic valve replacement: vascular outcomes with a fully percutaneous procedure. J Am Coll Cardiol. 2012;59(2):113–8.

97. Sharp AS, Michev I, Maisano F, Taramasso M, Godino C, Latib A, Denti P, Dorigo E, Giacomini A, Iaci G. A new technique for vascular access management in transcatheter aortic valve implantation. Catheter Cardiovasc Interv. 2010;75(5):784–93.

98. Hayashida K, Lefèvre T, Chevalier B, Hovasse T, Romano M, Garot P, Mylotte D, Uribe J, Farge A, Donzeau-Gouge P. Transfemoral aortic valve implantation: new criteria to predict vascular complications. JACC Cardiovasc Interv. 2011;4(8):851–8.

99. Kelm M, Perings SM, Jax T, Lauer T, Schoebel FC, Heintzen MP, Perings C, Strauer BE. Incidence and clinical outcome of iatrogenic femoral arteriovenous fistulas: implications for risk stratification and treatment. J Am Coll Cardiol. 2002;40(2):291–7.

100. Toggweiler S, Leipsic J, Binder RK, Freeman M, Barbanti M, Heijmen RH, Wood DA, Webb JG. Management of vascular access in transcatheter aortic valve replacement: part 2: vascular complications. JACC Cardiovasc Interv. 2013;6(8):767–76.

101. Stortecky S, Wenaweser P, Diehm N, Pilgrim T, Huber C, Rosskopf AB, Khattab AA, Buellesfeld L, Gloekler S, Eberle B, Schmidli J, Carrel T, Meier B, Windecker S. Percutaneous management of vascular complications in patients undergoing transcatheter aortic valve implantation. JACC Cardiovasc Interv. 2012;5(5):515–24.

102. Genereux P, Webb JG, Svensson LG, Kodali SK, Satler LF, Fearon WF, Davidson CJ, Eisenhauer AC, Makkar RR, Bergman GW, Babaliaros V, Bavaria JE, Velazquez OC, Williams MR, Hueter I, Xu K, Leon MB. Vascular complications after transcatheter aortic valve replacement: insights from the PARTNER (Placement of AoRTic TraNscathetER Valve) trial. J Am Coll Cardiol. 2012;60(12):1043–52.

103. Unzue L, Garcia E, Teijeiro R, Rubio-Alonso B. Percutaneous closure of a femoral arteriovenous fistula during transfemoral TAVI. J Invasive Cardiol. 2018;30(8):E67–e68.

104. Barbanti M, Binder RK, Freeman M, Wood DA, Leipsic J, Cheung A, Ye J, Tan J, Toggweiler S, Yang TH, Dvir D, Maryniak K, Lauck S, Webb JG. Impact of low-profile sheaths on vascular complications during transfemoral transcatheter aortic valve replacement. EuroIntervention. 2013;9(8):929–35.

105. Creager MA, Kaufman JA, Conte MS. Clinical practice. Acute limb ischemia. N Engl J Med. 2012;366(23):2198–206.

106. Schmidt AH. Acute compartment syndrome. Injury. 2017;48(Suppl 1):S22–s25.

107. McNally MM, Univers J. Acute limb ischemia. Surg Clin North Am. 2018;98(5):1081–96.

108. Conte JV, Hermiller J Jr, Resar JR, Deeb GM, Gleason TG, Adams DH, Popma JJ, Yakubov SJ, Watson D, Guo J, Zorn GL 3rd, Reardon MJ. Complications after self-expanding transcatheter or surgical aortic valve replacement. Semin Thorac Cardiovasc Surg. 2017;29(3):321–30.

109. Ong SH, Mueller R, Gerckens U. Iatrogenic dissection of the ascending aorta during TAVI sealed with the CoreValve revalving prosthesis. Catheter Cardiovasc Interv. 2011;77(6):910–4.

110. Berfield KK, Sweet MP, McCabe JM, Reisman M, Mackensen GB, Mokadam NA, Dean LS, Smith JW. Endovascular repair for type A aortic dissection after transcatheter aortic valve replacement with a Medtronic CoreValve. Ann Thorac Surg. 2015;100(4):1444–6.

111. Jacobzon E, Wolak A, Fink D, Silberman S. Delayed aortic dissection and valve thrombosis after transcatheter aortic valve implantation. Catheter Cardiovasc Interv. 2019;93(7):E391–3.

112. Nagasawa A, Shirai S, Hanyu M, Arai Y, Kamioka N, Hayashi M. Descending aortic dissection injured by tip of the sheath during transcatheter aortic valve implantation. Cardiovasc Interv Ther. 2016;31(2):122–7.

113. Lempel JK, Frazier AA, Jeudy J, Kligerman SJ, Schultz R, Ninalowo HA, Gozansky EK, Griffith B, White CS. Aortic arch dissection: a controversy of classification. Radiology. 2014;271(3):848–55.

114. Hayek SS, Corrigan FE 3rd, Condado JF, Lin S, Howell S, MacNamara JP, Zheng S, Keegan P, Thourani V, Babaliaros VC, Lerakis S. Paravalvular regurgitation after transcatheter aortic valve replacement: comparing transthoracic versus transesophageal echocardiographic guidance. J Am Soc Echocardiogr. 2017;30(6):533–40.

115. Thomas M, Schymik G, Walther T, Himbert D, Lefevre T, Treede H, Eggebrecht H, Rubino P, Michev I, Lange R, Anderson WN, Wendler O. Thirty-day results of the SAPIEN aortic Bioprosthesis European Outcome (SOURCE) Registry: a European registry of transcatheter aortic valve implantation using the Edwards SAPIEN valve. Circulation. 2010;122(1):62–9.

116. Shah P, Bajaj S, Shamoon F. Aortic dissection caused by percutaneous coronary intervention: 2 new case reports and detailed analysis of 86 previous cases. Tex Heart Inst J. 2016;43(1):52–60.

117. Dunning DW, Kahn JK, Hawkins ET, O'Neill WW. Iatrogenic coronary artery dissections extending into and involving the aortic root. Catheter Cardiovasc Interv. 2000;51(4):387–93.

118. Puippe GD. [Complicated acute type B aortic dissection-what does endovascular therapy contribute?]. Radiologe. 2018;58(9):822–8.

119. Nishimura RA, Otto CM, Bonow RO, Carabello BA, Erwin JP 3rd, Guyton RA, O'Gara PT, Ruiz CE, Skubas NJ, Sorajja P, Sundt TM 3rd, Thomas JD. 2014 AHA/ACC guideline for the management of patients with valvular heart disease: a report of the American College of Cardiology/American Heart Association Task Force on Practice Guidelines. J Am Coll Cardiol. 2014;63(22):e57–185.

120. Doherty JU, Kort S, Mehran R, Schoenhagen P, Soman P. ACC/AATS/AHA/ASE/ASNC/HRS/SCAI/SCCT/SCMR/STS 2017 appropriate use criteria for multimodality imaging in valvular heart disease: a Report of the American College of Cardiology Appropriate Use Criteria Task Force, American Association for Thoracic Surgery, American Heart Association, American Society of Echocardiography, American Society of Nuclear Cardiology, Heart Rhythm Society, Society for Cardiovascular Angiography and Interventions, Society of Cardiovascular Computed Tomography, Society for Cardiovascular Magnetic Resonance, and Society of Thoracic Surgeons. J Nucl Cardiol. 2017;24(6):2043–63.

121. Zoghbi WA, Adams D, Bonow RO, Enriquez-Sarano M, Foster E, Grayburn PA, Hahn RT, Han Y, Hung J, Lang RM, Little SH, Shah DJ, Shernan S, Thavendiranathan P, Thomas JD, Weissman NJ. Recommendations for noninvasive evaluation of native valvular regurgitation: a Report from the American Society of Echocardiography Developed in Collaboration with the Society for Cardiovascular Magnetic Resonance. J Am Soc Echocardiogr. 2017;30(4):303–71.

122. Mitchell C, Rahko PS, Blauwet LA, Canaday B, Finstuen JA, Foster MC, Horton K, Ogunyankin KO, Palma RA, Velazquez EJ. Guidelines for performing a comprehensive transthoracic echocardiographic examination in adults: recommendations from the American Society of Echocardiography. J Am Soc Echocardiogr. 2019;32(1):1–64.

123. Hahn RT, Abraham T, Adams MS, Bruce CJ, Glas KE, Lang RM, Reeves ST, Shanewise JS, Siu SC, Stewart W, Picard MH. Guidelines for performing a comprehensive transesophageal echocardiographic examination: recommendations from the American Society of Echocardiography and the Society of Cardiovascular Anesthesiologists. Anesth Analg. 2014;118(1):21–68.

124. Zoghbi WA, Asch FM, Bruce C, Gillam LD, Grayburn PA, Hahn RT, Inglessis I, Islam AM, Lerakis S, Little SH, Siegel RJ, Skubas N, Slesnick TC, Stewart WJ, Thavendiranathan P, Weissman NJ, Yasukochi S, Zimmerman KG. Guidelines for the evaluation of valvular regurgitation after percutaneous valve repair or replacement: a Report from the American Society of Echocardiography Developed in Collaboration with the Society for Cardiovascular Angiography and Interventions, Japanese Society of Echocardiography, and Society for Cardiovascular Magnetic Resonance. J Am Soc Echocardiogr. 2019;32(4):431–75.

Index